Recent Results in Cancer Research 186

Kerry S. Courneya • Christine M. Friedenreich
(Editors)

Physical Activity and Cancer

Springer

Editors
Kerry S. Courneya
Professor and Canada Research
Chair in Physical Activity and Cancer
Faculty of Physical Education
and Recreation
University of Alberta
E-488 Van Vliet Center
Edmonton, Alberta
T6G 2H9 CANADA
kerry.courneya@ualberta.ca

Christine M. Friedenreich
AHFMR Health Senior Scholar
Alberta Health Services
Adjunct Professor
University of Calgary
1331 29 St NW
Calgary, Alberta, Canada
T2N 4N2
christine.friedenreich@albertahealthservices.ca

ISBN 978-3-642-04230-0 e-ISBN 978-3-642-04231-7
DOI 10.1007/978-3-642-04231-7
Springer Heidelberg Dordrecht London New York

Library of Congress Control Number: 2010937975

Cover design: estudioCalamar Figueres/Berlin

Printed on acid-free paper

Springer is part of Springer Science + Business Media (www.springer.com)

Contents

Physical Activity and Cancer: An Introduction

1

Kerry S. Courneya and Christine M. Friedenreich

Abstract Physical activity (PA) is an important health behavior for many diseases, but its role in cancer control has been understudied and underappreciated. In this chapter, we introduce this volume on PA and cancer and provide an overview of its content and organization. We also review some of the methodological challenges in this field, summarize the key conclusions of each chapter, and offer some general directions for future research. The volume contains 16 chapters organized by the major cancer sites and the phases of the cancer control continuum. In addition to this introductory chapter, the volume includes six chapters on cancer prevention, six chapters on cancer survivorship, and three chapters on special topics. Overall, the research to date suggests that PA reduces the risk of developing some cancers, helps cancer survivors cope with and recover from treatments, improves the long-term health of cancer survivors, and possibly even reduces the risk of recurrence and extends survival in some cancer survivor groups. Much research remains to be done in this field, but the compelling data produced thus far suggests that PA has an important role to play in cancer prevention and survivorship.

Physical activity (PA) is an important health behavior for the prevention and management of many acute and chronic diseases; however, research in cancer has lagged behind other major chronic diseases. Nevertheless, the compelling data produced in this field over the past 2 decades has resulted in PA receiving a prominent place in many cancer control and exercise science guidelines including the American Cancer Society's guidelines for cancer prevention (Kushi et al. 2006) and survivorship (Doyle et al. 2006), the World Cancer Research Fund/American Institute for Cancer Research guidelines for cancer prevention (WCRF 2007), the Australian Association of Exercise and Sport Science's exercise guidelines for cancer survivors (Hayes et al. 2009), and the American College of Sports Medicine's exercise guidelines for cancer survivors (Schmitz et al. 2010). The purpose of this volume is to bring together some of the world's leading researchers to provide comprehensive and authoritative reviews on key topics related to PA and cancer. In this chapter, we introduce the topic of PA and cancer, provide an overview of the content and organization of this volume, review some

K.S. Courneya (✉)
University of Alberta, E-488 Van Vliet Center, Edmonton, Alberta, T6G 2H9 Canada
e-mail: kerry.courneya@ualberta.ca

C.M. Friedenreich
AHFMR Health Senior Scholar Alberta Health Services University of Calgary, 1331 29 St NW, Calgary, Alberta, Canada T2N 4N2
e-mail: christine.friedenreich@albertahealthservices.ca

K.S. Courneya and C.M. Friedenreich (eds.), *Physical Activity and Cancer*, Recent Results in Cancer Research 186, DOI: 10.1007/978-3-642-04231-7_1,

1

of the methodological challenges in this field, summarize the key conclusions of each chapter, and offer some directions for future research.

1.1 Physical Activity, Exercise, and Health-Related Fitness

PA is defined as any bodily movement produced by the skeletal muscles that results in a substantial increase in energy expenditure (Bouchard and Shepard 1994). Leisure-time PA refers to activity undertaken during discretionary time based on a personal choice and is usually contrasted with occupational and/or household activity. Exercise is a form of leisure-time PA that is performed on a repeated basis over an extended period of time with the intention of improving fitness, performance, or health. PA is often categorized by intensity levels using metabolic equivalent task (MET) units with 1 MET being equivalent to the amount of energy a person expends at rest. Activities requiring <1.5 METs (e.g., standing) are generally considered sedentary, whereas activities between 1.5 and 2.9 METs (e.g., casual walking) are light, activities between 3.0 and 5.9 METs (e.g., brisk walking) are moderate, and activities ≥6.0 METs are vigorous (e.g., jogging/running).

Health-related fitness (HRF) refers to the components of physical fitness that are directly related to the health of an individual and typically includes cardiorespiratory fitness, musculoskeletal fitness (strength, endurance, flexibility, and balance), and body composition (ACSM 2010). Cardiorespiratory fitness refers to the ability to perform dynamic exercise using relatively large muscle groups at a moderate to high intensity level for prolonged periods of time (ACSM 2010). Musculoskeletal fitness refers to the ability of the skeletal muscle system to generate force (strength), power (rate of force development) and maintain force (muscular endurance) as well as the capacity of the joints to move throughout a full range of motion (ACSM 2010). Body composition refers to the proportion of fat and fat-free tissue in the body (ACSM 2010) and often includes measurements of anthropometry which deal with the size, weight, and proportion of the body.

1.2 Content and Organization of the Volume

Research on PA and cancer can be organized in many different ways, but two of the most important distinctions are the particular cancer site being studied and the timing of the PA intervention along the cancer control continuum. Consequently, we organized this volume by these two factors. We divided the cancer sites by the major organ systems that comprise the most common cancers: breast, lung, genitourinary, gastrointestinal, gynecological, and hematological. This decision was made in order to include as many cancers as possible within the number of chapters available. We acknowledge, however, that not all cancers have been included in this volume. We divided the cancer control continuum into prediagnosis and postdiagnosis phases to reflect the different roles PA may serve in primary prevention and survivorship. We use the term "survivorship" in its broader sense to encompass the entire postdiagnosis time period rather than in its narrower sense referring to the period following first diagnosis and treatment, and prior to the development of a recurrence of cancer (Hewitt et al. 2006). Given the limited number of chapters, we were unable to further divide the survivorship chapters by treatment status (e.g., pretreatment, active treatment, posttreatment), treatment modality (e.g., chemotherapy, radiation therapy, hormone therapy), or primary endpoint (e.g., HRF, quality of life, biomarkers, disease outcomes). Consequently, we asked the authors of the survivorship chapters to include the entire postdiagnosis time period, all treatments, and all health outcomes. We asked the prevention chapter authors to focus on primary prevention, not secondary or tertiary prevention (i.e., recurrence), and to include the proposed biological mechanisms for disease prevention.

We also included three chapters on special topics, namely, pediatric cancer survivorship, palliative cancer care, and motivation and behavior change. The role of PA in pediatric cancer survivors (0–14 years) was considered to be unique and generally not included in the cancer site-specific chapters. We acknowledge that additional chapters may have been warranted on adolescent and young adult cancer survivors (15–39 years) and older adult cancer survivors (65+) but, again, space did not permit separate chapters. The chapter on palliative cancer care was considered important because of the unique challenges of PA interventions at the end of life. Finally, a chapter on PA motivation and behavior change in cancer survivors was considered critical given that the challenges of exercise adherence are likely exacerbated by a cancer diagnosis and its prolonged and difficult medical treatments. Given this special topic chapter, we asked the cancer site-specific survivorship authors to focus only on the outcomes of PA and not on its determinants.

1.3 Methodological Issues in Physical Activity and Cancer Research

In interpreting the studies in this volume, it is important to be aware of some of the common methodological limitations of this research. One issue relates to the temporal sequencing between the exposure (i.e., PA) and the outcome (i.e., disease outcomes) in observational studies. Some case-control studies of PA and cancer prevention captured only more recent or usual PA, while PA in the distant past or over the lifetime may be more etiologically relevant for some cancers. Moreover, in cancer survivorship studies, it is unclear how PA before diagnosis, during treatment, or after treatment influences recurrence and survival since relatively few studies have examined PA across these time periods.

A second factor that must be considered in observational studies is control for confounding of the association between PA and cancer outcomes and whether or not effect modification was adequately addressed. Important confounding factors such as other lifestyle or personal factors that may independently be associated with the disease outcomes need to be appropriately controlled for in these analyses. Moreover, consideration of potential effect modifiers like disease, medical, or demographic factors may be important for detecting any true benefit from PA, yet frequently these factors are not examined.

Another methodological challenge is the issue of selection bias which could arise if healthier, more active individuals are more likely to be screened for cancer, and hence more likely to be diagnosed, than less active people. In this scenario, a true inverse association between PA and cancer risk would be attenuated. In addition, for some cancers such as prostate cancer which are slow growing with a long latency period, a large percentage of men will die with evidence of undiagnosed prostate cancer. Therefore, associations may be diluted when comparing cancer cases to 'healthy' control populations because of latent, nonclinical prostate cancer among the controls.

Perhaps the most pressing issue in observational studies is how PA is measured. The heterogeneity of PA assessment methods across studies creates challenges for comparing and combining data in an effort to estimate overall risk reductions. Almost all studies have used self-report methods of data collection, primarily questionnaires, to ascertain estimates of PA. The greatest limitation is the validity of this method, particularly for assessing PA in the distant past, or PA of lighter intensity which may be more difficult to recall and is frequently omitted from questionnaires. Alternative methods such as behavioral observation, heart rate monitoring, motion sensors, and objective HRF measures can also be used; however, self-report is comparatively the most convenient and cost-effective way to collect PA data in large epidemiologic studies.

Some unique methodological challenges pertain specifically to randomized controlled trials (RCTs) of exercise in cancer survivors. One limitation of these RCTs is that many of the patient-reported outcomes (PROs) are often secondary outcomes to HRF outcomes. This situation means that survivors are rarely selected based on a patient-reported outcome (e.g., depressed, anxious, fatigued, poor quality of life, low physical functioning) which reduces the likelihood of finding an effect on such outcomes. Moreover, it also means that the trial is often underpowered for the PROs because of the greater variability and smaller anticipated effects of exercise on these outcomes compared to HRF outcomes. This lack of power also precludes subgroup analyses which can be very informative for clinical practice. Exercise RCTs are also limited in that most comparison groups receive no intervention at all rather than an intervention that attempts to control for attention and social interaction. Finally, few exercise RCTs have examined mediators of the effects of exercise on PROs which can be informative for the refinement of the exercise intervention.

1.4 Summary of Physical Activity and Cancer Prevention Chapters

PA may reduce the risk of developing a primary cancer. Cancer prevention remains the most studied and reviewed cancer control outcome. The association between PA and all cancer sites has been systematically reviewed by national (Physical Activity Guidelines Advisory Committee 2008) and international agencies including IARC (2002) and the World Cancer Research Fund/American Institute for Cancer Research (2007) and is the focus of the first section of this book. In general terms, the level of epidemiologic evidence varies by cancer site. There is *convincing* evidence for a beneficial effect of PA on risk of colon cancer; *probable* evidence for an effect on breast and endometrial cancers; *possible* evidence for cancers of the prostate, lung, and ovary; and *insufficient* or *null* evidence for most remaining cancer sites. With the rising prevalence of sedentary behavior occurring worldwide, these conclusions will have important and widespread public health implications.

Across cancer sites, some of the most compelling data for PA relates to breast cancer prevention. Lynch et al. (2011) reviewed 73 epidemiologic studies on PA and breast cancer prevention and estimate a 25% risk reduction from PA. They also discuss the type and dose of PA that might be most effective for breast cancer prevention. Associations were strongest for recreational PA, for PA sustained over the lifetime or done after menopause, and for PA of moderate to vigorous intensity. The review reveals greater benefit from PA for certain subgroups of women, namely those who are postmenopausal, parous, non-Caucasian, normal weight, or with no family history of breast cancer. Lynch et al. (2011) recommend future exercise RCTs to better understand the optimum type, dose, and timing of activity that may be required to lower risk, and the biologic mechanisms involved.

In contrast, the potential for PA to lower risk of genitourinary cancers is still questionable. Leitzmann (2011) reviews the epidemiologic literature on four genitourinary cancer sites but finds only weak inverse associations between PA and prostate cancer and renal cell cancer risks, and unclear associations with testicular and bladder cancer risk due to limited data. Clearly, most of the focus has been on prostate cancer. The review implied stronger effects on prostate cancer risk when studies considered PA intensity and when fatal prostate cancer was a study outcome. Inverse associations with renal cell cancer risk were more apparent among women and normal weight and older individuals. Leitzmann (2011) concludes that more research is needed to explore the role of physical fitness in genitourinary cancer, the effects of PA over the life course and in population subgroups, and to identify biologic pathways relating PA to cancer risk.

Associations between PA and gastrointestinal cancer risk are becoming increasingly clear. Wolin and Tuchman (2011) report consistent reductions in colon cancer risk with higher PA levels (average risk reduction of 25%), dose-response relations, and plausible biologic mechanisms. Future research is recommended to identify possible differences in PA-colon cancer associations across tumor subsites (distal vs. proximal) and population subgroups, the PA type, dose, and timing required to lower risk, and to better understand biologic mechanisms. The overall evidence surrounding PA and colon adenomas was limited but suggestive, and there was evidence for no association with rectal cancer. Studies relating PA to gastric cancer risk were too sparse to draw any conclusions.

The effect of PA on lung cancer prevention remains unclear. Emaus and Thune (2011) report a sizable 20–30% average decrease in lung cancer risk for women and a 20–50% decrease for men derived mainly from studies of total or recreational PA. These estimated decreases are comparable to those for breast and colon cancers. The crucial caveat to these data, however, is the lack of attention paid specifically to never smokers for whom there may be no benefit from PA in terms of lung cancer prevention. Furthermore, effect modification from smoking might only apply to certain histologic subtypes of lung cancer. More study is recommended by Emaus and Thune (2011) to clarify who benefits from PA (e.g., ever smokers) and to elucidate the biologic mechanisms involved.

Pan and Morrison (2011) provide a novel review of the epidemiologic literature on PA and four hematologic cancers: non-Hodgkin lymphoma (NHL), Hodgkin lymphoma, leukemia, and multiple myeloma. In essence, too few epidemiologic studies have been conducted to draw any conclusions about the influence of PA on hematologic cancer risk. The hypotheses surrounding these associations, therefore, are based largely on proposed biologic mechanisms which include enhancement of the immune system, prevention of overweight and obesity, improved antioxidant defense systems, decreased levels of insulin and insulin-like growth factors, and decreased inflammation (Pan and Morrison 2011). Recommendations are made for research into the role of PA in specific histologic subtypes of hematologic cancers and also for exercise RCTs to determine PA effects on the proposed biologic mechanisms (Pan and Morrison 2011).

Mounting evidence suggests preventive roles for PA in some gynecological cancers. Cust (2011) reviews the epidemiologic literature relating PA to risk of endometrial, ovarian, and cervical cancers and reveals, respectively, probable, possible, and insufficient evidence of a PA association. Endometrial cancer risk may be reduced on average by 20–30%, and ovarian cancer lowered by 20%, but about half of the ovarian studies found no association. Cust (2011) also discusses the possible detrimental role of sedentary behavior in endometrial and ovarian cancers and suggests that even light to moderate PA may be sufficient for reducing endometrial cancer risk. Hypothesized biologic mechanisms are described with the strongest biologic evidence supporting a PA-endometrial cancer association.

1

1.5 Summary of Physical Activity and Cancer Survivorship Chapters

Research into PA and cancer survivorship is a much more recent phenomenon that addresses a broad range of potential health outcomes. In the pretreatment phase, PA may: (a) help the person cope with the disease physically and emotionally while awaiting treatments, (b) improve HRF sufficiently to allow difficult treatments to go forward (e.g., lung surgery, cardiotoxic drugs), and (c) delay the need for treatment by managing the disease and its symptoms. During the active treatment phase, PA may help: (a) manage treatment side effects, maintain physical functioning, prevent muscle loss and fat gain, and improve mood states and quality of life, (b) facilitate completion of difficult treatments, and (c) potentiate the efficacy of cancer treatments. In the posttreatment phase, PA may help: (a) optimize recovery of physical functioning and quality of life, (b) manage any chronic and/or late-appearing effects of treatments (e.g., fatigue, lymphedema, fat gain, bone loss), (c) reduce the likelihood of disease recurrence, and (d) reduce the likelihood of developing other chronic diseases for which cancer survivors may be at increased risk (e.g., osteoporosis, heart disease, diabetes).

Most PA and cancer survivorship research has focused on breast cancer. Schmitz (2011) reports that PA is safe for most breast cancer survivors and, importantly, does not cause or exacerbate lymphedema. Moreover, there is good evidence from RCTs that PA can improve cardiorespiratory fitness, muscular strength, body composition, and important PROs such as quality of life, physical functioning, and fatigue in breast cancer survivors, especially during the posttreatment phase. Perhaps the most provocative research in PA and breast cancer survivorship is the recent observational studies suggesting that higher levels of postdiagnosis PA are associated with a lower risk of disease recurrence, breast cancer-specific mortality, and all-cause mortality. Schmitz (2011) concludes that, while much research remains to be done, the evidence is sufficient to warrant recommending exercise to breast cancer survivors both during and after adjuvant therapies.

Most research on PA and genitourinary cancer survivorship has focused on prostate cancer survivors receiving androgen deprivation therapy and/or radiation therapy. Galvao et al. (2011) report that, in this setting, well-conducted RCTs have shown compelling evidence that exercise improves muscular strength, lean body mass, physical functioning, fatigue, and quality of life, especially resistance exercise training. The trials have also shown no adverse effects of exercise training on prostate-specific antigen levels or testosterone levels. Galvao et al. (2011) conclude that exercise is safe for most prostate cancer survivors, even during treatments, and that both aerobic and resistance exercise should be recommended. They note that very little research has focused on other genitourinary cancers (e.g., bladder, kidney) and that the implications of exercise for disease outcomes in genitourinary cancers are unknown.

Somewhat surprisingly, comparatively little RCT data have focused on PA and supportive care outcomes in gastrointestinal cancer survivorship. Sellar and Courneya (2011) report that the limited research to date has either been observational or, if interventional, has focused on biomarker endpoints. Nevertheless, the observational research has shown consistent associations between higher levels of postdiagnosis PA and better quality of life, and lower risks of disease recurrence, cancer-specific mortality, and death from all causes in colorectal cancer survivors. Sellar and Courneya (2011) note that very little research has focused on other gastrointestinal cancers (e.g., esophageal, pancreas, liver) and much remains to be done in the area of PA and gastrointestinal cancer survivorship.

The role of PA in lung cancer survivorship is neither intuitive nor obvious. Nevertheless, Jones (2011) reports a growing interest in PA research in this survivor population and some preliminary positive findings. Appropriately, most of the early research has focused on the safety and feasibility of delivering exercise interventions in this population. These early findings have suggested that exercise training is safe and feasible for selected lung cancer survivors, especially those with operable disease, and that it may improve HRF and some PROs. Jones (2011) notes that additional feasibility and safety studies are warranted in this patient population given its heterogeneity and high-risk nature. Ultimately, larger RCTs are also needed to examine questions surrounding the effectiveness of exercise training for improving clinical outcomes in lung cancer survivors.

Most research in PA and hematological cancer survivorship has focused on recovery from bone marrow transplantation. Battaglini (2011) notes that these studies have demonstrated the safety and feasibility of exercise in this setting with very few adverse events. Moreover, positive changes have been observed for aerobic capacity, muscular strength, lean body mass, fatigue, depression, and quality of life. Nevertheless, many studies suffer from methodological limitations including small sample sizes and the absence of a comparison group. Battaglini (2011) notes that stronger methodological studies are needed to determine the effects of exercise on clinical outcomes in bone marrow transplant survivors and to extend this research to other hematological cancer survivor groups.

Another surprisingly understudied survivorship group is gynecological cancer. Gil and Von Gruenigen (2011) note that there is a strong rationale for examining PA in this cancer survivor group, but research to date is very limited. They also note that there are significant differences in the treatments, prognoses, and comorbidities of the two most common gynecologic cancers – ovarian and endometrial – and that these differences need to be taken into account when designing and testing PA interventions for these groups. At this early stage, Gil and Von Gruenigen (2011) suggest additional safety and feasibility studies prior to large RCTs addressing clinical outcomes.

1.6 Summary of Physical Activity and Cancer Special Topic Chapters

Improved treatments have resulted in excellent survival rates for various pediatric cancer groups. Unfortunately, these treatments can lead to significant chronic and late-appearing effects. San Juan et al. (2011) note that these side effects can be exacerbated by a lack of PA. In their review of this literature, they conclude that exercise interventions are safe in the pediatric population and have been shown to improve cardiorespiratory fitness and muscular strength. They also note that supervised exercise sessions may be necessary to achieve substantial improvements in these outcomes. San Juan et al. (2011) conclude by noting the many methodological limitations in this research and some of the unique challenges of conducting exercise research in pediatric cancer survivors.

The challenges facing people with advanced cancer can be significant. Lowe (2011) notes that PA may help palliative cancer patients manage symptoms, improve mobility, slow functional decline, and maintain quality of life at the end of life. As might be expected, however, few research studies have examined PA as a supportive care intervention in the palliative care setting. In summarizing the limited research to date, Lowe (2011) notes preliminary evidence that at least some palliative cancer patients are willing and able to participate in PA interventions, with some patients demonstrating improvements in select supportive

1

care outcomes. Once again, however, there are unique methodological challenges to conducting PA research in the palliative cancer setting.

PA motivation and behavior change is a challenge for any population, but it may be particularly difficult for cancer survivors. Pinto and Ciccolo (2011) review the burgeoning supportive literature on the determinants of exercise in cancer survivors and the various intervention strategies being developed to promote PA in this population. They provide a comprehensive review of the many theoretical models that have been used to guide this research and conclude that most of these theories have been helpful in identifying key determinants and informing behavior change interventions. They also note that several cancer- and treatment-related variables have been associated with PA in cancer survivors, highlighting some of the unique determinants of PA in this population. Finally, Pinto and Ciccolo (2011) conclude that more research is needed on intervention strategies that can target the well-established determinants of PA in cancer survivors across the entire cancer control continuum.

1.7 Future Research Directions for Physical Activity and Cancer Research

This volume highlights numerous important scientific advances in PA and cancer research but many questions remain. To this end, we provide general suggestions for future research efforts. First, there is a clear need for greater insight into the biologic mechanisms that relate PA to disease outcomes, ideally from exercise RCTs. Better understanding of these mechanisms will add plausibility to purported associations, guide future epidemiologic research, identify new targets for interventions, and inform public health and clinical recommendations for lowering cancer risk and recurrence. Across the cancer sites covered in this volume, many of the same mechanisms are proposed (e.g., insulin resistance, sex hormones, inflammation, immune function, vitamin D). Consequently, any RCT could potentially inform prevention strategies for multiple cancer sites.

Next, an important gap in the current knowledge is the PA type and minimum dose that is required for improved outcomes. Once again, exercise RCTs would inform future recommendations. Some relatively recent research suggests a preventive role for light intensity activity, which includes everyday household and occupational tasks, as well as potentially cancer-promoting effects from sedentary behaviour. Since past research has focused heavily on PA of moderate-to-vigorous intensity, these possibilities warrant attention in future research projects. There is also a need for valid and reliable instruments with which to measure these activities.

Another recurring recommendation in the cancer prevention chapters is for research to identify population subgroups that might benefit the most (or the least) from PA. Future etiologic studies must be sufficiently powered for subgroup analyses in order to illuminate important differences that might have been overlooked previously. Similarly, there is a need for future assessments of potential moderators of PA effectiveness that may influence cancer survivorship outcomes.

A number of additional recommendations pertaining specifically to exercise trials in cancer survivors are highlighted in the survivorship chapters. First, exercise intervention trials to understand the effectiveness of PA on cancer survivorship outcomes are needed for many understudied cancer sites. Second, most exercise RCTs in cancer survivors have focused on PA during or posttreatment as opposed to other points along the cancer continuum. More RCTs are needed to address the effects of PA on palliation of symptoms at the end of life and on survival after cancer has been eradicated. Third, a variety of psychosocial, physiologic, and other outcomes of potential importance have not been adequately assessed in past exercise RCTs in cancer survivors. Future exercise RCTs should investigate the effect of PA on these outcomes in patients who are at greatest need for improvement for those outcomes.

Finally, PA measurement is an ongoing methodological challenge that affects the integrity of all studies of PA and cancer. Objective monitoring of PA is a rapidly evolving field of research that holds promise for future epidemiologic research. Comprehensive PA questionnaires that measure all types and intensities of PA, including sedentary behaviour, over the lifetime are also recommended. A combined approach to PA measurement that relies on PA monitors to estimate PA dose and posture, and self-report methods to provide contextual information may become a future trend for PA and cancer research.

1.8 Overall Summary and Conclusions

PA and cancer research has increased exponentially over the past decade. Research to date suggests that PA may reduce the risk of developing some cancers, help cancer survivors cope with and recover from treatments, improve the health of long-term cancer survivors, and possibly even reduce the risk of recurrence and extend survival in some cancer survivor groups. Additional research in this field is likely to further reduce the burden of cancer. Consequently, there is a strong rationale for continued research on PA across the entire cancer control continuum that addresses the many unknown questions. Nevertheless, given the numerous cancer-related benefits already established for PA, there is a strong rationale for promoting PA for both cancer prevention and improved survivorship.

Acknowledgments Kerry S. Courneya is supported by the Canada Research Chairs Program. Christine M. Friedenreich is supported by a Health Senior Scholar Award from the Alberta Heritage Foundation for Medical Research.

References

ACSM (2010) ACSM's guidelines for exercise testing and prescription, 8th edn. Lippincott Williams & Wilkins, Philadelphia, PA

Battaglini CL (2011) Physical activity and hematologic cancer survivorship. In: Courneya KS, Friedenreich CM (eds) Physical activity and cancer. Recent results in cancer research, vol 186. Springer, Berlin Heidelberg

Bouchard C, Shepard RJ (1994) Physical activity, fitness and health: The model and key concepts. In: Bouchard C, Shephard RJ, Stephens T (eds) Physical activity, fitness and health. International Proceedings and Consensus Statement. Human Kinetics, Champaign, IL, pp 77–78

Cust AE (2011) Physical activity and gynecologic cancer prevention. In: Courneya KS, Friedenreich CM (eds) Physical activity and cancer: Recent results in cancer research, vol 186. Springer, Berlin Heidelberg

Doyle CL, Kushi LH, Byers T, Courneya KS, Demark-Wahnefried W, Grant B, McTiernan A, Rock CL, Thompson C, Gansler T, Andrews KS (2006) Nutrition and physical activity during and after cancer treatment: an American Cancer Society guide for informed choices. CA Cancer J Clin 56:323–353

Emaus A, Thune I (2011) Physical activity and lung cancer prevention. In: Courneya KS, Friedenreich CM (eds) Physical activity and cancer: Recent results in cancer research, vol 186. Springer, Berlin Heidelberg

Galvao DA, Taaffe DR, Spry N, Newton RU et al (2011) Physical activity and genitourinary cancer survivorship. In: Courneya KS, Friedenreich CM (eds) Physical activity and cancer: Recent results in cancer research, vol 186. Springer, Berlin Heidelberg

1

Gil KM, Von Gruenigen V (2011) Physical activity and gynecologic cancer survivorship. In: Courneya KS, Friedenreich CM (eds) Physical activity and cancer: Recent results in cancer research, vol 186. Springer, Berlin Heidelberg

Hayes SC, Spence RR, Galvao DA, Newton RU (2009) Australian Association for Exercise and Sport Science position stand: Optimising cancer outcomes through exercise. J Sci Med Sport 12:428–434

Hewitt M, Greenfield S, Stovall E (2006) From cancer patient to cancer survivor: Lost in transition. The National Academies Press, Washington, DC, p 536

IARC (2002) IARC Working Group 2002. IARC Handbook of Cancer Prevention: Weight control and physical activity, vol 6. IARC, Lyon

Jones LW (2011) Physical activity and lung cancer survivorship. In: Courneya KS, Friedenreich CM (eds) Physical activity and cancer: Recent results in cancer research, vol 186. Springer, Berlin Heidelberg

Kushi LH, Byers T, Doyle C, Bandera EV, McCullough M, Gansler T, Andrews KS, Thun MJ (2006) American Cancer Society Guidelines on Nutrition and Physical Activity for cancer prevention: reducing the risk of cancer with healthy food choices and physical activity. CA Cancer J Clin 56:254–281

Leitzmann MF (2011) Physical activity and genitourinary cancer prevention. In: Courneya KS, Friedenreich CM (eds) Physical activity and cancer: Recent results in cancer research, vol 186. Springer, Berlin Heidelberg

Lowe SS (2011) Physical activity and palliative cancer care. In: Courneya KS, Friedenreich CM (eds) Physical activity and cancer: Recent results in cancer research, vol 186. Springer, Berlin Heidelberg

Lynch BM, Neilson HK, Friedenreich C (2011) Physical activity and breast cancer prevention. In: Courneya KS, Friedenreich CM (eds) Physical activity and cancer: Recent results in cancer research, vol 186. Springer, Berlin Heidelberg

Pan SY, Morrison H (2011) Physical activity and hematologic cancer prevention. In: Courneya KS, Friedenreich CM (eds) Physical activity and cancer: Recent results in cancer research, vol 186. Springer, Berlin Heidelberg

Physical Activity Guidelines Advisory Committee (2008) Physical Activity Guidelines Advisory Committee Report. U.S. Department of Health and Human Services, Washington, DC

Pinto BM, Ciccolo JT (2011) Physical activity motivation and cancer survivorship. In: Courneya KS, Friedenreich CM (eds) Physical activity and cancer: Recent results in cancer research, vol 186. Springer, Berlin Heidelberg

San Juan AF, Wolin K, Lucia A (2011) Physical activity and pediatric cancer survivorship. In: Courneya KS, Friedenreich CM (eds) Physical activity and cancer: Recent results in cancer research, vol 186. Springer, Berlin Heidelberg

Schmitz K (2011) Physical activity and breast cancer survivorship. In: Courneya KS, Friedenreich CM (eds) Physical activity and cancer: Recent results in cancer research, vol 186. Springer, Berlin Heidelberg

Schmitz KH, Courneya KS, Matthews C, Demark-Wahnefried W, Galvao DA, Pinto BM, Irwin ML, Wolin KL, Segal RJ, Lucia A, Schneider CM, Von Greunigen VE, Schwartz AL (2010) American College of Sports Medicine roundtable on exercise guidelines for cancer survivors. Medicine & Science in Sports & Exercise, 42, 1409–1426

Sellar CM, Courneya KS (2011) Physical activity and gastrointestinal survivorship. In: Courneya KS, Friedenreich CM (eds) Physical activity and cancer: Recent results in cancer research, vol 186. Springer, Berlin Heidelberg

WCRF (2007) World Cancer research fund and the American institute for cancer research 2007 food, nutrition, physical activity, and the prevention of cancer: A global perspective. American Institute for Cancer Research, Washington, DC

Wolin KY, Tuchman H (2011) Physical activity and gastrointestinal cancer prevention. In: Courneya KS, Friedenreich CM (eds) Physical activity and cancer: Recent results in cancer research. Springer, Berlin Heidelberg

Part I

Physical Activity and Cancer Prevention

Physical Activity and Breast Cancer Prevention

2

Brigid M. Lynch, Heather K. Neilson, and Christine M. Friedenreich

Abstract Breast cancer is the most commonly diagnosed invasive malignancy and the second leading cause of cancer death in women. This chapter considers epidemiologic evidence regarding the association between physical activity and breast cancer risk from 73 studies conducted around the world. Across these studies there was a 25% average risk reduction amongst physically active women as compared to the least active women. The associations were strongest for recreational activity, for activity sustained over the lifetime or done after menopause, and for activity that is of moderate to vigorous intensity and performed regularly. There is also some evidence for a stronger effect of physical activity amongst postmenopausal women, women who are normal weight, have no family history of breast cancer, and are parous. It is likely that physical activity is associated with decreased breast cancer risk via multiple interrelated biologic pathways that may involve adiposity, sex hormones, insulin resistance, adipokines, and chronic inflammation. Future research should include prospective observational epidemiologic studies relating proposed biomarkers to breast cancer risk and also randomized controlled trials to examine how physical activity influences the proposed biomarkers. Exercise trials will provide more clarity regarding the appropriate type, dose, and timing of activity that relate to breast cancer risk reduction.

2.1 Introduction

Physical inactivity is one of the few established breast cancer risk factors amenable to intervention. Over 90 studies conducted worldwide have investigated some aspect of this association. In this chapter, we review the epidemiologic literature on physical activity and breast cancer risk, examining the effect of the different parameters of activity and effect modification within different population subgroups. We also review the biologic mechanisms whereby physical activity may influence the risk of breast cancer.

B.M. Lynch, H.K. Neilson,
Department of Population Health Research, Alberta Health Services-Cancer Care, 1331 29 St NW, Calgary, Alberta, Canada T2N 4N2

C.M. Friedenreich (✉)
AHFMR Health Senior Scholar Alberta Health Services, University of Calgary, 1331 29 St NW, Calgary, Alberta, Canada T2N 4N2
e-mail: christine.friedenreich@albertahealthservices.ca

K.S. Courneya and C.M. Friedenreich (eds.), *Physical Activity and Cancer*, Recent Results in Cancer Research 186, DOI: 10.1007/978-3-642-04231-7_2,

2

2.2 Epidemiologic Evidence

2.2.1 Background

Breast cancer is the most common invasive malignancy diagnosed in women, with 1,151,298 new cases estimated worldwide in 2002 (Ferlay et al. 2004). Female breast cancer represents 27% of all new female cancers in developed countries: estimates project 192,370 new cases in the U.S. and 22,700 cases in Canada in 2009 (Canadian Cancer Society 2009; Jemal et al. 2009). The lifetime risk of a woman being diagnosed with breast cancer is approximately one in eight in the United States (Jemal et al. 2009), and slightly lower in other developed countries (Australian Institute of Health and Welfare and National Breast and Ovarian Cancer Centre 2009; Canadian Cancer Society 2009; Cancer Research UK 2009).

Worldwide, breast cancer is the most common cause of cancer death among women; the number of estimated deaths in 2002 was 410,712 (Ferlay et al. 2004). In developed countries breast cancer is often the second leading cause of cancer death in women, following lung cancer (Canadian Cancer Society 2009; Jemal et al. 2009; Office for National Statistics 2008). A total of 40,170 and 5,400 breast cancer deaths are projected to occur in the U.S. and Canada, respectively, in 2009 (Canadian Cancer Society 2009; Jemal et al. 2009). However, 5-year relative survival is high, approaching 90% in developed countries (Australian Institute of Health and Welfare and National Breast and Ovarian Cancer Centre 2009; Canadian Cancer Society 2009; Jemal et al. 2009; Office for National Statistics 2008).

Most of the established risk factors for breast cancer are not easily modifiable. These include: age, race, a family history of breast cancer, genetic susceptibility, benign breast disease, early age at menarche, late age at menopause, and nulliparity (Bernstein 2009; Monninkhof et al. 2007a). Physical inactivity is one of the few behavioral risk factors amenable to change, and as such represents an opportunity to reduce the burden of disease from breast cancer.

There have been a number of reviews and reports written on the topic of physical activity and breast cancer prevention. These have generally concluded that the evidence supporting this association is convincing (Friedenreich and Cust 2008; Friedenreich and Orenstein 2002; IARC Working Group 2002; Monninkhof et al. 2007a); however the World Cancer Research Fund was more cautious, labeling the association probable (World Cancer Research Fund and the American Institute for Cancer Research 2007).

This chapter updates the review of physical activity and breast cancer risk provided by Friedenreich and Cust (2008). Here, we have incorporated the epidemiologic literature published to December 2009: 33 cohort studies and 40 case-control studies. Where multiple publications from the same study were found, the most recent publication (cohort studies), or the original publication (case-control studies), was selected for inclusion in our main results. We defined study results as null if the odds or hazard ratios fell between 0.9 and 1.1, inclusive. If the upper limit of the 95% confidence intervals (95% CI) was less than 1.05, we considered the results to be of borderline statistical significance.

2.2.2 Overall Associations Between Physical Activity and Breast Cancer Risk

Twenty-nine of the 73 studies reviewed (40%) found a statistically significant risk reduction for breast cancer when comparing the highest versus lowest level of physical activity (Bernstein et al. 2005; Breslow et al. 2001; Carpenter et al. 2003; Calle et al. 1998; Dallal et al. 2007; Dirx et al. 2001; Fraser and Shavlik 1997; Friedenreich et al. 2001; Kruk 2007a, b; Kruk and Aboul-

Enein 2003; Levi et al. 1999; Mathew et al. 2009; Matthews et al. 2001; Mezzetti et al. 1998; Moradi et al. 2000; Peplonska et al. 2008; Peters et al. 2009a; Rintala et al. 2002; Rockhill et al. 1999; Sesso et al. 1998; Shoff et al. 2000; Suzuki et al. 2008; Thune et al. 1997; Ueji et al. 1998; Verloop et al. 2000; Wyrwich and Wolinsky 2000; Wyshak and Frisch 2000; Yang et al. 2003). An additional eight studies (11%) had a borderline, statistically significant breast cancer risk reduction (Hirose et al. 2003; John et al. 2003; Lee et al. 2001b; Leitzmann et al. 2008; Maruti et al. 2008; McTiernan et al. 1996; McTiernan et al. 2003; Patel et al. 2003), and 14 (19%) observed a statistically nonsignificant reduction (Adams-Campbell et al. 2001; Chang et al. 2006; Dey et al. 2009; Dorn et al. 2003; Dosemeci et al. 1993; Friedenreich and Rohan 1995; Gilliland et al. 2001; Hu et al. 1997; Marcus et al. 1999; Moradi et al. 2002; Rintala et al. 2003; Shin et al. 2009; Slattery et al. 2007; Sprague et al. 2007). Nineteen (26%) studies produced null effects (Bardia et al. 2006; Calle et al. 1998; Chen et al. 1997; Colditz et al. 2003; Coogan and Aschengrau 1999; Gammon et al. 1998; Gao et al. 2009; Howard et al. 2009; Lahmann et al. 2007; Lee et al. 2001a; Luoto et al. 2000; Magnusson et al. 2005; Mertens et al. 2006; Nkondjock et al. 2006; Schmidt et al. 2008; Silvera et al. 2006; Steindorf et al. 2003; Taioli et al. 1995; Tehard et al. 2006), and three (4%) studies observed a statistically nonsignificant increased risk of breast cancer among the most physically active women (Dorgan et al. 1994; Margolis et al. 2005; Schnohr et al. 2005). Statistically significant risk reductions were reported as frequently in the case-control studies (16 studies from a total of 40; 40%) as in the cohort studies (13 from 33; 39%) (Figs. 2.1 and 2.2). Across all studies there was a 25% average risk reduction, with a stronger effect found in the case-control studies (an average risk reduction of 30%) than in the cohort studies (a 20% risk reduction). Of the 51 studies that found a decreased risk of breast cancer with increased levels of physical activity, 41 examined the trend of this relationship (Adams-Campbell et al. 2001; Bernstein et al. 2005; Breslow et al. 2001; Carpenter et al. 2003; Cerhan et al. 1998; Chang et al. 2006; Dallal et al. 2007; Dey et al. 2009; Dirx et al. 2001; Dorn et al. 2003; Dosemeci et al. 1993; Friedenreich et al. 2001; Friedenreich and Rohan 1995; Gilliland et al. 2001; Hirose et al. 2003; Hu et al. 1997; Kruk 2007a; b; Lee et al. 2001b; Leitzmann et al. 2008; Levi et al. 1999; Marcus et al. 1999; Maruti et al. 2008; Mathew et al. 2009; Matthews et al. 2001; McTiernan et al. 1996, 2003; Mezzetti et al. 1998; Moradi et al. 2000, 2002; Patel et al. 2003; Peplonska et al. 2008; Rockhill et al. 1999; Sesso et al. 1998; Shin et al. 2009; Shoff et al. 2000; Slattery et al. 2007; Sprague et al. 2007; Thune et al. 1997; Ueji et al. 1998; Yang et al. 2003). Thirty-three of these studies found evidence for a dose–response relation between increasing levels of physical activity and decreasing breast cancer risks (Adams-Campbell et al. 2001; Bernstein et al. 2005; Breslow et al. 2001; Carpenter et al. 2003; Cerhan et al. 1998; Dallal et al. 2007; Dey et al. 2009; Dirx et al. 2001; Friedenreich et al. 2001; Gilliland et al. 2001; Kruk 2007a; b; Lee et al. 2001b; Levi et al. 1999; Maruti et al. 2008; Mathew et al. 2009; Matthews et al. 2001; McTiernan et al. 1996, 2003; Mezzetti et al. 1998; Moradi et al. 2000, 2002; Patel et al. 2003; Peplonska et al. 2008; Rockhill et al. 1999; Sesso et al. 1998; Shin et al. 2009; Shoff et al. 2000; Slattery et al. 2007; Sprague et al. 2007; Thune et al. 1997; Ueji et al. 1998; Yang et al. 2003).

2.2.3 Type, Dose, and Timing of Activity

One of the difficulties inherent in reviewing the physical activity and breast cancer literature is the heterogeneity of methods used to assess physical activity. Some studies have utilized comprehensive assessments of lifetime physical activity, whereas others have used single-item measures.

2

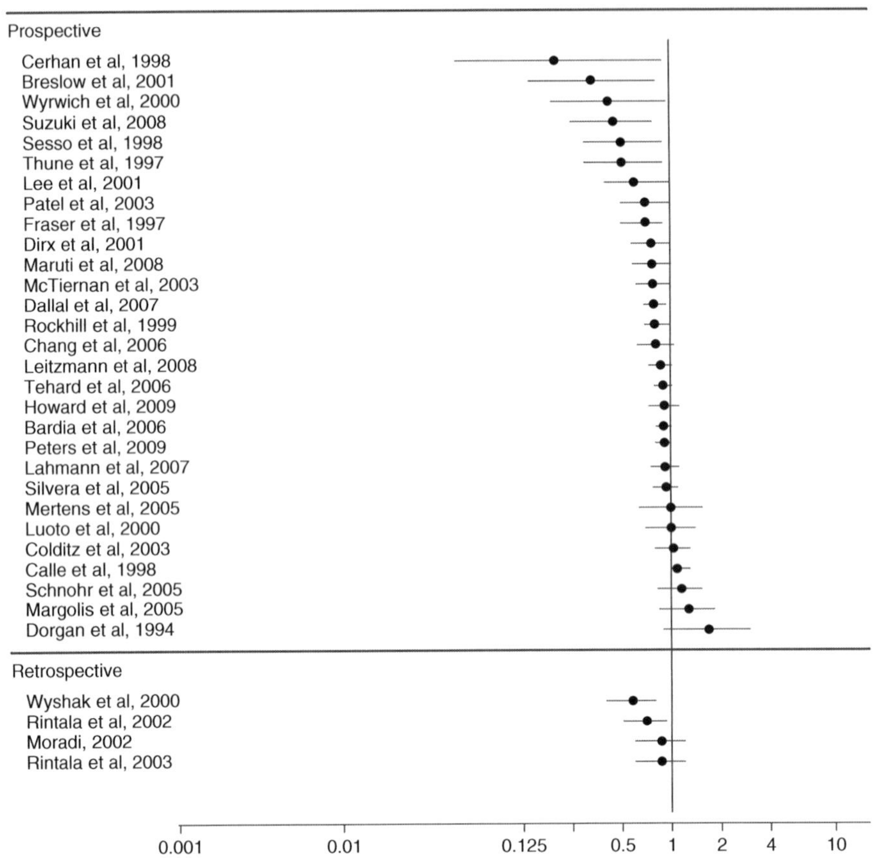

Fig. 2.1 Cohort studies of physical activity and breast cancer risk

Hence, we examined specific parameters of physical activity (i.e. type, dose, timing) and their association with breast cancer risk, separately.

Figures 2.3, 2.4, and 2.5 present study outcomes by type of physical activity: occupational, recreational, walking/cycling, and household activity. The greatest breast cancer risk reductions were found for recreational and household activity (average 21%), followed by walking/cycling (18%), and occupational activity (13%).

Dose refers to the combination of frequency, duration, and intensity of the activity performed. Frequency describes how many times a particular physical activity is undertaken, while duration describes the amount of time physical activity is undertaken for. Intensity describes the level of exertion required to perform a particular physical activity, and is often categorized as light, moderate, or vigorous, according to energy expenditure.

Few studies reported frequency of physical activity, hence no figure is presented. Participation in moderate intensity physical activity was associated with an average decreased risk of 15%. A slightly greater risk reduction was found for vigorous intensity physical activity, 18% (Fig. 2.6). Similarly, greater decreases in breast cancer risk were observed with greater duration of activity (moderate-to-vigorous intensity or recreational activity) (Fig. 2.7). Hence, while participation in 2–3 h per week was associated with an

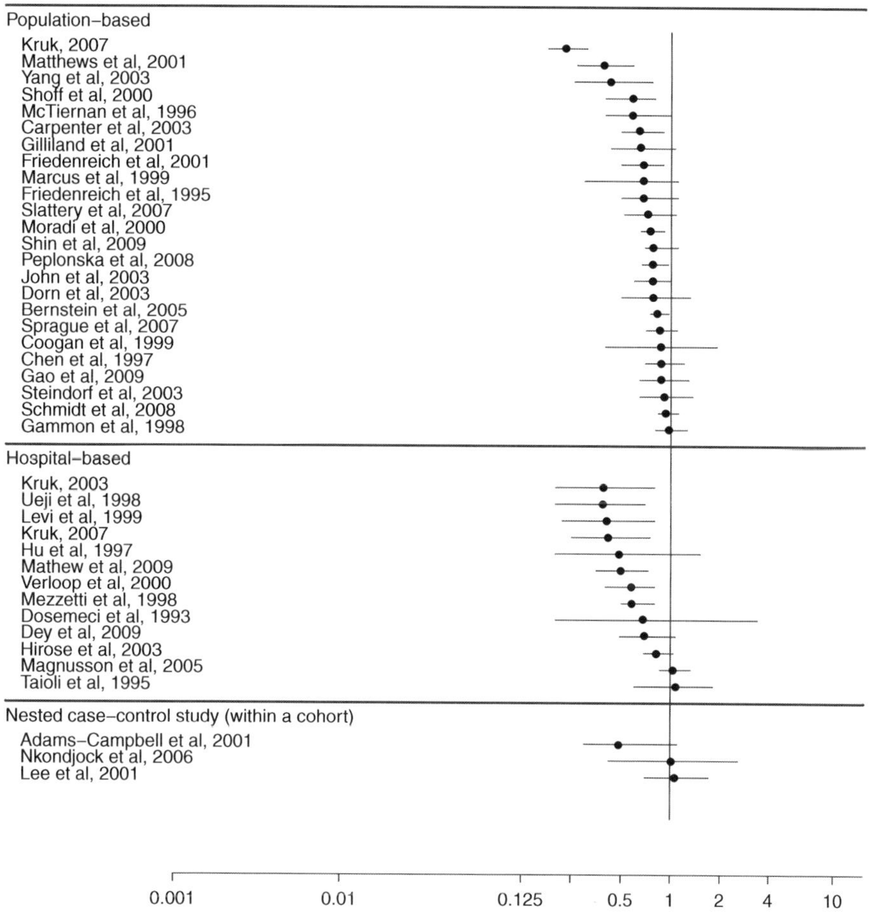

Fig. 2.2 Case–control studies of physical activity and breast cancer risk

average risk reduction of 9%, women who reported 6.5 h of activity per week or more had a decreased risk of 30%.

Studies also assessed physical activity performed during different periods of life: adolescence, early adulthood (20s), middle adulthood (30s/40s), and later adulthood (≥50 years) (Fig. 2.8). Although risk reductions were observed for physical activity performed at each age period, activity after age 50 seemed to have a slightly stronger effect than earlier periods of activity (an average risk reduction of 17%). The average decrease in breast cancer risk associated with physical activity performed during adolescence was 16%; during early adulthood it was 8%, and during middle adulthood it was 15%. Sixteen studies assessed physical activity over the adult lifetime and the average risk reduction was even greater at 27% (data not shown).

2.2.4 Population Subgroups

We also considered how the association between physical activity and breast cancer risk may vary between different population subgroups. There were sufficient data to examine effect modifica-

2

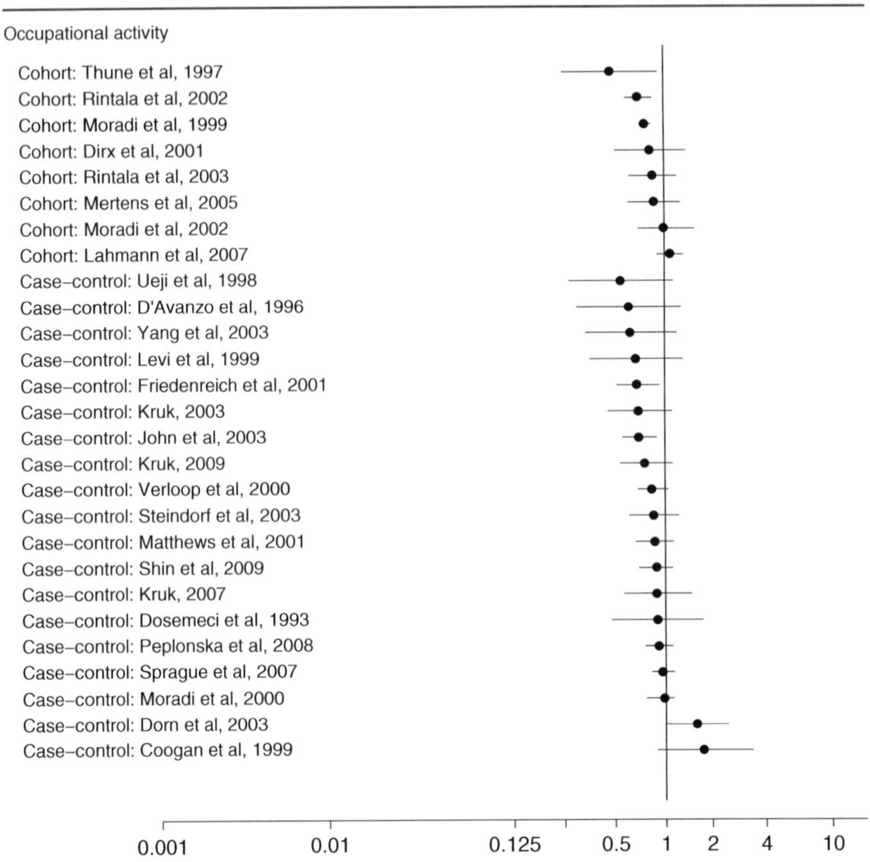

Fig. 2.3 Occupational physical activity and breast cancer risk

tion by menopausal status, body mass index (BMI; weight/height^2) race, family history of breast cancer, hormone receptor status, and parity.

A decrease in breast cancer risk was found for both pre- and postmenopausal women (Fig. 2.9); however, across all studies that reported on menopausal status, the average risk reduction was somewhat greater among postmenopausal women (31%) than among premenopausal women (27%). Twenty-five studies presented results stratified by menopausal status, i.e. both pre- and postmenopausal women in the same study population (Adams-Campbell et al. 2001; Dey et al. 2009; Dorn et al. 2003; Friedenreich et al. 2001; Friedenreich and Rohan 1995; Gammon et al. 1998; Gilliland et al. 2001; Hirose et al. 2003; Howard et al. 2009; Hu et al. 1997; John et al. 2003; Kruk 2007a, b; Lahmann et al. 2007; Mathew et al. 2009; Matthews et al. 2001; Mezzetti et al. 1998; Moradi et al. 1999; Shin et al. 2009; Silvera et al. 2006; Slattery et al. 2007; Suzuki et al. 2008; Thune et al. 1997; Ueji et al. 1998; Yang et al. 2003). Only three observed statistically significant decreases in breast cancer risk for both pre- and postmenopausal women (Kruk 2007a; Suzuki et al. 2008; Yang et al. 2003). From the 25 studies that examined breast cancer risk reductions of pre- and postmenopausal women separately, 13 studies found greater risk reductions among postmenopausal

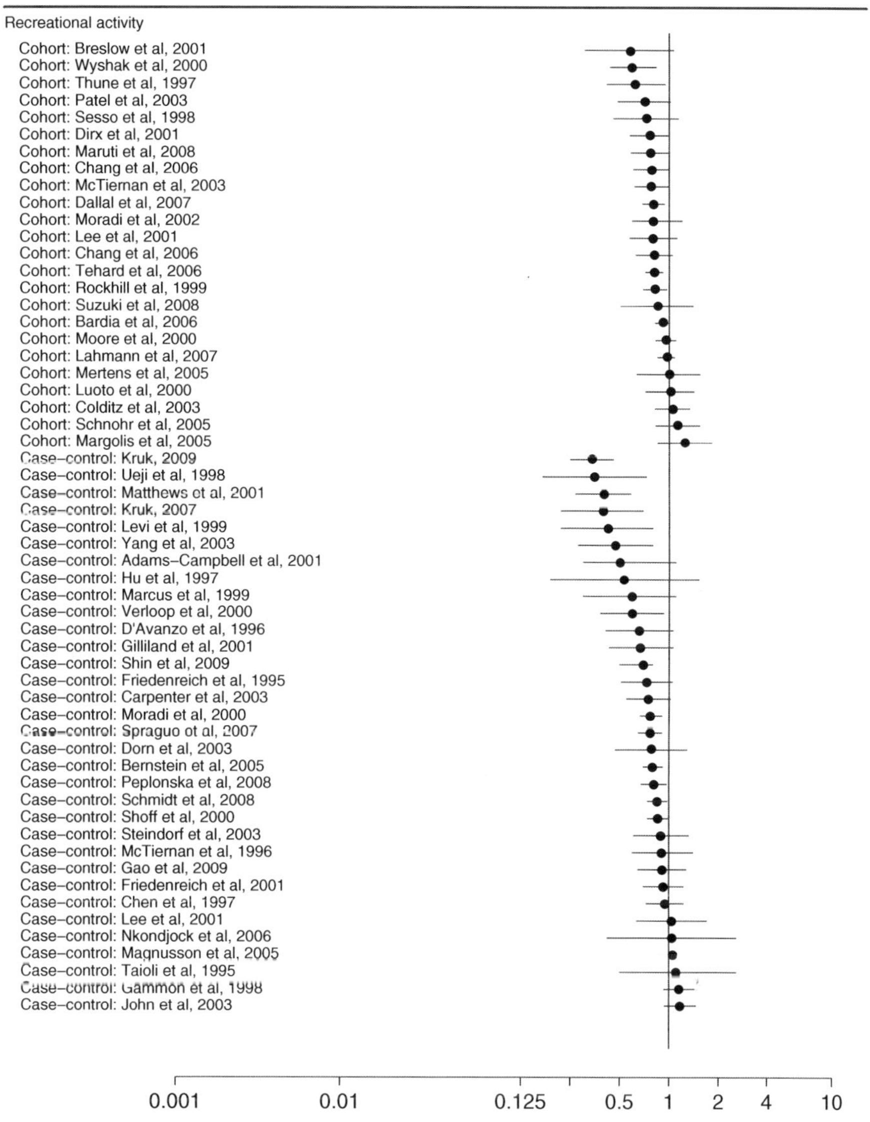

Fig. 2.4 Recreational physical activity and breast cancer risk

women (Adams-Campbell et al. 2001; Dey et al. 2009; Dorn et al. 2003; Friedenreich et al. 2001; Friedenreich and Rohan 1995; Gammon et al. 1998; Gilliland et al. 2001; Hirose et al. 2003; Howard et al. 2009; Hu et al. 1997; John et al. 2003; Kruk 2007a, b; Lahmann et al. 2007; Mathew et al. 2009; Matthews et al. 2001; Mezzetti et al. 1998; Moradi et al. 1999; Shin et al. 2009; Silvera et al. 2006; Slattery et al. 2007; Suzuki et al. 2008; Thune et al. 1997; Ueji et al. 1998; Yang et al. 2003), 11 studies found a stronger effect among premenopausal women (Dorn et al. 2003; Friedenreich and Rohan 1995; Hirose et al. 2003; John et al. 2003; Lahmann

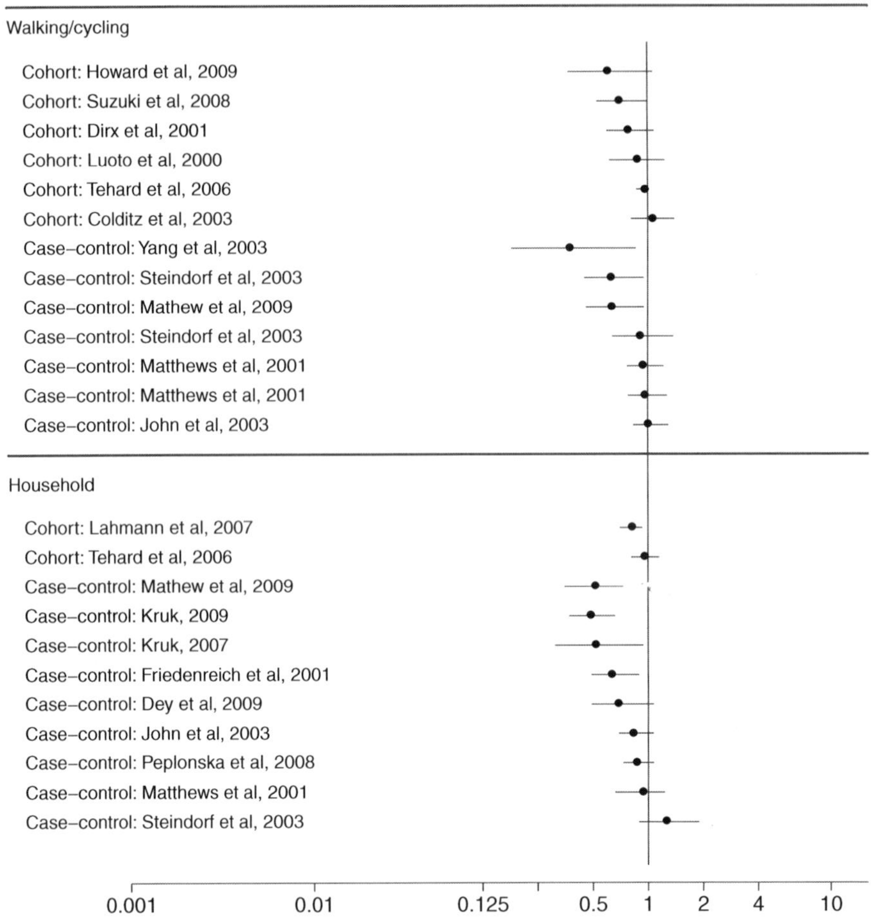

Fig. 2.5 Household physical activity, walking, cycling, and breast cancer risk

et al. 2007; Silvera et al. 2006; Slattery et al. 2007; Suzuki et al. 2008; Thune et al. 1997; Ueji et al. 1998; Yang et al. 2003), and one study found no difference by menopausal status (Shin et al. 2009). It is noteworthy, however, that of these 25 studies that stratified by menopausal status, 12 yielded statistically significant risk reductions in postmenopausal women, whereas for premenopausal women only three studies showed statistically significant risk reductions.

The second effect modifier, BMI, was examined in 22 studies (Breslow et al. 2001; Colditz et al. 2003; Dallal et al. 2007; Friedenreich et al. 2001; Gammon et al. 1998; Hirose et al. 2003; Kruk and Aboul-Enein 2003; Leitzmann et al. 2008; Luoto et al. 2000; Maruti et al. 2008; McTiernan et al. 2003; Moradi et al. 2002; Patel et al. 2003; Peplonska et al. 2008; Peters et al. 2009b; Schmidt et al. 2008; Sesso et al. 1998; Suzuki et al. 2008; Tehard et al. 2006; Thune et al. 1997; Verloop et al. 2000; Yang et al. 2003). Figure 2.10 presents the results of these studies categorized as low BMI (<22 kg/m^2), medium BMI (22–25 kg/m^2), high BMI (≥25 kg/m^2), and very high BMI (≥30 kg/m^2). Greater decreases in breast cancer risk for highest

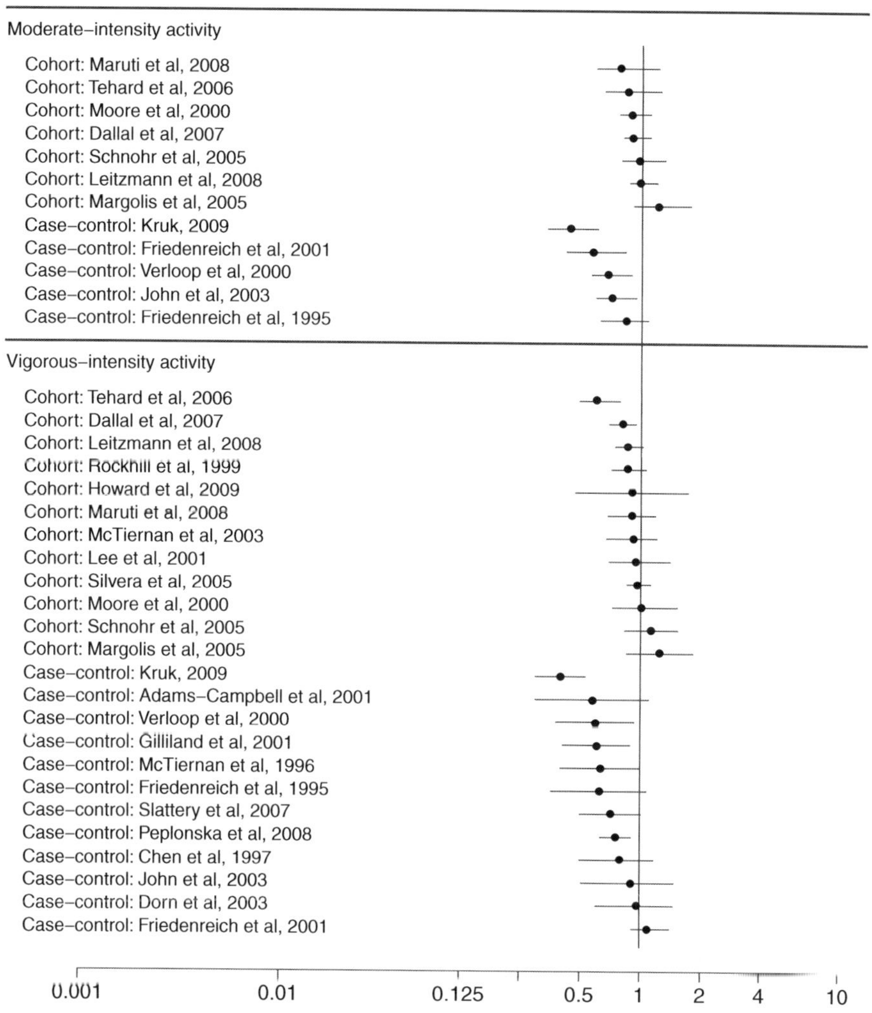

Fig. 2.6 Intensity of physical activity and breast cancer risk

versus lowest categories of physical activity were observed among women with lower BMI. The average risk reduction for low BMI was 27%; for medium BMI breast cancer risk was decreased by 24%; for high BMI it decreased by 18%; and, among women with very high BMI, the average risk reduction was less than 1%.

Only four studies calculated risk estimates separately for different racial/ethnic groups within their samples (Bernstein et al. 2005; Gilliland et al. 2001; John et al. 2003; Slattery et al. 2007) (Fig. 2.11). However, most of the studies included in this review could be classified according to the main racial group of their sample. An effect of physical activity on breast cancer risk was observed across all racial groups. Each of the three studies that included black women found a reduced risk (on average a relative decrease of 41%) (Adams-Campbell et al. 2001; Bernstein et al. 2005; John et al.

2

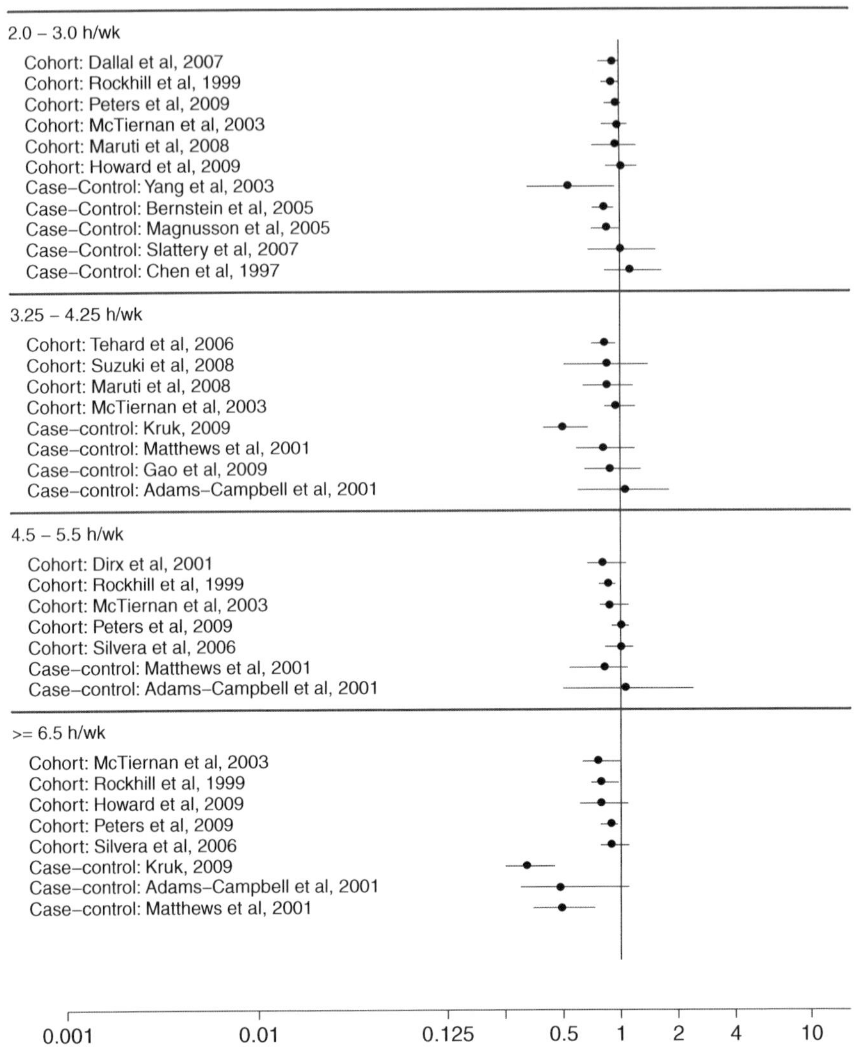

Fig. 2.7 Duration of physical activity and breast cancer risk

2003), two of the three studies of Hispanic women observed a reduced risk (average 28%) (Gilliland et al. 2001; John et al. 2003), and a decreased risk was found in both studies of Indian women (average 38%) (Dey et al. 2009; Mathew et al. 2009) and in the eight studies that included Asian women (average 41%) (Gao et al. 2009; Hirose et al. 2003; Hu et al. 1997; Matthews et al. 2001; Shin et al. 2009; Suzuki et al. 2008; Ueji et al. 1998; Yang et al. 2003). The average risk reduction for white women was somewhat lower (20%) (Bardia et al. 2006; Bernstein et al. 2005; Chang et al. 2006; Chen et al. 1997; Coogan and Aschengrau 1999; Dallal et al. 2007; Dirx et al. 2001; Fraser and Shavlik 1997; Friedenreich et al. 2001; Gilliland et al. 2001; Hofvind and Thoresen 2001; Howard et al. 2009; John et al. 2003; Kruk

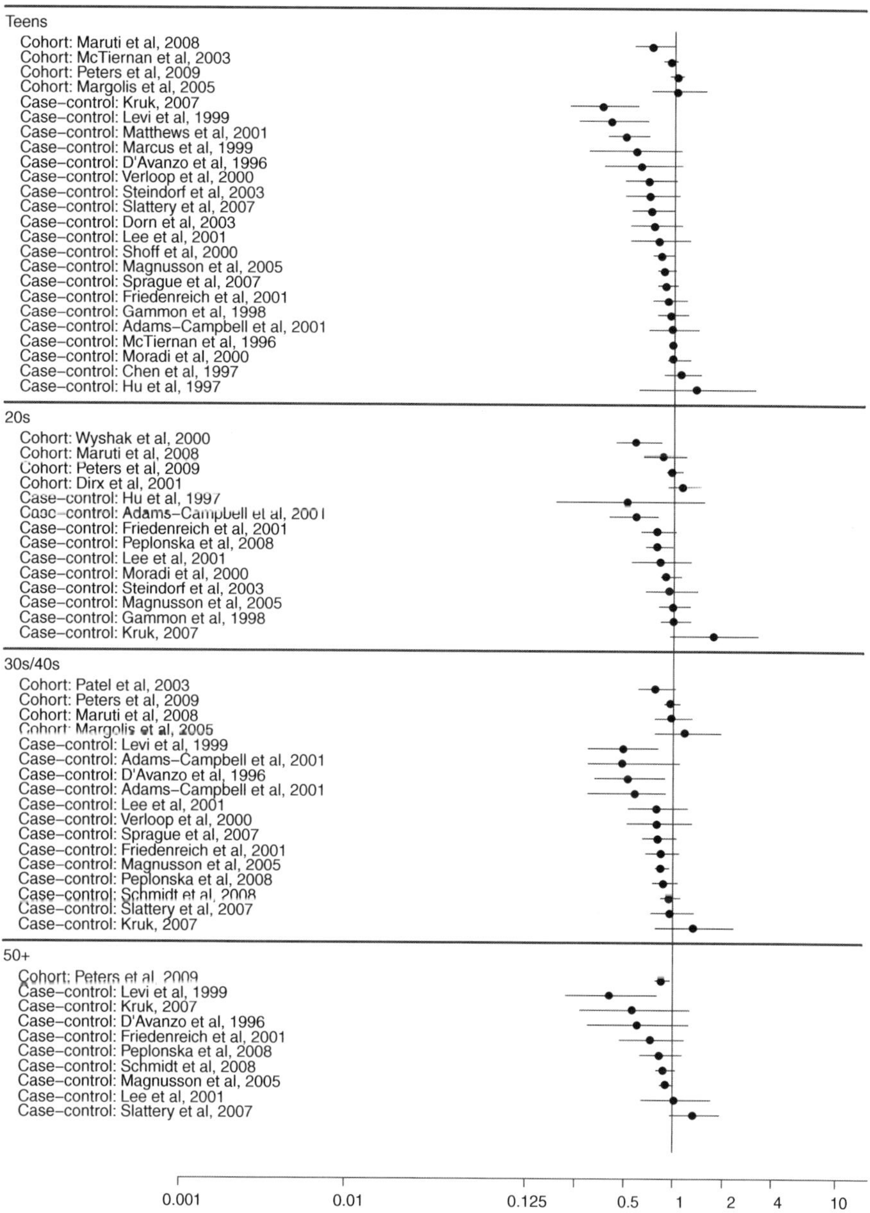

Fig. 2.8 Physical activity and breast cancer risk by decade of life

2007a; Kruk and Aboul-Enein 2003; Lahmann et al. 2007; Leitzmann et al. 2008; Levi et al. 1999; Luoto et al. 2000; Magnusson et al. 2005; Margolis et al. 2005; Maruti et al. 2008; Mezzetti et al. 1998; Moradi et al. 1999, 2000, 2002; Peplonska et al. 2008; Peters et al. 2009a; Rintala et al. 2002, 2003; Schmidt et al. 2008; Schnohr et al. 2005; Slattery et al. 2007;

2

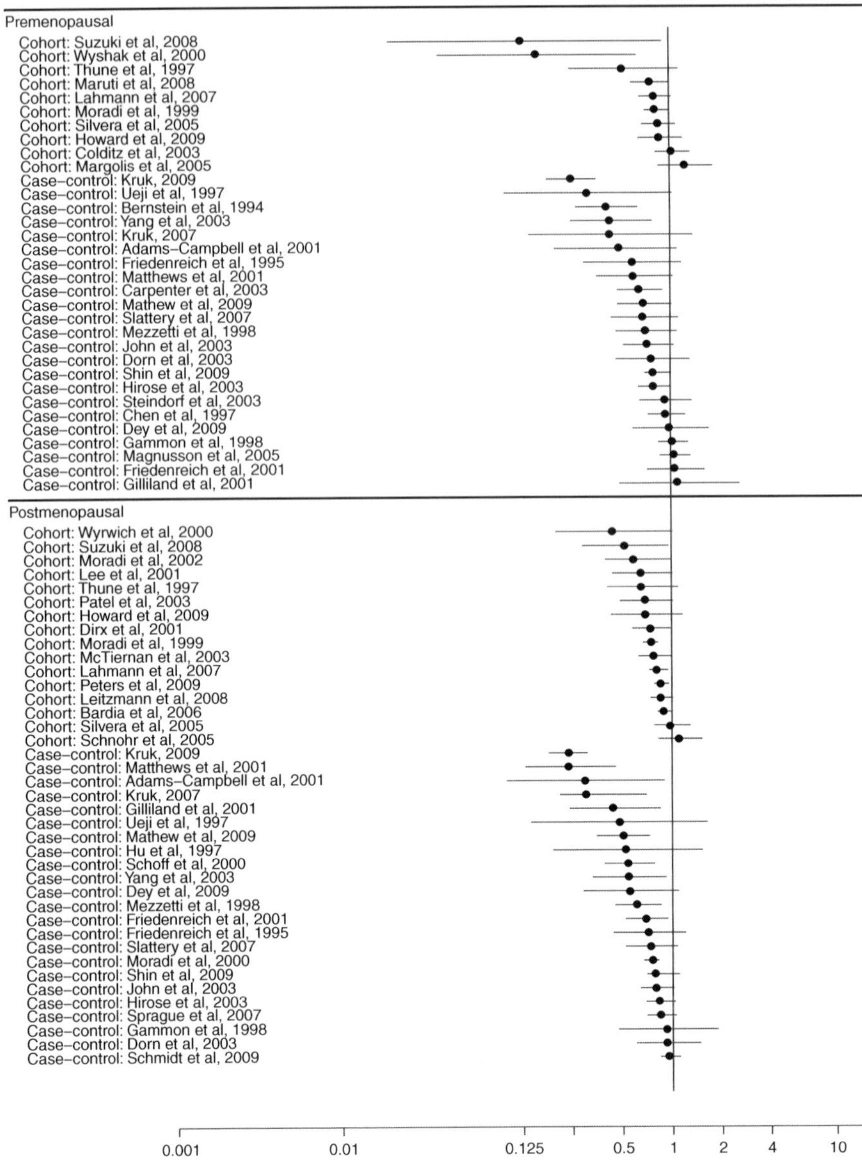

Fig. 2.9 Physical activity and breast cancer risk by menopausal status

Steindorf et al. 2003; Tehard et al. 2006; Thune et al. 1997; Verloop et al. 2000).

Nine studies included separate risk estimates for women with and without a family history of breast cancer (Bernstein et al. 2005; Carpenter et al. 2003; Dallal et al. 2007; Hirose et al. 2003; Magnusson et al. 2005; Peplonska et al. 2008; Peters et al. 2009b; Schmidt et al. 2008; Sprague et al. 2007). A strong risk reduction, on average 21%, was observed among women without a

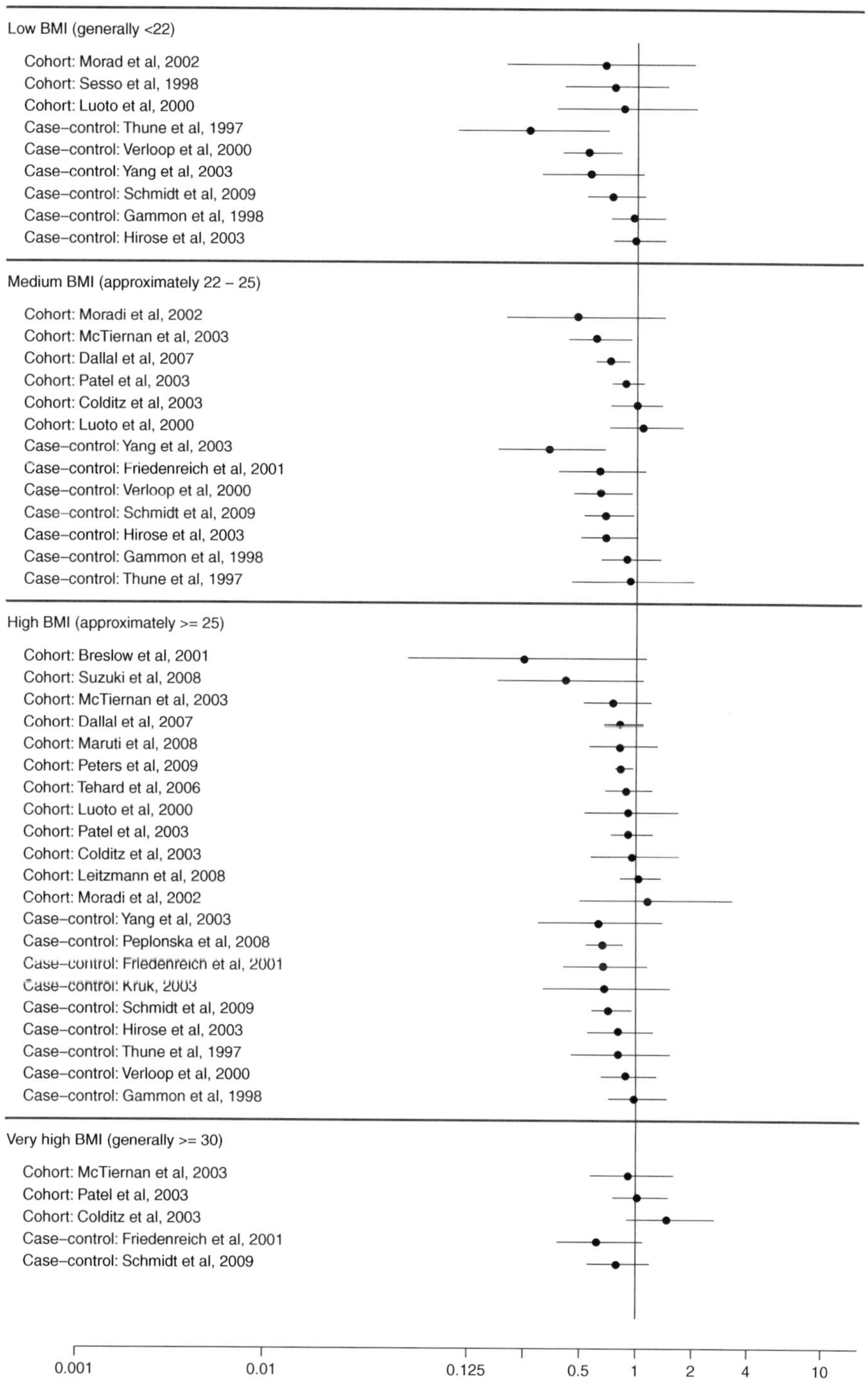

Fig. 2.10 Physical activity and breast cancer risk by body mass index

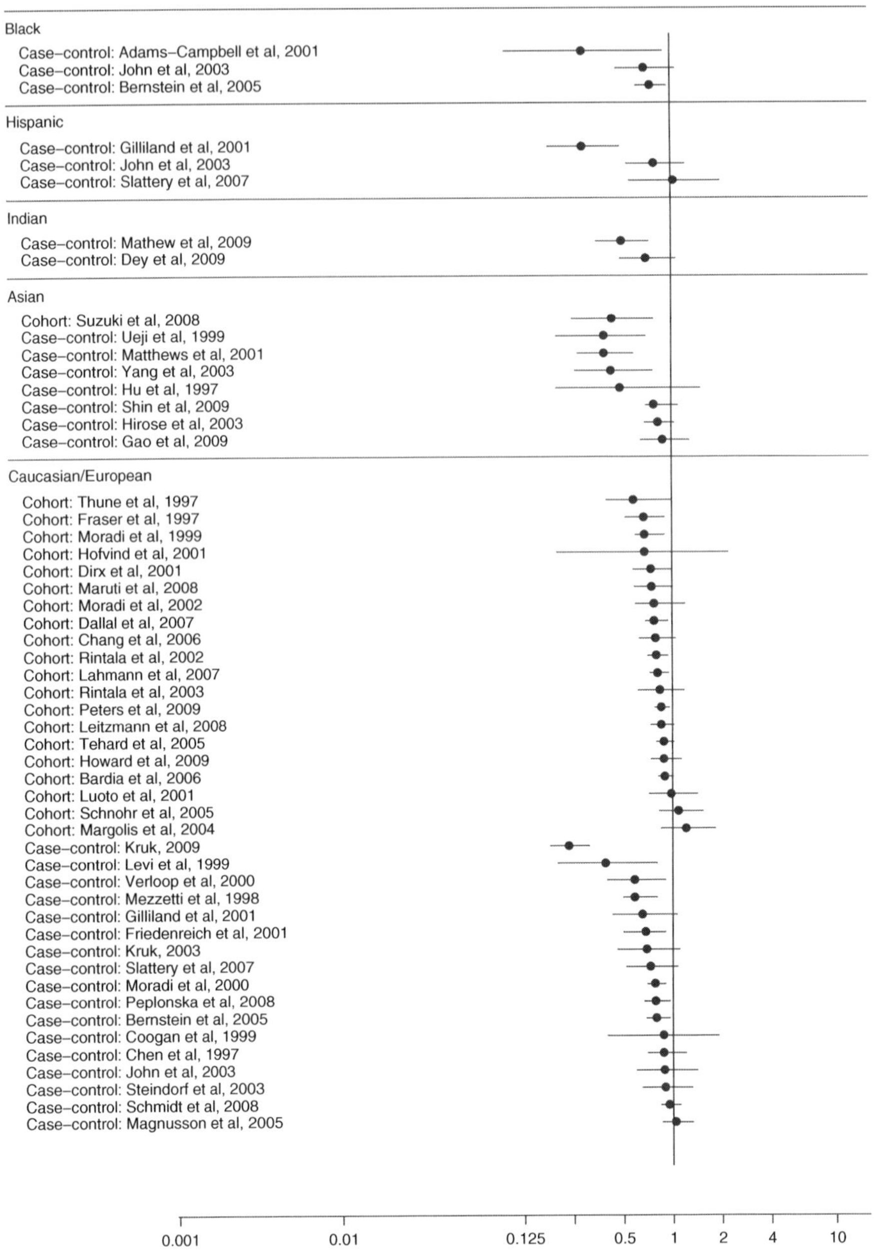

Fig. 2.11 Physical activity and breast cancer risk by race

family history of breast cancer while women with a family history experienced no breast cancer risk reduction with higher levels of physical activity (less than 1% on average). These risk decreases were statistically significant in all studies except for one that found no effect modification by family history of breast cancer (Magnusson et al. 2005).

Hormone receptor status was examined in 11 studies as a potential effect modifier (Bardia et al. 2006; Bernstein et al. 2005; Dallal et al. 2007; Dey et al. 2009; Enger et al. 2000; Lee et al. 2001b; Leitzmann et al. 2008; Maruti et al. 2008; Peplonska et al. 2008; Peters et al. 2009a; Schmidt et al. 2008). Seven studies examined the association between physical activity and breast cancer for estrogen positive (ER+) and negative (ER-) tumors (Bardia et al. 2006; Bernstein et al. 2005; Dallal et al. 2007; Dey et al. 2009; Peplonska et al. 2008; Peters et al. 2009a; Schmidt et al. 2008). Five studies observed statistically significant breast cancer risk reductions for higher levels of physical activity among women with ER+ tumors (Bardia et al. 2006; Bernstein et al. 2005; Peplonska et al. 2008; Peters et al. 2009a; Schmidt et al. 2008); two studies found significant reductions for ER- tumors (Dallal et al. 2007; Dey et al. 2009). The average risk reduction across all studies that examined the association for ER+ and ER- was the same for both groups (20%). Three studies compared the breast cancer risk reductions for highest versus lowest physical activity categories among women with progesterone positive (PR+) and negative (PR-) tumors (Bardia et al. 2006; Peplonska et al. 2008; Schmidt et al. 2008). Peplonska et al. (2008) and Schmidt et al. (2008) found statistically significant breast cancer risk reductions for higher physical activity among women with PR+ tumors, and no effect for PR- tumors. Bardia et al. (2006) observed the reciprocal – significant risk reductions for PR- and no effect for PR+. Eight studies compared women with estrogen- and progesterone- positive (ER+/PR+) tumors with women that had estrogen and progesterone negative (ER-/PR-) tumors (Bardia et al. 2006; Bernstein et al. 2005; Dallal et al. 2007; Enger et al. 2000; Lee et al. 2001b; Leitzmann et al. 2008; Maruti et al. 2008; Peters et al. 2009a; Schmidt et al. 2008), and an additional study considered women with ER-/PR- alone (Bernstein et al. 2005). Statistically significant risk reductions were found in only one ER+/PR+ study (Schmidt et al. 2008) and one ER-/PR- study (Dallal et al. 2007). Average risk reductions were greater for women with ER-/PR- tumors (27%) than for women with ER+/PR+ tumors (14%).

Parity was considered by seven studies (Bernstein et al. 2005; Dallal et al. 2007; Friedenreich et al. 2001; Magnusson et al. 2005; Maruti et al. 2008; Moradi et al. 2000; Tehard et al. 2006). A greater risk reduction was found for parous women (average decrease in breast cancer risk 38%) than for nulliparous women (average decrease 18%).

2.2.5 Summary of Epidemiologic Findings

In this review of 73 observational epidemiologic studies of physical activity and breast cancer risk, we found an average decrease in breast cancer risk of 25% when comparing the most physically active to the least active women. The risk reductions observed in studies assessing recreational and household activities were greater than for walking/cycling or occupational activity. Greater risk reductions were also observed for physical activity of longer than shorter duration. In terms of physical activity intensity, slightly stronger risk reductions were observed for women reporting participation in vigorous-intensity activities, in comparison with participation in moderate-intensity activities. We did not consider the associations of light-intensity activities or sedentary behavior separately in this review. Activity done after menopause appeared to have the greatest impact on the risk of breast cancer. However, risk reductions were apparent for physical activity performed across the lifespan. Within those studies that stratified by menopausal status, statistically significant risk reductions occurred more commonly amongst postmenopausal women than among premenopausal women. Physical activity reduced the risk of breast cancer within each BMI category except in obese women ($\geq$30 kg/m^2) with a clear dose–response in the breast cancer risk reduction across BMI categories with the

2

greatest decrease risk among lean women (<22 kg/m^2). Effect modification was also observed between race, family history of breast cancer, and parity subgroups with a stronger effect of physical activity observed amongst women of non-Caucasian backgrounds, without a family history of breast cancer and who were parous. Clear effect modification of the association between physical activity and breast cancer risk by hormone receptor status was not elucidated.

This review of the epidemiologic findings is limited, first and foremost, by the heterogeneity of methods used to assess physical activity. The vast majority of studies in our review used physical activity questionnaires, with some assessing lifetime physical activity and others using a single-item measure. Study quality also varied because of differences across these studies in sampling procedures and in reporting the results regarding the association between physical activity and breast cancer. Hence, direct comparisons across studies regarding these associations are difficult to interpret. We have presented average risk reductions, calculated as the mean of the point estimates, to allow comparisons between subgroups. However, average risk reduction is a crude measure that does not account for differences in study methods or the precision of the risk estimates. All risk reductions presented in this review represent the highest versus lowest category of physical activity assessed within a particular study. Physical activity categories may differ significantly between studies, and hence the strength of associations may be dependent somewhat on cutoffs used to define the most and least active participants.

Another factor for consideration is the validity of the physical activity questionnaires that were used. It is well recognized that physical activity questionnaires are prone to recall error and social desirability and other biases. In addition, many questionnaires focus on moderate- to vigorous-intensity activity, as it is difficult to capture light-intensity activities accurately by questionnaire. Hence, only a small fraction of an individual's total physical activity may be measured in a given study. Physical activity questionnaires are frequently validated against other criterion measures, but these validation studies are limited by the lack of a true gold standard criterion method for measuring habitual activity over the long term.

Finally observational studies, whilst providing etiological insights, are not able to establish a direct, causal link between physical activity and breast cancer risk (Friedenreich 2001). Three randomized, controlled trials (RCTs) that were specifically designed to examine the etiologic pathways between physical activity and postmenopausal breast cancer risk have been conducted (Friedenreich et al. 2010a; McTiernan et al. 1999; Monninkhof et al. 2007b). These studies have involved supervised, controlled exercise interventions in which several proposed breast cancer biomarkers were measured and compared between the exercise and control groups to assess the impact of exercise on these biomarkers. The Physical Activity for Total Health (PATH) study (n = 173) and the Alberta Physical Activity and Breast Cancer Prevention (ALPHA) trial (n = 320) administered a moderate- to vigorous-intensity physical activity intervention of approximately 225 min per week over 12 months (Friedenreich et al. 2010a; McTiernan et al. 1999); the Sex Hormones and Physical Exercise (SHAPE) study prescribed a combined strength and aerobic training program of approximately 150 min per week to 189 sedentary postmenopausal women over 12 months (Monninkhof et al. 2007b). The effects of exercise on a variety of proposed biomarkers of risk have been reported, with more published results anticipated in the future. Current findings are described in the sections below.

2.3 Biologic Mechanisms

Various biologic pathways relating physical activity to breast cancer risk have been proposed (McTiernan 2008; Neilson et al. 2009; Rogers et al. 2008; Thompson et al. 2009;

Wetmore and Ulrich 2006), but these pathways are still not well understood. It is likely that multiple interrelated pathways act cooperatively to decrease breast cancer risk. It is also possible that certain mechanisms predominate with specific doses or types of physical activity or perhaps in select subgroups of women, as implied earlier in this chapter.

One common theme of many hypotheses explaining the relation between physical activity and breast cancer risk is a mediation of the effect through body weight. Adiposity, frequently measured in terms of BMI, is now convincingly associated with increased breast cancer risk in postmenopausal women, and weight gain and abdominal fatness are probably also causally related (Renehan et al. 2008; World Cancer Research Fund and the American Institute for Cancer Research 2007). In premenopausal women there is no such association; in fact an inverse relation with BMI is probable (World Cancer Research Fund and the American Institute for Cancer Research 2007). Physical activity is recommended as a means for achieving modest weight loss in overweight and obese adults and also for weight maintenance (Donnelly et al. 2009; Lau et al. 2007). However, there is only limited evidence supporting the effectiveness of physical activity for abdominal fat loss (Lau et al. 2007; Ross and Janssen 1999). It remains plausible, however, that postmenopausal women could be amenable to significant abdominal fat loss given the right exercise prescription (e.g., Cuff et al. 2003; Giannopoulou et al. 2005; Irwin et al. 2003). The PATH and ALPHA trials demonstrated a clear exercise effect in a range of body composition measures (Friedenreich et al. 2010b; Irwin et al. 2003) including abdominal fat, whereas the SHAPE trial found that exercisers decreased body fat and waist circumference, but not weight, in comparison with controls (Velthuis et al. 2009). Therefore, fat loss is a logical explanation for the association between exercise and postmenopausal breast cancer risk.

One currently hypothesized biologic model for breast cancer risk, focusing mainly on the promotion and progression of initiated cells, implicates sex hormones, insulin resistance, adipokines, and chronic inflammation as possible mediators of physical activity (Neilson et al. 2009) (Fig. 2.12). While all of the proposed biomarkers in this model are associated with adiposity, and specifically abdominal fat, many of them are also influenced by exercise irrespective of body fat changes. Hence, the extent to which fat loss is necessary to derive a significant risk benefit from exercise remains a matter of controversy. Below we discuss these hypothesized mechanisms in more detail.

2.3.1 Sex Hormones

Endogenous estrogen status has been the predominant hypothesized mechanism relating physical activity to breast cancer risk for both pre- and postmenopausal women. Estrogens can inhibit apoptosis and act as mitogens in the breast, stimulating mammary cell proliferation through estrogen receptor-mediated transcriptional activity and by activation of intracellular signaling pathways (Lorincz and Sukumar 2006; Yager and Davidson 2006). In addition, oxidative estrogen metabolites with genotoxic and mutagenic potential could contribute to breast cancer initiation (Coyle 2008, Yager and Davidson 2006). The successful use of antiestrogenic drugs for reducing breast cancer risk serves as very strong evidence of the causal role for estrogens in women with ER+ breast tumors (Uray and Brown 2006).

Compelling evidence from observational studies supports a positive association between breast cancer risk and estrogens in postmenopausal women. In a pooled analysis of nine prospective studies in postmenopausal women (Key et al. 2002), the odds ratio for breast cancer was 2.00 (95% CI: 1.47–2.71) for the highest versus the lowest quintiles of total estradiol while for estrone the odds ratio was 2.19 (95% CI: 1.48–3.22). Given these findings and others

2

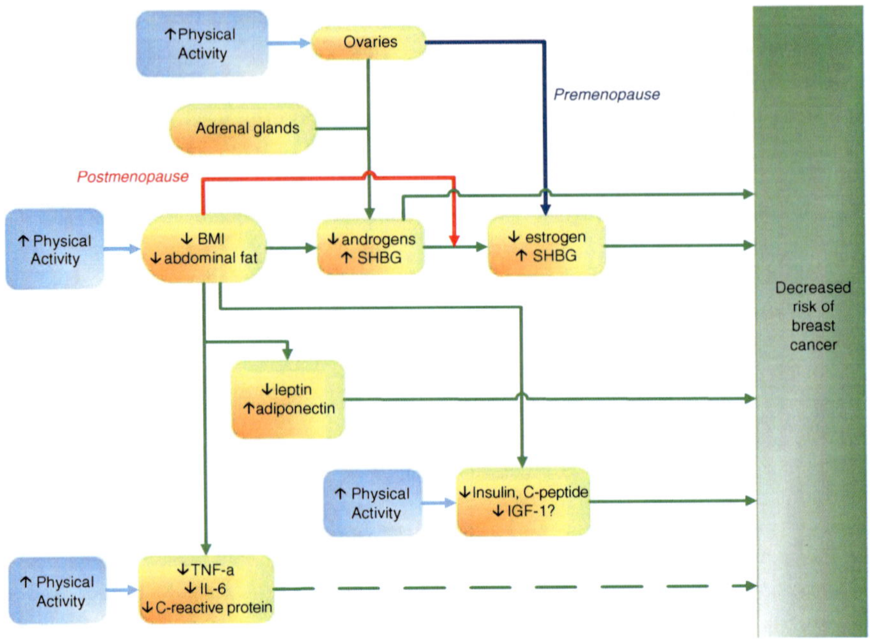

Fig. 2.12 Hypothesized biologic model relating proposed biomarkers of risk to long-term exercise in pre- and postmenopausal women (Adapted from Neilson et al. 2009)

(Cleary and Grossmann 2009), it is now widely accepted that estrogen status is associated with postmenopausal breast cancer. Fewer studies have examined this association in premenopausal women given the complexities of studying circulating hormone levels amidst menstrual cycles, and findings in general have been less consistent than for postmenopausal women (Eliassen and Hankinson 2008). Interestingly, one large cohort study conducted within the Nurses' Health Study II showed that estradiol levels collected in the follicular phase of the menstrual cycle (but not the luteal phase) were significantly associated with an increased risk of premenopausal breast cancer, both overall and for ER+/PR+ tumors (Eliassen et al. 2006).

Multiple mechanisms could explain associations between postmenopausal breast cancer, estrogen levels, and physical activity. The first relates to BMI, which increases breast cancer risk specifically in postmenopausal women (World Cancer Research Fund and the American Institute for Cancer Research 2007). This relation might exist in part because after menopause, ovarian estrogen production ceases and adipose tissue becomes a key endogenous source of circulating estrogens (Kendall et al. 2007; Lorincz and Sukumar 2006). Hence, by reducing body fat through exercise, estrogen levels may decrease resulting in a lower risk of breast cancer. Levels of adipokines that influence estrogen biosynthesis can also be altered with weight loss (Cleary and Grossmann 2009). Furthermore, physical activity can lower blood insulin levels thereby increasing circulating sex hormone binding globulin (SHBG) (Kaaks 1996; Pugeat et al. 1991) which binds reversibly to estrogens to affect their bioavailability.

In premenopausal women these biologic mechanisms are less well understood. Exercise has been linked to delayed menarche and menstrual dysfunction implying lower cumulative exposure to sex hormones and presumably lower risk of breast cancer; however, the level of activity needed to achieve these effects is probably high (reviewed in Bernstein 2009; Campbell and McTiernan 2007) and an energy deficit, rather than exercise per se, may be the predominant mechanism (Loucks 2003). In observational studies of highly active premenopausal women, blood estrogen levels have generally been inversely related to activity but in cross-sectional studies of nonathletes, the relation is more equivocal (Coyle 2008).

Breast cancer risk may also be affected by androgen levels. Androgens can act directly on breast cells by binding to the androgen receptor to influence cell growth (Nicolas Diaz-Chico et al. 2007) and/or they may act indirectly via estrogen production: the aromatase enzyme converts testosterone to estradiol, and androstenedione to estrone, within adipose and other tissues in postmenopausal women and principally in the ovaries of premenopausal women (Kendall et al. 2007). Testosterone, which is one of the most powerful natural forms of androgen, is derived from androstenedione in the ovaries and also in peripheral tissues such as adipose and breast (Nicolas Diaz-Chico et al. 2007). In a pooled analysis of prospective studies in postmenopausal women (Key et al. 2002) and in at least one other cohort study (Kaaks et al. 2005), adjustment for estradiol levels only slightly attenuated the relative risk associated with testosterone, thus supporting an independent mechanism for androgens. Physical activity might lower testosterone levels by decreasing adiposity, or possibly by increasing SHBG levels (and decreasing the bioavailability of testosterone) on account of lowered blood insulin levels (Kaaks 1996; Pugeat et al. 1991).

Epidemiologic evidence supports a positive association between serum androgen levels and postmenopausal (Key et al. 2002; Neilson et al. 2009) and, to a lesser extent, premenopausal breast cancer risk (Eliassen and Hankinson 2008). In a pooled analysis of prospective studies, postmenopausal women in the highest quintiles of serum testosterone and androstenedione concentrations, respectively, had more than double the risk of developing breast cancer compared to women in the lowest quintiles (RR = 2.22, 95% CI: 1.59–3.10 for testosterone; RR = 2.15, 95% CI: 1.44–3.21 for androstenedione) (Key et al. 2002). In premenopausal women, fewer studies have been conducted but findings have been fairly consistent, showing nonsignificantly and significantly increased risks for those with higher blood levels of testosterone (Eliassen and Hankinson 2008).

The effect of physical activity on sex hormones may vary according to hormone receptor status (Sieri et al. 2009), across the menopausal transition (Schmitz et al. 2007), and also with body fat (McTiernan et al. 2004a; McTiernan et al. 2004b). Three RCTs have examined the effect of exercise on sex hormone levels and weight change in postmenopausal women. In the PATH trial, women assigned to the exercise group who lost more than 2% body fat experienced significantly lower blood estrogen and androgen levels relative to controls after 12 months of exercise (McTiernan et al. 2004a; McTiernan et al. 2004b). Likewise, the SHAPE trial showed that relative to controls, androgen (but not estrogen) levels decreased significantly in exercisers who lost >2% body fat after 4 months of exercise (Monninkhof et al. 2009). In the ALPHA trial, estrogen levels decreased significantly more in exercisers than in controls after 12 months, even after adjusting for weight change, whereas androgen levels did not change significantly (Friedenreich et al. 2010a). Unlike the first two trials, the ALPHA trial findings for estrogen suggest an independent role for physical activity. Similarly, some cross-sectional studies (but not all, Bertone-Johnson et al. 2009; Van Gils et al. 2009) in postmenopausal women have found significant inverse associations between physical activity

2

and sex hormone levels even after controlling for BMI or adiposity (Cauley et al. 1989; Chan et al. 2007; Madigan et al. 1998; Verkasalo et al. 2001). Therefore, it remains unclear whether or not fat loss is needed to induce changes in sex hormones.

2.3.2 Insulin-Related Factors

A causal link between insulin resistance and breast cancer risk is biologically plausible. Insulin exerts mitotic, anti-apoptotic effects in breast cancer cells (Lann and LeRoith 2008; Osborne et al. 1976) and hyperinsulinemia increases the bioavailability of sex hormones by decreasing SHBG levels (Kaaks 1996; Pugeat et al. 1991). Insulin resistance and hyperinsulinemia are also strongly related to obesity (Haslam and James 2005) and particularly intraabdominal fat (Kaaks 1996), as well as various adipokines and inflammatory factors (Rose et al. 2004; Vona-Davis et al. 2007) that individually have been linked to breast cancer. Therefore, insulin may alter breast cancer risk independently or indirectly through other biomarkers of risk.

The epidemiologic evidence surrounding the role of insulin in breast cancer risk is growing but remains inconclusive. A modest causal association with breast cancer risk appears to exist with type 2 diabetes, specifically in postmenopausal women (Larsson et al. 2007; Xue and Michels 2007). Yet, while findings from retrospective studies have generally also shown positive associations between breast cancer risk and insulin and C-peptide (a marker of pancreatic insulin secretion (Bonser and Garcia-Webb 1984)) levels, cohort studies have typically produced null results (Pisani 2008). The effect may vary according to menopausal status. Yet within pre- and postmenopausal women, relations between breast cancer risk and insulin or C-peptide have been inconsistent (Neilson et al. 2009; Xue and Michels 2007). Recently, however, one cohort study of 5,450 postmenopausal women that employed serial measurements of glucose and insulin found a statistically significant positive association between breast cancer risk and insulin levels (Kabat et al. 2009) and a case-cohort study found the same association but only amongst non-users of hormone therapy (Gunter et al. 2009). Another recent prospective study (Cust et al. 2009) found no association with C-peptide in postmenopausal women but did observe decreased risk with increasing Hb_{AIC} levels, a measure of long-term blood glucose (Gabbay 1982).

Exercise combined with weight loss is generally accepted as an effective means for improving insulin sensitivity and preventing diabetes (Ivy 1997; Klein et al. 2004; Ryan 2000; Warburton et al. 2007). The effect of exercise may be strongest for those with impaired (versus normal) glucose tolerance (Ivy 1997), when as combined aerobic/resistance exercise versus aerobic exercise alone (Cuff et al. 2003), or at higher intensity (Gill 2007). In terms of abdominal fat loss (which correlates with insulin sensitivity), however, one 20-week exercise RCT in postmenopausal women on a calorie-restricted diet showed no difference whether moderate or vigorous aerobic exercise was undertaken (Nicklas et al. 2009). In the PATH trial, insulin levels decreased with moderate exercise and this change was significantly different from that of controls (Frank et al. 2005). Moreover, insulin change was modified by change in total fat mass: exercisers who lost >2 kg body fat over the year had a significantly larger decrease in insulin levels than those who gained fat mass. In addition, among those women who gained fat over the year, exercise prevented an increase in insulin levels. Hence, exercise appears to alter insulin levels through weight change but also independently of fat loss.

Higher levels of circulating insulin-like growth factor-1 (IGF) have also been hypothesized to increase breast cancer risk. IGF-1 may impact breast tissue directly by acting as a potent mitogen which increases cell proliferation and decreases apoptosis within the breast (Yu and Rohan 2000). The epidemiologic evidence for a positive association with breast cancer is stronger in pre- than in postmenopausal women (Fletcher et al. 2005), but is generally inconsistent (Eliassen and Hankinson 2008; Lann and LeRoith 2008). Furthermore, the evidence relating IGF-1 and IGF binding protein-3 (IGFBP-3) levels to physical activity in women has been inconsistent and generally unconvincing (McTiernan et al. 2005; Orenstein and Friedenreich 2004; Tworoger et al. 2007b). Thus, IGF-1 may not be an important intermediate factor in the proposed physical activity–breast cancer pathway.

2.3.3 Adipokines and Inflammation

Adipokines (adipocytokines) are a group of biologically active polypeptides produced by adipocytes or adipose tissue; they include leptin (Cirillo et al. 2008; Surmacz 2007), adiponectin (Barb et al. 2007; Wang et al. 2007), tumor necrosis factor-α (TNF-α) (Balkwill 2006; Szlosarek et al. 2006), and interleukin-6 (IL-6) (Knupfer and Preiss 2007). C-reactive protein (CRP) is not an adipokine, but an acute phase protein produced in the liver in response to TNF-α and IL-6 levels (Heikkila et al. 2007; Lee and Pratley 2005); all three are considered inflammatory markers. Obesity represents a chronic low-grade, systemic inflammatory state with elevated levels of inflammatory markers (Lee and Pratley 2005). Perpetual cell proliferation, microenvironmental changes and oxidative stress resulting from chronic inflammation could deregulate normal cell growth to promote initiated cells toward malignancy (Coussens and Werb 2002). Adipokines may also increase risk on account of their strong positive correlations with hyperinsulinemia, insulin resistance, and type 2 diabetes, by affecting estrogen biosynthesis and estrogen activity, or by directly altering cell growth and promoting metastases (reviewed in, Neilson et al. 2009).

While biologic plausibility exists, relatively little epidemiologic evidence has related elevated adipokines and inflammatory markers to a significantly increased risk of breast cancer in postmenopausal women (Neilson et al. 2009), for whom risk is most clearly associated with body fat. Among those studies that have examined these markers, most focused on leptin and adiponectin. Evidence was generally conflicting in the case of leptin and somewhat stronger for adiponectin (Barb et al. 2007), but for both of these proposed biomarkers only a few studies were of prospective design (Cust et al. 2009; Stattin et al. 2004; Tworoger et al. 2007a). The etiologic relevance of the adiponectin:leptin ratio also is now being considered (Cleary et al. 2009).

Exercise trials across various study populations have generally supported the absence of an effect of exercise on inflammatory markers, but differing study designs and study populations makes this overall finding difficult to interpret (Wetmore and Ulrich 2006). In fact recent RCT evidence from older type 2 diabetics implied that greater decreases in leptin, IL-6, TNF-α, and CRP and enhanced increases in adiponectin might be achieved with exercise of high intensity (versus low) and preferably using a combination of aerobic and resistance training (versus aerobic) (Balducci et al. 2009). In addition, the PATH trial in postmenopausal women demonstrated lowered leptin (Frank et al. 2005) and CRP (Campbell et al. 2009) levels after 12 months of exercise, but CRP was decreased only among women who were obese or had abdominal obesity.

Sustained physical activity probably lowers adipokine and CRP levels through several mechanisms. In one prospective cohort study, adipokine and inflammatory marker changes correlated significantly with changes in intraabdominal fat in women transitioning to menopause

2

(Lee et al. 2009), implying that biomarker decreases can be achieved through weight loss. Similarly, the PATH trial demonstrated significant decreases in CRP specifically in those who lost body fat (Campbell et al. 2009). Yet exercise RCTs have also shown decreases in adipokine and CRP levels that occurred independently of fat loss (Balducci et al. 2009; You et al. 2004). Such fat-independent mechanisms are generally not well understood, but hypotheses have been suggested (e.g., Mathur and Pedersen 2008).

2.3.4 Other Mechanisms

Other pathways relating physical activity to breast cancer almost certainly exist. Biologic pathways causing DNA damage, cancer initiation, or cancer promotion and progression (Rundle 2005) may interact with the mechanisms already discussed to increase breast cancer risk even further. With improved understanding regarding these interrelated mechanisms and their role in the causal pathways between physical activity and breast cancer risk, the biologic model depicted in Fig. 2.12 could be modified or expanded. Mammographic density was not included in this model since exercise has not been proven to lower the dense area or dense volume of the breast, which are positively associated with breast cancer risk (Woolcott et al. 2010). Likewise, the ratio of estrogen metabolites 2-hydroxyestrone:16α-hydroxyestrone has been hypothesized to increase breast cancer risk, but relatively strong epidemiologic evidence suggests no effect of physical activity on this ratio (Atkinson et al. 2004; Campbell et al. 2007; Schmitz et al. 2008). Other proposed mechanisms that might relate physical activity to breast cancer risk include the ability of exercise to decrease oxidative stress (e.g., as measured by F2-isoprostanes (Dai et al. 2009; Schmitz et al. 2008)) and enhance resting immune function (Campbell et al. 2008; Wetmore and Ulrich 2006). Moreover, by altering estrogen levels, exercise may reduce promoter hypermethylation of tumor suppressor genes (i.e., gene silencing by estrogens) and also genotoxicity from estrogen metabolite–DNA adducts formed in breast tissue (Coyle 2008). Other hypotheses suggest that certain intracellular signaling pathways are affected favorably by exercise, whereby procarcinogenic pathways are suppressed and anticarcinogenic pathways are promoted within the breast (Thompson et al. 2009). Across many proposed mechanisms, effect modification by genetic subtype might better our understanding of the etiologic importance of proposed biomarkers (Han et al. 2008; Kendall et al. 2007) and their responses to exercise (Gill 2007).

2.4 Conclusion

The criteria for causality for the association between physical activity and breast cancer risk are largely met with the evidence that has accumulated thus far from observational epidemiologic studies. There is consistent evidence from studies conducted around the world for a 25% risk reduction amongst physically active women as compared to the least active women. There is also evidence of a dose–response effect of decreasing risk with increasing levels of activity as well as mechanistic data from randomized exercise intervention trials that have examined intermediate biomarkers hypothesized to be part of the pathway between physical activity and breast cancer risk. The associations are strongest for recreational activity that is sustained over lifetime or at least after menopause, that is of moderate to vigorous intensity, and performed regularly. There is also emerging evidence that physical activity may have a differential effect amongst population subgroups with stronger effects found in postmenopausal women, normal weight women, non-Caucasians, parous women, and women without a family history of breast cancer.

Several areas for future research can be considered. These would include examining how sedentary behavior and light-intensity activity additionally contribute to breast cancer risk or risk reduction. More precision is needed in the assessment of physical activity including the type, dose, and timing of activity over the lifetime for these studies. Research that focuses on effect modification by factors such as menopausal status, tumor subtype, and other components of type, timing, and dose of activity would improve our understanding of the nature of the association between physical activity and breast cancer risk. Investigations of the related biologic mechanisms would also inform future epidemiologic research. There is a need for prospective observational epidemiologic studies relating new and proposed biomarkers to breast cancer risk (particularly pertaining to insulin resistance and inflammation). As well, additional randomized, controlled exercise intervention trials that evaluate biomarker changes with different types and doses of physical activity are needed to further elucidate how activity influences breast cancer risk.

References

Adams-Campbell LL, Rosenberg L, Rao RS et al (2001) Strenuous physical activity and breast cancer risk in African-American women. J Natl Med Assoc 93:267–275

Atkinson C, Lampe JW, Tworoger SS et al (2004) Effects of a moderate intensity exercise intervention on estrogen metabolism in postmenopausal women. Cancer Epidemiol Biomark Prev 13:868–874

Australian Institute of Health and Welfare, National Breast and Ovarian Cancer Centre (2009) Breast cancer in Australia: An overview. Cancer series no. 50, Cat. no. CAN 46, Canberra (in press)

Balducci S, Zanuso S, Nicolucci A et al (2009) Anti-inflammatory effect of exercise training in subjects with type 2 diabetes and the metabolic syndrome is dependent on exercise modalities and independent of weight loss. Nutr Metab Cardiovasc Dis DOI:10.1016/j.numecd.2009.04.015

Balkwill F (2006) TNF-alpha in promotion and progression of cancer. Cancer Metastasis Rev 25:409–416

Barb D, Williams CJ, Neuwirth AK et al (2007) Adiponectin in relation to malignancies: A review of existing basic research and clinical evidence. Am J Clin Nutr 86:s858–s866

Bardia A, Hartmann LC, Vachon CM et al (2006) Recreational physical activity and risk of postmenopausal breast cancer based on hormone receptor status. Arch Intern Med 166: 2478–2483

Bernstein L (2009) Exercise and breast cancer prevention. Curr Oncol Rep 11:490–496

Bernstein L, Patel AV, Ursin G et al (2005) Lifetime recreational exercise activity and breast cancer risk among black women and white women. J Natl Cancer Inst 97:1671–1679

Bertone-Johnson ER, Tworoger SS, Hankinson SE (2009) Recreational physical activity and steroid hormone levels in postmenopausal women. Am J Epidemiol 170:1095–1104

Bonser AM, Garcia-Webb P (1984) C-peptide measurement: Methods and clinical utility. Crit Rev Clin Lab Sci 19:297–352

Breslow RA, Ballard-Barbash R, Munoz K et al (2001) Long-term recreational physical activity and breast cancer in the National Health and Nutrition Examination Survey I epidemiologic follow-up study. Cancer Epidemiol Biomark Prev 10:805–808

Calle EE, Murphy TK, Rodriguez C et al (1998) Occupation and breast cancer mortality in a prospective cohort of US women. Am J Epidemiol 148:191–197

Campbell KL, McTiernan A (2007) Exercise and biomarkers for cancer prevention studies. J Nutr 137:161S–169S

Campbell KL, Westerlind KC, Harber VJ et al (2007) Effects of aerobic exercise training on estrogen metabolism in premenopausal women: A randomized controlled trial. Cancer Epidemiol Biomark Prev 16:731–739

Campbell PT, Wener MH, Sorensen B et al (2008) Effect of exercise on in vitro immune function: A 12-month randomized, controlled trial among postmenopausal women. J Appl Physiol 104: 1648–1655

2

Campbell PT, Campbell KL, Wener MH et al (2009) A yearlong exercise intervention decreases CRP among obese postmenopausal women. Med Sci Sports Exerc 41:1533–1539

Canadian Cancer Society (2009) Canadian Cancer Statistics 2009. Toronto

Cancer Research UK (2009) Breast cancer – UK incidence statistics. CancerStats http://info.cancerresearchuk.org/cancerstats/types/breast/incidence/index.htm#source5

Carpenter CL, Ross RK, Paganini-Hill A et al (2003) Effect of family history, obesity and exercise on breast cancer risk among postmenopausal women. Int J Cancer 106:96–102

Cauley JA, Gutai JP, Kuller LH et al (1989) The epidemiology of serum sex hormones in postmenopausal women. Am J Epidemiol 129: 1120–1131

Cerhan JR, Chiu BC et al (1998) Physical activity, physical function, and the risk of breast cancer in a prospective study among elderly women. J Gerontol A Biol Sci Med Sci 53A:M251–M256

Chan MF, Dowsett M, Folkerd E et al (2007) Usual physical activity and endogenous sex hormones in postmenopausal women: The European Prospective Investigation into Cancer-Norfolk population study. Cancer Epidemiol Biomark Prev 16:900–905

Chang SC, Ziegler RG, Dunn B et al (2006) Association of energy intake and energy balance with postmenopausal breast cancer in the prostate, lung, colorectal, and ovarian cancer screening trial. Cancer Epidemiol Biomark Prev 15: 334–341

Chen CL, White E, Malone KE et al (1997) Leisure-time physical activity in relation to breast cancer among young women (Washington, United States). Cancer Causes Control 8:77–84

Cirillo D, Rachiglio AM, la MR et al (2008) Leptin signaling in breast cancer: An overview. J Cell Biochem 105:956–964

Cleary MP, Grossmann ME (2009) Minireview: Obesity and breast cancer: the estrogen connection. Endocrinology 150:2537–2542

Cleary MP, Ray A, Rogozina OP et al (2009) Targeting the adiponectin:leptin ratio for postmenopausal breast cancer prevention. Front Biosci (Schol Ed) 1:329–357

Colditz GA, Feskanich D, Chen WY et al (2003) Physical activity and risk of breast cancer in premenopausal women. Br J Cancer 89:847–851

Coogan PF, Aschengrau A (1999) Occupational physical activity and breast cancer risk in the upper Cape Cod cancer incidence study. Am J Ind Med 36:279–285

Coussens LM, Werb Z (2002) Inflammation and cancer. Nature 420:860–867

Coyle YM (2008) Physical activity as a negative modulator of estrogen-induced breast cancer. Cancer Causes Control 19:1021–1029

Cuff DJ, Meneilly GS, Martin A et al (2003) Effective exercise modality to reduce insulin resistance in women with type 2 diabetes. Diab Care 26:2977–2982

Cust AE, Stocks T, Lukanova A et al (2009) The influence of overweight and insulin resistance on breast cancer risk and tumour stage at diagnosis: A prospective study. Breast Cancer Res Treat 113:567–576

Dai Q, Gao YT, Shu XO et al (2009) Oxidative stress, obesity, and breast cancer risk: Results from the Shanghai Women's Health Study. J Clin Oncol 27:2482–2488

Dallal CM, Sullivan-Halley J, Ross RK et al (2007) Long-term recreational physical activity and risk of invasive and in situ breast cancer: The California teachers study. Arch Intern Med 167: 408–415

Dey S, Boffetta P, Mathews A et al (2009) Risk factors according to estrogen receptor status of breast cancer patients in Trivandrum, South India. Int J Cancer 125:1663–1670

Dirx MJ, Voorrips LE, Goldbohm RA et al (2001) Baseline recreational physical activity, history of sports participation, and postmenopausal breast carcinoma risk in the Netherlands Cohort Study. Cancer 92:1638–1649

Donnelly JE, Blair SN, Jakicic JM et al (2009) American College of Sports Medicine Position Stand Appropriate physical activity intervention strategies for weight loss and prevention of weight regain for adults. Med Sci Sports Exerc 41:459–471

Dorgan JF, Brown C, Barrett M et al (1994) Physical activity and risk of breast cancer in the Framingham Heart Study. Am J Epidemiol 139: 662–669

Dorn J, Vena J, Brasure J et al (2003) Lifetime physical activity and breast cancer risk in pre- and postmenopausal women. Med Sci Sports Exerc 35:278–285

Dosemeci M, Hayes RB, Vetter R et al (1993) Occupational physical activity, socioeconomic status, and risks of 15 cancer sites in Turkey. Cancer Causes Control 4:313–321

Eliassen AH, Hankinson SE (2008) Endogenous hormone levels and risk of breast, endometrial and ovarian cancers: Prospective studies. Adv Exp Med Biol 630:148–165

Eliassen AH, Missmer SA, Tworoger SS et al (2006) Endogenous steroid hormone concentrations and risk of breast cancer among premenopausal women. J Natl Cancer Inst 98:1406–1415

Enger SM, Ross RK, Paganini-Hill A et al (2000) Body size, physical activity, and breast cancer hormone receptor status: Results from two case-control studies. Cancer Epidemiol Biomark Prev 9:681–687

Ferlay J, Bray F, Pisani P et al (2004) GLOBOCAN 2002: Cancer incidence, mortality and prevalence worldwide cancerbase no. 5. version 2.0. IARC Press, Lyon http://www-dep.iarc.fr

Fletcher O, Gibson L, Johnson N et al (2005) Polymorphisms and circulating levels in the insulin-like growth factor system and risk of breast cancer: A systematic review. Cancer Epidemiol Biomark Prev 14:2–19

Frank LL, Sorensen BE, Yasui Y et al (2005) Effects of exercise on metabolic risk variables in overweight postmenopausal women: A randomized clinical trial. Obes Res 13:615–625

Fraser GE, Shavlik D (1997) Risk factors, lifetime risk, and age at onset of breast cancer. Ann Epidemiol 7:375–382

Friedenreich CM (2001) Physical activity and cancer prevention: From observational to intervention research. Cancer Epidemiol Biomark Prev 10:287–301

Friedenreich CM, Cust AE (2008) Physical activity and breast cancer risk: Impact of timing, type and dose of activity and population subgroup effects. Brit J Sports Med 42:636–647

Friedenreich CM, Orenstein MR (2002) Physical activity and cancer prevention: Etiologic evidence and biological mechanisms. J Nutr 132: 3456S–3464S

Friedenreich CM, Rohan TE (1995) Physical activity and risk of breast cancer. Eur J Cancer Prev 4:145–151

Friedenreich CM, Bryant HE, Courneya KS (2001) Case-control study of lifetime physical activity and breast cancer risk. Am J Epidemiol 154: 336–347

Friedenreich CM, Woolcott CG, McTieman A et al (2010a) Alberta Physical Activity and Breast Cancer Prevention Trial: sex hormone changes in a year-long exercise intervention among postmenopausal women. J Clin Oncol 28: 1458–1466

Friedenreich C, Woolcott CG, McTiernan A et al (2010b) Adiposity changes after a one year aerobic exercise intervention among postmenopausal women: randomized controlled trial. Int J Obes (in press)

Gabbay KH (1982) Glycosylated hemoglobin and diabetes mellitus. Med Clin North Am 66: 1309–1315

Gammon MD, Schoenberg JB, Britton JA et al (1998) Recreational physical activity and breast cancer risk among women under age 45 years. Am J Epidemiol 147:273–280

Gao CM, Tajima K, Ding JH et al (2009) Body size, physical activity and risk of breast cancer. A case control study in Jangsu Province of China. Asian Pac J Cancer Prev 10:877–881

Giannopoulou I, Ploutz-Snyder LL, Carhart R et al (2005) Exercise is required for visceral fat loss in postmenopausal women with type 2 diabetes. J Clin Endocrinol Metab 90:1511–1518

Gill JM (2007) Physical activity, cardiorespiratory fitness and insulin resistance: A short update. Curr Opin Lipidol 18:47–52

Gilliland FD, Li YF, Baumgartner K et al (2001) Physical activity and breast cancer risk in hispanic and non-hispanic white women. Am J Epidemiol 154:442–450

Gunter MJ, Hoover DR, Yu H et al (2009) Insulin, insulin-like growth factor-I, and risk of breast cancer in postmenopausal women. J Natl Cancer Inst 101:48–60

Han CZ, Du LL, Jing JX et al (2008) Associations among lipids, leptin, and leptin receptor gene Gin223Arg polymorphisms and breast cancer in China. Biol Trace Elem Res 126:38–48

Haslam DW, James WP (2005) Obesity. Lancet 366:1197–1209

Heikkila K, Ebrahim S, Lawlor DA (2007) A systematic review of the association between circulating concentrations of C reactive protein and cancer. J Epidemiol Community Health 61: 824–833

Hirose K, Hamajima N, Takezaki T et al (2003) Physical exercise reduces risk of breast cancer in Japanese women. Cancer Sci 94:193–199

Hofvind SS, Thoresen SO (2001) Physical activity and breast cancer. Tidsskr Nor Laegeforen 121: 1892–1895

Howard RA, Leitzmann MF, Linet MS et al (2009) Physical activity and breast cancer risk among pre- and postmenopausal women in the U.S. Radiologic Technologists cohort. Cancer Causes Control 20:323–333

Hu YH, Nagata C, Shimizu H et al (1997) Association of body mass index, physical activity, and reproductive histories with breast cancer: A case-control study in Gifu, Japan. Breast Cancer Res Treat 43: 65–72

IARC Working Group (2002) IARC Handbook of Cancer Prevention, Volume 6: Weight control and physical activity. IARC, Lyon

Irwin ML, Yasui Y, Ulrich CM et al (2003) Effect of exercise on total and intra-abdominal body fat in postmenopausal women: A randomized controlled trial. JAMA 289:323–330

Ivy JL (1997) Role of exercise training in the prevention and treatment of insulin resistance and non-insulin-dependent diabetes mellitus. Sports Med 24:321–336

Jemal A, Siegel R, Ward E et al (2009) Cancer Statistics, 2009. Ca-A Cancer J Clin 59:225–249

John EM, Horn-Ross PL, Koo J (2003) Lifetime physical activity and breast cancer risk in a multiethnic population: The San Francisco Bay area breast cancer study. Cancer Epidemiol Biomark Prev 12:1143–1152

Kaaks R (1996) Nutrition, hormones, and breast cancer: Is insulin the missing link? Cancer Causes Control 7:605–625

Kaaks R, Rinaldi S, Key TJ et al (2005) Postmenopausal serum androgens, oestrogens and breast cancer risk: The European prospective investigation into cancer and nutrition. Endocr Relat Cancer 12:1071–1082

Kabat GC, Kim M, Caan BJ et al (2009) Repeated measures of serum glucose and insulin in relation to postmenopausal breast cancer. Int J Cancer 125:2704–2710

Kendall A, Folkerd EJ, Dowsett M (2007) Influences on circulating oestrogens in postmenopausal women: Relationship with breast cancer. J Steroid Biochem Mol Biol 103:99–109

Key T, Appleby P, Barnes I et al (2002) Endogenous sex hormones and breast cancer in postmenopausal women: Reanalysis of nine prospective studies. J Natl Cancer Inst 94:606–616

Klein S, Sheard NF, Pi-Sunyer X et al (2004) Weight management through lifestyle modification for the prevention and management of type 2 diabetes: Rationale and strategies: a statement of the American Diabetes Association, the North American Association for the Study of Obesity, and the American Society for Clinical Nutrition. Diab Care 27:2067–2073

Knupfer H, Preiss R (2007) Significance of interleukin-6 (IL-6) in breast cancer (review). Breast Cancer Res Treat 102:129–135

Kruk J (2007a) Lifetime physical activity and the risk of breast cancer: A case-control study. Cancer Detect Prev 31:18–28

Kruk J (2007b) Association of lifestyle and other risk factors with breast cancer according to menopausal status: A case-control study in the region of Western Pomerania (Poland). Asian Pacific J Cancer Prev 8:513–524

Kruk J, Aboul-Enein HY (2003) Occupational physical activity and the risk of breast cancer. Cancer Detect Prev 27:187–192

Lahmann PH, Friedenreich C, Schuit AJ et al (2007) Physical activity and breast cancer risk: The European prospective investigation into cancer and nutrition. Cancer Epidemiol Biomark Prev 16:36–42

Lann D, LeRoith D (2008) The role of endocrine insulin-like growth factor-I and insulin in breast cancer. J Mammary Gland Biol Neoplasia 13: 371–379

Larsson SC, Mantzoros CS, Wolk A (2007) Diabetes mellitus and risk of breast cancer: A meta-analysis. Int J Cancer 121:856–862

Lau DC, Douketis JD, Morrison KM et al (2007) 2006 Canadian clinical practice guidelines on the management and prevention of obesity in adults and children [summary]. CMAJ 176: S1–S13

Lee YH, Pratley RE (2005) The evolving role of inflammation in obesity and the metabolic syndrome. Curr Diab Rep 5:70–75

Lee IM, Cook NR, Rexrode KM et al (2001a) Lifetime physical activity and risk of breast cancer. Br J Cancer 85:962–965

Lee IM, Rexrode KM, Cook NR et al (2001b) Physical activity and breast cancer risk: The Women's Health Study (United States). Cancer Causes Control 12:137–145

Lee CG, Carr MC, Murdoch SJ et al (2009) Adipokines, inflammation, and visceral adiposity across the menopausal transition: A prospective study. J Clin Endocrinol Metab 94: 1104–1110

Leitzmann MF, Moore SC, Peters TM et al (2008) Prospective study of physical activity and risk of postmenopausal breast cancer. Breast Cancer Res 10:R92

Levi F, Pasche C, Lucchini F et al (1999) Occupational and leisure time physical activity and the risk of breast cancer. Eur J Cancer 35: 775–778

Lorincz AM, Sukumar S (2006) Molecular links between obesity and breast cancer. Endocr Relat Cancer 13:279–292

Loucks, AB (2003) Energy availability, not body fatness, regulates reproductive function in women. Exerc Sport Sci Rev 31:144–148.

Luoto R, Latikka P, Pukkala E et al (2000) The effect of physical activity on breast cancer risk: A cohort study of 30, 548 women. Eur J Epidemiol 16:973–980

Madigan MP, Troisi R, Potischman N et al (1998) Serum hormone levels in relation to reproductive and lifestyle factors in postmenopausal women (United States). Cancer Causes Control 9:199–207

Magnusson CM, Roddam AW, Pike MC et al (2005) Body fatness and physical activity at young ages and the risk of breast cancer in premenopausal women. Br J Cancer 93:817–824

Marcus PM, Newman B, Moorman PG et al (1999) Physical activity at age 12 and adult breast cancer risk (United States). Cancer Causes Control 10:293–302

Margolis KL, Mucci L, Braaten T et al (2005) Physical activity in different periods of life and the risk of breast cancer: The Norwegian-Swedish Women's Lifestyle and Health Cohort Study. Cancer Epidemiol Biomark Prev 14:27–32

Maruti SS, Willett WC, Feskanich D et al (2008) A prospective study of age-specific physical activity and premenopausal breast cancer. J Natl Cancer Inst 100:728–737

Mathew A, Gajalakshmi V, Rajan B et al (2009) Physical activity levels among urban and rural women in south India and the risk of breast cancer: A case-control study. Eur J Cancer Prev 18:368–376

Mathur N, Pedersen BK (2008) Exercise as a mean to control low-grade systemic inflammation. Mediat Inflamm 2008:1–6

Matthews CE, Shu XO, Jin F et al (2001) Lifetime physical activity and breast cancer risk in the Shanghai Breast Cancer Study. Br J Cancer 84:994–1001

McTiernan A (2008) Mechanisms linking physical activity with cancer. Nat Rev Cancer 8:205–211

McTiernan A, Stanford JL, Weiss NS et al (1996) Occurrence of breast cancer in relation to recreational exercise in women age 50-64 years. Epidemiology 7:598–604

McTiernan A, Ulrich CM, Yancey D et al (1999) The Physical Activity for Total Health (PATH) Study: Rationale and design. Med Sci Sports Exerc 31:1307–1312

McTiernan A, Kooperberg C, White E et al (2003) Recreational physical activity and the risk of breast cancer in postmenopausal women: The Women's Health Initiative Cohort Study. JAMA 290:1331–1336

McTiernan A, Tworoger SS, Rajan KB et al (2004a) Effect of exercise on serum androgens in postmenopausal women: A 12-month randomized clinical trial. Cancer Epidemiol Biomark Prev 13:1099–1105

McTiernan A, Tworoger SS, Ulrich CM et al (2004b) Effect of exercise on serum estrogens in postmenopausal women: A 12-month randomized clinical trial. Cancer Res 64:2923–2928

McTiernan A, Sorensen B, Yasui Y et al (2005) No effect of exercise on insulin-like growth factor 1 and insulin-like growth factor binding protein 3 in postmenopausal women: A 12-month randomized clinical trial. Cancer Epidemiol Biomark Prev 14:1020–1021

Mertens AJ, Sweeney C, Shahar E et al (2006) Physical activity and breast cancer incidence in middle-aged women: A prospective cohort study. Breast Cancer Res Treat 97:209–214

Mezzetti M, La Vecchia C, Decarli A et al (1998) Population attributable risk for breast cancer: Diet, nutrition, and physical exercise. J Natl Cancer Inst 90:389–394

Monninkhof EM, Elias SG, Vlems FA et al (2007a) Physical activity and breast cancer: A systematic review. Epidemiology 18:137–157

Monninkhof EM, Peeters PH, Schuit AJ (2007b) Design of the sex hormones and physical exercise (SHAPE) study. BMC Public Health 7

Monninkhof EM, Velthuis MJ, Peeters PH et al (2009) Effect of exercise on postmenopausal sex hormone levels and role of body fat: A randomized controlled trial. J Clin Oncol 27: 4492–4499

Moradi T, Adami HO, Bergstrom R et al (1999) Occupational physical activity and risk for breast cancer in a nationwide cohort study in Sweden. Cancer Causes Control 10:423–430

2

Moradi T, Nyren O, Zack M et al (2000) Breast cancer risk and lifetime leisure-time and occupational physical activity (Sweden). Cancer Causes Control 11:523–531

Moradi T, Adami HO, Ekbom A et al (2002) Physical activity and risk for breast cancer: A prospective cohort study among Swedish twins. Int J Cancer 100:76–81

Neilson HK, Friedenreich CM, Brockton NT et al (2009) Physical activity and postmenopausal breast cancer: Proposed biologic mechanisms and areas for future research. Cancer Epidemiol Biomark Prev 18:11–27

Nicklas BJ, Wang X, You T et al (2009) Effect of exercise intensity on abdominal fat loss during calorie restriction in overweight and obese postmenopausal women: A randomized, controlled trial. Am J Clin Nutr 89:1043–1052

Nicolas Diaz-Chico B, German RF, Gonzalez A et al (2007) Androgens and androgen receptors in breast cancer. J Steroid Biochem Mol Biol 105:1–15

Nkondjock A, Robidoux A, Paredes Y et al (2006) Diet, lifestyle and BRCA-related breast cancer risk among French-Canadians. Breast Cancer Res Treat 98:285–294

Office for National Statistics (2008) Annual Update: Cancer incidence and mortality in the United Kingdom and constituent countries, 2003–05. Health Stat Quart 40:91–97

Orenstein MR, Friedenreich CM (2004) Review of physical activity and the IGF family. J Phys Activ Health 1:291–320

Osborne CK, Bolan G, Monaco ME et al (1976) Hormone responsive human breast cancer in long-term tissue culture: Effect of insulin. Proc Natl Acad Sci USA 73:4536–4540

Patel AV, Callel EE, Bernstein L et al (2003) Recreational physical activity and risk of postmenopausal breast cancer in a large cohort of US women. Cancer Causes Control 14:519–529

Peplonska B, Lissowska J, Hartman TJ et al (2008) Adulthood lifetime physical activity and breast cancer. Epidemiology 19:226–236

Peters TM, Moore SC, Gierach GL et al (2009a) Intensity and timing of physical activity in relation to postmenopausal breast cancer risk: The prospective NIH-AARP Diet and Health Study. BMC Cancer 9(1):349

Peters TM, Schatzkin A, Gierach GL et al (2009b) Physical Activity and Postmenopausal Breast Cancer Risk in the NIH-AARP Diet and Health Study. Cancer Epidemiol Biomark Prev 18:289–296

Pisani P (2008) Hyper-insulinaemia and cancer, meta-analyses of epidemiological studies. Arch Physiol Biochem 114:63–70

Pugeat M, Crave JC, Elmidani M et al (1991) Pathophysiology of sex hormone binding globulin (SHBG): Relation to insulin. J Steroid Biochem Mol Biol 40:841–849

Renehan AG, Tyson M, Egger M et al (2008) Body-mass index and incidence of cancer: A systematic review and meta-analysis of prospective observational studies. Lancet 371:569–578

Rintala PE, Pukkala E, Paakkulainen HT et al (2002) Self-experienced physical workload and risk of breast cancer. Scand J Work Environ Health 28:158–162

Rintala P, Pukkala E, Laara E et al (2003) Physical activity and breast cancer risk among female physical education and language teachers: A 34-year follow-up. Int J Cancer 107:268–270

Rockhill B, Willett WC, Hunter DJ et al (1999) A prospective study of recreational physical activity and breast cancer risk. Arch Intern Med 159:2290–2296

Rogers CJ, Colbert LH, Greiner JW et al (2008) Physical activity and cancer prevention: Pathways and targets for intervention. Sports Med 38:271–296

Rose DP, Komninou D, Stephenson GD (2004) Obesity, adipocytokines, and insulin resistance in breast cancer. Obes Rev 5:153–165

Ross R, Janssen I (1999) Is abdominal fat preferentially reduced in response to exercise-induced weight loss? Med Sci Sports Exerc 31:S568–S572

Rundle A (2005) Molecular epidemiology of physical activity and cancer. Cancer Epidemiol Biomark Prev 14:227–236

Ryan AS (2000) Insulin resistance with aging: Effects of diet and exercise. Sports Med 30:327–346

Schmidt ME, Steindorf K, Mutschelknauss E et al (2008) Physical activity and postmenopausal breast cancer: Effect modification by breast cancer subtypes and effective periods in life. Cancer Epidemiol Biomark Prev 17:3402–3410

Schmitz KH, Lin H, Sammel MD et al (2007) Association of physical activity with reproductive hormones: The Penn Ovarian Aging Study. Cancer Epidemiol Biomark Prev 16: 2042–2047

Schmitz KH, Warren M, Rundle AG et al (2008) Exercise effect on oxidative stress is independent of change in estrogen metabolism. Cancer Epidemiol Biomark Prev 17:220–223

Schnohr P, Gronbaek M, Petersen L et al (2005) Physical activity in leisure-time and risk of cancer: 14-year follow-up of 28, 000 Danish men and women. Scand J Public Health 33: 244–249

Sesso HD, Paffenbarger RS Jr, Lee IM (1998) Physical activity and breast cancer risk in the College Alumni Health Study (United States). Cancer Causes Control 9:433–439

Shin A, Matthews CE, Shu XO et al (2009) Joint effects of body size, energy intake, and physical activity on breast cancer risk. Breast Cancer Res Treat 113:153–161

Shoff SM, Newcomb PA, Trentham-Dietz A et al (2000) Early-life physical activity and postmenopausal breast cancer: Effect of body size and weight change. Cancer Epidemiol Biomark Prev 9:591–595

Sieri S, Krogh V, Bolelli G et al (2009) Sex hormone levels, breast cancer risk, and cancer receptor status in postmenopausal women: The ORDET cohort. Cancer Epidemiol Biomark Prev 18:169–176

Silvera SA, Jain M, Howe GR et al (2006) Energy balance and breast cancer risk: A prospective cohort study. Breast Cancer Res Treat 97:97–106

Slattery ML, Edwards S, Murtaugh MA et al (2007) Physical activity and breast cancer risk among women in the southwestern United States. Ann Epidemiol 17:342–353

Sprague BL, Trentham-Dietz A, Newcomb PA et al (2007) Lifetime recreational and occupational physical activity and risk of in situ and invasive breast cancer. Cancer Epidemiol Biomark Prev 16:236–243

Stattin P, Soderberg S, Biessy C et al (2004) Plasma leptin and breast cancer risk: A prospective study in northern Sweden. Breast Cancer Res Treat 86:191–196

Steindorf K, Schmidt M, Kropp S et al (2003) Case-control study of physical activity and breast cancer risk among premenopausal women in Germany. Am J Epidemiol 157:121–130

Surmacz E (2007) Obesity hormone leptin: A new target in breast cancer? Breast Cancer Res 9(1):301

Suzuki S, Kojima S, Tokudome S et al (2008) Effect of physical activity on breast cancer risk: Findings of the Japan collaborative cohort study. Cancer Epidemiol Biomark Prev 17: 3396–3401

Szlosarek P, Charles KA, Balkwill FR (2006) Tumour necrosis factor-alpha as a tumour promoter. Eur J Cancer 42:745–750

Taioli E, Barone J, Wynder EL (1995) A case-control study on breast cancer and body mass. Eur J Cancer 31A:723–728

Tehard B, Friedenreich CM, Oppert JM et al (2006) Effect of physical activity on women at increased risk of breast cancer: Results from the E3N cohort study. Cancer Epidemiol Biomark Prev 15:57–64

Thompson HJ, Jiang W, Zhu Z (2009) Candidate mechanisms accounting for effects of physical activity on breast carcinogenesis. IUBMB Life 61:895–901

Thune I, Brenn T, Lund E et al (1997) Physical activity and the risk of breast cancer. NEJM 336:1269–1275

Tworoger SS, Eliassen AH, Kelesidis T et al (2007a) Plasma adiponectin concentrations and risk of incident breast cancer. J Clin Endocrinol Metab 92:1510–1516

Tworoger SS, Missmer SA, Eliassen AH et al (2007b) Physical activity and inactivity in relation to sex hormone, prolactin, and insulin-like growth factor concentrations in premenopausal women - exercise and premenopausal hormones. Cancer Causes Control 18:743–752

Ueji M, Ueno E, Osei-Hyiaman D et al (1998) Physical activity and the risk of breast cancer: A case-control study of Japanese women. J Epidemiol 8:116–122

Uray IP, Brown PH (2006) Prevention of breast cancer: Current state of the science and future opportunities. Expert Opin Investig Drugs 15:1583–1600

Van Gils CH, Peeters PH, Schoenmakers MC et al (2009) Physical activity and endogenous sex hormone levels in postmenopausal women: A cross-sectional study in the Prospect-EPIC Cohort. Cancer Epidemiol Biomark Prev 18:377–383

Velthuis MJ, Schuit AJ, Peeters PH et al (2009) Exercise program affects body composition but not weight in postmenopausal women. Menopause 16:777–784

Verkasalo PK, Thomas HV, Appleby PN et al (2001) Circulating levels of sex hormones and their relation to risk factors for breast cancer: A cross-sectional study in 1092 pre- and postmenopausal women (United Kingdom). Cancer Causes Control 12:47–59

2

Verloop J, Rookus MA, van der Kooy K et al (2000) Physical activity and breast cancer risk in women aged 20-54 years. J Natl Cancer Inst 92: 128–135

Vona-Davis L, Howard-McNatt M, Rose DP (2007) Adiposity, type 2 diabetes and the metabolic syndrome in breast cancer. Obes Rev 8: 395–408

Wang Y, Lam KS, Xu A (2007) Adiponectin as a negative regulator in obesity-related mammary carcinogenesis. Cell Res 17:280–282

Warburton DE, Katzmarzyk PT, Rhodes RE et al (2007) Evidence-informed physical activity guidelines for Canadian adults. Can J Public Health 98(Suppl 2):S16–S68

Wetmore CM, Ulrich CM (2006) Mechanisms associating physical activity with cancer incidence: Exercise and immune function. In: McTiernan A (ed) Cancer prevention and management through exercise and weight control. CRC Press Taylor & Francis, Boca Raton, FL

Woolcott CG, Courneya KS, Boyd NF et al (2010) Mammographic density change with one year of aerobic exercise among postmenopausal women: a randomized controlled trial. Cancer Epidemiol Biomark Prev 19:1112–1121

World Cancer Research Fund and the American Institute for Cancer Research (2007) Food, nutrition, physical activity, and the prevention of cancer: A Global perspective. American Institute for Cancer Research, Washington, DC

Wyrwich KW, Wolinsky FD (2000) Physical activity, disability, and the risk of hospitalization for breast cancer among older women. J Gerontol A Biol Sci Med Sci 55:M418–M421

Wyshak G, Frisch RE (2000) Breast cancer among former college athletes compared to non-athletes: A 15-year follow-up. Br J Cancer 82: 726–730

Xue F, Michels KB (2007) Diabetes, metabolic syndrome, and breast cancer: A review of the current evidence. Am J Clin Nutr 86:s823–s835

Yager JD, Davidson NE (2006) Estrogen carcinogenesis in breast cancer. N Engl J Med 354:270–282

Yang D, Bernstein L, Wu AH (2003) Physical activity and breast cancer risk among Asian-American women in Los Angeles: A case-control study. Cancer 97:2565–2575

You T, Berman DM, Ryan AS et al (2004) Effects of hypocaloric diet and exercise training on inflammation and adipocyte lipolysis in obese postmenopausal women. J Clin Endocrinol Metab 89:1739–1746

Yu H, Rohan T (2000) Role of the insulin-like growth factor family in cancer development and progression. J Natl Cancer Inst 92:1472–1489

Physical Activity and Genitourinary Cancer Prevention 3

Michael F. Leitzmann

Abstract The present review of epidemiologic studies of physical activity and genitourinary cancers (prostate, bladder, renal cell, and testicular cancers) suggests a weak inverse relation of physical activity to risk of prostate and renal cell cancer, with average risk decreases of less than 10% comparing high versus low levels of physical activity. For prostate cancer, studies that assessed activity intensity or those that considered fatal prostate cancer as a study endpoint produced the strongest inverse association. For renal cell cancer, the inverse relation with physical activity was more apparent among women than men, among normal weight than overweight or obese individuals, and among older than younger individuals. In contrast to prostate and renal cell cancer, available data show that physical activity is not associated with bladder or testicular cancer. Future research should include improvements in self-reported activity measures and incorporation of objective assessments of physical activity over the life course in order to more precisely characterize types, parameters, and timing of physical activity in relation to genitourinary cancers. Also, data are lacking regarding whether fitness potentially influences genitourinary cancer risk. The relation of physical activity and fitness to genitourinary cancer prognosis and survival requires specific attention. Mechanistic research should identify the underlying biologic pathways potentially linking physical activity to genitourinary cancers.

M.F. Leitzmann
Department of Epidemiology and Preventive Medicine, Regensburg University Medical Center, Franz-Josef-Strauss-Allee 11, 93053 Regensburg, Germany
e-mail: michael.leitzmann@klinik.uni-regensburg.de

3.1 Epidemiologic Evidence

3.1.1 Methods

A systematic review of the published literature was performed through March 2010 to identify all epidemiologic studies that examined an aspect of physical activity in relation to genitourinary cancer. No restrictions were made regarding language or year of publication. If more than one report from the same study was identified, the most recent or most complete publication was selected for review. The studies were classified according to type of study design and nature of physical activity

K.S. Courneya and C.M. Friedenreich (eds.), *Physical Activity and Cancer*,
Recent Results in Cancer Research 186, DOI: 10.1007/978-3-642-04231-7_3,

assessment and subsequently reviewed according to the direction and magnitude of the association and the presence or absence of a dose-response relationship. Potential methodological shortcomings of the studies were identified and considered as alternative explanations for the results observed. The potential biologic mechanisms linking physical activity to genitourinary cancer were examined separately by briefly reviewing pertinent literature on putative etiologic pathways, including those involving steroid hormones, chronic inflammation, growth factors, and insulin resistance.

The point estimate of a study was defined as suggestive if the 95% confidence interval included unity but the point estimate fell outside the range of 0.90 and 1.11. A study result was considered to be of borderline statistical significance if the upper bound of the 95% confidence interval was less than or equal to 1.05 or the lower bound of the 95% confidence interval was greater than or equal to 0.95 or the P value for the test for linear trend fell within the range of 0.05 and 0.09.

3.2 Prostate Cancer

3.2.1 Background

Prostate cancer is the most frequently diagnosed cancer and the second leading cause of cancer death among men in the United States (Jemal et al. 2009). Established risk factors include age, race, and family history; modifiable risk factors have not yet been established (Gronberg 2003). Among U.S. Black men, prostate cancer rates are particularly high, exceeding those of U.S. White men by 60% (Powell 2007).

3.2.2 Epidemiologic Studies of Physical Activity and Prostate Cancer

A total of 48 epidemiologic studies were identified that evaluated an aspect of physical activity in relation to prostate cancer. Among those publications there were several instances of multiple publications from the same study. Specifically, data from a cohort of former students from Harvard College and the University of Pennsylvania were published by Paffenbarger and colleagues in 1987 (Paffenbarger et al. 1987), by Lee and colleagues in 1992 (Lee et al. 1992), by Lee and colleagues in 1994 (Lee and Paffenbarger 1994), and once more by Lee and colleagues in 2001 (Lee et al. 2001). The current review contains the publication by Lee and colleagues in 1994 with follow-up of the cohort to 1988 and the publication by Lee and colleagues in 2001 with follow-up from 1988 to 1993. The publication by Paffenbarger and colleagues in 1987 is included in the current review because it also contains data from a cohort of longshoremen. Similarly, three publications examined data from the National Health and Nutrition Examination Survey (Albanes et al. 1989; Steenland et al. 1995; Clarke and Whittemore 2000). The current review includes only the most recent paper by Clarke and colleagues (Clarke and Whittemore 2000). Two publications presented data from the Health Professionals Follow-up Study (Giovannucci et al. 1998, 2005), only the latter of which was considered in the current review because it represents an updated analysis of the earlier paper. Likewise, two papers evaluated different lengths of follow-up of a cohort study from Norway (Lund Nilsen et al. 2000; Nilsen et al. 2006); only the second publication by Nilsen and colleagues (Nilsen et al. 2006) was evaluated here. Thus, a total of 42 studies, including 24 cohort studies (Cerhan et al. 1997; Clarke and Whittemore 2000; Giovannucci et al. 2005; Hartman et al. 1998; Hsing et al. 1994; Lee and

Paffenbarger 1994; Lee et al. 2001; Littman et al. 2006; Liu et al. 2000; Moore et al. 2008b, Moore et al. 2009; Nilsen et al. 2006; Norman et al. 2002; Oliveria et al. 1996; Patel et al. 2005; Pukkala et al. 2000; Putnam et al. 2000; Paffenbarger et al. 1987; Polednak 1976; Severson et al. 1989; Thune and Lund 1994; Vena et al. 1987; Wannamethee et al. 2001; Zeegers et al. 2005) and 18 case control studies (Andersson et al. 1995; Bairati et al. 2000; Brownson et al. 1991; Chen et al. 2005; Darlington et al. 2007; Dosemeci et al. 1993; Friedenreich et al. 2004; Gallus et al. 2007; Jian et al. 2005; Krishnadasan et al. 2008; Lacey et al. 2001; Le Marchand et al. 1991; Pierotti et al. 2005; Sung et al. 1999; Villeneuve et al. 1999; West et al. 1991; Whittemore et al. 1995; Yu et al. 1988) on physical activity and prostate cancer underwent review for the present chapter.

3.2.3 Overall Association Between Physical Activity and Total Prostate Cancer Risk

Two of the 42 studies reviewed in this chapter evaluated fatal prostate cancer only and are discussed separately in the section on physical activity and advanced prostate cancer Vena et al. 1987, Polednak 1976). In addition, one paper from the NIH-AARP Diet and Health Study (Moore et al. 2009) focused on a comparison of age-specific physical activity relations with prostate cancer between Black men and White men; the results of that paper are considered in the paragraphs on timing of physical activity and physical activity and prostate cancer risk in population subgroups. Thus, 39 studies were left for the first section of the review of total prostate cancer. A total of 21 studies, or 54% of the 39 studies, detected an inverse relation of physical activity to total prostate cancer. Of these, 11 publications noted a statistically significantly inverse association with total prostate cancer (Bairati et al. 2000; Brownson et al. 1991; Clarke and Whittemore 2000; Darlington et al. 2007; Gallus et al. 2007; Jian et al. 2005; Norman et al. 2002; Oliveria et al. 1996; Pierotti et al. 2005; Vena et al. 1987; Wannamethee et al. 2001). In two of those studies there was a statistically significant inverse relation with occupational activity only and there was a null association with recreational activity (Bairati et al. 2000; Pierotti et al. 2005). In addition, one of the inverse studies also found a statistically significant inverse relation between cardiorespiratory fitness and total prostate cancer (Oliveria et al. 1996). One study found a borderline statistically significantly inverse relation between physical activity and total prostate cancer (Krishnadasan et al. 2008), and nine studies reported a statistically nonsignificant inverse association (Andersson et al. 1995; Dosemeci et al. 1993; Friedenreich et al. 2004; Lee and Paffenbarger 1994; Littman et al. 2006; Nilsen et al. 2006; Thune and Lund 1994; Villeneuve et al. 1999; Yu et al. 1988). An overall null association between physical activity and total prostate cancer was reported in 14 studies, or 36% of publications (Giovannucci et al. 2005; Hartman et al. 1998; Hsing et al. 1994; Lee et al. 2001; Le Marchand et al. 1991; Liu et al. 2000; Moore et al. 2008b; Patel et al. 2005; Pukkala et al. 2000, Putnam et al. 2000; Severson et al. 1989; West et al. 1991; Whittemore et al. 1995; Zeegers et al. 2005). In contrast, four studies or 10% of studies reported a positive relation of physical activity to total prostate cancer, two of which were statistically significantly positive (Chen et al. 2005; Sung et al. 1999), one of which was borderline statistically significantly positive (Cerhan et al. 1997), and one of which was statistically nonsignificantly positive (Lacey et al. 2001). In addition, one of the null studies observed a statistically nonsignificant positive association between time spent sitting and total prostate cancer (Hsing et al. 1994), whereas

3

one of the statistically nonsignificant inverse studies found a statistically nonsignificant inverse relation with time spent sitting (Dosemeci et al. 1993). One of the null studies also examined resting heart rate in relation to total prostate cancer risk and found no association between the two (Severson et al. 1989).

The magnitude of the relation between physical activity and risk of total prostate cancer ranged from a 75% decrease in risk (Wannamethee et al. 2001) to a 116% increase in risk (Sung et al. 1999) for the highest versus the lowest level of activity. Across all studies, there was an estimated 9% decrease in total prostate cancer risk with high versus low overall physical activity, with a similar magnitude of risk reduction in the cohort studies (average risk reduction of 9%) and the case control studies (average risk reduction of 10%). Although the cohort studies produced a similar average risk reduction than the case control studies, inverse associations were noted in a smaller proportion of the cohort studies (nine of 21 studies; 43%) than the case control studies (12 of 18 studies; 67%).

Among the 21 publications that observed an inverse relation of overall physical activity to total prostate cancer risk (Andersson et al. 1995; Bairati et al. 2000; Brownson et al. 1991; Clarke and Whittemore 2000; Darlington et al. 2007; Dosemeci et al. 1993; Friedenreich et al. 2004; Gallus et al. 2007; Jian et al. 2005; Krishnadasan et al. 2008; Lee and Paffenbarger 1994; Littman et al. 2006; Nilsen et al. 2006; Norman et al. 2002; Oliveria et al. 1996; Pierotti et al. 2005; Thune and Lund 1994; Vena et al. 1987; Villeneuve et al. 1999; Wannamethee et al. 2001;Yu et al. 1988), 20 studies performed an evaluation of the linear trend and of those, eight studies found a statistically significant decreasing risk of total prostate cancer with increasing physical activity level (Bairati et al. 2000; Brownson et al. 1991; Darlington et al. 2007; Gallus et al. 2007; Norman et al. 2002; Pierotti et al. 2005; Vena et al. 1987; Yu et al. 1988). In contrast, among the four studies that reported a positive relation of physical activity to total prostate cancer (Cerhan et al. 1997; Chen et al. 2005; Lacey et al. 2001; Sung et al. 1999), three investigations conducted an analysis of the linear trend and of those, only one study detected a statistically significant increasing total prostate cancer risk (Sung et al. 1999) and another study reported a borderline statistically significant increasing total prostate cancer risk (Cerhan et al. 1997) with increasing physical activity level.

3.2.4 Type of Physical Activity and Total Prostate Cancer Risk

An analysis of the type of physical activity revealed that recreational activity was related to total prostate cancer risk reduction in 12 of 25 or 48% of publications that assessed recreational activity (Andersson et al. 1995; Clarke and Whittemore 2000; Darlington et al. 2007; Friedenreich et al. 2004; Lee and Paffenbarger 1994; Littman et al. 2006; Nilsen et al. 2006; Oliveria et al. 1996; Thune and Lund 1994; Villeneuve et al. 1999; Wannamethee et al. 2001; Yu et al. 1988) (Fig. 3.1). Similarly, occupational activity was related to a reduction in total prostate cancer risk in eight of 18 or 44% of studies that inquired about occupational activity (Bairati et al. 2000; Brownson et al. 1991; Clarke and Whittemore 2000; Dosemeci et al. 1993; Gallus et al. 2007; Krishnadasan et al. 2008; Pierotti et al. 2005; Thune and Lund 1994) (Fig. 3.2). High versus low levels of recreational activity displayed less pronounced inverse associations with total prostate cancer risk than did high versus low levels of occupational activity. There was an average decrease in total prostate cancer risk with high versus low activity of 5% for recreational activity and 22% for occupational activity.

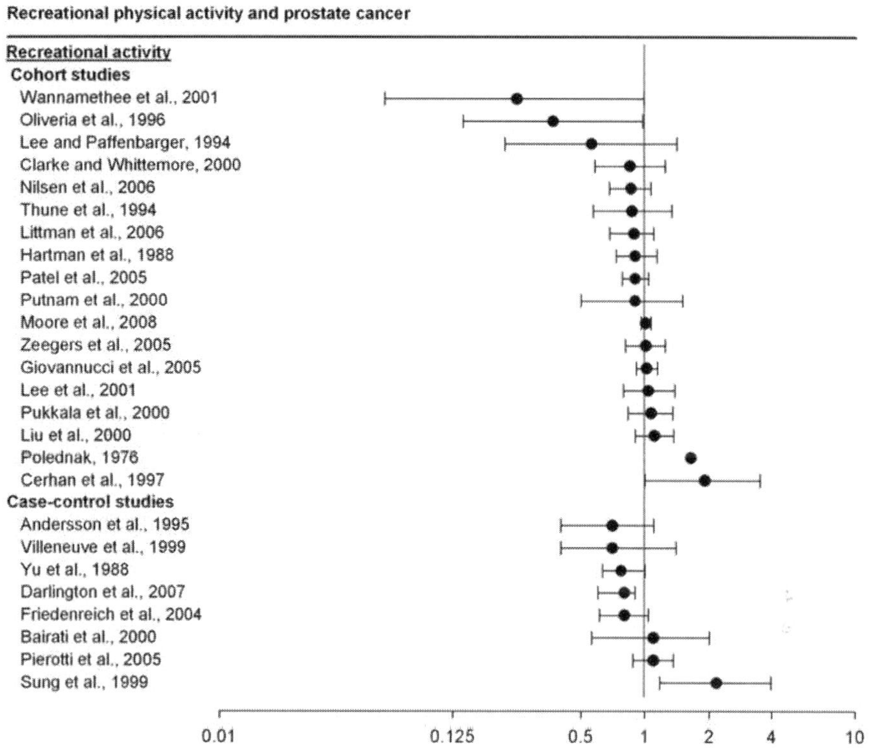

Fig. 3.1 Epidemiologic studies of recreational physical activity and prostate cancer risk

When activity type was analyzed according to study design, recreational activity was assessed in a larger number of cohort studies (n = 17 studies) than case control studies (n = 8 studies). Despite their larger number, a smaller proportion of cohort than case control studies showed an inverse relation of recreational activity to total prostate cancer. Specifically, only seven of 17 cohort studies (41%) on recreational activity showed an inverse relation with total prostate cancer (i.e., point estimate of less than 0.90). In contrast, five of eight case control studies (63%) on recreational activity produced an inverse association with total prostate cancer. Although a smaller proportion of cohort studies showed an inverse relation with recreational activity than case control studies, cohort studies of recreational activity created an overall decrease in risk of total prostate cancer (average risk reduction of 8%), whereas case control studies of recreational activity generated an average null association with total prostate cancer (average risk increase of 1%).

As compared with recreational activity, occupational activity was assessed in a slightly smaller number of cohort studies (n = 8 studies) than case control studies (n = 10 studies). Moreover, only two of eight cohort studies (25%) on occupational activity showed an inverse relation with total prostate cancer, whereas six of ten case control studies (60%) on occupational activity produced an inverse association with total prostate cancer. In addition, cohort studies of occupational activity generated a less pronounced total prostate cancer risk

3

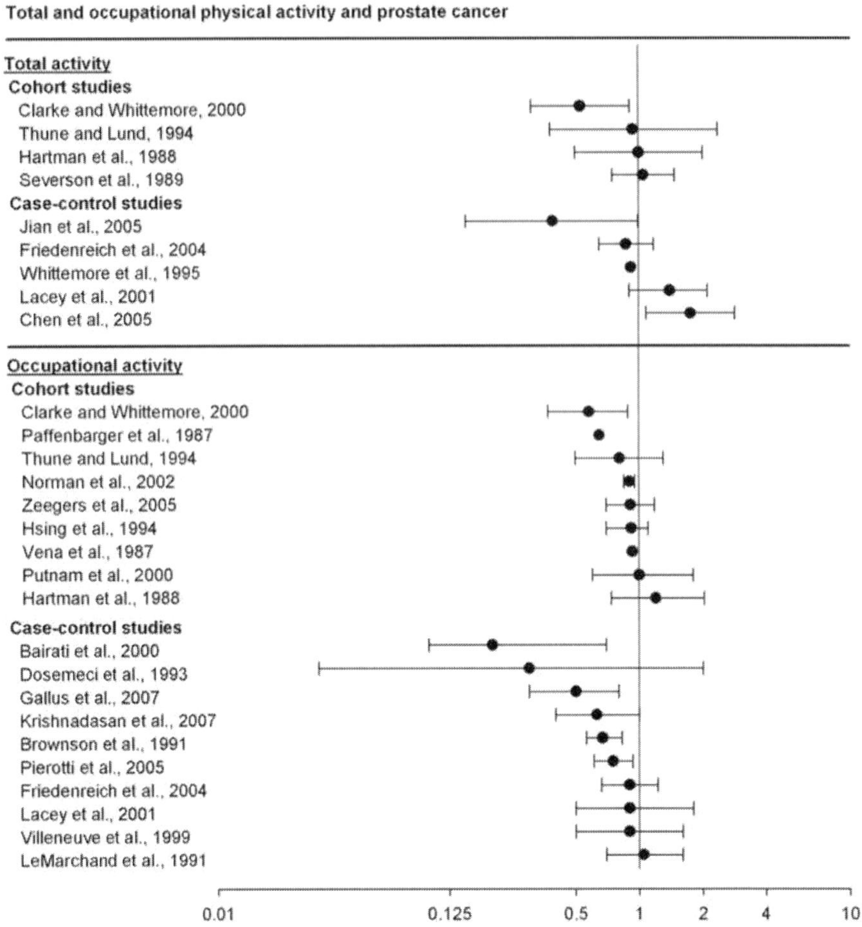

Fig. 3.2 Epidemiologic studies of occupational physical activity and prostate cancer risk

reduction (average risk reduction of 9%) than case control studies of occupational activity (average risk reduction of 32%). Five studies did not present separate data on recreational and occupational activity but provided information on total activity and reported a wide range of associations with total prostate cancer, ranging from a 61% decrease in risk to a 75% increase in risk (Chen et al. 2005; Jian et al. 2005; Severson et al. 1989; West et al. 1991; Whittemore et al. 1995).

3.2.5 Dose of Physical Activity in Relation to Total Prostate Cancer Risk

Dose is defined as the frequency, duration, and intensity of physical activity. In particular, frequency refers to the number of times a certain activity is performed, while duration portrays the amount of time an activity is done, and intensity expresses the level of effort necessary to carry out a certain activity. The latter is frequently expressed as light, moderate, or vigorous, depending upon the amount of energy expended to perform a particular activity.

Thirty-six of 39 studies of total prostate cancer described their assessment of physical activity dose by providing information on individual dose parameters (i.e., activity intensity, duration, and frequency). Most studies performed a joint assessment of activity intensity, duration, and frequency (n = 13 studies), followed by studies that conducted an assessment of activity intensity and duration (n = 10 studies), and studies that included an assessment of activity intensity only (n = 8 studies). A small number of studies conducted an assessment of activity intensity and frequency (n = 3 studies), activity duration and frequency (one study), and activity frequency only (one study). Studies that included an assessment of activity intensity and duration generated the most pronounced decrease in risk of total prostate cancer (average risk reduction of 16%), followed by studies that assessed activity intensity only (average risk reduction of 13%). By comparison, studies that included an assessment of activity intensity, duration, and frequency showed a small decrease in risk (average risk reduction of 3%). Taken together, the assessment of the combination of activity intensity and duration or the assessment of activity intensity only generated the strongest reduction in risk of total prostate cancer.

As compared with studies that presented data on total physical activity, eight investigations that used physical activity of vigorous intensity or heavy exercise as one of their areas of interest (Giovannucci et al. 2005; Lee et al. 2001; Liu et al. 2000; Friedenreich et al. 2004; Villeneuve et al. 1999; Yu et al. 1988; Patel et al. 2005; Moore et al. 2008 generated risk estimates that were of comparable magnitude to those that examined total activity (average risk reduction for high versus low vigorous activity = 9%). However, when evaluated by study design, cohort studies on vigorous activity generated an average risk increase of total prostate cancer of 4% (Giovannucci et al. 2005; Lee et al. 2001; Liu et al. 2000; Patel et al. 2005; Moore et al. 2008b), whereas case control studies on vigorous activity produced an average risk reduction of total prostate cancer of 30% (Friedenreich et al. 2004; Villeneuve et al. 1999; Yu et al. 1988).

3.2.6 Timing of Physical Activity in Relation to Total Prostate Cancer Risk

The relation of physical activity to prostate cancer showed little variation regarding the assessment of activities performed at different periods of life. Of the eight studies that evaluated total or recreational activity during adolescence in relation to total prostate cancer, (Andersson et al. 1995; Darlington et al. 2007; Friedenreich et al. 2004; Littman et al. 2006; Moore et al. 2008b; Pierotti et al. 2005; Pukkala et al. 2000; Villeneuve et al. 1999), two showed inverse risk estimates (Andersson et al. 1995; Friedenreich et al. 2004), five presented null risk estimates (Darlington et al. 2007; Littman et al. 2006; Moore et al. 2008b; Pierotti et al. 2005; Pukkala et al. 2000), and one found a positive risk estimate (Villeneuve et al. 1999). These studies collectively generated a weak average risk decrease of 2% for high versus low adolescent physical activity. All but one (Pukkala et al. 2000) presented an estimate of the linear trend of the association and of those that did, one study found a statistically significant inverse trend with recreational activity (Moore et al. 2008b) and another study observed a statistically borderline significant inverse trend with total adolescent physical activity (Friedenreich et al. 2004).

Three studies of recreational or total physical activity carried out in young adulthood (Friedenreich et al. 2004; Lacey et al. 2001;

3

Littman et al. 2006) and seven studies of recreational or total activity performed during middle adulthood (Darlington et al. 2007; Friedenreich et al. 2004; Lacey et al. 2001; Littman et al. 2006; Patel et al. 2005; Pierotti et al. 2005; Villeneuve et al. 1999) generated average risk increases of 7% and 2%, respectively. In contrast, eight studies that presented data on physical activity during different life periods produced an average risk reduction of 5% with high versus low late adulthood recreational or total physical activity (Darlington et al. 2007; Friedenreich et al. 2004; Lacey et al. 2001; Littman et al. 2006; Moore et al. 2008b; Patel et al. 2005; Pierotti et al. 2005; Villeneuve et al. 1999). By comparison, studies that assessed current recreational or total activity only and did not assess physical activity performed at different life periods (n = 21 studies) generated a null association with total prostate cancer (average risk reduction of 1%).

In contrast, three investigations of occupational activity performed in adolescence, during middle adulthood, and during late adulthood produced average total prostate cancer risk decreases of 23%, 34%, and 17% for those time periods, respectively (Gallus et al. 2007; Pierotti et al. 2005; Villeneuve et al. 1999). One study assessed lifetime recreational, occupational, and total activity and reported statistically nonsignificant decreases in risk of 20%, 10%, and 13%, respectively (Friedenreich et al. 2004). In contrast, that study observed a 36% increase of total prostate cancer associated with lifetime household activity (Friedenreich et al. 2004). Taken together, available data do not strongly support a relation of earlier life recreational activity to risk of total prostate cancer, but studies indicate a small possible benefit from recreational activity performed during late adulthood. In addition, data based on a small number of studies suggest a benefit from occupational activity performed in adolescence and throughout adulthood.

3.2.7 Physical Activity and Total Prostate Cancer Risk in Population Subgroups

Seven studies (Giovannucci et al. 2005; Lee et al. 2001; Le Marchand et al. 1991; Liu et al. 2000; Moore et al. 2008b; Norman et al. 2002; Pierotti et al. 2005) presented data regarding the relation of physical activity to prostate cancer according to age at study baseline (with varying age cutoff points that ranged from 65 to 70 years between studies) and found that the association between physical and total prostate cancer tended to be inverse among younger men (ages less than or equal to 65–70 years; average risk reduction of 15%), whereas the relation had a tendency to be positive among older men (ages greater than 65–70 years; average risk increase of 12%). Three additional investigations noted a lack of heterogeneity of the physical activity and prostate cancer association according to age but did not tabulate data (Lacey et al. 2001; Lee et al. 2001; Nilsen et al. 2006).

Race/ethnicity as a potential effect modifier of the physical activity and prostate cancer association was considered by five studies (Clarke and Whittemore 2000; Le Marchand et al. 1991; Moore et al. 2009; Whittemore et al. 1995; Yu et al. 1988). Notably, the studies tended to produce an increase in prostate cancer risk associated with greater physical activity within the strata of race/ethnicity. A greater risk increase associated with high versus low physical activity was found among Black men (average risk increase of 116%) than among White men (average risk increase of 20%), whereas there was a decrease in risk associated with physical activity among Asian men (average risk decrease of 6%). However, one of those studies (Moore et al. 2009) reported a pronounced inverse association between physical activity performed during ages 19 to 29 years and total prostate cancer among Black men younger than 65 years old at baseline (risk reduction of 56%).

Data regarding a positive family history of prostate cancer as a potential effect modifier of the physical activity and prostate cancer association were reported in only one investigation (Friedenreich et al. 2004). That study noted a pronounced prostate cancer risk reduction associated with high versus low lifetime total physical activity among men with a positive family history (52% decrease in risk), whereas a null association with physical activity was found among men without a family history of prostate cancer. Another study reported the absence of effect modification of the physical activity and prostate cancer relation by family history of prostate cancer but did not present risk estimates (Littman et al. 2006).

Six studies (Chen et al. 2005; Littman et al. 2006; Liu et al. 2000; Moore et al. 2009; Pierotti et al. 2005; Zeegers et al. 2005) presented data on the relation of physical activity to prostate cancer stratified by BMI and produced null relations between high versus low physical activity among normal weight individuals (BMI < 25.0 kg/m^2; null average risk) and overweight individuals (BMI = 25.0–29.9 kg/m^2; null average risk), whereas the physical activity relation was positive among obese individuals (BMI ≥ 30.0 kg/m^2; average risk increase of 32%; based on n = 2 studies). Two additional studies reported the absence of effect modification of physical activity and prostate cancer association by BMI but did not show data (Lee et al. 2001; Littman et al. 2006).

One study considered whether the relation of physical activity to prostate cancer risk potentially varied across subgroups of individuals defined by socioeconomic status (SES) and found a strong inverse relation with physical activity among men in the low SES category (53% decrease in risk), a modest inverse association among men in the intermediate SES group (29% decrease in risk), and a null association among men with a high SES level (Pierotti et al. 2005). However, neither this study nor that of Nilsen et al. (2006) observed evidence of the heterogeneity of physical activity and prostate cancer association by education level (Pierotti et al. 2005).

One study reported a null association between physical activity and prostate cancer within numerous population subgroups, including those defined by alcohol intake, multivitamin use, and histories of hypertension, hypercholesterolemia, and diabetes (Liu et al. 2000). This study (Liu et al. 2000) and an additional study (Nilsen et al. 2006) also found no effect modification by smoking. In addition, one study found no effect modification by total energy intake (Bairati et al. 2000), whereas another study noted a positive relation with high versus low physical activity among men with intermediate and high total energy intake levels, but found no association between physical activity and prostate cancer among men with low intake of total energy (Zeegers et al. 2005).

Studies conducted in Europe showed a more consistent reduction in prostate cancer risk with high versus low physical activity than studies carried out in North America. Specifically, European studies generated an average prostate cancer risk reduction of 25% with high versus low physical activity, whereas North American studies produced an average risk decrease of only 11%. One possible explanation is greater variation or a greater magnitude of activity levels among European than North American men resulting in greater statistical power to detect an association in the European studies, if one existed.

An alternative possibility is that North American studies included as cases a greater proportion of screen-detected, early-stage prostate cancers than European studies, a disease entity that may not be as strongly inversely associated with physical activity than late stage or advanced prostate cancers. However, that possibility is not strongly supported by a joint evaluation of studies by continent and calendar time, which revealed an average prostate cancer risk reduction of 6% in North American studies

3

conducted before 1990 (the approximate time period PSA tests for prostate cancer screening were introduced in North America) as opposed to an average risk reduction of 13% in North American studies conducted in 1990 or later. By comparison, European studies carried out before 1990 and those performed in 1990 or later showed average prostate cancer risk reductions with high versus low physical activity levels of 26% and 21%, respectively.

Two studies formally presented data regarding whether the physical activity and prostate cancer relation differed according to the presence or absence of an individual man's history of PSA testing (Littman et al. 2006; Moore et al. 2008b). The first study found a strong inverse relation of physical activity to prostate cancer among men with no recent history of PSA testing but observed no association among men with a recent PSA test (Littman et al. 2006). The second study reported no difference in the physical activity and prostate cancer association by history of screening with PSA (Moore et al. 2008b).

Eight investigations found no difference in the relation of physical activity to total prostate cancer compared to that with advanced prostate cancer, generating an average risk increase of 3% for high versus low physical activity with either endpoint (Cerhan et al. 1997; Gallus et al. 2007; Giovannucci et al. 2005; Littman et al. 2006; Moore et al. 2008b; Nilsen et al. 2006; Patel et al. 2005; Zeegers et al. 2005). A ninth study reported no effect modification of the physical activity and prostate cancer association by disease stage but did not present risk estimates (Lacey et al. 2001).

However, a subset of three of the former group of studies (Giovannucci et al. 2005; Moore et al. 2008b; Nilsen et al. 2006) and one other study (Norman et al. 2002) considered fatal prostate cancer as an alternative study endpoint and produced average decreases in risk of total and fatal prostate cancer of 2% and 29%, respectively. In addition, two studies examined physical activity and fatal prostate cancer only and generated an average increase in risk of fatal disease of 29% with high versus low activity levels (Vena et al. 1987; Polednak 1976). Two studies addressed whether the association between physical activity and fatal prostate cancer was further modified by age (Giovannucci et al. 2005; Moore et al. 2008b). The first study (Giovannucci et al. 2005) found a strong inverse relation between vigorous recreational activity and fatal prostate cancer among older men (i.e., aged 65 years or more) but detected a suggestive positive association with vigorous activity among younger men (i.e., men less than 65 years of age); the second study (Moore et al. 2008b) found the opposite: an inverse association between vigorous recreational activity and fatal prostate cancer among younger men and no relation among older men. Another study (West et al. 1991) published findings that appear compatible with those found in the study by Giovannucci and colleagues (2005), namely a positive association between physical activity and aggressive prostate cancer among younger but not older men.

3.2.8 Summary of Epidemiologic Findings on Physical Activity and Prostate Cancer

The present review of 39 epidemiologic studies of physical activity and risk of prostate cancer generated an average 9% decrease in prostate cancer risk when comparing high versus low levels of physical activity. A somewhat stronger average risk reduction was seen with occupational than recreational activity, particularly when considering results from case control studies. Studies that assessed activity intensity or those that considered fatal prostate cancer as a study endpoint produced the strongest inverse association. Based on a limited number of studies, there was no strong apparent protective effect of earlier life physical activity on risk for prostate cancer. Likewise, the association between physical activity and prostate cancer did not vary markedly between population subgroups, including subgroups of men defined by differences in the frequency of screening for elevated PSA.

3.3 Bladder Cancer

3.3.1 Background

Bladder cancer is the fourth most common malignancy in men and the ninth most common in women in the United States (American Cancer Society 2008). Established risk factors for bladder cancer include occupational exposure to certain carcinogenic substances such as aromatic amines, schistosomiasis, tobacco use, drinking tap water containing arsenic, certain drugs such as phenacetin-containing analgesics, and a positive family history of bladder cancer (Pelucchi et al. 2006).

3.3.2 Epidemiologic Studies of Physical Activity and Bladder Cancer

Ten epidemiologic studies, including eight cohort studies (Holick et al. 2007; Koebnick et al. 2008; Paffenbarger et al. 1987; Schnohr et al. 2005; Severson et al. 1989; Soll-Johanning and Bach 2004; Tripathi et al. 2002; Wannamethee et al. 2001) and two case-control studies (Brownson et al. 1991; Dosemeci et al. 1993) examined the association between physical activity and risk of bladder cancer and are reviewed in this chapter.

3.3.3 Overall Association Between Physical Activity and Bladder Cancer Risk

Four or 40% (Koebnick et al. 2008; Paffenbarger et al. 1987; Schnohr et al. 2005; Tripathi et al. 2002) of the ten studies that examined physical activity in relation to bladder cancer found a statistically nonsignificant inverse association between an aspect of physical activity and bladder cancer, in two of which the relation was borderline statistically significantly inverse (Koebnick et al. 2008; Tripathi et al. 2002). Five studies (50%) observed a null association (Brownson et al. 1991; Dosemeci et al. 1993; Holick et al. 2007; Severson et al. 1989; Soll-Johanning and Bach 2004), and one study (10%) reported a statistically significant, strong positive relation between physical activity and bladder cancer (Wannamethee et al. 2001). In addition, one study found a statistically nonsignificant positive relation between resting heart rate and bladder cancer (Severson et al. 1989). One study observed a statistically nonsignificant positive association between time spent sitting and bladder cancer (Dosemeci et al. 1993), and another study found no relation between time spent sedentarily and bladder cancer risk (Koebnick et al. 2008) (Fig. 3.3).

The magnitude of the association between physical activity and bladder cancer ranged from a 34% decrease in risk (Tripathi et al. 2002) to a 106% increase in risk (Wannamethee et al. 2001) for the highest versus the lowest level of activity. Across all studies there was an estimated 2% increase in bladder cancer risk with high versus low physical activity. When the positive study by Wannamethee and colleagues (Wannamethee et al. 2001) was removed, there was an overall 9% decrease in bladder cancer risk across all studies, with a somewhat more pronounced magnitude of risk reduction in the cohort studies (average risk reduction of 12%) than in the case control studies (overall null association). Based on small numbers, inverse relations were

3

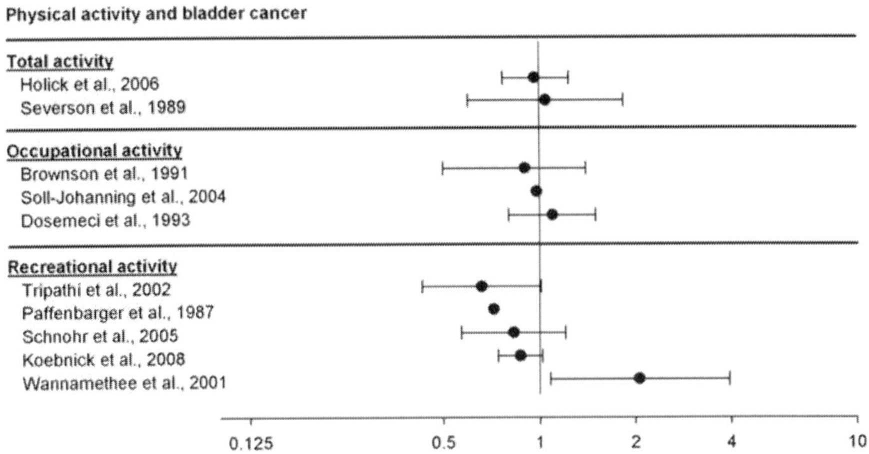

Fig. 3.3 Epidemiologic studies of physical activity and bladder cancer risk

observed in an identical proportion of the cohort studies (four of eight studies; 50%) and the case control studies (one of two studies; 50%); the risk estimates were above unity in two (25%) of the eight cohort studies and one (50%) of the two case control studies.

Of the four studies that reported an inverse association between physical activity and bladder cancer (Koebnick et al. 2008; Paffenbarger et al. 1987; Schnohr et al. 2005; Tripathi et al. 2002), three studies conducted an analysis of the linear trend of the association between the two and did not detect a statistically significant decreasing risk of bladder cancer with increasing physical activity level (Koebnick et al. 2008; Paffenbarger et al. 1987; Schnohr et al. 2005). In contrast, the single study that observed a statistically significant positive association between physical activity and bladder cancer in the categorical analysis also found a statistically significant trend of an increasing bladder cancer risk with increasing activity (Wannamethee et al. 2001).

3.3.4 Type of Physical Activity and Bladder Cancer Risk

An evaluation of physical activity type indicated null relations of both recreational activity and occupational activity to bladder cancer risk. The average change in risk with high versus low activity was a 3% average increase in risk for recreational activity and a 1% average decrease in risk for occupational activity. When the study by Wannamethee and colleagues (Wannamethee et al. 2001) was not included in the estimation for recreational activity, there was an average bladder cancer risk reduction of 17% for high versus low recreational activity. Recreational activity was related to bladder cancer risk reduction in four or 67% (Koebnick et al. 2008; Paffenbarger et al. 1987; Schnohr et al. 2005; Tripathi et al. 2002) of the six studies that assessed recreational activity (Holick et al. 2007; Koebnick et al. 2008; Paffenbarger et al. 1987; Schnohr et al. 2005; Tripathi et al. 2002; Wannamethee et al. 2001). In contrast, occupational activity showed a null association in all or 100% of studies that inquired about occupational activity (Brownson et al. 1991; Dosemeci et al. 1993; Soll-Johanning and Bach 2004). One study (Severson et al. 1989) did not present separate data on recreational and occupational activity but provided information on total activity and reported a null association with bladder cancer.

3.3.5 Dose of Physical Activity in Relation to Bladder Cancer Risk

Two studies assessed activity duration only, one of which observed an inverse relation (Paffenbarger et al. 1987) while the other found no association with bladder cancer (Soll-Johanning and Bach 2004). Another study examined activity intensity only and reported a null relation with bladder cancer (Brownson et al. 1991). Two studies assessed the combination of activity frequency and intensity, one of which reported an inverse association (Tripathi et al. 2002) and the other a positive relation with bladder cancer (Wannamethee et al. 2001). Three studies inquired about the combination of activity duration and intensity, one of which detected an inverse relation (Schnohr et al. 2005) whereas two reported a null association with bladder cancer (Dosemeci et al. 1993; Severson et al. 1989). Two studies (Holick et al. 2007; Koebnick et al. 2008) measured the frequency, duration, and intensity of physical activity, one of which reported an inverse relation with bladder cancer (Koebnick et al. 2008). Studies using physical activity assessments that offered numerous examples of activities did not show a more pronounced inverse association between activity dose and bladder cancer than studies that provided none or few specific activity examples.

3.3.6 Timing of Physical Activity in Relation to Bladder Cancer Risk

There was little variation in available studies regarding the assessment of activities performed at different periods of life in relation to bladder cancer risk. Four studies evaluated current activity (Holick et al. 2007; Koebnick et al. 2008; Schnohr et al. 2005; Tripathi et al. 2002), two studies did not state explicitly which time period in life their physical activity assessment referred to although the wording implied it was current activity (Severson et al. 1989; Wannamethee et al. 2001), three studies assessed lifetime occupational activity (Brownson et al. 1991; Dosemeci et al. 1993; Soll-Johanning and Bach 2004), and one study assessed physical activity performed during young adulthood (Paffenbarger et al. 1987). In one study (Paffenbarger et al. 1987), physical activity carried out in young adulthood showed a stronger inverse relation with bladder cancer risk (risk reduction of 28%) than activity performed during middle to late adulthood (average risk increase of 9% based on studies by Holick et al. 2007; Koebnick et al. 2008; Severson et al. 1989; Schnohr et al. 2005; Tripathi et al. 2002; and Wannamethee et al. 2001; after exclusion of Wannamethee et al. 2001 average risk reduction of 11%). Three studies that assessed lifetime physical activity produced a 1% average bladder cancer risk reduction (Brownson et al. 1991; Dosemeci et al. 1993; Soll-Johanning and Bach 2004)

3.3.7 Physical Activity and Bladder Cancer Risk in Population Subgroups

Of the ten studies that examined physical activity in relation to bladder cancer risk (Brownson et al. 1991; Dosemeci et al. 1993; Holick et al. 2007; Koebnick et al. 2008; Paffenbarger et al. 1987; Schnohr et al. 2005; Severson et al. 1989; Soll-Johanning and Bach 2004; Tripathi et al. 2002; Wannamethee et al. 2001), five studies (50%) were conducted in men only (Brownson et al. 1991; Dosemeci et al. 1993; Schnohr et al. 2005; Severson et al. 1989; Wannamethee et al. 2001) four studies (40%) included both women and men (Holick et al. 2007; Koebnick et al. 2008) (Paffenbarger et al. 1987; Soll-Johanning and Bach 2004) and one study (10%) was conducted among women only (Tripathi et al. 2002). Thus, the average risk estimate for bladder cancer from all available studies combined is based primarily

3

on data from men. When the data were evaluated according to gender, there was an inverse association between physical activity and bladder cancer among women (average risk reduction of 19%), whereas the relation of physical activity to bladder cancer was null among men (average risk increase of 4%). When the study of men by Wannamethee and colleagues (Wannamethee et al. 2001) was excluded there was an average risk reduction of 8% in men.

Two studies considered whether the relation of physical activity to bladder cancer risk potentially varies across additional subgroups of individuals (Holick et al. 2007; Koebnick et al. 2008). The first study detected no heterogeneity of the physical activity and bladder cancer association across tertiles of BMI but did not tabulate data (Holick et al. 2007). The second study reported null associations between physical activity and bladder cancer within numerous population subgroups, including those defined by BMI, age, race, and intakes of fruits, vegetables, and beverages study (Koebnick et al. 2008). Of note, the latter study reported a statistically significant inverse relation of physical activity to bladder cancer among participants who formerly smoked, those who consumed alcohol, and subjects with regular NSAID use. In addition, a borderline statistically significant inverse association was found among men, those with Caucasian race/ethnicity, and individuals with college or postgraduate education (Koebnick et al. 2008). Whether some or all of those subgroup findings are the result of chance due to multiple testing needs to be clarified in future epidemiologic investigations of physical activity and bladder cancer.

3.3.8 Summary of Epidemiologic Findings on Physical Activity and Bladder Cancer

Available data from ten epidemiologic studies show that physical activity is not independently associated with bladder cancer risk. Essentially null findings emerged from both cohort and case control studies and in studies that considered recreational activity and occupational activity. Studies using more refined physical activity assessments did not show relations that differed from those of studies that used crude physical activity assessments. There was little variation regarding activities performed at different periods of life in relation to bladder cancer risk. Data from a single study suggest that increased physical activity may indirectly protect against bladder cancer development through a mechanism involving body weight control. Because very few studies have examined physical activity in relation to bladder cancer risk among women, the epidemiologic basis for a largely null relation of physical activity to bladder cancer is based primarily on data from men.

3.4 Renal Cell Cancer

3.4.1 Background

Renal cell carcinoma (RCC) represents the seventh leading cause of cancer incidence among men and the 12th leading cancer among women in the United States (Cohen and McGovern 2005). The incidence rate of RCC increases with age and is greater for men than women (Cohen and McGovern 2005). Established risk factors for RCC include smoking, adiposity, and hypertension (Scelo and Brennan 2007).

3.4.2 Epidemiologic Studies of Physical Activity and RCC

A total of 16 epidemiologic investigations (Bergstrom et al. 1999, 2001; Chiu et al. 2006; Goodman et al. 1986; Lindblad et al. 1994; Mahabir et al. 2004; Mellemgaard et al. 1994,

1995; Menezes et al. 2003; Moore et al. 2008a; Nicodemus et al. 2004; Paffenbarger et al. 1987; Pan et al. 2006; Setiawan et al. 2007; Tavani et al. 2007; van Dijk et al. 2004) were identified that evaluated the relation between physical activity and RCC risk. Of those 16 investigations, one report (Mellemgaard et al. 1995) included data from a previous publication (Mellemgaard et al. 1994) and the earlier study was not included in the current review. Thus, a total of 15 publications, including eight cohort studies (Bergstrom et al. 1999, 2001; Mahabir et al. 2004; Moore et al. 2008a; Nicodemus et al. 2004; Paffenbarger et al. 1987; Setiawan et al. 2007; van Dijk et al. 2004) and seven case-control studies (Chiu et al. 2006; Goodman et al. 1986; Lindblad et al. 1994; Mellemgaard et al. 1995; Menezes et al. 2003; Pan et al. 2006; Tavani et al. 2007) could be reviewed.

3.4.3 Overall Association Between Physical Activity and RCC Risk

A statistically significant inverse association between a measure of physical activity and RCC was reported in eight or 53% (Bergstrom et al. 1999; Chiu et al. 2006; Lindblad et al. 1994; Menezes et al. 2003; Moore et al. 2008a; Nicodemus et al. 2004; Setiawan et al. 2007; Tavani et al. 2007) of the 15 RCC studies discussed in this chapter (Fig. 3.4) One study (7%) observed a statistically nonsignificant inverse relation (Mahabir et al. 2004), three studies (21%) produced a null association (Goodman et al. 1986; Paffenbarger et al. 1987; Pan et al. 2006), one study (7%) reported a statistically nonsignificant positive relation (Mellemgaard et al. 1995), and one study (7%) found a statistically borderline significant positive relation (Bergstrom et al. 2001) between physical activity and RCC risk. One study (7%) reported a statistically nonsignificant relation of physical activity to RCC that was inverse among men and positive among women (van Dijk et al. 2004).

The magnitude of the relation between physical activity and RCC was distributed between a 63% decrease in risk (Nicodemus et al. 2004) and a 67% increase in risk (Bergstrom et al. 2001) for the highest versus the lowest level of activity. Across all studies there was an estimated 8% RCC risk reduction with high versus low physical activity, with a somewhat more pronounced magnitude of risk reduction in the case control studies (average risk reduction of 11%) than in the cohort studies (average risk reduction of 6%). Likewise, statistically significant inverse relations were observed in a slightly higher proportion of the case control studies (four of seven studies; 57%) than the cohort studies (four of eight studies; 50%).

Among the eight studies that observed a statistically significant inverse relation (Bergstrom et al. 1999; Chiu et al. 2006; Lindblad et al. 1994; Menezes et al. 2003; Moore et al. 2008a; Nicodemus et al. 2004; Setiawan et al. 2007; Tavani et al. 2007) and the two studies that found a statistically nonsignificant inverse relation (Mahabir et al. 2004; van Dijk et al. 2004) of physical activity to risk of RCC, nine evaluated the trend of this association (Bergstrom et al. 1999; Chiu et al. 2006; Lindblad et al. 1994; Mahabir et al. 2004; Moore et al. 2008a; Nicodemus et al. 2004; Setiawan et al. 2007; Tavani et al. 2007; van Dijk et al. 2004) and of those, six studies reported a statistically significant decreasing risk of RCC with increasing level of physical activity (Bergstrom et al. 1999; Lindblad et al. 1994; Moore et al. 2008a; Nicodemus et al. 2004; Setiawan et al. 2007; Tavani et al. 2007). In contrast, one study found a borderline statistically significant trend of an increasing RCC risk with increasing activity (Bergstrom et al. 2001).

3.4.4 Type of Physical Activity and RCC Risk

An analysis of the type of physical activity revealed that recreational activity showed a slightly stronger RCC risk reduction (average

3

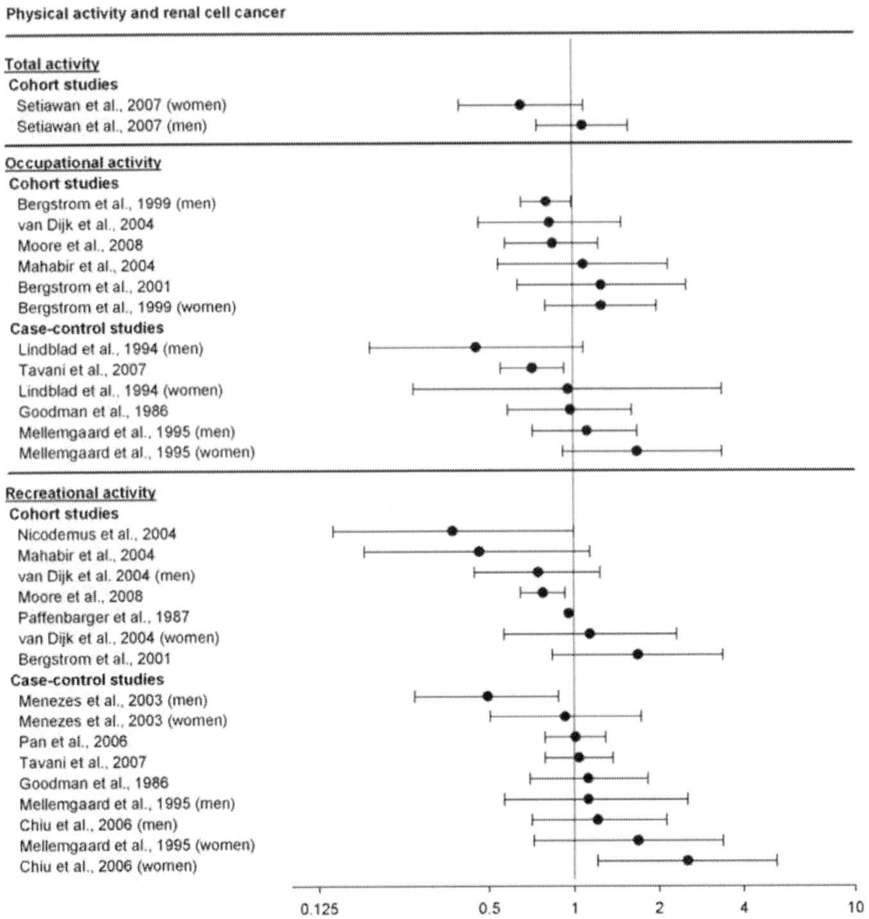

Fig. 3.4 Epidemiologic studies of physical activity and renal cancer risk

risk reduction of 9%) than occupational activity (average risk reduction of 6%). Specifically, recreational activity was related to a RCC risk reduction in six or 46% (Chiu et al. 2006; Mahabir et al. 2004; Menezes et al. 2003; Moore et al. 2008a; Nicodemus et al. 2004; van Dijk et al. 2004) of the 13 available studies that assessed recreational activity (Bergstrom et al. 1999; Chiu et al. 2006; Goodman et al. 1986; Lindblad et al. 1994; Mahabir et al. 2004; Mellemgaard et al. 1995; Menezes et al. 2003; Moore et al. 2008a; Nicodemus et al. 2004; Paffenbarger et al. 1987; Pan et al. 2006; Tavani et al. 2007; van Dijk et al. 2004). By comparison, occupational activity was associated with decreased risk in four or 40% (Lindblad et al. 1994; Moore et al. 2008a; Tavani et al. 2007; van Dijk et al. 2004) of the ten studies that assessed occupational activity (Bergstrom et al. 1999; Bergstrom et al. 2001; Goodman et al. 1986; Lindblad et al. 1994; Mahabir et al. 2004; Mellemgaard et al. 1995; Menezes et al. 2003; Moore et al. 2008a; Tavani et al. 2007; van Dijk et al. 2004).

Seven studies (Bergstrom et al. 2001; Goodman et al. 1986; Mahabir et al. 2004;

Mellemgaard et al. 1995; Moore et al. 2008a; Tavani et al. 2007; van Dijk et al. 2004) presented data on both recreational and occupational or daily routine activity. Of those, two studies (Moore et al. 2008a; van Dijk et al. 2004) observed inverse relations of both recreational and occupational/daily routine activity to RCC risk that were somewhat more pronounced for recreational than occupational/daily routine activity. One study (Mahabir et al. 2004) found an inverse association with recreational activity but detected no association with occupational activity, and one study (Tavani et al. 2007) found the opposite: an inverse association with occupational activity and no association with recreational activity. One study (Goodman et al. 1986) found no association with either recreational or occupational activity. One study (Setiawan et al. 2007) presented the combination of recreational and occupational activity only and did not produce a more pronounced decrease in RCC risk than studies that conducted separate analyses of recreational and occupational activity. In contrast, two studies (Bergstrom et al. 2001; Mellemgaard et al. 1995) reported positive relations of both recreational and occupational activity to RCC risk that were slightly more pronounced for recreational than occupational activity.

3.4.5 Dose of Physical Activity in Relation to RCC Risk

One study that inquired solely about the frequency of physical activity observed an inverse association with RCC (Chiu et al. 2006). In contrast, one study that assessed activity duration only found no relation with RCC (Paffenbarger et al. 1987). Three studies inquired about activity intensity only, one of which detected an inverse relation (Mahabir et al. 2004); the second found no association (Goodman et al. 1986) and the third produced a positive relation (Bergstrom et al. 2001). No study queried about the combination of activity frequency and duration, two studies assessed the combination of activity frequency and intensity and reported an inverse association with RCC (Menezes et al. 2003; Nicodemus et al. 2004), and two studies inquired about the combination of activity duration and intensity and detected an inverse relation (Setiawan et al. 2007; Tavani et al. 2007) with RCC. Two (Moore et al. 2008a; van Dijk et al. 2004) of three studies (Moore et al. 2008a; Pan et al. 2006; van Dijk et al. 2004) that measured the frequency, duration, and intensity of physical activity reported an inverse relation with RCC.

Studies using physical activity assessments that provided numerous examples of activities tended to observe a more pronounced inverse association between activity dose and RCC than studies that offered few or no specific activity examples. For instance, the physical activity instruments used in the seven studies that detected an inverse relation of recreational activity to RCC (Chiu et al. 2006; Mahabir et al. 2004; Menezes et al. 2003; Moore et al. 2008a; Nicodemus et al. 2004; Setiawan et al. 2007; van Dijk et al. 2004) allowed for three to seven response options per physical activity question, with between three and 11 examples of specific activities for each response option. In contrast, two studies that did not specify the number of questions or response options to assess recreational physical activity produced a null (Goodman et al. 1986) and a statistically nonsignificant positive finding (Mellemgaard et al. 1995). However, three other studies that did provide detailed response options and also included examples regarding specific recreational activities were either unable to detect an association if one existed (Pan et al. 2006; Tavani et al. 2007) or found a statistically nonsignificant positive relation with RCC (Bergstrom et al. 2001).

3

3.4.6 Timing of Physical Activity in Relation to RCC Risk

An evaluation of the timing of physical activity in life in relation to risk of RCC showed risk reductions for physical activity performed at each period of life: adolescence (ages 12–19 years), early to middle adulthood (age 20–49 years), and later adulthood (ages 50 years or older). Physical activity carried out in later adulthood showed a stronger inverse relation with RCC risk (average risk reduction of 27%) than activity performed during early to middle adulthood (average risk reduction of 6–7%). Physical activity conducted during adolescence was also associated with RCC risk reduction (average risk reduction of 17%).

3.4.7 Physical Activity and RCC Risk in Population Subgroups

Of the ten studies that observed an inverse relation of physical activity to RCC risk (Bergstrom et al. 1999; Chiu et al. 2006; Lindblad et al. 1994; Mahabir et al. 2004; Menezes et al. 2003; Moore et al. 2008a; Nicodemus et al. 2004; Setiawan et al. 2007; Tavani et al. 2007; van Dijk et al. 2004), the relative risk estimates were based on analyses of the total study population in four studies (Mahabir et al. 2004; Moore et al. 2008a; Nicodemus et al. 2004; Tavani et al. 2007). Three of those studies presented additional results of a subanalysis by gender, the first of which showed a stronger inverse relation of adolescent physical activity to RCC among women than men (Moore et al. 2008a); the second reported an inverse relation among women and a positive relation among men (Pan et al. 2006), and the third found a stronger inverse relation of physical activity at ages 30–39 years to RCC among men than women (Tavani et al. 2007).

In the current review, the evaluation of the primary results from six other studies was based on combining subgroups of gender (Bergstrom et al. 1999; Chiu et al. 2006; Lindblad et al. 1994; Menezes et al. 2003; Setiawan et al. 2007; van Dijk et al. 2004). When the findings of the latter six studies were considered according to gender, an inverse association between physical activity and RCC for both men and women was noted in three studies (Chiu et al. 2006; Lindblad et al. 1994; Menezes et al. 2003). Of these, the inverse relation was more pronounced in men than in women in two studies (Lindblad et al. 1994; Menezes et al. 2003), whereas inverse the association was stronger in women than in men in the remaining study (Chiu et al. 2006). In contrast, the relation of physical activity to RCC was qualitatively heterogeneous by gender in three studies (Bergstrom et al. 1999; Setiawan et al. 2007; van Dijk et al. 2004). Of these, two studies showed a risk estimate that was above unity among men and below unity in women (Bergstrom et al. 1999; Setiawan et al. 2007), whereas the third study demonstrated a risk estimate that was above unity for women and below unity for men (van Dijk et al. 2004). The degree of heterogeneity by gender was not quantified using formal tests for interaction in those studies. The results of the nine studies that presented physical activity and RCC risk data according to gender (Bergstrom et al. 1999; Chiu et al. 2006; Lindblad et al. 1994; Menezes et al. 2003; Moore et al. 2008a; Pan et al. 2006; Setiawan et al. 2007; Tavani et al. 2007; van Dijk et al. 2004) were suggestive of a stronger inverse association between physical activity and RCC among women (average risk reduction of 24%) than men (average risk reduction of 14%).

Four studies (Mahabir et al. 2004; Moore et al. 2008a; Pan et al. 2006; Tavani et al. 2007) presented data on the relation of physical activity to RCC stratified by BMI and showed that the relation of physical activity to RCC tended to be more strongly inverse among normal weight individuals (BMI ≤ 25.0 kg/m^2; average risk reduction of 27%) than among overweight (BMI = 25.0–29.9 kg/m^2; average risk reduction of 18%) or obese individuals (BMI ≥ 30.0 kg/m^2; average risk reduction of 5%). However, the studies did not always conduct formal tests for interaction and those that did revealed that apparent differences in the activity and RCC relation according to BMI were not statistically significant.

The same four studies (Mahabir et al. 2004; Moore et al. 2008a; Pan et al. 2006; Tavani et al. 2007) analyzed physical activity in relation to RCC stratified by age and found that the association between physical activity and RCC tended to be more strongly inverse among older than younger individuals (with varying age cutoff points between studies that ranged from 50 to 65 years). The average risk reduction associated with high versus low physical activity among older subjects was 25%, whereas the average risk reduction for physical activity among younger subjects was 17%.

Three studies included separate risk estimates for physical activity and RCC within strata of smoking status or smoking intensity (Mahabir et al. 2004; Moore et al. 2008a; Tavani et al. 2007). The association between physical activity and RCC did not vary according to smoking status or intensity, showing a 22% average risk reduction for physical activity among persons who never smoked, among those with past or current smoking, and among those with low or high numbers of cigarettes smoked per day.

Alcohol consumption as a potential effect modifier of the physical activity and RCC relation was considered by one study (Tavani et al. 2007). A greater risk reduction associated with high versus low physical activity was found among persons who reported never consuming alcohol (44% decrease in risk) than among those who reported 'ever consuming' alcohol (25% decrease in risk).

A history of hypertension was examined in one study as a potential effect modifier (Moore et al. 2008a). That study observed no material difference in the RCC risk reduction associated with physical activity between individuals with a history of hypertension (33% decrease in risk) and those without a history of hypertension (36% decrease in risk).

3.4.8 Summary of Epidemiologic Findings on Physical Activity and RCC

In this review of 15 studies of physical activity and RCC, there was an estimated average 8% RCC risk reduction with high versus low physical activity. A somewhat more pronounced magnitude of risk reduction was observed in case control than cohort studies, for recreational than occupational activity, and for physical activity performed during late than early adulthood. In addition, physical activity conducted during adolescence was also related to RCC risk reduction. Studies that employed numerous specific examples of activities revealed a more pronounced inverse association than investigations that provided few or no activity examples. Analyses according to population subgroups suggest a stronger inverse association between physical activity and RCC among women than men, among normal weight than overweight or obese individuals, and among older than younger individuals.

3.5 Testicular Cancer

3.5.1 Background

Testicular cancer is the most common malignancy in younger men. Risk factors for testicular cancer include age, history of undescended testes, family history of testicular cancer, and race/ethnicity (McGlynn 2001).

3

3.5.2 Epidemiologic Studies of Physical Activity and Testicular Cancer

Ten epidemiologic investigations examined the relation of physical activity to testicular cancer, including two cohort studies (Paffenbarger et al. 1987; Thune and Lund 1994) and eight case-control studies (Brownson et al. 1991; Coldman et al. 1982; Cook et al. 2008; Dosemeci et al. 1993; Gallagher et al. 1995; Littman et al. 2009; Srivastava and Kreiger 2000; U.K. Testicular Cancer Study Group 1994). One early case-control study evaluated three individual sports activities, namely cycling, horseback-riding, and soccer (Coldman et al. 1982). That study reported strong positive relations of cycling and horseback-riding to testicular cancer, with relative risk estimates ranging from a 99% to 356% increased testicular cancer risk, but did not present additional data regarding recreational physical activity and was not further considered in the present chapter. Thus, a total of nine studies remained for review here (Brownson et al. 1991; Cook et al. 2008; Dosemeci et al. 1993; Gallagher et al. 1995; Littman et al. 2009; Paffenbarger et al. 1987; Srivastava and Kreiger 2000; Thune and Lund, 1994; U.K. Testicular Cancer Study Group).

3.5.3 Overall Association Between Physical Activity and Testicular Cancer Risk

Three (Brownson et al. 1991; Gallagher et al. 1995; U.K. Testicular Cancer Study Group 1994) of the nine studies (Brownson et al. 1991; Cook et al. 2008; Dosemeci et al. 1993; Gallagher et al. 1995; Littman et al. 2009; Paffenbarger et al. 1987; Srivastava and Kreiger 2000; Thune and Lund, 1994; U.K. Testicular Cancer Study Group 1994) that examined physical activity in relation to testicular cancer observed a statistically inverse association between a measure of physical activity and testicular cancer (Fig. 3.5). Four studies (Cook et al. 2008; Dosemeci et al. 1993; Littman et al. 2009; Srivastava and

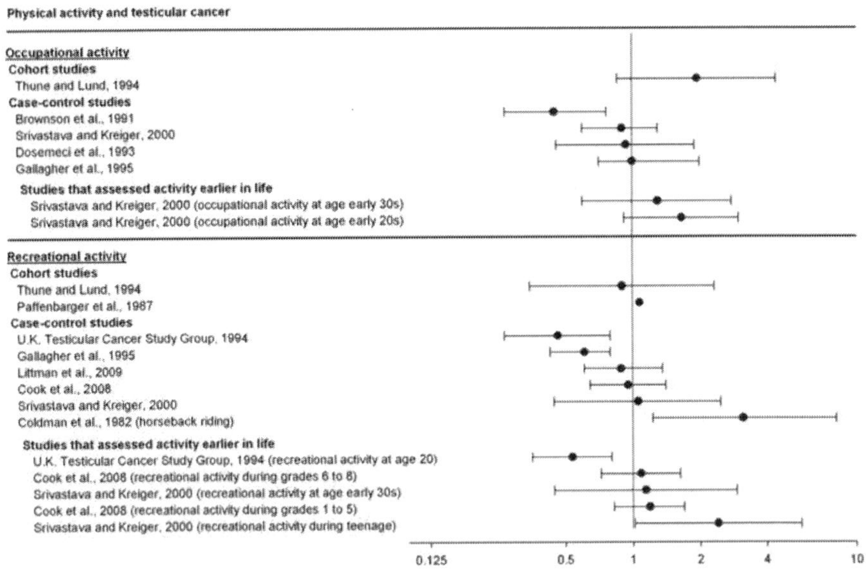

Fig. 3.5 Epidemiologic studies of physical activity and testicular cancer risk

Kreiger 2000) reported a null association and two studies found a statistically nonsignificant positive relation between physical activity and testicular cancer (Paffenbarger et al. 1987; Thune and Lund 1994). One study noted a statistically nonsignificant inverse association between time spent sitting and testicular cancer (Dosemeci et al. 1993).

The magnitude of the relation of physical activity to risk of testicular cancer extended from a 55% decrease in risk (Brownson et al. 1991) to a 95% increase in risk (Thune and Lund 1994) for the highest versus the lowest level of activity. There was an overall estimated 4% decrease in testicular cancer risk with high versus low physical activity across all studies. Inverse associations were noted in four case control studies, but not in any of the cohort studies; the risk estimates for overall physical activity were above unity in two cohort studies, but in none of the case control studies.

All three investigations that observed an inverse association between physical activity and testicular cancer conducted an analysis of the linear trend of the association between the two and found a statistically significant decreasing risk of testicular cancer with increasing physical activity level (Brownson et al. 1991; Gallagher et al. 1995; U.K. Testicular Cancer Study Group 1994). One study that was classified as a null study because of the lack of an association with vigorous activity noted a borderline statistically significant positive trend of the relation of moderate activity to testicular cancer (Cook et al. 2008). No study reported a statistically significant positive trend between physical activity and testicular cancer.

3.5.4 Type of Physical Activity and Testicular Cancer Risk

An assessment of the type of physical activity suggested null relations of both recreational activity and occupational activity to testicular cancer risk, although risk estimates were heterogeneous by type of activity. Comparing high to low levels of physical activity there was an average 4% decrease in risk for recreational activity and an average 5% increase in risk for occupational activity. Accordingly, recreational activity was associated with a reduction in testicular cancer risk in two or 29% (Gallagher et al. 1995; U.K. Testicular Cancer Study Group 1994) of the seven studies that requested information on recreational activity (Cook et al. 2008; Gallagher et al. 1995; Littman et al. 2009; Paffenbarger et al. 1987; Srivastava and Kreiger 2000; Thune and Lund 1994; U.K. Testicular Cancer Study Group 1994). By comparison, occupational activity was related to a decrease in testicular cancer risk in only one or 20% (Brownson et al. 1991) of the five studies that queried about occupational activity (Brownson et al. 1991; Dosemeci et al. 1993; Gallagher et al. 1995; Srivastava and Kreiger 2000; Thune and Lund 1994).

3.5.5 Dose of Physical Activity in Relation to Testicular Cancer Risk

Three studies evaluated activity duration only (Cook et al. 2008; Paffenbarger et al. 1987; U.K. Testicular Cancer Study Group 1994): the first noted a null association (Cook et al. 2008), the second a positive relation (Paffenbarger et al. 1987), and the third reported an inverse relation with testicular cancer (U.K. Testicular Cancer Study Group 1994). One study examined activity intensity only and found an inverse association (Brownson et al. 1991). One study assessing the combination of activity frequency and intensity (Srivastava and Kreiger 2000) and another study inquiring about the combination of activity duration and intensity (Dosemeci et al. 1993) both noted a null association with testicular cancer. Two studies measured the frequency, duration, and intensity of physical activity

3

(Gallagher et al. 1995; Littman et al. 2009): one reported an inverse relation (Gallagher et al. 1995) and the other observed no association with testicular cancer (Littman et al. 2009).

3.5.6 Timing of Physical Activity in Relation to Testicular Cancer Risk

Two studies (Cook et al. 2008; Srivastava and Kreiger 2000) that assessed physical activity performed during childhood and adolescence tended to observe positive relations with testicular cancer risk, one of which was statistically significant (Srivastava and Kreiger 2000) while the other was statistically nonsignificant (Cook et al. 2008). These two studies generated an average 55% increase in testicular cancer risk with high versus low childhood and adolescent recreational activity (Cook et al. 2008; Srivastava and Kreiger 2000). Additionally, one of the studies (Srivastava and Kreiger 2000) reported that recreational activity performed during the early 30s and occupational activity carried out in the early 20s and early 30s was associated with a statistically nonsignificant increased risk of testicular cancer. In contrast, another study observed a statistically significant 38% decreased risk of testicular cancer with high versus low recreational activity performed at age 20 years (U.K. Testicular Cancer Study Group 1994).

3.5.7 Physical Activity and Testicular Cancer Risk by Tumor Histology

Two studies considered whether the relation of physical activity to testicular cancer risk potentially varies across histological subgroups of testicular cancer (Cook et al. 2008; Littman et al. 2009). The first study detected a borderline significant positive association with recreational activity performed at ages 12–14 years that was restricted to seminoma, suggesting a possible adverse effect of high versus low adolescent physical activity to seminoma risk. However, the mother's responses to the adolescent physical activity question did not confirm the suggestive positive relation of physical activity to seminoma risk seen with the son's responses. In contrast, but the physical activity responses provided by the mothers showed an apparent protective effect of adolescent physical activity on risk of nonseminoma (Cook et al. 2008). The second study reported inconsistent findings of a statistically significant positive association between moderate recreational activity and risk of nonseminoma but no relation of vigorous activity to nonseminoma (Littman et al. 2009).

3.5.8 Summary of Epidemiologic Findings on Physical Activity and Testicular Cancer

The present review of nine studies of physical activity and testicular cancer shows very limited support for a relationship. There was an estimated average 4% decrease in testicular cancer risk with high versus low current or adulthood physical activity, with similar relations noted for recreational and occupational activity. Inverse associations are based on data from case control studies; the risk estimates were above unity but lacked a positive trend in the two available cohort studies of testicular cancer. Inconsistent data from a very small number of case control studies suggest a positive relation of adolescent or young adulthood physical activity to testicular cancer risk.

3.6 Limitations of Epidemiologic Studies of Physical Activity and Genitourinary Cancers

Several possible limitations of observational epidemiologic studies of physical activity and genitourinary cancers exist. Many of the available studies did not permit detailed analyses of physical activity because they were not designed to adequately assess the combinations of type, frequency, duration, and intensity of activity. Most studies used self-reported assessments of physical activity, which may have resulted in various degrees of measurement error and misclassification of physical activity levels. In addition, studies that queried about physical activity during adolescence required participants to recall their physical activity level from a period many decades in the past. Such distant recall may have resulted in imprecise assessments of actual physical activity levels during adolescence and could have generated errors in estimating relative risks. Questions concerning routine activities may not have captured activity from housework, which is common in women and may explain why observed relations of physical activity to bladder or renal cell cancer in some studies have been weaker in women than men. Furthermore, residual confounding may explain some or all of the associations observed between physical activity and genitourinary cancers. Case control studies are prone to selection and recall biases, possibly contributing to inconsistent findings in the existing literature.

Apart from the possibility of a true lack of an association between physical activity and genitourinary cancers, an additional possible explanation for the weak or null results observed in previous studies is the inability to assess relations by histologic tumor grade or tumor stage as additional endpoints. For example, prostate cancer represents a heterogeneous endpoint that shows etiologic differences by different groups of men (e.g., younger versus older men) or by types of endpoints (e.g., incident versus fatal disease). In addition, studies on prostate cancer often were unable to account for PSA screening frequency. The diagnosis of prostate cancer is largely determined by screening for PSA, a behavioral characteristic that may be associated with increased levels of physical activity. This circumstance could potentially bias the relation of physical activity to prostate cancer.

3.7 Biologic Mechanisms Relating Physical Activity to Genitourinary Cancers

3.7.1 Prostate Cancer

The mechanisms through which physical activity may decrease the risk of prostate cancer are speculative. Potential etiologic pathways include certain hormones and growth factors, such as insulin, IGF-1, leptin, vitamin D, and testosterone. Physical activity enhances insulin sensitivity and decreases circulating insulin (Lindgarde and Saltin 1981), and although the association between physical activity and IGF-1 is inconsistent, the decrease in insulin increases circulating levels of IGFBP-1, which lowers free IGF-1 (Giovannucci 2003). IGF-1 increases prostate tumor cell growth (Iwamura et al. 1993) and predicts future increased risk of prostate cancer (Chan et al. 1998). Moreover, physical activity is related to higher 25(OH) vitamin D levels due to greater outdoor exposure to UV radiation (Giovannucci et al. 2006), which may favorably impact prostate carcinogenesis. Although circulating levels of testosterone

3

appear to be unrelated to prostate cancer risk (Roddam et al. 2008), androgens induce prostate cancer cell proliferation in vitro (Webber et al. 1996) and an inhibition of androgen activity (through finasteride) decreases prostate cancer risk (Thompson et al. 2003). Thus, whether physical activity impacts prostate cancer risk through a mechanism involving testosterone remains unclear. Likewise, physical activity may reduce prostate cancer risk through its effects on enhancing immune function and antioxidant defense mechanisms, although evidence relating exercise-mediated enhancements in immunity and oxidative defense to decreased prostate cancer risk is lacking. In theory, physical activity may reduce prostate cancer incidence or progression by decreasing chronic low-grade inflammation, a factor that is directly related to prostate cancer development (De Marzo et al. 2007). Physical activity may also indirectly affect prostate carcinogenesis by preventing adiposity and weight gain, factors that have been positively associated with fatal prostate cancer (Wright et al. 2007).

3.7.2 Bladder Cancer

Few potential biologic mechanisms exist that potentially link increased physical activity to decreased risk of bladder cancer, and those that can be identified likely operate indirectly by preventing adiposity. Overweight and obesity are related to enhanced insulin production and type 2 diabetes is positively related to bladder cancer (Larsson et al. 2006), providing indirect support for an insulin mechanism. In addition, insulin acts as a mitogen that may affect bladder cancer development by increasing IGF-1 (Suikkari et al. 1988), which has also been positively associated with bladder cancer (Zhao et al. 2003). Apart from an insulin pathway, adiposity may also be associated with bladder cancer through a mechanism involving chronic inflammation (Festa et al. 2001) because inflammatory markers such as C-reactive protein (CRP) and interleukin (IL)-6 are positively associated with bladder cancer mortality (Andrews et al. 2002; Hilmy et al. 2005).

3.7.3 Renal Cell Cancer

Few biologic mechanisms have been hypothesized through which enhanced physical activity may be associated with decreased RCC risk. Factors linking increased physical activity to decreased risk of RCC operate indirectly through avoidance of overweight and obesity, including reduced levels of insulin and circulating IGF-1 (Kellerer et al. 1995), decreased lipid peroxidation (Gago-Dominguez et al. 2002), and prevention of renal atherosclerosis (Chade et al. 2005), factors that may be related to RCC risk (Chow et al. 2000).

3.7.4 Testicular Cancer

Two main biologic mechanisms have been proposed regarding the association between physical activity and testicular cancer. One mechanism involves an alteration in androgen levels, which have been found to increase (Mantzoros and Georgiadis 1995), decrease (Hackney et al. 1998), and remain unchanged (Ukkola et al. 2001) in relation to physical activity levels. Thus, whether a potential association between physical activity and testicular cancer is mediated by androgens remains poorly understood. The second mechanism is that physical activity such as horseback riding or cycling possibly causes testicular trauma sufficient to result in testicular atrophy, a potential testicular cancer risk factor (Gallagher et al. 1995). However, the etiologic role for trauma in testicular cancer is uncertain.

3.8 Future Directions

The current review of physical activity and genitourinary cancer points toward the need for improvements in self-reported and objective measurements of physical activity in order to more precisely characterize different types and parameters of physical activity in relation to genitourinary cancer risk. More information is also needed regarding how physical activity over the life course potentially influences risk of genitourinary cancer. In addition, little is known about the impact of fitness on genitourinary cancer. The sparse data available suggest that fitness is inversely related to risk of prostate cancer. Moreover, the potentially beneficial impact of exercise on genitourinary cancer prognosis and survival is poorly understood and requires specific attention. The identification of the underlying biologic mechanisms potentially linking physical activity to the incidence and prognosis of genitourinary cancer may assist in identifying appropriate future molecular targets for cancer prevention. Importantly, further research is needed to determine whether physical activity more strongly affects genitourinary cancer risk among specific subgroups of the population, which forms the basis for the future development of personalized strategies for prevention.

References

Albanes D, Blair A, Taylor PR (1989) Physical activity and risk of cancer in the NHANES I population. Am J Public Health 6:744–750

American Cancer Society (2008) Cancer facts and figures 2008

Andersson SO, Baron J, Wolk A et al (1995) Early life risk factors for prostate cancer: a population-based case- control study in Sweden. Cancer Epidemiol Biomark Prev 3:187–192

Andrews B, Shariat SF, Kim JH et al (2002) Preoperative plasma levels of interleukin-6 and its soluble receptor predict disease recurrence and survival of patients with bladder cancer. J Urol 3:1475–1481

Bairati I, Larouche R, Meyer F et al (2000) Lifetime occupational physical activity and incidental prostate cancer (Canada). Cancer Causes Control 8:759–764

Bergstrom A, Moradi T, Lindblad P et al (1999) Occupational physical activity and renal cell cancer: a nationwide cohort study in Sweden. Int J Cancer 2:186–191

Bergstrom A, Terry P, Lindblad P et al (2001) Physical activity and risk of renal cell cancer. Int J Cancer 1:155–157

Brownson RC, Chang JC, Davis JR et al (1991) Physical activity on the job and cancer in Missouri. Am J Public Health 5:639–642

Cerhan JR, Torner JC, Lynch CF et al (1997) Association of smoking, body mass, and physical activity with risk of prostate cancer in the Iowa 65+ Rural Health Study (United States). Cancer Causes Control 2:229–238

Chade AR, Lerman A, Lerman LO (2005) Kidney in early atherosclerosis. Hypertension 6:1042–1049

Chan JM, Stampfer MJ, Giovannucci E et al (1998) Plasma insulin-like growth factor-I and prostate cancer risk: a prospective study. Science 5350: 563–566

Chen YC, Chiang CI, Lin RS et al (2005) Diet, vegetarian food and prostate carcinoma among men in Taiwan. Br J Cancer 9:1057–1061

Chiu BC, Gapstur SM, Chow WH et al (2006) Body mass index, physical activity, and risk of renal cell carcinoma. Int J Obes (Lond) 6: 940–947

3

Chow WH, Gridley G, Fraumeni JF Jr et al (2000) Obesity, hypertension, and the risk of kidney cancer in men. N Engl J Med 18:1305–1311

Clarke G, Whittemore AS (2000) Prostate cancer risk in relation to anthropometry and physical activity: the National Health and Nutrition Examination Survey I Epidemiological Follow-Up Study. Cancer Epidemiol Biomark Prev 9: 875–881

Cohen HT, McGovern FJ (2005) Renal-cell carcinoma. N Engl J Med 23:2477–2490

Coldman AJ, Elwood JM, Gallagher RP (1982) Sports activities and risk of testicular cancer. Br J Cancer 5:749–756

Cook MB, Zhang Y, Graubard BI et al (2008) Risk of testicular germ-cell tumours in relation to childhood physical activity. Br J Cancer 1: 174–178

Darlington GA, Kreiger N, Lightfoot N et al (2007) Prostate cancer risk and diet, recreational physical activity and cigarette smoking. Chron Dis Can 4:145–153

De Marzo AM, Platz EA, Sutcliffe S et al (2007) Inflammation in prostate carcinogenesis. Nat Rev Cancer 4:256–269

Dosemeci M, Hayes RB, Vetter R et al (1993) Occupational physical activity, socioeconomic status, and risks of 15 cancer sites in Turkey. Cancer Causes Control 4:313–321

Festa A, D'Agostino R Jr, Williams K et al (2001) The relation of body fat mass and distribution to markers of chronic inflammation. Int J Obes Relat Metab Disord 10:1407–1415

Friedenreich CM, McGregor SE, Courneya KS et al (2004) Case-control study of lifetime total physical activity and prostate cancer risk. Am J Epidemiol 8:740–749

Gago-Dominguez M, Castelao JE, Yuan JM et al (2002) Lipid peroxidation: a novel and unifying concept of the etiology of renal cell carcinoma (United States). Cancer Causes Control 3:287–293

Gallagher RP, Huchcroft S, Phillips N et al (1995) Physical activity, medical history, and risk of testicular cancer (Alberta and British Columbia, Canada). Cancer Causes Control 5: 398–406

Gallus S, Foschi R, Talamini R et al (2007) Risk factors for prostate cancer in men aged less than 60 years: a case-control study from Italy. Urology 6:1121–1126

Giovannucci E (2003) Nutrition, insulin, insulin-like growth factors and cancer. Horm Metab Res 11–12:694–704

Giovannucci E, Leitzmann M, Spiegelman D et al (1998) A prospective study of physical activity and prostate cancer in male health professionals. Cancer Res 22:5117–5122

Giovannucci EL, Liu Y, Leitzmann MF et al (2005) A prospective study of physical activity and incident and fatal prostate cancer. Arch Intern Med 9:1005–1010

Giovannucci E, Liu Y, Rimm EB et al (2006) Prospective study of predictors of vitamin D status and cancer incidence and mortality in men. J Natl Cancer Inst 7:451–459

Goodman MT, Morgenstern H, Wynder EL (1986) A case-control study of factors affecting the development of renal cell cancer. Am J Epidemiol 6:926–941

Gronberg H (2003) Prostate cancer epidemiology. Lancet 9360:859–864

Hackney AC, Fahrner CL, Gulledge TP (1998) Basal reproductive hormonal profiles are altered in endurance trained men. J Sports Med Phys Fitness 2:138–141

Hartman TJ, Albanes D, Rautalahti M et al (1998) Physical activity and prostate cancer in the Alpha-Tocopherol, Beta-Carotene (ATBC) Cancer Prevention Study (Finland). Cancer Causes Control 1:11–18

Hilmy M, Bartlett JM, Underwood MA et al (2005) The relationship between the systemic inflammatory response and survival in patients with transitional cell carcinoma of the urinary bladder. Br J Cancer 4:625–627

Holick CN, Giovannucci EL, Stampfer MJ et al (2007) Prospective study of body mass index, height, physical activity and incidence of bladder cancer in US men and women. Int J Cancer 1:140–146

Hsing AW, McLaughlin JK, Zheng W et al (1994) Occupation, physical activity, and risk of prostate cancer in Shanghai, People's Republic of China. Cancer Causes Control 2: 136–140

Iwamura M, Sluss PM, Casamento JB et al (1993) Insulin-like growth factor I: action and receptor characterization in human prostate cancer cell lines. Prostate 3:243–252

Jemal A, Siegel R, Ward E et al (2009) Cancer statistics, 2009. CA Cancer J Clin 4:225–249

Jian L, Shen ZJ, Lee AH et al (2005) Moderate physical activity and prostate cancer risk: a case-control study in China. Eur J Epidemiol 2: 155–160

Kellerer M, von Eye CH, Muhlhofer A et al (1995) Insulin- and insulin-like growth-factor-I receptor tyrosine-kinase activities in human renal carcinoma. Int J Cancer 5:501–507

Koebnick C, Michaud D, Moore SC et al (2008) Body mass index, physical activity, and bladder cancer in a large prospective study. Cancer Epidemiol Biomark Prev 5:1214–1221

Krishnadasan A, Kennedy N, Zhao Y et al (2008) Nested case-control study of occupational physical activity and prostate cancer among workers using a job exposure matrix. Cancer Causes Control 1:107–114

Lacey JV Jr, Deng J, Dosemeci M et al (2001) Prostate cancer, benign prostatic hyperplasia and physical activity in Shanghai, China. Int J Epidemiol 2:341–349

Larsson SC, Orsini N, Brismar K et al (2006) Diabetes mellitus and risk of bladder cancer: a meta-analysis. Diabetologia 12:2819–2823

Le Marchand L, Kolonel LN, Yoshizawa CN (1991) Lifetime occupational physical activity and prostate cancer risk. Am J Epidemiol 2:103–111

Lee IM, Paffenbarger RS Jr (1994) Physical activity and its relation to cancer risk: a prospective study of college alumni. Med Sci Sports Exerc 7:831–837

Lee IM, Paffenbarger RS Jr, Hsieh CC (1992) Physical activity and risk of prostatic cancer among college alumni. Am J Epidemiol 2:169–179

Lee IM, Sesso HD, Paffenbarger RS Jr (2001) A prospective cohort study of physical activity and body size in relation to prostate cancer risk (United States). Cancer Causes Control 2:187–193

Lindblad P, Wolk A, Bergstrom R et al (1994) The role of obesity and weight fluctuations in the etiology of renal cell cancer: a population-based case-control study. Cancer Epidemiol Biomark Prev 8:631–639

Lindgarde F, Saltin B (1981) Daily physical activity, work capacity and glucose tolerance in lean and obese normoglycaemic middle-aged men. Diabetologia 2:134–138

Littman AJ, Kristal AR, White E (2006) Recreational physical activity and prostate cancer risk (United States). Cancer Causes Control 6:831–841

Littman AJ, Doody DR, Biggs ML et al (2009) Physical activity in adolescence and testicular germ cell cancer risk. Cancer Causes Control 20:1281–1290

Liu S, Lee IM, Linson P et al (2000) A prospective study of physical activity and risk of prostate cancer in US physicians. Int J Epidemiol 1:29–35

Lund Nilsen TI, Johnsen R, Vatten LJ (2000) Socio-economic and lifestyle factors associated with the risk of prostate cancer. Br J Cancer 7:1358–1363

Mahabir S, Leitzmann MF, Pietinen P et al (2004) Physical activity and renal cell cancer risk in a cohort of male smokers. Int J Cancer 4:600–605

Mantzoros CS, Georgiadis EI (1995) Body mass and physical activity are important predictors of serum androgen concentrations in young healthy men. Epidemiology 4:432–435

McGlynn KA (2001) Environmental and host factors in testicular germ cell tumors. Cancer Invest 8:842–853

Mellemgaard A, Engholm G, McLaughlin JK et al (1994) Risk factors for renal-cell carcinoma in Denmark. III. Role of weight, physical activity and reproductive factors. Int J Cancer 1:66–71

Mellemgaard A, Lindblad P, Schlehofer B et al (1995) International renal-cell cancer study. III. Role of weight, height, physical activity, and use of amphetamines. Int J Cancer 3:350–354

Menezes RJ, Tomlinson G, Kreiger N (2003) Physical activity and risk of renal cell carcinoma. Int J Cancer 4:642–646

Moore SC, Chow WH, Schatzkin A et al (2008a) Physical activity during adulthood and adolescence in relation to renal cell cancer. Am J Epidemiol 2:149–157

Moore SC, Peters TM, Ahn J et al (2008b) Physical activity in relation to total, advanced, and fatal prostate cancer. Cancer Epidemiol Biomark Prev 9:2458–2466

Moore SC, Peters TM, Ahn J et al (2009) Age-specific physical activity and prostate cancer risk among white men and black men. Cancer 21:5060–5070

Nicodemus KK, Sweeney C, Folsom AR (2004) Evaluation of dietary, medical and lifestyle risk factors for incident kidney cancer in postmenopausal women. Int J Cancer 1:115–121

Nilsen TI, Romundstad PR, Vatten LJ (2006) Recreational physical activity and risk of prostate cancer: A prospective population-based

3

study in Norway (the HUNT study). Int J Cancer 12:2943–2947

Norman A, Moradi T, Gridley G et al (2002) Occupational physical activity and risk for prostate cancer in a nationwide cohort study in Sweden. Br J Cancer 1:70–75

Oliveria SA, Kohl HW 3rd, Trichopoulos D et al (1996) The association between cardiorespiratory fitness and prostate cancer. Med Sci Sports Exerc 1:97–104

Paffenbarger RS Jr, Hyde RT, Wing AL (1987) Physical activity and incidence of cancer in diverse populations: a preliminary report. Am J Clin Nutr 1(Suppl):312–317

Pan SY, DesMeules M, Morrison H et al (2006) Obesity, high energy intake, lack of physical activity, and the risk of kidney cancer. Cancer Epidemiol Biomark Prev 12:2453–2460

Patel AV, Rodriguez C, Jacobs EJ et al (2005) Recreational physical activity and risk of prostate cancer in a large cohort of U.S. men. Cancer Epidemiol Biomark Prev 1:275–279

Pelucchi C, Bosetti C, Negri E, et al. Mechanisms of disease: the epidemiology of bladder cancer. Nat Clin Pract Urol 2006;3:327–340.

Pierotti B, Altieri A, Talamini R et al (2005) Lifetime physical activity and prostate cancer risk. Int J Cancer 4:639–642

Polednak AP (1976) College athletics, body size, and cancer mortality. Cancer 1:382–387

Powell IJ (2007) Epidemiology and pathophysiology of prostate cancer in African-American men. J Urol 2:444–449

Pukkala E, Kaprio J, Koskenvuo M et al (2000) Cancer incidence among Finnish world class male athletes. Int J Sports Med 3:216–220

Putnam SD, Cerhan JR, Parker AS et al (2000) Lifestyle and anthropometric risk factors for prostate cancer in a cohort of Iowa men. Ann Epidemiol 6:361–369

Roddam AW, Allen NE, Appleby P et al (2008) Endogenous sex hormones and prostate cancer: a collaborative analysis of 18 prospective studies. J Natl Cancer Inst 3:170–183

Scelo G, Brennan P (2007) The epidemiology of bladder and kidney cancer. Nat Clin Pract Urol 4:205–217

Schnohr P, Gronbaek M, Petersen L et al (2005) Physical activity in leisure-time and risk of cancer: 14-year follow-up of 28,000 Danish men and women. Scand J Public Health 4: 244–249

Setiawan VW, Stram DO, Nomura AM et al (2007) Risk factors for renal cell cancer: the multiethnic cohort. Am J Epidemiol 8:932–940

Severson RK, Nomura AM, Grove JS et al (1989) A prospective analysis of physical activity and cancer. Am J Epidemiol 3:522–529

Soll-Johanning H, Bach E (2004) Occupational exposure to air pollution and cancer risk among Danish urban mail carriers. Int Arch Occup Environ Health 5:351–356

Srivastava A, Kreiger N (2000) Relation of physical activity to risk of testicular cancer. Am J Epidemiol 1:78–87

Steenland K, Nowlin S, Palu S (1995) Cancer incidence in the National Health and Nutrition Survey I. Follow-up data: diabetes, cholesterol, pulse and physical activity. Cancer Epidemiol Biomark Prev 8:807–811

Suikkari AM, Koivisto VA, Rutanen EM et al (1988) Insulin regulates the serum levels of low molecular weight insulin-like growth factor-binding protein. J Clin Endocrinol Metab 2:266–272

Sung JF, Lin RS, Pu YS et al (1999) Risk factors for prostate carcinoma in Taiwan: a case-control study in a Chinese population. Cancer 3: 484–491

Tavani A, Zucchetto A, Dal Maso L et al (2007) Lifetime physical activity and the risk of renal cell cancer. Int J Cancer 9:1977–1980

Thompson IM, Goodman PJ, Tangen CM et al (2003) The influence of finasteride on the development of prostate cancer. N Engl J Med 3:215–224

Thune I, Lund E (1994) Physical activity and the risk of prostate and testicular cancer: a cohort study of 53, 000 Norwegian men. Cancer Causes Control 6:549–556

Tripathi A, Folsom AR, Anderson KE (2002) Risk factors for urinary bladder carcinoma in postmenopausal women. The Iowa women's health study. Cancer 11:2316–2323

UK Testicular Cancer Study Group (1994) Aetiology of testicular cancer: association with congenital abnormalities, age at puberty, infertility, and exercise. United Kingdom Testicular Cancer Study Group. BMJ 6941:1393–1399

Ukkola O, Gagnon J, Rankinen T et al (2001) Age, body mass index, race and other determinants of steroid hormone variability: the HERITAGE Family Study. Eur J Endocrinol 1:1–9

van Dijk BA, Schouten LJ, Kiemeney LA et al (2004) Relation of height, body mass, energy intake, and physical activity to risk of renal cell carcinoma: results from the Netherlands Cohort Study. Am J Epidemiol 12:1159–1167

Vena JE, Graham S, Zielezny M et al (1987) Occupational exercise and risk of cancer. Am J Clin Nutr 1(Suppl):318–327

Villeneuve PJ, Johnson KC, Kreiger N et al (1999) Risk factors for prostate cancer: results from the Canadian National Enhanced Cancer Surveillance System. The Canadian Cancer Registries Epidemiology Research Group. Cancer Causes Control 5:355–367

Wannamethee SG, Shaper AG, Walker M (2001) Physical activity and risk of cancer in middle-aged men. Br J Cancer 9: 1311–1316

Webber MM, Bello D, Quader S (1996) Immortalized and tumorigenic adult human prostatic epithelial cell lines: characteristics and applications. Part I. Cell markers and immortalized nontumorigenic cell lines. Prostate 6:386–394

West DW, Slattery ML, Robison LM et al (1991) Adult dietary intake and prostate cancer risk in Utah: a case-control study with special emphasis on aggressive tumors. Cancer Causes Control 2:85–94

Whittemore AS, Kolonel LN, Wu AH et al (1995) Prostate cancer in relation to diet, physical activity, and body size in blacks, whites, and Asians in the United States and Canada. J Natl Cancer Inst 9:652–661

Wright ME, Chang SC, Schatzkin A et al (2007) Prospective study of adiposity and weight change in relation to prostate cancer incidence and mortality. Cancer 4:675–684

Yu H, Harris RE, Wynder EL (1988) Case-control study of prostate cancer and socioeconomic factors. Prostate 4:317–325

Zeegers MP, Dirx MJ, van den Brandt PA (2005) Physical activity and the risk of prostate cancer in the Netherlands cohort study, results after 9.3 years of follow-up. Cancer Epidemiol Biomark Prev 6:1490–1495

Zhao H, Grossman HB, Spitz MR et al (2003) Plasma levels of insulin-like growth factor-1 and binding protein-3, and their association with bladder cancer risk. J Urol 2: 714–717

Physical Activity and Gastrointestinal Cancer Prevention 4

Kathleen Y. Wolin and Hallie Tuchman

Abstract Colorectal cancer is the third most common cancer globally and is a leading cause of cancer death. Gastric cancer contributes significantly to the global cancer burden, particularly in low- and middle-income countries. We reviewed the literature for studies on physical activity or exercise and colon, rectal, and gastric cancers as well as colonic adenomatous pol yps. We identified 52 studies of colon cancer, 31 studies of rectal cancer, 23 studies of colon polyps, and 16 studies of gastric cancer. Of the 52 studies of physical activity and colon cancer, 37 found a statistically significant association between increased levels of physical activity and decreased colon cancer risk in at least one comparison. Accumulated evidence suggests that physical activity is associated with a 25% reduction in colon cancer risk. In line with previous reports, we found no indication that the association was more pronounced for occupational versus recreational physical activity, with both resulting in a risk reduction of about 22%. Evidence for other domains of physical activity (i.e., transportation or household physical activity) is limited. Evidence is emerging that individuals who are consistently active across the lifetime may obtain greater risk reductions than those who are only active in recent years. Despite consistent associations with colon cancer, evidence is more limited though suggestive that physical activity reduces risk of colon adenomas or adenoma recurrence. There is clear evidence that physical activity is not associated with rectal or gastric cancers.

K.Y. Wolin (✉) and H. Tuchman
Department of Surgery, Washington University School of Medicine, St. Louis, MO, USA

4.1 Introduction

Colon cancer is the third most commonly occurring cancer in men and women in the USA (American Cancer Society 2007; Howe et al. 2001). Globally, colorectal cancer incidence ranks behind lung, stomach, and liver cancer in men and breast, lung, and stomach in women (World Health Organization 2008) and is a leading cause of cancer death (Danaei et al. 2005). It is the second leading cause of cancer death in high socioeconomic countries (Danaei et al. 2005). Gastric cancer, which accounts for 12% of cancer deaths, contributes significantly to the global cancer burden, particularly in low- and middle-income countries (Danaei et al. 2005; Parkin et al. 2005). Gastric cancer is the second leading cause of cancer death worldwide (Danaei et al. 2005).

K.S. Courneya and C.M. Friedenreich (eds.), *Physical Activity and Cancer*, Recent Results in Cancer Research 186, DOI: 10.1007/978-3-642-04231-7_4,

4

Nearly 90% of colorectal tumors are adenocarcinomas (International Agency for Research on Cancer 2003). Studies of migrants from low- to high-incidence countries have shown that these individuals rapidly acquire the level of risk of the new location, suggesting that environmental factors have a large role in colorectal cancer epidemiology (International Agency for Research on Cancer 2003). Only about 5% of colon cancer cases are believed to be inherited (International Agency for Research on Cancer 2003). As evidence-based colorectal cancer screening programs have grown, tumors are detected at earlier stages and survival rates have improved (International Agency for Research on Cancer 2003). Established risk factors for colon cancer include excess body weight and a high intake of red and processed meat (World Cancer Research Fund/American Institute for Cancer Research 2007). There is reliable evidence that physical activity, calcium, and nonsteroidal anti-inflammatory drugs (NSAIDs) and postmenopausal hormones reduce risk (Potter and Hunter 2002). Data on modifiable risk factors for rectal cancer are less clear (Wei et al. 2004).

The majority of gastric cancers are carcinomas, while nonepithelial tumors include lymphomas and mesenchymal tumors (International Agency for Research on Cancer 2003). Nearly two-thirds of gastric cancers occur in developing countries. Migration studies have indicated that risk of gastric cancer shifts within two generations when individuals move from a high-incidence (e.g., Japan) to a low-incidence (e.g., USA) country (International Agency for Research on Cancer 2003). Probable risk factors for gastric cancer include salt (and salty foods), while fruit and vegetable intake likely decreases risk. Perhaps the leading known risk factor for gastric cancer is infection with *Helicobacter pylori* (*H. pylori*) bacteria, which is thought to be associated with 40–70% of gastric cancer (International Agency for Research on Cancer 2003). Gastric cancer typically presents in the late stages and has a poor prognosis. Nearly 80% of individuals presenting with gastric cancer in developed countries present with advanced tumors (International Agency for Research on Cancer 2003). While Japan has a large gastric cancer screening program in place, it is costly and a survival benefit has not been conclusively demonstrated (International Agency for Research on Cancer 2003).

4.2 Methods

We searched the literature using PubMed for all studies on physical activity or exercise and colon, rectal, and gastric cancers through February 2010. We employed the terms exercise and physical activity in combination with each cancer of interest (i.e., colon cancer, rectal cancer, and gastric or stomach cancer). We searched for studies of colon polyps using the terms colon polyp, colon adenoma, colorectal polyp, colorectal adenoma, and adenomatous polyps. We also relied on previous qualitative and quantitative reviews of the available data (Lee and Oguma 2006; Samad et al. 2005; World Cancer Research Fund/American Institute for Cancer Research 2007) and manual searches of the reference lists of identified manuscripts. We included case-control and cohort studies whose endpoint was incident cancer. For colon polyps, we included incident and prevalent cases. Given the small number of studies, we also included studies of cancer-specific mortality in our gastric cancer review. We did not limit studies by type of physical activity or study sample demographics. We excluded manuscripts not in English. We relied on the most recent report from studies with multiple manuscripts, except in cases where earlier reports included subanalyses not included in later reports or when later reports did not present multivariable analyses. In our review of colon cancer, we focused almost exclusively on papers with a colon cancer endpoint (excluding those that only examined colorectal cancer as an endpoint).

Our PubMed search for colon cancer yielded 667 potential articles. We excluded reviews, studies in nonhumans, editorials/comments/letters to the editor, studies without colon cancer incidence as an outcome, and studies where physical activity was only included as a covariate (and thus no relative risk was presented). This research, combined with searches from the references sections of manuscripts and previous reviews, yielded 52 separate studies of colon cancer incidence and physical activity (as noted above, in some cases, multiple publications from a single study were included since different results were presented in separate publications). Our strategy yielded 89 potential papers for colon polyps, 204 articles for rectal cancer, and 144 on gastric cancer. Of these, we included 23 papers on colon polyps, 31 on rectal cancer, and 16 for gastric cancer.

4.3 Colon Cancer

A substantial body of epidemiologic evidence exists that consistently has demonstrated that increased levels of physical activity are associated with a reduced risk of colon cancer (International Agency for Research on Cancer 2002; Samad et al. 2005; Slattery 2004; Wolin et al. 2009; World Cancer Research Fund/American Institute for Cancer Research 2007). This body of evidence includes studies published across a span of more than 30 years and that were conducted with a wide array of different study designs, study populations, and physical activity assessment methods. Previous reviews have estimated that physical activity reduces colon cancer risk by one-fourth to one-third (Lee and Oguma 2006; Wolin et al. 2009). It has been further estimated that physical inactivity causes 16% of colon and rectal cancers and 15% of colorectal cancer mortality globally (Bull et al. 2004).

Early observational epidemiologic studies examined the association between physical activity and lower gastrointestinal cancers (colon and rectal) combined. However, over time, evidence emerged to suggest that risk factors differed between these two cancer sites; hence, subsequent studies have examined these outcomes separately. This approach is more appropriate since these two sites have different natural histories and etiologies (Wei et al. 2004). Consequently, we examined the association of physical activity separately for colon and rectal tumors and focused our review on studies that examined colon cancer separately.

There is now consistent evidence from observational epidemiologic studies that physical activity reduces colon cancer risk (International Agency for Research on Cancer 2002; Samad et al. 2005; Slattery 2004; Wolin et al. 2009). A recent meta-analysis of studies on colon cancer and physical activity estimated a 25% risk reduction for the most physically active populations as compared to the least active (Wolin et al. 2009). For this review, we identified 52 studies of physical activity and colon cancer, of which 37 found a statistically significant association between physical activity and colon cancer in at least one comparison. Evidence for a dose response between increasing levels of physical activity and decreasing colon cancer risk was found in 24 out of 35 studies that formally tested for this trend. For example, Chao et al. reported a statistically significant trend ($p = 0.006$) of decreasing risk with increasing physical activity (Chao et al. 2004). In the 16 studies that tested a dose response for both men and women (Chao et al. 2004; Hou et al. 2004; Howard et al. 2008; Isomura et al. 2006; Johnsen et al. 2006; Lee et al. 2007; Moradi et al. 2008; Nilsen et al. 2008; Schnohr et al. 2005; Takahashi et al. 2007;

Tang et al. 1999; Tavani et al. 1999; Thune and Lund 1996; Wei et al. 2004; White et al. 1996; Zhang et al. 2006), separately, five found evidence of a trend only among men (Howard et al. 2008; Lee et al. 2007; Takahashi et al. 2007; Tang et al. 1999; White et al. 1996), three found evidence only among women (Hou et al. 2004; Nilsen et al. 2008; Thune and Lund 1996), four found evidence in both men and women (Chao et al. 2004; Moradi et al. 2008; Tavani et al. 1999; Wei et al. 2004), and four found no evidence in either (Isomura et al. 2006; Johnsen et al. 2006; Schnohr et al. 2005; Zhang et al. 2006) (Figs. 4.1 and 4.2).

4.3.1 Type of Physical Activity

The association between physical activity and colon cancer has been seen for studies measuring all types of physical activity. In a 2007 meta-analyses of cohort-only data published between 1997 and 2005, the World Cancer Research

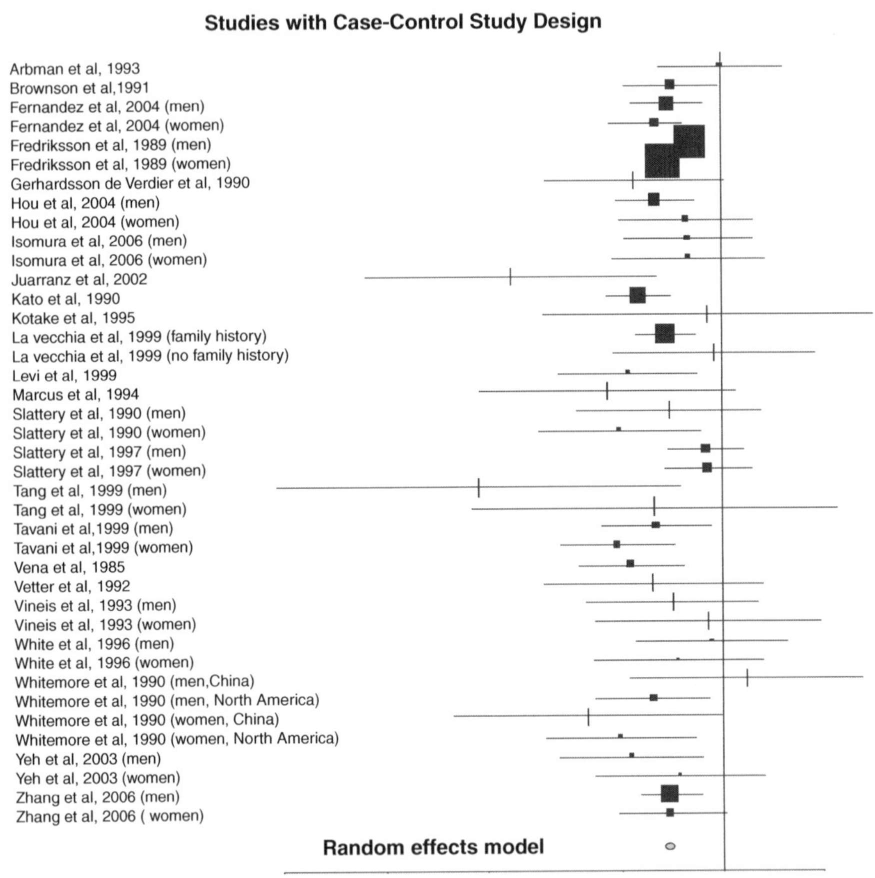

Fig. 4.1 Meta-analysis of case-control studies of physical activity and colon cancer (Reprinted with permission from original publication in the British Journal of Cancer 2009 (Wolin et al. 2009)

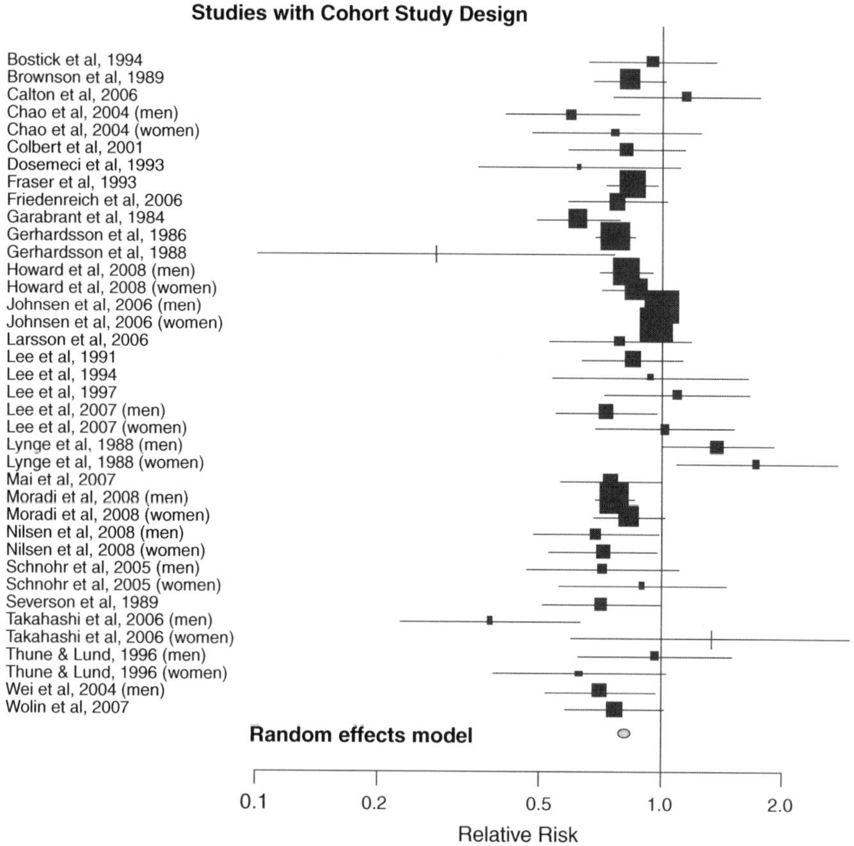

Fig. 4.2 Meta-analysis of cohort studies of physical activity and colon cancer (Reprinted with permission from original publication in the British Journal of Cancer 2009 (Wolin et al. 2009)

Fund/American Institute for Cancer Research (WCRF/AICR) report found slightly stronger associations for occupational physical activity (RR = 0.71, 95% CI 0.60–0.83) than recreational physical activity (RR = 0.82, 95% CI 0.72–0.94) and colon cancer (World Cancer Research Fund/ American Institute for Cancer Research 2007). However, a meta-analysis by Wolin et al. found no difference in the association for occupational (RR = 0.78, 95% CI 0.74–0.83) as compared to recreational (RR = 0.77, 95% CI 0.72–0.82) physical activity (Wolin et al. 2009). We identified 32 studies that examined occupational physical activity independent of other activity domains, of which 16 reported a statistically significant reduction in colon cancer risk (Brownson et al. 1991, 1989; Colbert et al. 2001; Fernandez et al. 2004; Fraser and Pearce 1993; Garabrant et al. 1984; Gerhardsson et al. 1986; Kato et al. 1990; La Vecchia et al. 1999; Levi et al. 1999; Lynge and Thygesen 1988; Moradi et al. 2008; Severson et al. 1989; Tavani et al. 1999; Vena et al. 1985; Whittemore et al. 1990). We identified 33 studies that examined recreational physical activity independent of other activity domains, of which 15 reported a significant association. (The 15 significant studies are: Chao et al. 2004; Gerhardsson et al. 1988;

Howard et al. 2008; Juarranz et al. 2002; Larsson et al. 2006; Lee et al. 2007; Levi et al. 1999; Nilsen et al. 2008; Severson et al. 1989; Slattery et al. 1990; Tan et al. 1999; Whittemore et al. 1990; Wei et al. 2004; Yeh et al. 2003; Zhang et al. 2006).

Only two studies examined transportation as a separate type of physical activity and both reported statistically significant colon cancer risk reductions (Hou et al. 2004; Takahashi et al. 2007). Household physical activity has not been examined frequently independently of other types of physical activity, possibly because of the belief that these activities are more difficult to measure accurately through self-report. White et al. (1996) and Friedenreich et al. (2006) both found no association between household activities and colon cancer risk, while Larsson and colleagues (Larsson et al. 2006) and Severson et al. (1989) both observed significantly significant risk reductions with increasing levels of household activity. Sedentary behavior, often defined in these studies as time spent sitting, has also been associated with increased risk of physical activity in the occupational setting (Gerhardsson et al. 1986) as well as in a study measuring global sedentary time (Howard et al. 2008).

Few studies have examined specific recreational physical activities as they relate to colon cancer. Wolin et al. found that walking alone was sufficient to significantly reduce risk of colon cancer in a sample of US women (Wolin et al. 2007). This finding is important as walking is the most commonly reported activity, particularly among women (Brownson et al. 2000; Crespo et al. 1996). Wannamethee et al. also found duration of walking to be associated with a reduced risk of colorectal cancer in a sample of British men (Wannamethee et al. 2001). However, Takahashi et al. found the association between walking and colon cancer risk was only present in men, while Chao et al. found no such association in US men or women (Chao et al. 2004; Takahashi et al. 2007). Walking pace was not associated with risk in either study that evaluated it separately (Wannamethee et al. 2001; Wolin et al. 2007). Hou et al. found commuting (which could include walking or cycling) to be associated with a significantly reduced risk of colon cancer (Hou et al. 2004).

4.3.2 Dose of Physical Activity

The three components of dose of activity (i.e., duration, frequency, and intensity) have been examined separately and in combination in some of these studies. A 2007 WCRF/AICR meta-analysis found a statistically significant inverse association for high- versus low-intensity recreational physical activity with colon cancer (RR = 0.80, 95% CI 0.68–0.95) (World Cancer Research Fund/American Institute for Cancer Research 2007). When considering the duration of activity needed for a risk reduction, Martinez et al. (1997) observed that women who participated in more than 1 h per day of moderate intensity recreational activity had a significantly lower risk of colon cancer (RR = 0.59, 95% CI 0.52–0.91) than women who participated in less than 1 h. The WCRF/AICR also reported a borderline significant association for the highest versus lowest category of frequency of any physical activity (RR = 0.87, 95% CI 0.72–1.06) (World Cancer Research Fund/American Institute for Cancer Research 2007). Intensity of total physical activity was also associated with a lower risk of colon cancer in the WCRF/AICR meta-analysis, with a 17% lower risk in the highest versus lowest category reported (RR = 0.83, 95% CI 0.69–1.01) (World Cancer Research Fund/American Institute for Cancer Research 2007).

While some have suggested that participation in vigorous intensity activity may be necessary to alter risk (Chao et al. 2004; Slattery 2004), previous studies have also reported a reduced risk of colon cancer with engagement in moderate (Cronin et al. 2001; Lee et al. 1991) and low intensity (Howard et al. 2008) physical activity. It has been hypothesized that moderate intensity physical activity may be sufficient to reduce risk if it is of sufficient duration. Recent analyses in the Nurses' Health Study found a significant risk reduction among women who walked at least 2 h per week (Wolin et al. 2007), approximately equivalent to the latest US physical activity recommendations for health (Physical Activity Guidelines Advisory Committee 2008), suggesting vigorous physical activity is not necessary to reduce risk as these women did not participate in other, more vigorous, forms of physical activity. It is also possible that stronger associations are seen for vigorous activity because this level of activity is easier to recall (Yore et al. 2007) and less prone to random measurement error that would result in attenuation of the associations.

4.3.3 Timing of Physical Activity

It is also of interest to determine how the association of physical activity with colon cancer varies over the lifetime. Several studies have examined how physical activity levels across the life course are associated with risk of colon cancer (Chao et al. 2004; Hou et al. 2004; Howard et al. 2008; Le Marchand et al. 1997; Lee et al. 1991; Levi et al. 1999; Mai et al. 2007; Slattery et al. 1997, 2003b; Tavani et al. 1999; Vena et al. 1985; Vetter et al. 1992; Wolin et al. 2007; Zhang et al. 2006). Four studies (Levi et al. 1999; Mai et al. 2007; Tavani et al. 1999; Zhang et al. 2006) have examined the association of early life physical activity and risk of colon cancer. Two of these (Mai et al. 2007; Tavani et al. 1999) found that early life physical activity was significantly associated with a decreased risk of colon cancer, but recent physical activity was not. In contrast, Levi et al. reported significant associations for recreational physical activity from age 30–39 and 50–59, but not age 15–19 (Levi et al. 1999) and Zhang et al. found no association of occupational physical activity from age 20–40 and risk of colon cancer (Zhang et al. 2006).

Eight studies evaluated summary indictors of lifetime physical activity (Hou et al. 2004; Howard et al. 2008; Le Marchand et al. 1997; Mai et al. 2007; Slattery et al. 1997, 2003b; Vena et al. 1985; Vetter et al. 1992) and all reported significant colon cancer risk reductions with higher levels of lifetime physical activity associations, though Howard et al. and Le Marchand et al. found these associations only amongst men.

Three studies examined change in physical activity during adulthood using prospectively collected data (Chao et al. 2004; Lee et al. 1991; Wolin et al. 2007). Lee et al. found that men who were highly active at two time points 11 15 years apart had a statistically significantly lower risk of colon cancer than those who were sedentary at both time points (RR = 0.50, 95% CI 0.27–0.93) (Lee et al. 1991). In contrast, Wolin et al. found that change in physical activity over a 10-year period (represented as a Z-score of change) was not associated with colon cancer risk, though the study may have been underpowered for this outcome (Wolin et al. 2007). Similarly, Chao and colleagues found physical activity 10 years earlier did not modify the association of recent physical activity and colon cancer (Chao et al. 2004).

The lack of associations seen for recent change in activity despite consistent associations for lifetime and adult only activity may be attributable to several factors. First, these studies relied on the self-report of physical activity, which is known to be subject to measurement error. This error becomes compounded when the measures are combined into an indicator of change of physical activity over time. Adult physical activity levels may undergo substantial fluctuations because of changing life circumstances and increasing risk of injury with age. Maintaining an increased physical activity level may be necessary to decrease colon cancer risk and the studies above did not evaluate maintenance of change over the life course. Their reliance on a limited number of measures of physical activity may not capture sustained changes accurately. Finally, we do not know how long the increased physical activity levels need to be maintained to decrease risk. Future research in this area is needed to address these questions of timing of physical activity over lifetime and its impact on colon cancer risk.

4.3.4 Population Subgroup Analyses

Despite the consistency of the evidence overall, many aspects of the relationship between physical activity and colon cancer remain to be elucidated. Recent analyses have begun to examine population subgroups that may particularly benefit from increased physical activity as a means of colon cancer risk reduction. However, only a few studies have examined data stratified by factors of interest, which limits definitive summaries of results across factors such as ethnic origin or race, dietary or alcohol intake, exogenous hormone use, smoking habits, and anthropometric characteristics.

The effect of physical activity on colon cancer risk exists amongst both men and women. Early studies suggested that the benefits of physical activity might be limited to men or be less pronounced in women, but a recent meta-analysis indicated that men (RR = 0.76, 95% CI 0.71, 0.82) and women (RR = 0.79, 95% CI: 0.71, 0.88) benefitted similarly from a physically active lifestyle for colon cancer risk reduction (Wolin et al. 2009).

Early observational epidemiologic studies did not assess a wide range of lifestyle factors and often only adjusted for age or gender; hence, there was the possibility of residual uncontrolled confounding that may have influenced the magnitude of the associations reported. More recent studies, particularly those in large prospective cohort studies (Chao et al. 2004; Friedenreich et al. 2006; Wolin et al. 2007), have controlled for most known risk factors for colon cancer (including body mass index (BMI)) and hence the magnitude of the associations between physical activity and colon cancer risk can be ascertained with more certainty. These studies have found that the associations between colon cancer and physical activity remain, suggesting that this association is attributable to physical activity and not to another healthy lifestyle factor that was uncontrolled in the analysis.

One of the most important risk factors for colon cancer that has been examined as an effect modifier of the association between physical activity and colon cancer is (BMI). The effect of physical activity on colon cancer risk has been observed across categories of BMI in most studies (Giovannucci et al. 1995; Lee et al. 1997; Wolin et al. 2007); however, some data also suggest that the effect of physical activity on colon cancer risk may vary by BMI level. For example, Hou et al. reported a statistically significant interaction between commuting physical activity and BMI ($p < 0.001$) (Hou et al. 2004). Among women with a BMI <19 kg/m^2, those with a low physical activity level had no statistically significant increased risk for colon cancer relative to women with high physical activity (OR = 1.42, 95% CI 0.47–2.35). Among women who were highly active, those who were overweight (BMI > 23.6 kg/m^2) were not at increased risk of colon cancer relative to those who were lean (BMI < 19 kg/m^2) (RR = 1.17, 95%CI 0.7–1.89). However, women who were both overweight and had low activity were at significantly higher risk of colon cancer (RR = 7.42, 95%CI 2.84–10.01) than women who were lean and had high activity.

Two studies have examined risk separately for those with and without a family history of colon cancer. Slattery et al. 1997 reported a statistically significant risk reduction for physical activity among those without a family history (RR = 0.59, 95% CI 0.49–0.72), but none for those with a family history (RR = 0.89, 95% CI 0.52–1.53) (Slattery et al. 1997). These are similar to results from La Vecchia et al. who found an increased risk of colon cancer among those with lower physical activity levels only among those with no family history of colon cancer (La Vecchia et al. 1999).

4.3.5 Colon Sub-site

There is some indication that tumor biology may differ for tumors in the proximal versus distal colon (Iacopetta 2002). Specifically, experimental data have suggested that the tumor carcinogenesis pathway and molecular changes undergone during carcinogenesis differ by subsite. This finding may arise since proximal and distal colon tissues have different embryonic origins and functional structures (e.g., different capillary network structures, different crypt lengths) (Iacopetta 2002).

We identified 30 studies that examined the association of physical activity by tumor subsite (Arbman et al. 1993; Brownson et al. 1991, 1989; Calton et al. 2006; Chao et al. 2004; Colbert et al. 2001; Fraser and Pearce 1993; Fredriksson et al. 1989; Friedenreich et al. 2006; Garabrant et al. 1984; Gerhardsson de Verdier et al. 1990; Gerhardsson et al. 1986; Howard et al. 2008; Isomura et al. 2006; Kato et al. 1990; Larsson et al. 2006; Le Marchand et al. 1997; Lee et al. 2007; Levi et al. 1999; Mai et al. 2007; Marcus et al. 1994; Moradi et al. 2008; Nilsen et al. 2008; Severson et al. 1989; Tavani et al. 1999; Thune and Lund 1996; Vena et al. 1985; White et al. 1996; Wolin et al. 2007; Zhang et al. 2006). Of these 28 studies, nine found a significant association between physical activity and risk of distal colon cancer (Colbert et al. 2001; Garabrant et al. 1984; Gerhardsson de Verdier et al. 1990; Isomura et al. 2006; Kato et al. 1990; Moradi et al. 2008; Nilsen et al. 2008; Tavani et al. 1999; Wolin et al. 2007) and 14 found a significant association in the proximal colon (Brownson et al. 1991, 1989; Chao et al. 2004; Fraser and Pearce 1993; Friedenreich et al. 2006; Garabrant et al. 1984; Gerhardsson et al. 1986; Kato et al. 1990; Lee et al. 2007; Levi et al. 1999; Moradi et al. 2008; Nilsen et al. 2008; Vena et al. 1985; Zhang et al. 2006). Nine studies found no association in either subsite (Arbman et al. 1993; Calton et al. 2006; Fredriksson et al. 1989; Howard et al. 2008; Larsson et al. 2006; Mai et al. 2007; Marcus et al. 1994; Severson et al. 1989; Thune and Lund 1996). The analysis of cohort study data published between 1997 and 2005 by WCRF/AICR reported similar effect estimates for the association of total physical activity and both proximal (RR = 0.77, 95% CI 0.52–1.15) and distal (RR = 0.72, 95%CI 0.50–1.05) tumors (World Cancer Research Fund/American Institute for Cancer Research 2007). However, in their meta-analysis, Wolin et al. found the association was stronger for distal (RR = 0.54, 95% CI 0.34–0.84) than proximal (RR = 0.97, 95% CI 0.68–1.38) tumors (Wolin et al. 2007). This difference could have implications for future studies as screening rates increase since colonoscopy is more likely to remove distal adenomas, resulting in attenuation of the association between physical activity and colon cancer in future studies. It is worth noting, however, that several studies reported stronger associations in the proximal colon (Chao et al. 2004; Le Marchand et al. 1997; Thune and Lund 1996) and other found no differences by subsite; (White et al. 1996).

As previously noted, there is strong biologic rationale for examining colon and rectal tumors separately (Wei et al. 2004). However, several epidemiologic investigations have combined these tumors in the analyses. Despite the lack of association between physical activity and rectal cancer (detailed below), a substantial literature reports a significant association between physical activity and colorectal cancer, likely driven by the higher prevalence of colon than rectal tumors. A meta-analysis of cohort studies reported effects of physical activity on colorectal cancer risk that were similar to those in studies of only colon cancer (World Cancer Research Fund / American Institute for Cancer Research 2007). However, a recent systematic review found there was insufficient evidence to support a *convincing* relation between physical activity and risk of colorectal cancer (Spence et al. 2009). While many studies reported a statistically significant inverse association between physical activity and colorectal cancer risk (Ballard-Barbash et al. 1990; Benito et al. 1990; Boutron-Ruault et al. 2001; Huang et al. 2004; Le Marchand et al. 1997; Longnecker et al. 1995; Lund Nilsen and Vatten 2002; Markowitz et al. 1992; Nilsen and Vatten 2001; Russo et al. 1998; Steindorf et al. 2005; Wohlleb et al. 1990; Wu et al. 1987), several reported no association (Albanes et al. 1989; Jarebinski et al. 1988; Kune et al. 1990; Peters et al. 1989). Interestingly, several of the studies that found a statistically significant association observed it only among men (Ballard-Barbash et al. 1990; Le Marchand et al. 1997; Lund Nilsen and Vatten 2002; Nilsen and Vatten 2001; Wu et al. 1987). Together, these data may explain why earlier reviews of colorectal cancer suggested that the association was limited to men (McTiernan et al. 2006), in contrast with more recent reports of colon cancer that demonstrate a benefit for both genders (Wolin et al. 2009). As with analyses of colon cancer alone, studies of colorectal cancer note associations for both occupational and recreational activity (Samad et al. 2005), though the association may be stronger for occupational activity (World Cancer Research Fund/American Institute for Cancer Research 2007).

4.3.6 Colonic Adenomas

We identified 23 studies of the association between physical activity and colon adenomas, 11 case-control studies (Boutron-Ruault et al. 2001; Chiu and Gapstur 2004; Hauret et al. 2004; Kono et al. 1999; Kono et al. 1991; Little et al. 1993; Lubin et al. 1997; Sandler et al. 1995; Terry et al. 2002; Tiemersma et al. 2003; Wallace et al. 2005), eight cohort studies (Colbert et al. 2002; Enger et al. 1997; Giovannucci et al. 1995; Giovannucci et al. 1996; Hermann et al. 2009; Kahn et al. 1998; Neugut et al. 1996; Rosenberg et al. 2006), and four cross-sectional studies (Larsen et al. 2006; Lieberman et al. 2003; Shinchi et al. 1994; Stemmermann et al. 1988). Observational data from the eight cohort studies have suggested a protective effect of physical activity on colon polyps; four studies found a statistically significant inverse association (Giovannucci et al. 1996; Kahn et al. 1998; Neugut et al. 1996; Rosenberg et al. 2006), and two reported a dose-response effect (Giovannucci et al. 1996; Neugut et al. 1996). Giovannucci et al. found physical activity was statistically nonsignificantly associated with large (>1 cm) (RR = 0.63, 95% CI 0.36–1.10), but not small adenomas in a sample of US male health professionals (Giovannucci et al. 1995). In a cohort of US female nurses, Giovannucci et al. reported a significant overall risk reduction (RR = 0.58, 95% CI 0.40–0.86) that was also stronger for larger than smaller adenomas (Giovannucci et al. 1996). A large US cohort found physical activity decreased risk of polyp occurrence in men and women (RR_{men} = 0.83, 95% CI 0.76, 0.91; RR_{women} = 0.90, 95% CI 0.78, 1.03) (Kahn et al. 1998). In contrast, Rosenberg et al. noted a nearly 30% risk reduction in Black women who had the highest level of physical activity (vigorous plus walking) as compared to the least active women (Rosenberg et al. 2006). In a cohort of men and women in Los Angeles,

Enger et al. found a marginally statistically non-significant association between vigorous recent physical activity and prevalence of adenomas (RR = 0.7, 95% CI 0.4–1.1), but past recreational physical activity was not associated with adenoma prevalence, nor was recent or past total physical activity (Enger et al. 1997). Neugut and colleagues found recreational activity was not associated with adenoma, but occupational activity was associated with a large risk reduction (RR = 0.2, 95% CI 0.0–0.9) in men, but not women (Neugut et al. 1996).

Case-control studies were more likely than cohort studies to find a statistically significant association between physical activity and colonic polyps with six (Hauret et al. 2004; Kono et al. 1991; Little et al. 1993; Lubin et al. 1997; Terry et al. 2002; Wallace et al. 2005) of the 11 case- control studies (Boutron-Ruault et al. 2001; Chiu and Gapstur 2004; Sandler et al. 1995; Tiemersma et al. 2003;Kono et al. 1999) reporting a significant inverse association in at least one subgroup of their study population. There was a tendency for the effect of physical activity to be isolated to advanced adenomas and not low grade ones. In a US case-control study, Wallace and colleagues reported a statistically significant risk reduction among men (RR = 0.35, 95% CI 0.17–0.72) but not women (RR = 1.21, 95% CI 0.36–4.03) for advanced polyps, and no association for hyperplastic or tubular adenomas (Wallace et al. 2005). Similarly, Terry et al. in a pooled analysis of case-control studies found the association existed only for advanced adenomas in men (RR = 0.4, 95% CI 0.2–1.0) (Terry et al. 2002). Hauret et al. found the inverse association between physical activity and adenoma was present only among those not taking NSAIDs (RR = 0.49, 95% CI 0.25–0.94) (Hauret et al. 2004).

Not all studies found an effect of physical activity on risk of colonic adenomas. Hermann et al. found no association of total physical activity with adenomas in a European cohort (Hermann et al. 2009). Polyp recurrence as assessed in the Polyp Prevention Trial was not associated with recent physical activity (Colbert et al. 2002). In contrast, two recent studies of prevalent adenomas found physical activity was significantly associated with advanced adenomas (Larsen et al. 2006; Lieberman et al. 2003). Combined, the data indicate that physical activity likely reduces risk of adenomatous polyps.

4.4 Rectal Cancer

In contrast with the evidence for colorectal cancer, and colon cancer in particular, there has been little evidence for an association of rectal cancer with physical activity. Research studies have consistently reported no association between physical activity and rectal cancer, and the consensus is that one is unlikely to exist (International Agency for Research on Cancer 2002). Far fewer studies (31 in total) have examined rectal cancer separately from colon cancer, with the majority reporting no relation. A meta-analysis of 18 studies found no association between physical activity and rectal cancer (Samad et al. 2005). The summary relative risk for cohort studies was similar in men (RR = 1.01, 95% CI 0.78–1.30) and women (RR = 1.00, 95% CI 0.54–1.88). The summary relative risk in case-control studies was lower, but still null. Similarly, a 2007 WCRF/AICR meta-analysis reported no association between total physical activity and rectal cancer (RR = 0.97, 95% CI 0.68–1.40) (World Cancer Research Fund/American Institute for Cancer Research 2007) and a systematic review noted that none of the studies included reported a statistically significant association (Spence et al. 2009). Since the 2005 meta-analysis by Samad et al., which included publications through 2001, we identified 13

4

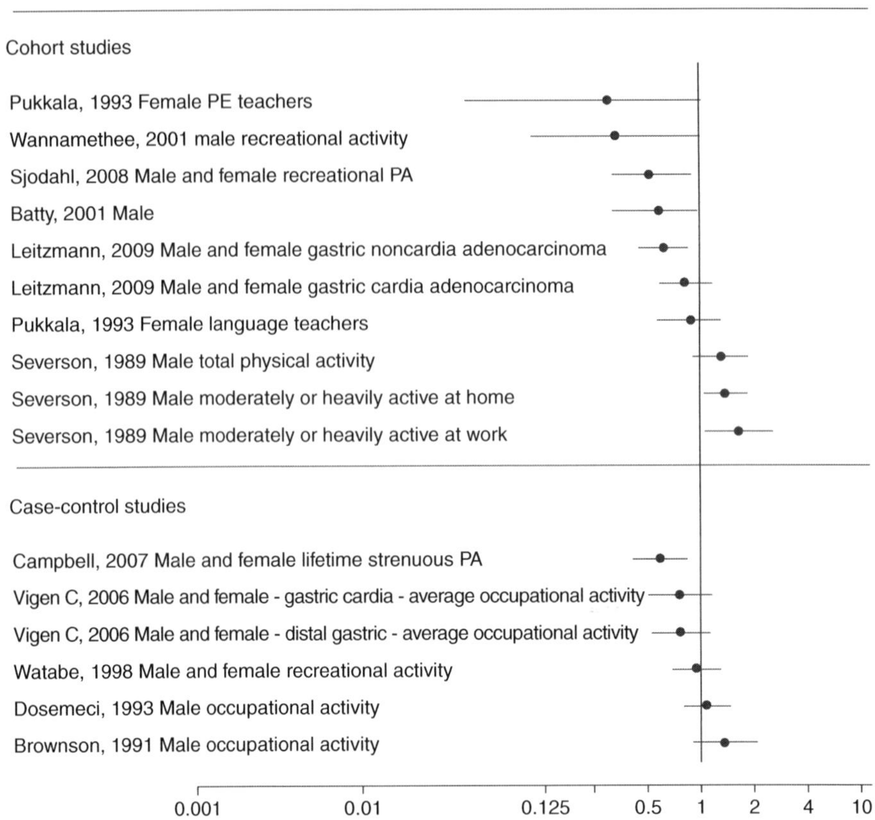

Fig. 4.3 Epidemiologic studies of physical activity and rectal cancer

additional publications (four case-control (Mao et al. 2003; Slattery et al. 2003a, b; Steindorf et al. 2005) and nine cohort studies (Chao et al. 2004; Friedenreich et al. 2006; Howard et al. 2008; Larsson et al. 2006; Lee et al. 2007; Moradi et al. 2008; Nilsen et al. 2008; Schnohr et al. 2005; Wei et al. 2004) that reported on associations between physical activity and rectal cancer. Consistent with previous reviews, these studies almost universally reported no association with rectal cancer. The one exception was a study that examined long term participation in vigorous physical activity in men and women and reported statistically significant risk reductions (Slattery et al. 2003a). The null associations in the other studies were consistent across all types and doses of physical activity (Fig. 4.3).

4.5 Gastric Cancer

Research on the association of physical activity and gastric cancer is extremely limited; we identified only 16 studies that had examined this association to date (Batty et al. 2001; Boccia et al. 2005; Brownson et al. 1991; Campbell et al. 2007; Dosemeci et al. 1993; Leitzmann et al. 2009; Nomura et al. 1995; Pukkala et al. 1993; Severson et al. 1989; Sjodahl et al. 2008; Stukonis and Doll 1969; Vigen et al. 2006; Wannamethee et al. 2001; Watabe et al. 1998; Whittemore et al. 1985; Zhang et al. 1996). The WCRF/AICR concluded that there was currently insufficient evidence to evaluate the association (World Cancer Research Fund/American Institute for Cancer Research 2007). The first cohort study to examine the relation was in men in England and Wales in the 1940s and 1950s (Stukonis and Doll 1969). This study reported that occupational activity was associated with gastric cancer mortality. More recent evidence regarding the association between physical activity and gastric cancer incidence has been inconsistent. Of the 16 studies, only four (Boccia et al. 2005; Campbell et al. 2007; Leitzmann et al. 2009; Sjodahl et al. 2008) reported a statistically significant decrease in gastric cancer risk and one study (Severson et al. 1989) observed a statistically significant increased risk associated with higher levels of physical activity, suggesting that physical activity is likely not related to risk of gastric cancer. However, all four studies that reported statistically significant inverse risks used more detailed physical activity measures of all types of activity including recreational (Sjodahl et al. 2008), occupational (Severson et al. 1989), total physical activity (Leitzmann et al. 2009), and also lifetime activity (Campbell et al. 2007). In a Canadian case-control study, frequent strenuous lifetime physical activity decreased risk of stomach cancer (RR = 0.58; 95% CI: 0.40–0.84) (Campbell et al. 2007). A prospective cohort study of men and women in Norway found a 40–50% decrease in risk of gastric cancer in people who had at least a moderate level of recreational physical activity when compared to people with no physical activity (RR = 0.5; 95% CI, 0.3–0.9) with evidence of a dose–response relation (*P* for trend = 0.01) (Sjodahl et al. 2008). A US cohort study found a significant risk reduction with higher physical activity only for gastric noncardia adenocarcinoma (RR = 0.62, 95% CI 0.44–0.87) (Leitzmann et al. 2009). Boccia found a significant association (*p* = 0.01) between physical activity and gastric cancer (Boccia et al. 2005). In addition, Wannamethee found physical activity of moderate or vigorous intensity was marginally associated with a reduced risk of stomach cancer (RR = 0.32, 95% CI 0.10–1.01) in a cohort study of British men (Wannamethee et al. 2001) (Fig. 4.4).

4.5.1 Type of Physical Activity

Most studies did not assess specific types of activity and instead used a global or total physical activity index. Among those that examined the effect of type of physical activity, most found no association for occupational physical activity. Occupational activity has not been found to be significantly associated with stomach cancer risk in four (Brownson et al. 1991; Dosemeci et al. 1993; Stukonis and Doll 1969; Vigen et al. 2006) of the six (Brownson et al. 1991; Dosemeci et al. 1993; Pukkala et al. 1993; Severson et al. 1989; Stukonis and Doll 1969; Vigen et al. 2006) studies that examined occupational activity. However, in a cohort of Finnish female teachers no difference was found in the standardized incidence rates of stomach cancer for physical education teachers versus language teachers (Pukkala et al. 1993). A Japanese cohort study found no association of total physical activity with stomach cancer (RR = 1.34, 95%CI 0.92–1.95), but noted statistically significant increased risk among those moderately or heavily active at home (RR = 1.45, 95% CI 1.07–1.97) or work (RR = 1.74, 95% CI 1.08–2.81) as compared to those who engaged mostly in sedentary activities (Severson et al. 1989). Recreational activity was similarly not associated with stomach cancer in a

4

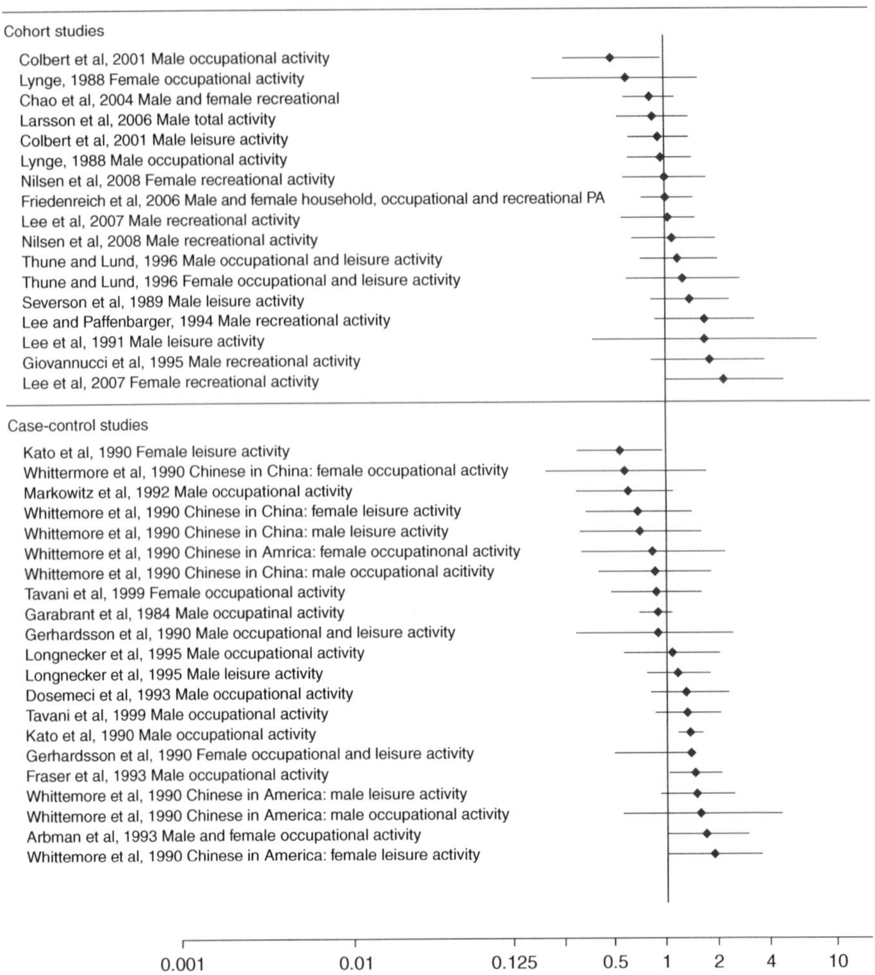

Fig. 4.4 Epidemiologic studies of physical activity and gastric cancer

case-control study (Watabe et al. 1998) or a study of endoscopy/gastroscopy patients who participated in active sports and exercise more than once a week (Zhang et al. 1996). Cohort studies that used general definitions of physical activity tended not to find any association between physical activity and gastric cancer risk (Nomura et al. 1995; Whittemore et al. 1985) or gastric cancer mortality (Batty et al. 2001).

4.5.2 Dose of Physical Activity

Despite the limited number of studies that have reported a beneficial effect of physical activity on gastric cancer risk, there is some evidence for a dose-response effect in those studies that did observe an inverse association (Campbell et al. 2007; Leitzmann et al. 2009; Sjodahl et al. 2008; Wannamethee et al. 2001).

4.5.3 Gastric Subsite

Few studies of gastric cancer and physical activity have examined the data separately by anatomic subsite or tumor histology. Epidemiologic evidence has suggested that risk factors may differ for proximal and distal gastric cancers. A US-based case-control study found no association of occupational physical activity and gastric cardia or distal cardia cancers (Vigen et al. 2006). The one cohort study to examine this association comprehensively observed a statistically significant inverse association for gastric noncardia adenocarcinoma (RR = 0.62; 95% CI = 0.44, 0.87) that persisted after adjustment for BMI (RR = 0.62; 95% CI = 0.44, 0.87) (Leitzmann et al. 2009). In contrast, the association for gastric cardia adenocarcinoma became statistically nonsignificant when the multivariate model included BMI (RR = 0.83; 95% CI = 0.58, 1.19). There was no statistically significant association found for squamous cell carcinoma. In their case-control study, Campbell et al. reported associations that were similar between the two subsites, though the number of cardia cases was less than one half of the noncardia cases (Campbell et al. 2007).

4.6 Biologic Mechanisms

The association between physical activity and colon cancer is plausibly supported by several biologic mechanisms (see Fig. 4.5), including decreased inflammation, reduced intestinal transit time, decreased insulin-like growth factor (IGF) levels, reduced hyperinsulinemia, modulated immune function (Harriss et al. 2007; Rogers et al. 2008), and increased vitamin D levels (Gorham et al. 2005). While some of the association between physical activity and colon cancer may be mediated through energy balance and obesity, since these mechanisms are also associated with colon cancer (International Agency for Research on Cancer 2002; Wolin and Colditz 2008; World Cancer Research Fund/American Institute for Cancer Research 2007), physical activity has an association with colon cancer that is independent of obesity, since studies that control for body composition continue to observe a statistically significant association between physical activity and colon cancer.

Insulin and insulin-like growth factors (IGF) are believed to play a key role in colon cell proliferation and apoptosis (Giovannucci 1995;

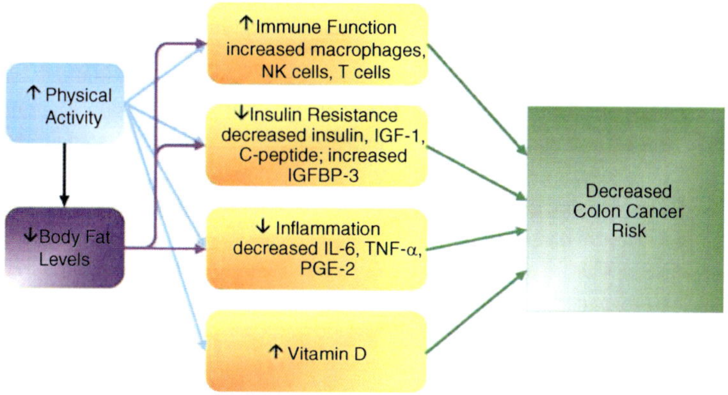

Fig. 4.5 Hypothesized biologic mechanisms involved in the association between physical activity and colon cancer risk

Kim 1998; McKeown-Eyssen 1994). Consequently, the role of insulin in carcinogenesis has received considerable research attention. Several lines of evidence have supported the hypothesis that hyperinsulinemia promotes the growth of colon tumors. Colon tissue has insulin receptors (MacDonald et al. 1993) and insulin stimulates the growth of both normal and colon cancer cells in vitro (Calle and Kaaks 2004; Koenuma et al. 1989; Watkins et al. 1990). Animal studies also support a role for insulin (Tran et al. 1996). The association seen between type II diabetes, which often results in hyperinsulinemia because of insulin resistance, and colon cancer provides additional support for the role of hyperinsulinemia in colon carcinogenesis (Hu et al. 1999; La Vecchia et al. 1991; Le Marchand et al. 1997; Will et al. 1998). Observational studies have found associations between insulin and both risk of colon cancer (Limburg et al. 2006; Schoen et al. 1999) and risk of colon polyps (Keku et al. 2005; Schoen et al. 2005; Yoshida et al. 2006). Individuals in the highest quartile for insulin had a twofold increased risk for colon cancer compared to those in the lowest quartile (Schoen et al. 1999). C-peptide is an insulin production by-product created when proinsulin is cleaved into insulin and C-peptide. C-peptide is more stable and, therefore, a better marker of insulin secretion; levels reflect how much insulin the body is producing. Recent research (Kaaks et al. 2000; Ma et al. 2004; Otani et al. 2007; Wei et al. 2005) has found a positive association between C-peptide levels and risk of colon cancer as well as risk of colorectal adenoma (Wei et al. 2006), further supporting the hypothesis that hyperinsulinemia may play an important role in colon carcinogenesis.

Physical activity may act on this pathway as it increases insulin sensitivity, (Aldred et al. 1995; Hasson et al. 2006; Holt et al. 2007; Houmard et al. 2004; Koivisto et al. 1986; Moore et al. 1998; O'Donovan et al. 2005; Weiss and Holloszy 2007; Weiss et al. 2006) with the effects of a single exercise bout potentially lasting for several days, (Burstein et al. 1985; Schneider et al. 1984) resulting in decreased plasma insulin levels (Campbell and McTiernan 2007; Dowse et al. 1991; Fontana et al. 2006; Frank et al. 2005; Lindgarde and Saltin 1981; O'Donovan et al. 2005; Pischon et al. 2003; Regensteiner et al. 1991; Schmitz et al. 2002; Wang et al. 1989). Physical activity is also inversely associated with C-peptide levels (Allen et al. 2003; Fung et al. 2000; Giovannucci et al. 2004; Ma et al. 2004; Major et al. 2005; Regensteiner et al. 1991; Voskuil et al. 2001).

High levels of IGF-1 have also been associated with colorectal cancer as have low levels of insulin-like growth factor binding protein (IGFBP-3) (Giovannucci et al. 2000; Kaaks et al. 2000; Ma et al. 1999). The effects of IGF-1 on colorectal cancer risk are more pronounced after adjusting for IGFBP-3 levels (Giovannucci et al. 2000). Exercise bouts result in acute and transient increases in IGF-1(Kaaks and Lukanova 2001), and exercise training results in increased IGF-1 and IGFBP-3(Koziris et al. 1999).While physical activity may be associated with lower levels of IGF-1 and higher levels of IGFBP-3 (Kaaks and Lukanova 2001), not all data support this and a systematic review was unable to show this association definitively (Orenstein and Friedenreich 2004). However, the effect of IGF-1 on tumors is supported by in vitro data (Singh and Rubin 1993).

Several lines of research have suggested a role for inflammation in colon carcinogenesis. Nonsteroidal anti-inflammatory drugs (NSAIDs) have shown promise as chemopreventive agents, but concerns exist regarding the side effects associated with long term use (O'Dwyer et al. 2007). COX-2 specific inhibitors have shown protection against colon polyps, but have been found to have adverse cardiovascular effects (Baron et al. 2003; O'Dwyer et al. 2007; Sandler et al. 2003). The mechanism behind the protective effect of NSAID use is hypothesized to be in part due to the inhibition of COX-derived prostaglandin E2 (PGE-2), which promotes tumor carcinogenesis (Friedenreich and Orenstein 2002). PGE-2 is the most abundant prostaglandin in colorectal cancer (Rigas et al. 1993) and promotes tumor progression by stimulating cell proliferation and angiogenesis, inhibiting apoptosis, and modulating immunosuppression (Rhodes and Campbell 2002). Research has also demonstrated a key role for interleukin-6 (IL-6) in the inflammation–colon cancer relationship. IL-6 is a proinflammatory cytokine secreted by T-cells and macrophages. IL-6 promotes the transition from acute to chronic inflammation (Rose-John et al. 2006). Emerging research indicates a predominant role for the IL-6 pathway in bowel inflammation (Atreya and Neurath 2005). Men and women demonstrating IL-6 associated genetic polymorphisms have shown an increased risk of colon cancer (Landi et al. 2003). The polymorphisms are associated with alterations in transcription which change the overall level of IL-6 released. An observational case-series has provided preliminary support for this model, demonstrating a positive association between serum IL-6 levels and colon cancer tumor size and stage (Chung and Chang 2003). IL-6 levels were also correlated with larger tumor size, and metastasis and levels increased in a stage-related manner. Finally, there is some indication that IL-6 may be positively related to insulin resistance in cancer patients (Makino et al. 1998).

Observational studies have found inverse relations between physical activity and inflammatory markers, independent of body composition (Abramson and Vaccarino 2002; Ford 2002; Geffken et al. 2001; Hamer 2007; King et al. 2003), though the exact mechanism is unclear (Robinson and Graham 2004; Shephard 2002). In cross-sectional analyses of several populations, physical activity was inversely associated with IL-6 (Colbert et al. 2004; Elosua et al. 2005; Pischon et al. 2003; Taaffe et al. 2000). In addition, a review of exercise intervention trial data indicated decreases in inflammatory marker levels with physical activity (Woods et al. 2009). A significant decrease in IL-6 was found following a 12-week aerobic training intervention in 24 men (Dekker et al. 2007) and a separate 10-week intervention in 20 men and women (Starkweather 2007). In a 10-month study of older adults, Kohut and colleagues found that thrice weekly aerobic training, but not thrice weekly flexibility training, reduced IL-6 levels (Kohut et al. 2006). Finally, a 6-month intervention in women found significant decreases in inflammatory markers (CRP, IL-6) in the arm prescribed reduced calorie diet and exercise, but not in the diet only arm (You et al. 2004). Physical activity appears to inhibit PGE2 synthesis (Bennett et al. 1977; Tutton and Barkla 1980) and is inversely associated with rectal mucosal levels of PGE2 (Martinez et al. 1999). However, a 12-month randomized controlled trial of middle-aged men and women found no effect of moderate to vigorous aerobic exercise on colon mucosal PGE-2 concentration (Abrahamson et al. 2007).

There are limited data to support a role for immune function as a pathway linking physical activity and colon cancer. Macrophages mediate the immune response and are recruited through the inflammatory response. Some macrophages can be proinflammatory and may accelerate tumor growth (Goerdt et al. 1999). Physical activity may boost immune response – specifically by increasing natural killer cell and modulating macrophage activity (Nieman and Henson 1994; Pedersen et al. 1988). Exercise may decrease expression of chemokines that attract macrophages (Troseid et al. 2004). Exercise also enhances lymphocyte proliferation and increases lymphokine-activated killer cell levels (Harriss et al. 2007).

More active individuals are also likely to have more opportunity for sun exposure and, therefore, higher vitamin D levels (Scragg and Camargo 2008; Zittermann et al. 2000), which may also be associated with a reduced risk of

4

colon polyps (Platz et al. 2000), colon cancer (Martinez et al. 1996; Martinez and Willett 1998) and colon cancer mortality (Giovannucci et al. 2006). In fact a meta-analysis found a significant decrease in incidence of colon cancer with increasing vitamin D levels (Gorham et al. 2005). Vitamin D may modulate cell growth and reduce angiogenesis by modulating signaling cascades (Deeb et al. 2007). Treating colon cancers with vitamin D induces cell differentiation (Chen et al. 1999; Palmer et al. 2001). Vitamin D may induce apoptosis by repressing anti-apoptotic proteins or inducing proapoptotic proteins (Deeb et al. 2007).

4.7 Conclusion

While accumulated evidence has not included randomized controlled trials of exercise and cancer incidence, the strength and consistency of the data from observational epidemiologic studies, combined with plausible mechanistic data, provides sufficient evidence to conclude that physical activity decreases risk of colon cancer. The majority of the observational studies to date demonstrated a statistically significant risk reduction of approximately 25%, with evidence of a dose-response relation. To date, there is no suggestion that one type of physical activity provides greater benefit than another. There is evidence that physical activity may be more strongly associated with distal than proximal tumors. Future research will likely continue to elucidate differences by tumor site and the type, dose, and timing of physical activity needed to obtain and maximize risk reduction. Understanding the mechanistic pathways may also facilitate answering these questions and point to the importance of transdisciplinary research in cancer prevention. In contrast, there is little evidence for an association between physical activity and rectal or gastric cancers. Cancer prevention efforts on these cancers may best be directed at other, more established, risk factors. Progress in this field will be possible with on-going advances in physical activity measurement, additional studies focusing on the underlying biologic mechanisms, studies on colonic adenomas, and exercise intervention trials. Finally, improved understanding of strategies to sustain the types of physical activity that reduce risk throughout the appropriate time of life remains an important public health priority.

References

Abrahamson PE, King IB, Ulrich CM, Rudolph RE, Irwin ML, Yasui Y et al (2007) No effect of exercise on colon mucosal prostaglandin concentrations: a 12-month randomized controlled trial. Cancer Epidemiol Biomark Prev 16(11): 2351–2356

Abramson JL, Vaccarino V (2002) Relationship between physical activity and inflammation among apparently healthy middle-aged and older US adults. Arch Intern Med 162(11): 1286–1292

Albanes D, Blair A, Taylor PR (1989) Physical activity and risk of cancer in the NHANES I population. Am J Public Health 79(6):744–750

Aldred HE, Hardman AE, Taylor S (1995) Influence of 12 weeks of training by brisk walking on post-prandial lipemia and insulinemia in sedentary middle-aged women. Metabolism 44(3): 390–397

Allen NE, Appleby PN, Kaaks R, Rinaldi S, Davey GK, Key TJ (2003) Lifestyle determinants of serum insulin-like growth-factor-I (IGF-I), C-peptide and hormone binding protein levels in British women. Cancer Causes Control 14(1): 65–74

American Cancer Society (2007) Cancer facts and figures 2007. American Cancer Society, Atlanta, GA

Arbman G, Axelson O, Fredriksson M, Nilsson E, Sjodahl R (1993) Do occupational factors influence the risk of colon and rectal cancer in different ways? Cancer 72(9):2543–2549

Atreya R, Neurath MF (2005) Involvement of IL-6 in the pathogenesis of inflammatory bowel disease and colon cancer. Clin Rev Allergy Immunol 28(3):187–196

Ballard-Barbash R, Schatzkin A, Albanes D, Schiffman MH, Kreger BE, Kannel WB et al (1990) Physical activity and risk of large bowel cancer in the Framingham Study. Cancer Res 50(12):3610–3613

Baron JA, Cole BF, Sandler RS, Haile RW, Ahnen D, Bresalier R et al (2003) A randomized trial of aspirin to prevent colorectal adenomas. N Engl J Med 348(10):891–899

Batty GD, Shipley MJ, Marmot M, Smith GD (2001) Physical activity and cause-specific mortality in men: further evidence from the Whitehall study. Eur J Epidemiol 17(9):863–869

Benito E, Obrador A, Stiggelbout A, Bosch FX, Mulet M, Munoz N et al (1990) A population-based case-control study of colorectal cancer in Majorca I. Dietary factors. Int J Cancer 45(1): 69–76

Bennett A, Tacca MD, Stamford IF, Zebro T (1977) Prostaglandins from tumours of human large bowel. Br J Cancer 35(6):881–884

Boccia S, Persiani R, La Torre G, Rausei S, Arzani D, Gianfagna F et al (2005) Sulfotransferase 1A1 polymorphism and gastric cancer risk: a pilot case-control study. Cancer Lett 229(2): 235–243

Boutron-Ruault MC, Senesse P, Meance S, Belghiti C, Faivre J (2001) Energy intake, body mass index, physical activity, and the colorectal adenoma-carcinoma sequence. Nutr Cancer 39(1): 50–57

Brownson RC, Chang JC, Davis JR, Smith CA (1991) Physical activity on the job and cancer in Missouri. Am J Public Health 81(5):639–642

Brownson RC, Eyler AA, King AC, Brown DR, Shyu YL, Sallis JF (2000) Patterns and correlates of physical activity among US women 40 years and older. Am J Public Health 90(2): 264–270

Brownson RC, Zahm SH, Chang JC, Blair A (1989) Occupational risk of colon cancer. An analysis by anatomic subsite. Am J Epidemiol 130(4): 675–687

Bull FC, Armstrong TP, Dixon T, Ham S, Neiman A, Pratt M (2004) Physical inactivity. In: Ezzati M, Lopez AD, Rodgers A, Murray CJL (eds) Comparative quantification of health risks: global and regional burden of disease attributable to select major risk factors, vol 1. World Health Organization, Geneva

Burstein R, Polychronakos C, Toews CJ, MacDougall JD, Guyda HJ, Posner BI (1985) Acute reversal of the enhanced insulin action in trained athletes. Association with insulin receptor changes. Diabetes 34(8):756–760

Calle EE, Kaaks R (2004) Overweight, obesity and cancer: epidemiological evidence and proposed mechanisms. Nat Rev Cancer 4(8):579–591

Calton BA, Lacey JV Jr, Schatzkin A, Schairer C, Colbert LH, Albanes D et al (2006) Physical activity and the risk of colon cancer among women: a prospective cohort study (United States). Int J Cancer 119(2):385–391

Campbell KL, McTiernan A (2007) Exercise and biomarkers for cancer prevention studies. J Nutr 137(1 Suppl):161S–169S

Campbell PT, Sloan M, Kreiger N (2007) Physical activity and stomach cancer risk: the influence of intensity and timing during the lifetime. Eur J Cancer 43(3):593–600

Chao A, Connell CJ, Jacobs EJ, McCullough ML, Patel AV, Calle EE et al (2004) Amount, type, and timing of recreational physical activity in relation to colon and rectal cancer in older adults: the Cancer Prevention Study II Nutrition Cohort. Cancer Epidemiol Biomark Prev 13(12): 2187–2195

Chen A, Davis BH, Bissonnette M, Scaglione-Sewell B, Brasitus TA (1999) 1, 25-Dihydroxyvitamin D(3) stimulates activator protein-1-dependent Caco-2 cell differentiation. J Biol Chem 274(50): 35505–35513

Chiu BC, Gapstur SM (2004) Changes in diet during adult life and risk of colorectal adenomas. Nutr Cancer 49(1):49–58

Chung YC, Chang YF (2003) Serum interleukin-6 levels reflect the disease status of colorectal cancer. J Surg Oncol 83(4):222–226

Colbert LH, Hartman TJ, Malila N, Limburg PJ, Pietinen P, Virtamo J et al (2001) Physical activity in relation to cancer of the colon and rectum in a cohort of male smokers. Cancer Epidemiol Biomark Prev 10(3):265–268

Colbert LH, Lanza E, Ballard-Barbash R, Slattery ML, Tangrea JA, Caan B et al (2002) Adenomatous polyp recurrence and physical activity in the Polyp Prevention Trial (United States). Cancer Causes Control 13(5): 445–453

Colbert LH, Visser M, Simonsick EM, Tracy RP, Newman AB, Kritchevsky SB et al (2004) Physical activity, exercise, and inflammatory markers in older adults: findings from the health, aging and body composition study. J Am Geriatr Soc 52(7):1098–1104

4

Crespo CJ, Keteyian SJ, Heath GW, Sempos CT (1996) Leisure-time physical activity among US adults. Results from the Third National Health and Nutrition Examination Survey. Arch Intern Med 156(1):93–98

Cronin KA, Krebs-Smith SM, Feuer EJ, Troiano RP, Ballard-Barbash R (2001) Evaluating the impact of population changes in diet, physical activity, and weight status on population risk for colon cancer (United States). Cancer Causes Control 12(4):305–316

Danaei G, Vander Hoorn S, Lopez AD, Murray CJL, Ezzati M (2005) Causes of cancer in the world: comparative risk assessment of nine behavioural and environmental risk factors. Lancet 366(9499):1784–1793

Deeb KK, Trump DL, Johnson CS (2007) Vitamin D signalling pathways in cancer: potential for anticancer therapeutics. Nat Rev Cancer 7(9): 684–700

Dekker MJ, Lee S, Hudson R, Kilpatrick K, Graham TE, Ross R et al (2007) An exercise intervention without weight loss decreases circulating interleukin-6 in lean and obese men with and without type 2 diabetes mellitus. Metabolism 56(3): 332–338

Dosemeci M, Hayes RB, Vetter R, Hoover RN, Tucker M, Engin K et al (1993) Occupational physical activity, socioeconomic status, and risks of 15 cancer sites in Turkey. Cancer Causes Control 4(4):313–321

Dowse GK, Zimmet PZ, King H (1991) Relationship between prevalence of impaired glucose tolerance and NIDDM in a population. Diab Care 14(11):968–974

Elosua R, Bartali B, Ordovas JM, Corsi AM, Lauretani F, Ferrucci L (2005) Association between physical activity, physical performance, and inflammatory biomarkers in an elderly population: the InCHIANTI study. J Gerontol A Biol Sci Med Sci 60(6):760–767

Enger SM, Longnecker MP, Lee ER, Frankl HD, Haile RW (1997) Recent and past physical activity and prevalence of colorectal adenomas. Br J Cancer 75(5):740–745

Fernandez E, Gallus S, La Vecchia C, Talamini R, Negri E, Franceschi S (2004) Family history and environmental risk factors for colon cancer. Cancer Epidemiol Biomark Prev 13(4): 658–661

Fontana L, Klein S, Holloszy JO (2006) Long-term low-protein, low-calorie diet and endurance exercise modulate metabolic factors associated with cancer risk. Am J Clin Nutr 84(6): 1456–1462

Ford ES (2002) Does exercise reduce inflammation? Physical activity and C-reactive protein among U.S. adults. Epidemiology 13(5): 561–568

Frank LL, Sorensen BE, Yasui Y, Tworoger SS, Schwartz RS, Ulrich CM et al (2005) Effects of exercise on metabolic risk variables in overweight postmenopausal women: a randomized clinical trial. Obes Res 13(3):615–625

Fraser G, Pearce N (1993) Occupational physical activity and risk of cancer of the colon and rectum in New Zealand males. Cancer Causes Control 4(1):45–50

Fredriksson M, Bengtsson NO, Hardell L, Axelson O (1989) Colon cancer, physical activity, and occupational exposures. A case-control study. Cancer 63(9):1838–1842

Friedenreich C, Norat T, Steindorf K, Boutron-Ruault MC, Pischon T, Mazuir M et al (2006) Physical activity and risk of colon and rectal cancers: the European prospective investigation into cancer and nutrition. Cancer Epidemiol Biomark Prev 15(12):2398–2407

Friedenreich CM, Orenstein MR (2002) Physical activity and cancer prevention: etiologic evidence and biological mechanisms. J Nutr 132(11 Suppl):3456S–3464S

Fung TT, Hu FB, Yu J, Chu NF, Spiegelman D, Tofler GH et al (2000) Leisure-time physical activity, television watching, and plasma biomarkers of obesity and cardiovascular disease risk. Am J Epidemiol 152(12): 1171–1178

Garabrant DH, Peters JM, Mack TM, Bernstein L (1984) Job activity and colon cancer risk. Am J Epidemiol 119(6):1005–1014

Geffken DF, Cushman M, Burke GL, Polak JF, Sakkinen PA, Tracy RP (2001) Association between physical activity and markers of inflammation in a healthy elderly population. Am J Epidemiol 153(3):242–250

Gerhardsson de Verdier M, Steineck G, Hagman U, Rieger A, Norell SE (1990) Physical activity and colon cancer: a case-referent study in Stockholm. Int J Cancer 46(6):985–989

Gerhardsson M, Floderus B, Norell SE (1988) Physical activity and colon cancer risk. Int J Epidemiol 17(4):743–746

Gerhardsson M, Norell SE, Kiviranta H, Pedersen NL, Ahlbom A (1986) Sedentary jobs and colon cancer. Am J Epidemiol 123(5):775–780

Giovannucci E (1995) Insulin and colon cancer. Cancer Causes Control 6(2):164–179

Giovannucci E, Ascherio A, Rimm EB, Colditz GA, Stampfer MJ, Willett WC (1995) Physical activity, obesity, and risk for colon cancer and adenoma in men. Ann Intern Med 122(5): 327–334

Giovannucci E, Colditz GA, Stampfer MJ, Willett WC (1996) Physical activity, obesity, and risk of colorectal adenoma in women (United States). Cancer Causes Control 7(2):253–263

Giovannucci E, Liu Y, Willett WC (2006) Cancer incidence and mortality and vitamin D in black and white male health professionals. Cancer Epidemiol Biomark Prev 15(12):2467–2472

Giovannucci E, Pollak MN, Platz EA, Willett WC, Stampfer MJ, Majeed N et al (2000) A prospective study of plasma insulin-like growth factor-1 and binding protein-3 and risk of colorectal neoplasia in women. Cancer Epidemiol Biomark Prev 9(4):345–349

Giovannucci E, Rimm EB, Liu Y, Willett WC (2004) Height, predictors of C-peptide and cancer risk in men. Int J Epidemiol 33(1):217–225

Goerdt S, Politz O, Schledzewski K, Birk R, Gratchev A, Guillot P et al (1999) Alternative versus classical activation of macrophages. Pathobiology 67(5–6):222–226

Gorham ED, Garland CF, Garland FC, Grant WB, Mohr SB, Lipkin M et al (2005) Vitamin D and prevention of colorectal cancer. J Steroid Biochem Mol Biol 97(1–2):179–194

Hamer M (2007) The relative influences of fitness and fatness on inflammatory factors. Prev Med 44(1):3–11

Harriss DJ, Cable NT, George K, Reilly T, Renehan AG, Haboubi N (2007) Physical activity before and after diagnosis of colorectal cancer: disease risk, clinical outcomes, response pathways and biomarkers. Sports Med 37(11):947–960

Hasson RE, Freedson PS, Braun B (2006) Post-exercise insulin action in African-American women. J Natl Med Assoc 98(11):1832–1839

Hauret KG, Bostick RM, Matthews CE, Hussey JR, Fina MF, Geisinger KR et al (2004) Physical activity and reduced risk of incident sporadic colorectal adenomas: observational support for mechanisms involving energy balance and inflammation modulation. Am J Epidemiol 159(10): 983–992

Hermann S, Rohrmann S, Linseisen J (2009) Lifestyle factors, obesity and the risk of colorectal adenomas in EPIC-Heidelberg. Cancer Causes Control 20(8):1397–1408

Holt HB, Wild SH, Wareham N, Ekelund U, Umpleby M, Shojaee-Moradie F et al (2007) Differential effects of fatness, fitness and physical activity energy expenditure on whole-body, liver and fat insulin sensitivity. Diabetologia 50(8):1698–1706

Hou L, Ji BT, Blair A, Dai Q, Gao YT, Chow WH (2004) Commuting physical activity and risk of colon cancer in Shanghai, China. Am J Epidemiol 160(9):860–867

Houmard JA, Tanner CJ, Slentz CA, Duscha BD, McCartney JS, Kraus WE (2004) Effect of the volume and intensity of exercise training on insulin sensitivity. J Appl Physiol 96(1): 101–106

Howard RA, Freedman DM, Park Y, Hollenbeck A, Schatzkin A, Leitzmann MF (2008) Physical activity, sedentary behavior, and the risk of colon and rectal cancer in the NIH-AARP Diet and Health Study. Cancer Causes Control 19(9): 939–953

Howe HL, Wingo PA, Thun MJ, Ries LA, Rosenberg HM, Feigal EG et al (2001) Annual report to the nation on the status of cancer (1973 through 1998), featuring cancers with recent increasing trends. J Natl Cancer Inst 93(11):824–842

Hu FB, Manson JE, Liu S, Hunter D, Colditz GA, Michels KB et al (1999) Prospective study of adult onset diabetes mellitus (type 2) and risk of colorectal cancer in women. J Natl Cancer Inst 91(6):542–547

Huang XE, Hirose K, Wakai K, Matsuo K, Ito H, Xiang J et al (2004) Comparison of lifestyle risk factors by family history for gastric, breast, lung and colorectal cancer. Asian Pac J Cancer Prev 5(4):419–427

Iacopetta B (2002) Are there two sides to colorectal cancer? Int J Cancer 101(5):403–408

International Agency for Research on Cancer, W. H. O (2002) IARC handbooks of cancer prevention: weight control and physical activity, vol 6. International Agency for Research on Cancer, Lyon, France

4

International Agency for Research on Cancer, W. H. O (2003) World Cancer Report. International Agency for Research on Cancer, Lyon, France

Isomura K, Kono S, Moore MA, Toyomura K, Nagano J, Mizoue T et al (2006) Physical activity and colorectal cancer: the Fukuoka Colorectal Cancer Study. Cancer Sci 97(10): 1099–1104

Jarebinski M, Vlajinac H, Adanja B (1988) Biosocial and other characteristics of the large bowel cancer patients in Belgrade (Yugloslavia). Arch Geschwulstforsch 58(6):411–417

Johnsen NF, Christensen J, Thomsen BL, Olsen A, Loft S, Overvad K et al (2006) Physical activity and risk of colon cancer in a cohort of Danish middle-aged men and women. Eur J Epidemiol 21(12):877–884

Juarranz M, Calle-Puron ME, Gonzalez-Navarro A, Regidor-Poyatos E, Soriano T, Martinez-Hernandez D et al (2002) Physical exercise, use of Plantago ovata and aspirin, and reduced risk of colon cancer. Eur J Cancer Prev 11(5): 465–472

Kaaks R, Lukanova A (2001) Energy balance and cancer: the role of insulin and insulin-like growth factor-I. Proc Nutr Soc 60(1):91–106

Kaaks R, Toniolo P, Akhmedkhanov A, Lukanova A, Biessy C, Dechaud H et al (2000) Serum C-peptide, insulin-like growth factor (IGF)-I, IGF-binding proteins, and colorectal cancer risk in women. J Natl Cancer Inst 92(19): 1592–1600

Kahn HS, Tatham LM, Thun MJ, Heath CW Jr (1998) Risk factors for self-reported colon polyps. J Gen Intern Med 13(5):303–310

Kato I, Tominaga S, Ikari A (1990) A case-control study of male colorectal cancer in Aichi Prefecture, Japan: with special reference to occupational activity level, drinking habits and family history. Jpn J Cancer Res 81(2):115–121

Keku TO, Lund PK, Galanko J, Simmons JG, Woosley JT, Sandler RS (2005) Insulin resistance, apoptosis, and colorectal adenoma risk. Cancer Epidemiol Biomark Prev 14(9): 2076–2081

Kim YI (1998) Diet, lifestyle, and colorectal cancer: is hyperinsulinemia the missing link? Nutr Rev 56(9):275–279

King DE, Carek P, Mainous AG 3rd, Pearson WS (2003) Inflammatory markers and exercise: differences related to exercise type. Med Sci Sports Exerc 35(4):575–581

Koenuma M, Yamori T, Tsuruo T (1989) Insulin and insulin-like growth factor 1 stimulate proliferation of metastatic variants of colon carcinoma 26. Jpn J Cancer Res 80(1):51–58

Kohut ML, McCann DA, Russell DW, Konopka DN, Cunnick JE, Franke WD et al (2006) Aerobic exercise, but not flexibility/resistance exercise, reduces serum IL-18, CRP, and IL-6 independent of beta-blockers, BMI, and psychosocial factors in older adults. Brain Behav Immun 20(3):201–209

Koivisto VA, Yki-Jarvinen H, DeFronzo RA (1986) Physical training and insulin sensitivity. Diab Metab Rev 1(4):445–481

Kono S, Handa K, Hayabuchi H, Kiyohara C, Inoue H, Marugame T et al (1999) Obesity, weight gain and risk of colon adenomas in Japanese men. Jpn J Cancer Res 90(8):805–811

Kono S, Shinchi K, Ikeda N, Yanai F, Imanishi K (1991) Physical activity, dietary habits and adenomatous polyps of the sigmoid colon: a study of self-defense officials in Japan. J Clin Epidemiol 44(11):1255–1261

Koziris LP, Hickson RC, Chatterton RT Jr, Groseth RT, Christie JM, Goldflies DG et al (1999) Serum levels of total and free IGF-I and IGFBP-3 are increased and maintained in long-term training. J Appl Physiol 86(4):1436–1442

Kune GA, Kune S, Watson LF (1990) Body weight and physical activity as predictors of colorectal cancer risk. Nutr Cancer 13(1–2):9–17

La Vecchia C, D'Avanzo B, Negri E, Franceschi S (1991) History of selected diseases and the risk of colorectal cancer. Eur J Cancer 27(5): 582–586

La Vecchia C, Gallus S, Talamini R, Decarli A, Negri E, Franceschi S (1999) Interaction between selected environmental factors and familial propensity for colon cancer. Eur J Cancer Prev 8(2): 147–150

Landi S, Moreno V, Gioia-Patricola L, Guino E, Navarro M, de Oca J et al (2003) Association of common polymorphisms in inflammatory genes interleukin (IL)6, IL8, tumor necrosis factor alpha, NFKB1, and peroxisome proliferator-activated receptor gamma with colorectal cancer. Cancer Res 63(13):3560–3566

Larsen IK, Grotmol T, Almendingen K, Hoff G (2006) Lifestyle as a predictor for colonic neoplasia in asymptomatic individuals. BMC Gastroenterol 6:5

Larsson SC, Rutegard J, Bergkvist L, Wolk A (2006) Physical activity, obesity, and risk of colon and rectal cancer in a cohort of Swedish men. Eur J Cancer 42(15):2590–2597

Le Marchand L, Wilkens LR, Kolonel LN, Hankin JH, Lyu LC (1997) Associations of sedentary lifestyle, obesity, smoking, alcohol use, and diabetes with the risk of colorectal cancer. Cancer Res 57(21):4787–4794

Lee IM, Manson JE, Ajani U, Paffenbarger RS Jr, Hennekens CH, Buring JE (1997) Physical activity and risk of colon cancer: the Physicians' Health Study (United States). Cancer Causes Control 8(4):568–574

Lee IM, Oguma Y (2006) Physical Activity. In: Schottenfeld D, Fraumeni JF Jr (eds) Cancer epidemiology and prevention, 3rd edn. Oxford University Press, New York, pp 449–467

Lee IM, Paffenbarger RS Jr, Hsieh C (1991) Physical activity and risk of developing colorectal cancer among college alumni. J Natl Cancer Inst 83(18):1324–1329

Lee KJ, Inoue M, Otani T, Iwasaki M, Sasazuki S, Tsugane S (2007) Physical activity and risk of colorectal cancer in Japanese men and women: the Japan Public Health Center-based prospective study. Cancer Causes Control 18(2): 199–209

Leitzmann MF, Koebnick C, Freedman ND, Park Y, Ballard-Barbash R, Hollenbeck A et al (2009) Physical activity and esophageal and gastric carcinoma in a large prospective study. Am J Prev Med 36(2):112–119

Levi F, Pasche C, La Vecchia C, Lucchini F, Franceschi S (1999) Food groups and colorectal cancer risk. Br J Cancer 79(7–8):1283–1287

Lieberman DA, Prindiville S, Weiss DG, Willett W (2003) Risk factors for advanced colonic neoplasia and hyperplastic polyps in asymptomatic individuals. JAMA 290(22):2959–2967

Limburg PJ, Stolzenberg-Solomon RZ, Vierkant RA, Roberts K, Sellers TA, Taylor PR et al (2006) Insulin, glucose, insulin resistance, and incident colorectal cancer in male smokers. Clin Gastroenterol Hepatol 4(12):1514–1521

Lindgarde F, Saltin B (1981) Daily physical activity, work capacity and glucose tolerance in lean and obese normoglycaemic middle-aged men. Diabetologia 20(2):134–138

Little J, Logan RF, Hawtin PG, Hardcastle JD, Turner ID (1993) Colorectal adenomas and energy intake, body size and physical activity: a case-control study of subjects participating in the Nottingham faecal occult blood screening programme. Br J Cancer 67(1):172–176

Longnecker MP, Gerhardsson le Verdier M, Frumkin H, Carpenter C (1995) A case-control study of physical activity in relation to risk of cancer of the right colon and rectum in men. Int J Epidemiol 24(1):42–50

Lubin F, Rozen P, Arieli B, Farbstein M, Knaani Y, Bat L et al (1997) Nutritional and lifestyle habits and water-fiber interaction in colorectal adenoma etiology. Cancer Epidemiol Biomark Prev 6(2): 79–85

Lund Nilsen TI, Vatten LJ (2002) Colorectal cancer associated with BMI, physical activity, diabetes, and blood glucose. IARC Sci Publ 156: 257–258

Lynge E, Thygesen L (1988) Use of surveillance systems for occupational cancer: data from the Danish National system. Int J Epidemiol 17(3): 493–500

Ma J, Giovannucci E, Pollak M, Leavitt A, Tao Y, Gaziano JM et al (2004) A prospective study of plasma C-peptide and colorectal cancer risk in men. J Natl Cancer Inst 96(7):546–553

Ma J, Pollak MN, Giovannucci E, Chan JM, Tao Y, Hennekens CH et al (1999) Prospective study of colorectal cancer risk in men and plasma levels of insulin-like growth factor (IGF)-I and IGF-binding protein-3. J Natl Cancer Inst 91(7): 620–625

MacDonald RS, Thornton WH Jr, Bean TL (1993) Insulin and IGE-1 receptors in a human intestinal adenocarcinoma cell line (CACO-2): regulation of Na+ glucose transport across the brush border. J Recept Res 13(7):1093–1113

Mai PL, Sullivan-Halley J, Ursin G, Stram DO, Deapen D, Villaluna D et al (2007) Physical activity and colon cancer risk among women in the California Teachers Study. Cancer Epidemiol Biomark Prev 16(3):517–525

Major GC, Piche ME, Bergeron J, Weisnagel SJ, Nadeau A, Lemieux S (2005) Energy expenditure from physical activity and the metabolic risk profile at menopause. Med Sci Sports Exerc 37(2):204–212

Makino T, Noguchi Y, Yoshikawa T, Doi C, Nomura K (1998) Circulating interleukin 6 concentrations and insulin resistance in patients with cancer. Br J Surg 85(12):1658–1662

Mao Y, Pan S, Wen SW, Johnson KC (2003) Physical inactivity, energy intake, obesity and the risk of rectal cancer in Canada. Int J Cancer 105(6): 831–837

4

Marcus PM, Newcomb PA, Storer BE (1994) Early adulthood physical activity and colon cancer risk among Wisconsin women. Cancer Epidemiol Biomark Prev 3(8):641–644

Markowitz S, Morabia A, Garibaldi K, Wynder E (1992) Effect of occupational and recreational activity on the risk of colorectal cancer among males: a case-control study. Int J Epidemiol 21(6): 1057–1062

Martinez ME, Giovannucci E, Spiegelman D, Hunter DJ, Willett WC, Colditz GA (1997) Leisure-time physical activity, body size, and colon cancer in women Nurses' Health Study Research Group. J Natl Cancer Inst 89(13): 948–955

Martinez ME, Giovannucci EL, Colditz GA, Stampfer MJ, Hunter DJ, Speizer FE et al (1996) Calcium, vitamin D, and the occurrence of colorectal cancer among women. J Natl Cancer Inst 88(19):1375–1382

Martinez ME, Heddens D, Earnest DL, Bogert CL, Roe D, Einspahr J et al (1999) Physical activity, body mass index, and prostaglandin E2 levels in rectal mucosa. J Natl Cancer Inst 91(11): 950–953

Martinez ME, Willett WC (1998) Calcium, vitamin D, and colorectal cancer: a review of the epidemiologic evidence. Cancer Epidemiol Biomark Prev 7(2):163–168

McKeown-Eyssen G (1994) Epidemiology of colorectal cancer revisited: are serum triglycerides and/or plasma glucose associated with risk? Cancer Epidemiol Biomark Prev 3(8):687–695

McTiernan A, Yasui Y, Sorensen B, Irwin ML, Morgan A, Rudolph RE et al (2006) Effect of a 12-month exercise intervention on patterns of cellular proliferation in colonic crypts: a randomized controlled trial. Cancer Epidemiol Biomark Prev 15(9):1588–1597

Moore MA, Park CB, Tsuda H (1998) Physical exercise: a pillar for cancer prevention? Eur J Cancer Prev 7(3):177–193

Moradi T, Gridley G, Bjork J, Dosemeci M, Ji BT, Berkel HJ et al (2008) Occupational physical activity and risk for cancer of the colon and rectum in Sweden among men and women by anatomic subsite. Eur J Cancer Prev 17(3): 201–208

Neugut AI, Terry MB, Hocking G, Mosca L, Garbowski GC, Forde KA et al (1996) Leisure and occupational physical activity and risk of colorectal adenomatous polyps. Int J Cancer 68(6):744–748

Nieman DC, Henson DA (1994) Role of endurance exercise in immune senescence. Med Sci Sports Exerc 26(2):172–181

Nilsen TI, Romundstad PR, Petersen H, Gunnell D, Vatten LJ (2008) Recreational physical activity and cancer risk in subsites of the colon (the Nord-Trondelag Health Study). Cancer Epidemiol Biomark Prev 17(1):183–188

Nilsen TI, Vatten LJ (2001) Prospective study of colorectal cancer risk and physical activity, diabetes, blood glucose and BMI: exploring the hyperinsulinaemia hypothesis. Br J Cancer 84(3):417–422

Nomura AM, Stemmermann GN, Chyou PH (1995) Gastric cancer among the Japanese in Hawaii. Jpn J Cancer Res 86(10):916–923

O'Donovan G, Kearney EM, Nevill AM, Woolf-May K, Bird SR (2005) The effects of 24 weeks of moderate- or high-intensity exercise on insulin resistance. Eur J Appl Physiol 95(5–6): 522–528

O'Dwyer PJ, Eckhardt SG, Haller DG, Tepper J, Ahnen D, Hamilton S et al (2007) Priorities in colorectal cancer research: recommendations from the Gastrointestinal Scientific Leadership Council of the Coalition of Cancer Cooperative Groups. J Clin Oncol 25(16):2313–2321

Orenstein MR, Friedenreich CM (2004) Review of physical activity and the IGF family. J Phys Activ Health 1:291–320

Otani T, Iwasaki M, Sasazuki S, Inoue M, Tsugane S (2007) Plasma C-peptide, insulin-like growth factor-I, insulin-like growth factor binding proteins and risk of colorectal cancer in a nested case-control study: the Japan public health center-based prospective study. Int J Cancer 120(9): 2007–2012

Palmer HG, Gonzalez-Sancho JM, Espada J, Berciano MT, Puig I, Baulida J et al (2001) Vitamin D(3) promotes the differentiation of colon carcinoma cells by the induction of E-cadherin and the inhibition of beta-catenin signaling. J Cell Biol 154(2):369–387

Parkin DM, Bray F, Ferlay J, Pisani P (2005) Global cancer statistics, 2002. CA Cancer J Clin 55(2): 74–108

Pedersen BK, Tvede N, Hansen FR, Andersen V, Bendix T, Bendixen G et al (1988) Modulation of natural killer cell activity in peripheral blood by physical exercise. Scand J Immunol 27(6): 673–678

Peters RK, Garabrant DH, Yu MC, Mack TM (1989) A case-control study of occupational and dietary factors in colorectal cancer in young men by subsite. Cancer Res 49(19): 5459–5468

Physical Activity Guidelines Advisory Committee (2008) Physical activity guidelines advisory committee report, 2008. U.S. Department of Health and Human Services, Washington, DC

Pischon T, Hankinson SE, Hotamisligil GS, Rifai N, Rimm EB (2003) Leisure-time physical activity and reduced plasma levels of obesity-related inflammatory markers. Obes Res 11(9): 1055–1064

Platz EA, Hankinson SE, Hollis BW, Colditz GA, Hunter DJ, Speizer FE et al (2000) Plasma 1, 25-dihydroxy- and 25-hydroxyvitamin D and adenomatous polyps of the distal colorectum. Cancer Epidemiol Biomark Prev 9(10): 1059–1065

Potter JD, Hunter D (2002) Colorectal Cancer. In: Adami HO, Hunter D, Trichopoulos D (eds) Textbook of cancer epidemiology. Oxford University Press, New York, pp 188–211

Pukkala E, Poskiparta M, Apter D, Vihko V (1993) Life-long physical activity and cancer risk among Finnish female teachers. Eur J Cancer Prev 2(5):369–376

Regensteiner JG, Mayer EJ, Shetterly SM, Eckel RH, Haskell WL, Marshall JA et al (1991) Relationship between habitual physical activity and insulin levels among nondiabetic men and women. San Luis Valley Diabetes Study. Diab Care 14(11):1066–1074

Rhodes JM, Campbell BJ (2002) Inflammation and colorectal cancer: IBD-associated and sporadic cancer compared. Trends Mol Med 8(1): 10–16

Rigas B, Goldman IS, Levine L (1993) Altered eicosanoid levels in human colon cancer. J Lab Clin Med 122(5):518–523

Robinson LE, Graham TE (2004) Metabolic syndrome, a cardiovascular disease risk factor: role of adipocytokines and impact of diet and physical activity. Can J Appl Physiol 29(6): 808–829

Rogers CJ, Colbert LH, Greiner JW, Perkins SN, Hursting SD (2008) Physical activity and cancer prevention: pathways and targets for intervention. Sports Med 38(4):271–296

Rose-John S, Scheller J, Elson G, Jones SA (2006) Interleukin-6 biology is coordinated by membrane-bound and soluble receptors: role in inflammation and cancer. J Leukoc Biol 80(2): 227–236

Rosenberg L, Boggs D, Wise LA, Palmer JR, Roltsch MH, Makambi KH et al (2006) A follow-up study of physical activity and incidence of colorectal polyps in African-American women. Cancer Epidemiol Biomark Prev 15(8):1438–1442

Russo A, Franceschi S, La Vecchia C, Dal Maso L, Montella M, Conti E et al (1998) Body size and colorectal-cancer risk. Int J Cancer 78(2): 161–165

Samad AK, Taylor RS, Marshall T, Chapman MA (2005) A meta-analysis of the association of physical activity with reduced risk of colorectal cancer. Colorectal Dis 7(3):204–213

Sandler RS, Halabi S, Baron JA, Budinger S, Paskett E, Keresztes R et al (2003) A randomized trial of aspirin to prevent colorectal adenomas in patients with previous colorectal cancer. N Engl J Med 348(10):883–890

Sandler RS, Pritchard ML, Bangdiwala SI (1995) Physical activity and the risk of colorectal adenomas. Epidemiology 6(6):602–606

Schmitz KH, Ahmed RL, Yee D (2002) Effects of a 9-month strength training intervention on insulin, insulin-like growth factor (IGF)-I, IGF-binding protein (IGFBP) 1, and IGFBP-3 in 30-50-year-old women. Cancer Epidemiol Biomark Prev 11(12):1597–1604

Schneider SH, Amorosa LF, Khachadurian AK, Ruderman NB (1984) Studies on the mechanism of improved glucose control during regular exercise in type 2 (non-insulin-dependent) diabetes. Diabetologia 26(5):355–360

Schnohr P, Gronbaek M, Petersen L, Hein HO, Sorensen TI (2005) Physical activity in leisure-time and risk of cancer: 14-year follow-up of 28, 000 Danish men and women. Scand J Public Health 33(4):244–249

Schoen RE, Tangen CM, Kuller LH, Burke GL, Cushman M, Tracy RP et al (1999) Increased blood glucose and insulin, body size, and incident colorectal cancer. J Natl Cancer Inst 91(13): 1147–1154

Schoen RE, Weissfeld JL, Kuller LH, Thaete FL, Evans RW, Hayes RB et al (2005) Insulin-like

4

growth factor-I and insulin are associated with the presence and advancement of adenomatous polyps. Gastroenterology 129(2):464–475

Scragg R, Camargo CA Jr (2008) Frequency of leisure-time physical activity and serum 25-hydroxyvitamin D levels in the US population: results from the Third National Health and Nutrition Examination Survey. Am J Epidemiol 168(6):577–586, discussion 587–591

Severson RK, Nomura AM, Grove JS, Stemmermann GN (1989) A prospective analysis of physical activity and cancer. Am J Epidemiol 130(3): 522–529

Shephard RJ (2002) Cytokine responses to physical activity, with particular reference to IL-6: sources, actions, and clinical implications. Crit Rev Immunol 22(3):165–182

Shinchi K, Kono S, Honjo S, Todoroki I, Sakurai Y, Imanishi K et al (1994) Obesity and adenomatous polyps of the sigmoid colon. Jpn J Cancer Res 85(5):479–484

Singh P, Rubin N (1993) Insulinlike growth factors and binding proteins in colon cancer. Gastroenterology 105(4):1218–1237

Sjodahl K, Jia C, Vatten L, Nilsen T, Hveem K, Lagergren J (2008) Body mass and physical activity and risk of gastric cancer in a population-based cohort study in Norway. Cancer Epidemiol Biomark Prev 17(1):135–140

Slattery ML (2004) Physical activity and colorectal cancer. Sports Med 34(4):239–252

Slattery ML, Abd-Elghany N, Kerber R, Schumacher MC (1990) Physical activity and colon cancer: a comparison of various indicators of physical activity to evaluate the association. Epidemiology 1(6):481–485

Slattery ML, Caan BJ, Benson J, Murtaugh M (2003a) Energy balance and rectal cancer: an evaluation of energy intake, energy expenditure, and body mass index. Nutr Cancer 46(2): 166–171

Slattery ML, Edwards S, Curtin K, Ma K, Edwards R, Holubkov R et al (2003b) Physical activity and colorectal cancer. Am J Epidemiol 158(3): 214–224

Slattery ML, Edwards SL, Ma KN, Friedman GD, Potter JD (1997) Physical activity and colon cancer: a public health perspective. Ann Epidemiol 7(2):137–145

Spence RR, Heesch KC, Brown WJ (2009) A systematic review of the association between physical activity and colorectal cancer risk. Scand J Med Sci Sports 19:764–781

Starkweather AR (2007) The effects of exercise on perceived stress and IL-6 levels among older adults. Biol Res Nurs 8(3):186–194

Steindorf K, Jedrychowski W, Schmidt M, Popiela T, Penar A, Galas A et al (2005) Case-control study of lifetime occupational and recreational physical activity and risks of colon and rectal cancer. Eur J Cancer Prev 14(4): 363–371

Stemmermann GN, Heilbrun LK, Nomura AM (1988) Association of diet and other factors with adenomatous polyps of the large bowel: a prospective autopsy study. Am J Clin Nutr 47(2): 312–317

Stukonis M, Doll R (1969) Gastric cancer in man and physical activity at work. Int J Cancer 4(2): 248–254

Taaffe DR, Harris TB, Ferrucci L, Rowe J, Seeman TE (2000) Cross-sectional and prospective relationships of interleukin-6 and C-reactive protein with physical performance in elderly persons: MacArthur studies of successful aging. J Gerontol A Biol Sci Med Sci 55(12): M709–715

Takahashi H, Kuriyama S, Tsubono Y, Nakaya N, Fujita K, Nishino Y et al (2007) Time spent walking and risk of colorectal cancer in Japan: the Miyagi Cohort study. Eur J Cancer Prev 16(5):403–408

Tang R, Wang JY, Lo SK, Hsieh LL (1999) Physical activity, water intake and risk of colorectal cancer in Taiwan: a hospital-based case-control study. Int J Cancer 82(4):484–489

Tavani A, Braga C, La Vecchia C, Conti E, Filiberti R, Montella M et al (1999) Physical activity and risk of cancers of the colon and rectum: an Italian case-control study. Br J Cancer 79(11–12): 1912–1916

Terry MB, Neugut AI, Bostick RM, Sandler RS, Haile RW, Jacobson JS et al (2002) Risk factors for advanced colorectal adenomas: a pooled analysis. Cancer Epidemiol Biomark Prev 11(7):622–629

Thune I, Lund E (1996) Physical activity and risk of colorectal cancer in men and women. Br J Cancer 73(9):1134–1140

Tiemersma EW, Wark PA, Ocke MC, Bunschoten A, Otten MH, Kok FJ et al (2003) Alcohol consumption, alcohol dehydrogenase 3 polymorphism, and colorectal adenomas. Cancer Epidemiol Biomark Prev 12(5):419–425

Tran TT, Medline A, Bruce WR (1996) Insulin promotion of colon tumors in rats. Cancer Epidemiol Biomark Prev 5(12):1013–1015

Troseid M, Lappegard KT, Claudi T, Damas JK, Morkrid L, Brendberg R et al (2004) Exercise reduces plasma levels of the chemokines MCP-1 and IL-8 in subjects with the metabolic syndrome. Eur Heart J 25(4):349–355

Tutton PJ, Barkla DH (1980) Influence of prostaglandin analogues on epithelial cell proliferation and xenograft growth. Br J Cancer 41(1): 47–51

Vena JE, Graham S, Zielezny M, Swanson MK, Barnes RE, Nolan J (1985) Lifetime occupational exercise and colon cancer. Am J Epidemiol 122(3):357–365

Vetter R, Dosemeci M, Blair A, Wacholder S, Unsal M, Engin K et al (1992) Occupational physical activity and colon cancer risk in Turkey. Eur J Epidemiol 8(6):845–850

Vigen C, Bernstein L, Wu AH (2006) Occupational physical activity and risk of adenocarcinomas of the esophagus and stomach. Int J Cancer 118(4): 1004–1009

Voskuil DW, Bueno de Mesquita HB, Kaaks R, van Noord PA, Rinaldi S, Riboli E et al (2001) Determinants of circulating insulin-like growth factor (IGF)-I and IGF binding proteins 1–3 in premenopausal women: physical activity and anthropometry (Netherlands). Cancer Causes Control 12(10):951–958

Wallace K, Baron JA, Karagas MR, Cole BF, Byers T, Beach MA et al (2005) The association of physical activity and body mass index with the risk of large bowel polyps. Cancer Epidemiol Biomark Prev 14(9):2082–2086

Wang JT, Ho LT, Tang KT, Wang LM, Chen YD, Reaven GM (1989) Effect of habitual physical activity on age-related glucose intolerance. J Am Geriatr Soc 37(3):203–209

Wannamethee SG, Shaper AG, Walker M (2001) Physical activity and risk of cancer in middle-aged men. Br J Cancer 85(9):1311–1316

Watabe K, Nishi M, Miyake H, Hirata K (1998) Lifestyle and gastric cancer: a case-control study. Oncol Rep 5(5):1191–1194

Watkins LF, Lewis LR, Levine AE (1990) Characterization of the synergistic effect of insulin and transferrin and the regulation of their receptors on a human colon carcinoma cell line. Int J Cancer 45(2):372–375

Wei EK, Giovannucci E, Wu K, Rosner B, Fuchs CS, Willett WC et al (2004) Comparison of risk factors for colon and rectal cancer. Int J Cancer 108(3):433–442

Wei EK, Ma J, Pollak MN, Rifai N, Fuchs CS, Hankinson SE et al (2005) A prospective study of C-peptide, insulin-like growth factor-I, insulin-like growth factor binding protein-1, and the risk of colorectal cancer in women. Cancer Epidemiol Biomark Prev 14(4):850–855

Wei EK, Ma J, Pollak MN, Rifai N, Fuchs CS, Hankinson SE et al (2006) C-peptide, insulin-like growth factor binding protein-1, glycosylated hemoglobin, and the risk of distal colorectal adenoma in women. Cancer Epidemiol Biomark Prev 15(4):750–755

Weiss EP, Holloszy JO (2007) Improvements in body composition, glucose tolerance, and insulin action induced by increasing energy expenditure or decreasing energy intake. J Nutr 137(4): 1087–1090

Weiss EP, Racette SB, Villareal DT, Fontana L, Steger-May K, Schechtman KB et al (2006) Improvements in glucose tolerance and insulin action induced by increasing energy expenditure or decreasing energy intake: a randomized controlled trial. Am J Clin Nutr 84(5): 1033–1042

White E, Jacobs EJ, Daling JR (1996) Physical activity in relation to colon cancer in middle-aged men and women. Am J Epidemiol 144(1): 42–50

Whittemore AS, Wu-Williams AH, Lee M, Zheng S, Gallagher RP, Jiao DA et al (1990) Diet, physical activity, and colorectal cancer among Chinese in North America and China. J Natl Cancer Inst 82(11):915–926

Whittemore AS, Zheng S, Wu A, Wu ML, Fingar T, Jiao DA et al (1985) Colorectal cancer in Chinese and Chinese Americans. Natl Cancer Inst Monogr 69:43–46

Will JC, Galuska DA, Vinicor F, Calle EE (1998) Colorectal cancer: another complication of diabetes mellitus? Am J Epidemiol 147(9): 816–825

Wohlleb JC, Hunter CF, Blass B, Kadlubar FF, Chu DZ, Lang NP (1990) Aromatic amine acetyltransferase as a marker for colorectal cancer: environmental and demographic associations. Int J Cancer 46(1):22–30

Wolin KY, Colditz GA (2008) Can weight loss prevent cancer? Br J Cancer 99(7):995–999

Wolin KY, Lee IM, Colditz GA, Glynn RJ, Fuchs C, Giovannucci E (2007) Leisure-time physical activity patterns and risk of colon cancer in women. Int J Cancer 121(12):2776–2781

4

Wolin KY, Yan Y, Colditz GA, Lee IM (2009) Physical activity and colon cancer prevention: a meta-analysis. Br J Cancer 100(4):611–616

Woods JA, Vieira VJ, Keylock KT (2009) Exercise, inflammation, and innate immunity. Immunol Allergy Clin North Am 29(2):381–393

World Cancer Research Fund/American Institute for Cancer Research (2007) Food, Nutrition, Physical Activity and the Prevention of Cancer: a Global Perspective. AICR, Washington DC

World Health Organization. (2008). Cancer. http://www.who.int/mediacentre/factsheets/fs297/en/index.html. Accessed 10 Aug 2008

Wu AH, Paganini-Hill A, Ross RK, Henderson BE (1987) Alcohol, physical activity and other risk factors for colorectal cancer: a prospective study. Br J Cancer 55(6):687–694

Yeh CC, Hsieh LL, Tang R, Chang-Chieh CR, Sung FC (2003) Risk factors for colorectal cancer in Taiwan: a hospital-based case-control study. J Formos Med Assoc 102(5):305–312

Yore MM, Ham S, Ainsworth B, Kruger J, Reis JP, Kohl HW 3rd et al (2007) Reliability and validity of the instrument used in BRFSS to assess physical activity. Med Sci Sports Exerc 39(8):1267–1274

Yoshida I, Suzuki A, Vallee M, Matano Y, Masunaga T, Zenda T et al (2006) Serum insulin levels and the prevalence of adenomatous and hyperplastic polyps in the proximal colon. Clin Gastroenterol Hepatol 4(10):1225–1231

You T, Berman DM, Ryan AS, Nicklas BJ (2004) Effects of hypocaloric diet and exercise training on inflammation and adipocyte lipolysis in obese postmenopausal women. J Clin Endocrinol Metab 89(4):1739–1746

Zhang Y, Cantor KP, Dosemeci M, Lynch CF, Zhu Y, Zheng T (2006) Occupational and leisure-time physical activity and risk of colon cancer by subsite. J Occup Environ Med 48(3): 236–243

Zhang ZF, Kurtz RC, Sun M, Karpeh M Jr, Yu GP, Gargon N et al (1996) Adenocarcinomas of the esophagus and gastric cardia: medical conditions, tobacco, alcohol, and socioeconomic factors. Cancer Epidemiol Biomark Prev 5(10): 761–768

Zittermann A, Sabatschus O, Jantzen S, Platen P, Danz A, Dimitriou T et al (2000) Exercise-trained young men have higher calcium absorption rates and plasma calcitriol levels compared with age-matched sedentary controls. Calcif Tissue Int 67(3):215–219

Physical Activity and Lung Cancer Prevention

5

Aina Emaus and Inger Thune

Abstract Since lung cancer is among the cancers with the highest incidence and has the highest mortality rate of cancer worldwide, the means of reducing its impact are urgently needed. Emerging evidence shows that physical activity plays an etiological role in lung cancer risk reduction. The majority of studies support the fact that total and recreational physical activity reduces lung cancer risk by 20–30% for women and 20–50% for men, and there is evidence of a dose–response effect. The biological mechanisms operating between physical activity and lung cancer are likely complex and influenced by many factors including inherited or acquired susceptibility genes, gender, smoking, and other environmental factors. Several plausible biological factors and mechanisms have been hypothesized linking physical activity to reduced lung cancer risk including: improved pulmonary function, reduced concentrations of carcinogenic agents in the lungs, enhanced immune function, reduced inflammation, enhanced DNA repair capacity, changes in growth factor levels and possible gene–physical activity interactions. Future research should target the possible subgroup effects and the biologic mechanisms that may be involved.

A. Emaus (✉)
Division of Cancer Etiology, Department of Population Science, City of Hope National Medical Center, CA, USA and
Department of Oncology,
Oslo University Hospital, Norway
e-mail: aina.emaus@medisin.uio.no

I. Thune
Department of Oncology,
Oslo University Hospital, Norway

5.1 Introduction

Lung cancer is one of the most common incident forms of cancer worldwide and is the leading cause of cancer-related deaths among men and women (Parkin et al. 2006; WCRF/AICR 2007). In Europe, lung cancer accounted for 12% of new cancer cases in 2006 and represented approximately 20% of the total number of cancer deaths (Ferlay et al. 2007). In the United States, 15% of cancer diagnosed and about 28% of all cancer deaths in 2009 were attributable to lung cancer (American Cancer Society 2009; Jemal et al. 2009). Globally, there is a rise in lung cancer incidence; however, the incidence varies among different populations throughout the world (Parkin et al. 2006). It is most common in high socioeconomic status countries, is increasing in some

K.S. Courneya and C.M. Friedenreich (eds.), *Physical Activity and Cancer*,
Recent Results in Cancer Research 186, DOI: 10.1007/978-3-642-04231-7_5,

developing countries, and is higher in males than in females (Sano and Marugame 2006). Lung cancer treatment depends on the type and stage of the disease. Treatment may include surgery and/or radiation therapy and chemotherapy (DeVita et al. 2008). Even if treatment options have been improved, lung cancer has, in general, low survival rates and the overall five-year survival of patients with this disease is less than 15% (WCRF/AICR 2007), pointing to the importance of possible modifiable risk factors, such as physical activity.

Lung cancer usually develops in the cells lining bronchial passages, reflecting the cells' susceptibility for malignant transformation in a vital part of the respiratory system. The lungs contain hundreds of lobules, and each lobule contains a bronchiole, its branches, and a cluster of alveoli (Fig. 5.1). Malignant cells develop through a series of progressive pathological changes occurring in the respiratory epithelium, which may vary by their embryologic, morphologic, physiologic and biochemical differences and, additionally, between central or peripheral locations in the lung. The main histological subtypes of lung cancer are categorized by cell type into small cell (SCLC) and nonsmall cell (NSCLC) carcinomas (DeVita et al. 2008). The latter is further divided into adenocarcinoma, squamous carcinoma, and large cell carcinoma and accounts for approximately 30–40%, 30%, and 10% of the total number of lung cancer cases, respectively, while small cell carcinoma accounts for 15–20% (DeVita et al. 2008). These different histologic subtypes may also have varying susceptibility for carcinogenes.

Active tobacco smoking accounts for an estimated 80–90% of lung cancer and passive smoking for 3–5%. Additionally, carcinogens in the workplace and ambient environment such as radon, polycyclic aromatic hydrocarbons (PAHs), and asbestos also cause lung cancer (Bruske-Hohlfeld 2009), alone or through interactions with smoking (Alberg et al. 2007). Thus, lung

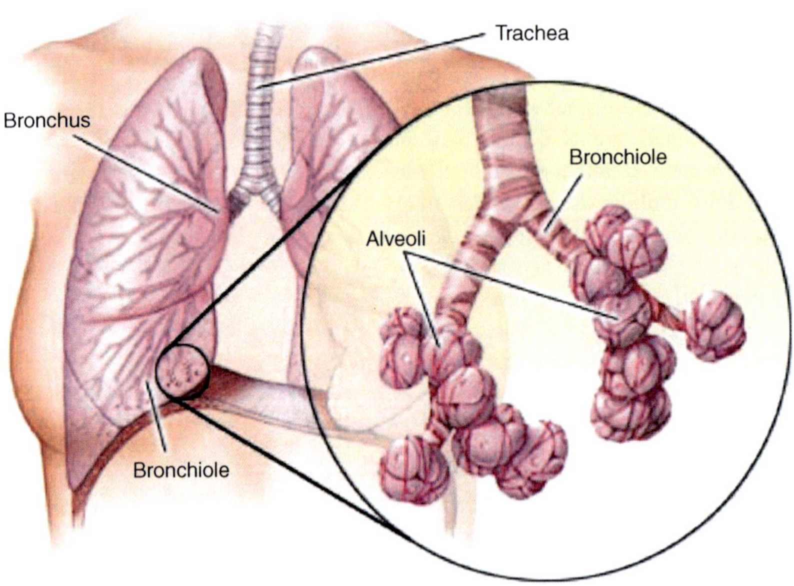

Fig. 5.1 Anatomic structure of the lungs. The major features of the lungs include the bronchus, the bronchiole, and the alveoli. (By permission of Mayo Foundation for Medical Education and Research. All rights reserved)

cancer incidence may reflect gene–environment interactions as well as historical differences in cigarette smoking habits. While smoking prevalence has declined in many developed countries, it is increasing in developing countries and also among women. Importantly, although it is generally accepted that tobacco smoke causes lung cancer, not everyone who smokes develops lung cancer. Studies have shown that smokers are 14 times more likely to develop lung cancer than nonsmokers, but only about 11% of heavy smokers develop lung cancer in their lifetime (Amos et al. 1999), suggesting substantial individual variation in susceptibility to smoke-associated respiratory carcinogens and, additionally, pointing to modifiable factors influencing lung cancer risk.

The favorable effects of physical activity on, in particular, pulmonary function and physical functioning, and later against the risk of developing several chronic diseases, including other site-specific cancers, and improved knowledge of several biological mechanisms' operating, have been well documented (Blair et al. 1993; Bouchard 2001). In spite of this mounting evidence of the beneficial effects of physical activity on health, high and increasing rates of a sedentary lifestyle are observed worldwide (Knuth and Hallal 2009). Thus, if there is an association between physical activity and lung cancer risk, physical activity may act as a risk factor and/or effect modifier and be an important potential modifiable factor influencing lung cancer risk and incidence.

Importantly, knowledge regarding whether or not physical activity influences lung cancer risk is warranted, and this association has only been studied for a short time and in a few studies (WCRF/AICR 2007). The current chapter will present the most recent studies focusing on the impact of physical activity in preventing lung cancers and then highlight some of the possible biological mechanisms operating between physical activity and lung cancer risk.

5.2 Epidemiological Studies of Physical Activity and Lung Cancer

A review of the published literature through December 2009 was conducted on PubMed to identify epidemiological studies that reported measures of physical activity in relation to lung cancer risk. In addition, previous reviews (IARC 2002; WCRF/AICR 2007), a meta-analysis (Tardon et al. 2005), and the reference lists of the included studies were examined. A total of 27 studies were identified that examined the association between physical activity and lung cancer risk, including mainly cohort studies and some case control studies (Table 5.1). Some of them were multiple publications from the same population; namely, the Iowa Women's Health Study (Olson et al. 2002; Sellers et al. 1991; Sinner et al. 2006), the National Health and Nutrition Examination Survey (NHANES) (Albanes et al. 1989; Steenland et al. 1995), and a series of studies from the Czech Republic (Kubik et al. 2008; Kubik et al. 2007; Kubik et al. 2004; Kubik et al. 2002. Among these studies, including multiple publications, only one publication representing each study was included; the latest publication or the publication with the most complete data was chosen. The studies were conducted in different countries worldwide using a wide range of unique study populations, designs, endpoints, and methods for assessing physical activity, which complicated the interpretation of the association between physical activity and lung cancer risk.

5.2.1 Overall Results

Most of the studies (Albanes et al. 1989; Kubik et al. 2007; Lee et al. 1999; Lee et al. 2002; Leitzmann et al. 2009; Mao et al. 2003; Severson et al. 1989; Sinner et al. 2006; Sprague et al.

2008; Thune and Lund 1997; Yun et al. 2008), but not all (Bak et al. 2005; Colbert et al. 2002; Dosemeci et al. 1993; Inoue et al. 2008; Schnohr et al. 2005; Steenland et al. 1995; Steindorf et al. 2006; Wannamethee et al. 2001) have demonstrated decreased risk of lung cancer among the most physically active subjects compared with the least physically active subjects. Overall, the studies that show an inverse graded dose–response association between physical activity and lung cancer risk suggest that physical activity decreases lung cancer risk by 20–50% (Table 5.1).

Interestingly, in 2002, an International Agency for Research on Cancer (IARC) report concluded that the evidence for an association between physical activity and decreased lung cancer risk remained inconclusive because of the uncertainty of the association and the limited amount of data available (IARC 2002). However, a subsequent meta-analysis, including studies upto October 2003 concluded that higher levels of recreational physical activity protected against lung cancer (Tardon et al. 2005). Furthermore, in 2007, the report from World Cancer Research Fund/American Institute for Cancer Research concluded there is limited evidence suggesting that physical activity protects against lung cancer (WCRF/AICR 2007).

5.2.2 Subgroup Results

5.2.2.1 Type of Physical Activity Measurement and Lung Cancer Risk

Figure 5.2 shows the main results for lung cancer risk organized by different types of physical activity measurements and gender. Six cohort studies have investigated total physical activity and lung cancer risk (Inoue et al. 2008; Lee et al. 1999; Leitzmann et al. 2009; Severson et al. 1989; Sprague et al. 2008; Thune and Lund 1997). For men, four of six studies reported statistically significant reduced risks (Lee et al. 1999; Leitzmann et al. 2009; Sprague et al. 2008; Thune and Lund 1997), while only one of four studies reported a statistically significant decreased risk among women (Leitzmann et al. 2009).

Most of the studies in this field have elucidated the association between recreational physical activity and lung cancer risk. Among men, all (Colbert et al. 2002; Knekt et al. 1996; Lee et al. 2002; Schnohr et al. 2005; Thune and Lund 1997; Wannamethee et al. 2001; Yun et al. 2008) except two studies (Albanes et al. 1989; Steindorf et al. 2006) reported decreased risk for lung cancer with increasing recreational physical activity, but only three studies (Lee et al. 2002; Thune and Lund 1997; Yun et al. 2008) reported statistically significantly reduced risks. Among women, only four studies have been conducted. All of them (Inoue et al. 2008; Leitzmann et al. 2009; Sinner et al. 2006; Thune and Lund 1997) reported decreased risks for lung cancer with increasing recreational physical activity, but only one study (Sinner et al. 2006) reported a statistically significant decreased risk.

Nonrecreational activity has been studied in relation to lung cancer risk in two studies from the same cohort (Albanes et al. 1989; Steenland et al. 1995). Albanes et al. (Albanes et al. 1989) reported significantly decreased lung cancer risk with increased physical activity.

The studies published with respect to occupational physical activity and lung cancer risk yielded inconclusive results (Bak et al. 2005; Colbert et al. 2002; Severson et al. 1989; Steindorf et al. 2006; Thune and Lund 1997). Two studies (Severson et al. 1989; Thune and Lund 1997) reported statistically nonsignificant decreases in risk with increasing occupational activity, while the other three studies reported the opposite; a statistically nonsignificant increased risk for increasing occupational

Table 5.1 Main results of epidemiological studies of physical activity and lung cancer

Author, publication year, country, study, follow-up time	Total (n), cases (n)	Physical activity (PA) assessment	Exposure level	Results RR (95% CI)	Subgroup analysis; By smoking and or histology	Adjustments, comments
COHORT STUDIES						
Albanes et al., 1989, USA, National Health and Nutrition Survey (NHANES I), 1971/75-82/84	*Men* Cohort 5138 Cases 114	Recreational exercise	Little or no Moderate Much	0.9 (0.6, 1.5) 1.0 (0.6, 1.6) 1.0 (ref) P trend 0.80		Age, smoking, BMI, race economic status, energy
		Nonrecreational activity	Quite inactive Moderate Very active	2.0 (1.2, 3.5) 1.3 (0.9, 2.0) 1.0 (ref) P trend 0.02		
Severson et al., 1989, Japan, Honolulu Heart Study, 1965/68-86	*Men* Cohort 8006 Cases 192	24-h PA summary index	1sttertile (low) 2sttertile (medium) 3sttertile (high)	1.00 (ref) 1.06 (0.76, 1.48) 0.70 (0.48, 1.01) P trend 0.04		Age, BMI, smoking
Sellers et al., 1991, USA, Iowa Women's Health Study, 1986	*Women* Control 1900 Cases 152	Leisure time PA	Low or moderate High	1.0 (ref) 0.4 (0.3, 0.5)		Unadjusted. Same cohort reported in Sinner et al., 2006. Nested case-control.
Steenland et al., 1995,USA, NHANES I, 1971/75-1987	Cohort 14407, both gender *Men* Cases 151	Nonrecreational PA	Lots of PA Some Little	1.00 1.12 (0.77, 1.63) 1.26 (0.71, 2.24)		Age, BMI, smoking, alcohol, income, recreational PA. Longer FUP of same cohort
	Women Cases 59	Nonrecreational PA	Lots of PA Some Little	1.00 (ref) 0.95 (0.52, 1.75) 1.41 (0.59, 3.35)		

(*continued*)

5

Table 5.1 (continued)

COHORT STUDIES							
Author, publication year, country, study, follow-up time	Total (n), cases (n)	Physical activity (PA) assessment	Exposure level	Results RR (95% CI)	Subgroup analysis: By smoking and or histology		Adjustments, comments
							reported in Al-banes et al., 1989
Knekt et al., 1996, Finland, 1978/80-91	*Men* Cohort 3245 Cases 70	Leisure time exercise	Low Moderate High	1.00 (ref) 0.93 (0.57, 1.53) 0.45 (0.17, 1.18)			Unadjusted
Thune and Lund, 1997, Norway, 1972/78-91	*Men* Cohort 53242 Cases 413	Recreational PA	Sedentary Moderate Regular training	1.00 (ref) 0.75 (0.60, 0.94) 0.71 (0.52, 0.97) P trend 0.01	< 15 cig 1.00 (ref) 0.77 (0.53, 1.11) 0.79 (0.49, 1.26)	15 cig + 1.00 (ref) 0.71 (0.52, 0.96) 0.59 (0.35, 0.97)	Age, geo-graphical area, smoking, BMI
		Recreational PA	Sedentary Moderate and regular		*Squamous-cell* 1.00 (ref) 0.97 (0.65, 1.44)	*Adenocarcinoma* 1.00 (ref) 0.65 (0.41, 1.05) Small-cell 1.00 (ref) 0.59 (0.38, 0.94)	
		Occupational PA	Sedentary Walking Lifting Heavy manual	1.00 (ref) 1.15 (0.90, 1.47) 1.13 (0.87, 1.47) 0.99 (0.70, 1.41) P trend 0.71			
		Total PA (occupational + recreational)	Sedentary Active	1.00 (ref) 0.73 (0.54, 0.98)			

	Women	Recreational PA	Sedentary	1.00 (ref)			
	Cohort		Moderate	0.91 (0.48, 1.71)			
	28274		Regular training	0.99 (0.35, 2.78)			
	Cases 51			P trend 0.88			
		Occupational PA	Sedentary	1.00 (ref)			
			Walking	0.81 (0.37, 1.76)			
			Lifting	0.79 (0.30, 2.12)			
				P trend 0.30			
		Total PA (occupational + recreational)	Sedentary	1.00 (ref)			
			Active	0.87 (0.21, 3.62)			
Lee et al., 1999,	*Men*	Total energy expended in PA (kJ/week)	<4200	1.00 (ref)	*Non-former smokers*	*Heavy smokers*	Age, smoking, BMI
USA, Harvard	Cohort				1.00	1.00	
Alumni,	13905		4200-8399	0.87 (0.64, 1.18)	0.88	0.91	
1977-88/93	Cases 245		8400-12599	0.76 (0.52, 1.11)	0.83	0.92	
			≥ 12600	0.61 (0.41, 0.89)	0.54	0.61	
				P trend 0.01	P trend 0.03	P trend 0.24	
		Distance walked (km/week)	<5	1.00 (ref)			
			5 to < 10	0.76 (0.54, 1.07)			
			10 to < 20	0.71 (0.51, 0.99)			
			≥ 20	0.65 (0.45, 0.94)			
				P trend 0.01			
		Stair climbed (storeys/week)	<10	1.00 (ref)			
			10 to < 20	0.63 (0.44, 0.92)			
			20 to < 35	0.64 (0.44, 0.93)			
			≥ 35	0.74 (0.54, 1.02)			
				P trend 0.08			
		Activities at <4.5 MET (kJ/week)	None	1.00 (ref)			
			1 to <1050	1.20 (0.79, 1.83)			
			1050 to <2520	0.92 (0.57, 1.48)			
			2520 to <5880	0.81 (0.50, 1.32)			
			≥5880	0.99 (0.66, 1.48)			
				P trend 0.62			

(*continued*)

Table 5.1 (continued)

COHORT STUDIES						
Author, publication year, country, study, follow -up time	Total (n), cases (n)	Physical activity (PA) assessment	Exposure level	Results RR (95% CI)	Subgroup analysis; By smoking and or histology	Adjustments, comments
		Activities at ≥ 4.5 MET (kJ/week)	None 1 to <1050 1050 to <2520 2520 to <5880 ≥5880	1.00 (ref) 0.84 (0.58, 1.22) 0.64 (0.39, 1.04) 0.93 (0.62, 1.39) 0.60 (0.38, 0.96) P trend 0.046		
Wannamethee et al., 2001, UK, British Regional Heart Study (BRHS), 1978/80-97	*Men* Cohort 7588 Cases 265	Leisure time PA	None to moderate Moderate-vigorous Vigorous	1.00 (ref) 0.77 (0.49, 1.21) 0.76 (0.40, 1.43) P trend 0.19		Age, smoking, BMI, alcohol. social class
		Sporting activity > 1 month	No Yes	1.00 (ref) 0.81 (0.58, 1.14)		
		Regular walking (min/day)	<20 20–40 40–60 >60	1.00 0.90 (0.62, 1.30) 1.04 (0.70, 1.55) 0.77 (0.38, 1.56)		
Colbert et al., 2002, Finland, ATBC study, 1985/88-97	*Men* Cohort 27087 Cases 1442	Leisure time PA	Sedentary Active	1.00 (ref) 0.97 (0.87, 1.07)	*Squamous* 0.93 (0.79, 1.10) *Adenocarcinoma* 0.96 (0.73, 1.25) Small cell 1.05 (0.84, 1.31)	Age, BMI, smoking, education, energy intake, vegetable intake

		Occupational PA	Non-worker Sedentary Light Moderate Heavy	1.27 (1.04, 1.56) 1.00 (ref) 1.01 (0.81, 1.27) 1.09 (0.86, 1.37) 1.23 (0.95, 1.59) P trend 0.12		
Olson et al., 2002, USA, Iowa Women's Health Study, 1986-98	*Women* Cohort 41836 Cases 596	Leisure time PA (score)	Low Medium High	1.00 (ref) 0.86 (0.70, 1.06) 0.74 (0.59, 0.93) P trend 0.01		Age, smoking. Longer FUP of same cohort reported in Sinner et al., 2006
Lee et al., 2002, Korea, 1992/94-99	*Men* Cohort 452645 Cases 833	Exercise	Yes No	1.00 0.8 (0.7, 0.9)		Age
Alfano et al., 2004, USA, CARET RCT, 1985-2002	Both genders: Cohort 7045 Cases 263	Total PA	Moderate-vigorous PA Vigorous PA	HRR for 1 SD increase in PA: 0.99 (0.87, 1.11) 1.00 (0.88, 1.12)		Gender
Bak et al., 2005, Denmark, 1993/97-2002	*Men* Cohort 26070 Cases 194	Occupational PA	Sitting Standing Light activity Heavy activity Not working	1.00 (ref) 1.71 (1.07, 2.73) 1.24 (0.76, 2.01) 1.30 (0.75, 4.31) 1.07 (0.69, 1.64)		Smoking, education, fruit and vegetables, occupational exposure, occupational activity or leisure activity
		Sport	Non-active Active	1.00 (ref) 0.60 (0.42, 0.84)		
		Cycling	Non-active Active	1.00 (ref) 1.01 (0.75, 1.35)		
		Walking	Non-active Active	1.00 (ref) 1.09 (0.66, 1.79)		

(*continued*)

Table 5.1 (continued)

COHORT STUDIES						
Author, publication year, country, study, follow -up time	Total (n), cases (n)	Physical activity (PA) assessment	Exposure level	Results RR (95% CI)	Subgroup analysis; By smoking and or histology	Adjustments, comments
		Gardening	Non-active Active	1.00 (ref) 0.85 (0.61, 1.19)		
		Housework	Non-active Active	1.00 (ref) 1.32 (0.84, 2.08)		
		Do-it-yourself work	Non-active Active	1.00 (ref) 1.08 (0.72, 1.04)		
	Women Cohort 28352 Cases 175	Occupational PA	Sitting Standing Light activity Heavy activity Not working	1.00 (ref) 1.71 (1.07, 2.73) 1.24 (0.76, 2.01) 1.80 (0.75, 4.31) 1.07 (0.69, 1.64)		
		Sport	Non-active Active	1.00 (ref) 0.92 (0.67, 1.27)		
		Cycling	Non-active Active	1.00 0.65 (0.48, 0.89)		
		Walking	Non-active Active	1.00 (ref) 0.76 (0.46, 1.25)		
		Gardening	Non-active Active	1.00 (ref) 0.91 (0.67, 1.25)		
		Housework	Non-active Active	1.00 (ref) 1.02 (0.74, 1.41)		
		Do-it-yourself work	Non-active Active	1.00 (ref) 0.86 (0.76, 0.97)		

Schnohr et al.,	*Men*	Leisure time PA	Low	1.00 (ref)			Age, birth
2005,	Cohort 15043		Moderate	0.88 (0.70, 1.10)			cohort, occupa-
Denmark,	Cases 545		Vigorous	0.92 (0.72, 1.18)			tional PA,
1984-1998				P trend 0.63			smoking,
	Women	Leisure time PA	Low	1.00 (ref)			education,
	Cohort		Moderate	0.99 (0.71, 1.37)			alcohol
	13216		Vigorous	1.06 (0.71, 1.60)			
	Cases 228			P trend 0.78			
Steindorf et al.,	*Men*	Recreational PA	0–<13.5	1.0 (ref)	Squamous	Adenocarcinoma	Age Centre
2006, Europe,	Cohort	(METs-hours/wk)	13.5–<27.5	1.09 (0.88, 1.35)	1.00 (ref)	1.00 (ref)	Smoking,
EPIC,	130438		27.5–<45.0	0.85 (0.67, 1.08)	0.75 (0.49, 1.14)	1.44 (0.94, 2.21)	weight, height,
1992/2000-	Cases 607		≥ 45.0	1.00 (0.79, 1.27)	0.84 (0.55, 1.29)	0.97 (0.60, 1.56)	education, total
1999/2003					0.94 (0.60, 1.45)	0.92 (0.55, 1.53)	energy intake,
						Small cell	alcohol, fruits,
						1.00 (ref)	vegetables, red
						0.91 (0.54, 1.55)	and processed
						0.74 (0.42, 1.32)	meat, occu-
						0.95 (0.54, 1.67)	pational
							exposure
		Non-occupational	0–<33.7	1.00 (ref)	Squamous	Adenocarcinoma	
		PA (METs-	33.7–56.6	0.39 (0.70, 1.13)	1.00 (ref)	1.00 (ref)	
		hours/wk)	56.6–86.6	1.20 (0.96, 1.51)	0.73 (0.45, 1.16)	1.04 (0.65, 1.67)	
			≥86.6	0.97 (0.76, 1.25)	1.29 (0.84, 1.98)	1.43 (0.91, 2.26)	
					1.17 (0.75, 1.83)	0.90 (0.53, 1.52)	
						Small cell	
						1.00 (ref)	
						0.70 (0.40, 1.25)	
						0.80 (0.46, 1.39)	
						0.84 (0.48, 1.46)	

(*continued*)

Table 5.1 (continued)

COHORT STUDIES							
Author, publication year, country, study, follow -up time	Total (n). cases (n)	Physical activity (PA) assessment	Exposure level	Results RR (95% CI)	Subgroup analysis: By smoking and or histology		Adjustments, comments
		Vigorous non-occupational PA (METs-hours/wk)	None	1.00 (ref)	Squamous	Adenocarcinoma	
			>0–<15	0.94 (0.69, 1.28)	1.00 (ref)	1.00 (ref)	
			15–<40	0.86 (0.65, 1.15)	1.13 (0.64, 2.01)	1.06 (0.58, 1.94)	
			≥40	0.87 (0.65, 1.16)	0.91 (0.53, 1.55)	1.04 (0.59, 1.82)	
					0.73 (0.41, 1.28)	0.98 (0.55, 1.75)	
						Small cell	
						1.00 (ref)	
						1.17 (0.61, 2.23)	
						0.68 (0.34, 1.37)	
						0.59 (0.28, 1.27)	
		Household physical activity (MET-hours/week)	0–<11	1.00 (ref)	Squamous	Adenocarcinoma	
			11–<23.8	0.77 (0.60, 1.01)	1.00 (ref)	1.00 (ref)	
			23.8–<43.6	0.86 (0.67, 1.10)	0.60 (0.35–1.01)	0.82 (0.50, 1.35)	
			≥43.6	1.04 (0.82, 1.31)	0.99 (0.62–1.59)	0.73 (0.44, 1.22)	
					1.25 (0.80–1.95)	1.03 (0.64, 1.65)	
						Small cell	
						1.00 (ref)	
						0.80 (0.44, 1.48)	
						0.86 (0.48, 1.57)	
						0.94 (0.53, 1.67)	
		Occupational (PA)	Sitting	1.00 (ref)			
			Unemployed	1.57 (1.20, 2.05)			
			Standing	1.35 (1.02, 1.79)			
			Heavy manual	1.25 (0.94, 1.66)			
		Sport	None	1.00 (ref)			
			0–<9.0	0.82 (0.61, 1.10)			
			9.0–<18.0	0.77 (0.59, 1.02)			
			≥18.0	0.71 (0.50, 0.98)			

	Also reported results for: walking, cycling, gardening, housework, climbing stairs and do-it-yourself work. No association found.				
Women	Recreational PA	0–<12.0	1.00 (ref)	Squamous	Adenocarcinoma
Cohort	(METs-hours/wk)	12.0– <24.0	0.99 (0.77, 1.28)	1.00 (ref)	1.00 (ref)
285789		24.0– <42.0	0.99 (0.76, 1.30)	1.22 (0.60, 2.48)	0.87 (0.58, 1.32)
Cases 476		≥ 42.0	0.99 (0.76, 1.30)	0.96 (0.43, 2.10)	0.79 (0.51, 1.23)
				1.16 (0.55, 2.44)	0.77 (0.50, 1.19)
					Small cell
					1.00 (ref)
					0.60 (0.29, 1.26)
					1.15 (0.59, 2.25)
					1.43 (0.76, 2.69)
	Non-occupational	0–<51.1	1.00 (ref)	Squamous	Adenocarcinoma
	PA (METs-	51.1–<82.2	0.99 (0.77, 1.26)	1.00 (ref)	1.00 (ref)
	hours/wk)	82.2–<123.0	0.93 (0.71, 1.21)	1.06 (0.53, 2.11)	0.81 (0.54, 1.21)
		≥123.0	1.00 (0.75, 1.35)	0.79 (0.37, 1.68)	0.74 (0.48, 1.15)
				0.81 (0.36, 1.83)	0.80 (0.51, 1.28)
					Small cell
					1.00 (ref)
					1.14 (0.62, 2.08)
					0.80 (0.39, 1.62)
					1.26 (0.61, 2.57)
	Vigorous	None	1.00 (ref)	Squamous	Adenocarcinoma
	non-occupational	>0 –<13.5	0.65 (0.43, 0.98)	1.00 (ref)	1.00 (ref)
	PA (METs-	13.5–<33.5	0.60 (0.40, 0.98)	1.31 (0.39, 4.36)	0.75 (0.40, 1.41)
	hours/wk)	≥33.5	0.92 (0.65, 1.32)	1.38 (0.37, 5.12)	0.62 (0.33, 1.19)
				2.03 (0.67, 6.16)	1.09 (0.61, 1.92)
					Small cell
					1.00 (ref)
					0.69 (0.24, 1.93)
					0.50 (0.18, 1.42)
					0.81 (0.30, 2.16)

(*continued*)

5

Table 5.1 (continued)

COHORT STUDIES							
Author, publication year, country, study, follow -up time	Total (n), cases (n)	Physical activity (PA) assessment	Exposure level	Results RR (95% CI)	Subgroup analysis; By smoking and or histology		Adjustments, comments
		Household overall	0–<26.0	1.00 (ref)	Squamous	Adenocarcinoma	
		(METs-hours/wk)	26.0 –<49.3	1.04 (0.81, 1.33)	1.00 (ref)	1.00 (ref)	
			49.3–<86.3	0.90 (0.68, 1.18)	0.99 (0.50, 1.95)	1.00 (0.66, 1.51)	
			≥86.3	0.95 (0.70, 1.30)	0.53 (0.23, 1.19)	1.02 (0.66, 1.58)	
					0.70 (0.30, 1.64)	0.84 (0.50, 1.40)	
						Small cell	
						1.00 (ref)	
						0.91 (0.51, 1.62)	
						0.37 (0.17, 0.82)	
						0.69 (0.33, 1.48)	
		Occupational	Sitting	1.00 (ref)			
			Unemployed	1.25 (0.94, 1.66)			
			Standing	1.14 (0.83, 1.57)			
			Heavy manual	1.09 (0.76, 1.56)			
		Sport	None	1.00 (ref)			
			0–<6.0	0.95 (0.73, 1.23)			
			6.0–<15.0	0.81 (0.58, 1.12)			
			≥15.0	1.14 (0.87, 1.50)			
		Cycling	None	1.00 (ref)			
			>0–<6.0	0.84 (0.62, 1.12)			
			6.0–<18.0	0.77 (0.58, 1.02)			
			≥18.0	0.73 (0.54, 0.99)			
		Also reported results for: walking, gardening, housework, climbing stairs and do-it-yourself work. No association found.					

Sinner et al., 2006, USA, Iowa Women's Health Study, 1986-2002	*Women* Cohort 36410 Cases 777	Leisure time PA	Low Medium High	1.00 (ref) 0.84 (0.70, 1.00) 0.77 (0.64, 0.94)	Never Smokers 1.00 (ref) 1.83 (1.21, 2.78) 1.32 (0.83, 2.10) Former Smokers 1.00 (ref) 0.72 (0.50, 1.04) 0.63 (0.43, 0.92) Current Smokers 1.00 (ref) 0.65 (0.51, 0.83) 0.72 (0.55, 0.94)	Squamous cell 1.00 (ref) 1.01 (0.68, 1.50) 0.77 (0.48, 1.24) Adenocarcinoma 1.00 (ref) 0.95 (0.72, 1.26) 0.86 (0.64, 1.16) Small cell 1.00 (ref) 0.70 (0.45, 1.08) 0.91 (0.58, 1.43)	BMI, smoking, education Marital status Alcohol Vegetable intake
		Regular PA	No Yes	1.00 (ref) 0.92 (0.79, 1.07)			
		Moderate PA (per week)	Never ≤1 >1	1.00 (ref) 0.90 (0.75, 1.09) 0.79 (0.66, 0.94)			
		Vigorous PA (per week)	Never ≤1 >1	1.00 (ref) 0.80 (0.60, 1.07) 0.71 (0.51, 0.99)			
Sprague et al., 2008, USA, 1987/88-2004	*Men* Cohort 2166 Cases 79	Total PA index (kcal/week)	0–174 175–874 ≥ 875	1.0 (ref) 0.56 (0.33, 0.97) 0.50 (0.29, 0.87) P trend 0.01	Both gender: Current smokers 1.00 (ref) 0.48 (0.26, 0.91) 0.49 (0.25, 0.97)	Both gender: Never/former smokers 1.00 (ref) 0.97 (0.55, 1.71) 0.60 (0.33, 1.11)	Age, smoking, BMI, alcohol, education
	Women Cohort: 2760 Cases: 55	Total PA index (kcal/week)	0–174 175–874 ≥ 875	1.0 (ref) 1.02 (0.54, 1.95) 0.66 (0.30, 1.44) P trend 0.35			

(*continued*)

Table 5.1 (continued)

COHORT STUDIES						
Author, publication year, country, study, follow -up time	Total (n), cases (n)	Physical activity (PA) assessment	Exposure level	Results RR (95% CI)	Subgroup analysis: By smoking and or histology	Adjustments, comments
Inoue et al., 2008, Japan, The Japan Public Health Center-based Prospective Study, 1995/99-2004	*Men* Cohort 37898 Cases 388	Total PA	Lowest Q1 Second Q2 Third Q3 Highest Q4	1.00 (ref) 1.22 (0.91, 1.63) 1.44 (1.09, 1.90) 1.10 (0.83, 1.45) Ptrend 0.494		Age, area, total energy intake, history of diabetes, smoking, alcohol, BMI
	Women Cohort 41873 Cases 144	Total PA	Lowest Q1 Second Q2 Third Q3 Highest Q4	1.00 (ref) 0.90 (0.58, 1.38) 0.90 (0.57, 1.42) 0.92 (0.56, 1.49) P trend 0.69		
Yun et al., 2008, Korea The National Health Insurance corporation, 1996-2002	*Men* Cohort 444963 Cases 1574	Leisure time PA	Low Moderate-High	1.00 (ref) 0.83 (0.75, 0.92)		Age, dietary pref, smoking, alcohol, BMI, employment, fasting blood sugar

Leitzmann et	*Men*	Total PA (above 20	0	1.0 (ref)	Both sexes:	Both sexes:	BMI, smoking,
al., 2009, USA,	Cohort	minutes, times/	<1	0.92 (0.84, 1.02)	Squamous cell	Never Smokers	race/ethnicity,
NIH AARP	303892	week)	1–2	0.85 (0.78, 0.93)	1.00 (ref)	1.00 (ref)	education,
Diet and Health	Cases 4419		3–4	0.80 (0.74, 0.88)	0.95 (0.80, 1.13)	1.02 (0.81, 1.86)	marital status,
Study,			≥ 5	0.77 (0.70, 0.85)	0.82 (0.70, 0.97)	1.28 (0.89, 1.84)	family history
1995/96-2003				P trend <0.001	0.87 (0.74, 1.02)	1.08 (0.75, 1.56)	of cancer,
	Women	Total PA (above 20	0 times/week	1.0 (ref)	0.78 (0.65, 0.93)	1.02 (0.69, 1.52)	fruit/ veg
	Cohort	minutes, times/	<1 times/week	0.88 (0.77, 1.00)	P trend 0.01	P trend 0.50	intake, red
	197253	week)	1–2 times/week	0.95 (0.84, 1.07)	Adenocarcinoma	Former Smokers	meat, alcohol
	Cases 2326		3–4 times/week	0.90 (0.80, 1.01)	1.00 (ref)	1.00 (ref)	
			≥ 5 times/week	0.80 (0.69, 0.92)	0.97 (0.86, 1.10)	0.94 (0.83, 1.05)	
				P trend 0.01	0.94 (0.84, 1.05)	0.87 (0.79, 0.97)	
					0.84 (0.75, 0.94)	0.82 (0.74, 0.91)	
					0.80 (0.71, 0.91)	0.78 (0.70, 0.87)	
					P trend 0.001	P trend <0.001	
					Small cell	Current Smokers	
					1.00 (ref)	1.00 (ref)	
					0.80 (0.66, 0.98)	0.88 (0.78, 0.88)	
					0.82 (0.68, 0.98)	0.88 (0.80, 0.97)	
					0.86 (0.72, 1.03)	0.84 (0.76, 0.94)	
					0.82 (0.67, 1.01)	0.77 (0.68, 0.87)	
					P trend 0.190	P trend <0.001	

(*continued*)

5

Table 5.1 (continued)

CASE CONTROL STUDIES							
Author, publication year, country, study, follow -up time	Total (n), cases (n)	Physical activity (PA) assessment	Exposure level	Results RR (95% CI)	Subgroup analysis; By smoking and or histology		Adjustments, comments
Population based case-control							
Brownson et al., 1991, USA, 1984-89	*Men* Cases 509	Occupational PA	Low Moderate High	0.8 (0.6, 0.9) 0.9 (0.8, 1.0) 1.0 (ref) P trend <0.01			Age, geographical area, smoking, BMI
Dosemeci et al., 1993, Turkey, 1979-84	*Men* Cases 1148	Occupational PA	Sedentary Moderate Active	1.1 (0.9, 1.3) 1.0 (0.8, 1.2) 1.0 (ref)			Age, smoking
Mao et al., 2003, Canada, Canadian National Enhanced Cancer Surveillance System (NECSS), 1994-97	*Men* Cases 1131	Recreational (Moderate + Strenuous, MET hrs/wk)	<6.4 6.3–<19.1 19.1–<37.4 ≥37.4	1.00 (ref) 0.91 (0.71, 1.17) 0.84 (0.65, 1.09) 0.74 (0.57, 0.99) P trend 0.04	Never Smokers 1.00 (ref) 0.53 (0.17, 1.63) 0.87 (0.29, 2.62) 0.31 (0.08, 1.14) P trend 0.15 Former Smokers 1.00 (ref) 1.07 (0.74, 1.53) 0.93 (0.65, 1.34) 0.81 (0.61, 1.30) P for trend 0.16 Current Smokers 1.00 (ref) 0.83 (0.57, 1.21) 0.69 (0.46, 1.03) 0.65 (0.42, 1.02) P for trend 0.03	Squamous cell 1.00 (ref) 0.95 (0.67, 1.34) 0.82 (0.57, 1.19) 0.96 (0.66, 1.41) P trend 0.63 Small cell 1.00 (ref) 0.69 (0.44, 1.09) 0.68 (0.42, 1.10) 0.52 (0.30, 0.91) P trend 0.019 Adenocarcinoma 1.00 (ref) 0.83 (0.57, 1.20) 0.80 (0.54, 1.09) 0.80 (0.53, 1.21) P trend 0.27	Age, residence, education, BMI, caloric intake, vegetable intake, smoking, occupational exposure, alcohol,

		Moderate (Met hrs/wk)	<3.9	1.00 (ref)		
			3.9–11.6	0.84 (0.65, 1.09)		
			11.6–25.5	0.89 (0.69, 1.16)		
			≥25.5	0.81 (0.62, 1.06)		
				P trend 0.18		
		Vigorous (MET hrs/wk)	0	1.00 (ref)		
			<3.3	0.88 (0.68, 1.13)		
			3.3–<16.4	0.86 (0.66, 1.14)		
			≥16.4	0.69 (0.51, 0.94)		
				P trend 0.02		
	Women Cases 997	Recreational (Moderate + Strenuous, MET hrs/wk)	<6.1	1.00 (ref)	Never Smokers	Squamous cell
			6.1–<15.2	0.73 (0.55, 0.98)	1.00 (ref)	1.00 (ref)
			15.2–<31.4	0.66 (0.49, 0.89)	0.70 (0.37, 1.32)	0.86 (0.50, 1.45)
			≥31.4	0.72 (0.53, 0.98)	0.82 (0.55, 1.90)	0.60 (0.33, 0.99)
				P trend 0.02	0.80 (0.54, 1.83)	0.51 (0.27, 0.94)
					P trend 0.25	P trend 0.01
					Former	Small cell
					1.00 (ref)	1.00 (ref)
					0.46 (0.27, 0.79)	0.87 (0.52, 1.42)
					0.50 (0.30, 0.85)	0.73 (0.44, 1.20)
					0.56 (0.34, 0.91)	0.65 (0.37, 1.13)
					P trend 0.02	P trend 0.09
					Current	Adenocarcinoma
					1.00 (ref)	1.00 (ref)
					1.03 (0.68, 1.56)	0.74 (0.51, 1.07)
					0.66 (0.44, 1.00)	0.63 (0.44, 0.92)
					0.72 (0.46, 1.11)	0.84 (0.58, 1.22)
					P trend 0.04	P trend 0.25
		Moderate (METhrs/wk)	<4.7	1.00 (ref)		
			4.7–<12.1	0.67 (0.50, 0.89)		
			12.1–<23.1	0.60 (0.44, 0.82)		
			≥23.1	0.73 (0.54, 0.98)		
				P trend 0.03		

(*continued*)

Table 5.1 (continued)

CCASE CONTROL STUDIES							
Author, publication year, country, study, follow -up time	Total (n), cases (n)	Physical activity (PA) assessment	Exposure level	Results RR (95% CI)	Subgroup analysis; By smoking and or histology		Adjustments, comments
		Vigorous (MET hrs/wk)	0 <1.5 1.5–<7.3 ≥7.3	1.00 (ref) 0.93 (0.69, 1.24) 0.64 (0.47, 0.89) 0.82 (0.66, 1.25) P trend 0.13			
Hospital-based case-control							
Kubik et al., 2002, Czech Republic	*Women* Cases 269	Leisure time PA (hours/week)	0 1–5 >5	1.00 (ref) 0.62 (0.42, 0.92) 0.42 (0.29, 0.62)			Age, residence, education
Kubik et al., 2004, Czech Republic, 1998-2002	*Women* Cases 419	Physical Exercise (within recent 10 years, hrs/week)	0–2 3–6 >6		Never Smokers 1.00 (ref) 1.08 (0.67, 1.73) 0.74 (0.45, 1.22) P trend 0.21	Ever Smokers 1.00 (ref) 0.70 (0.47, 1.03) 0.48 (0.32, 0.71) P trend <0.001	Age, residence, education. Longer FUP of same case-control reported in Kubik et al., 2002
		Other PA (within recent 10 years, hrs/week)	0–2 3–6 >6		Never smokers 1.00 (ref) 0.83 (0.48, 1.44) 1.22 (0.77, 1.92) P trend 0.36	Ever Smokers 1.00 (ref) 0.82 (0.54, 1.25) 0.71 (0.49, 1.04) P trend 0.074	
		Physical Exercise (1 year before baseline, hrs/week)	0–2 3–6 >6		Never smokers 1.00 (ref) 1.00 (0.57, 1.77) 1.01 (0.54, 1.86) P trend 0.98	Ever smokers 1.00 (ref) 0.78 (0.46, 1.31) 0.63 (0.37, 1.05) P trend 0.07	

		Other PA (1 year before baseline, hrs/week)	0–2 3–6 >6		Never smokers 1.00 (ref) 1.06 (0.53, 2.11) 1.04 (0.56, 1.94) P trend 0.91	Ever smokers 1.00 (ref) 0.89 (0.51, 1.55) 0.73 (0.44, 1.23) P trend 0.23	
Kubik et al., 2007, Czech Republic, 1998-2005	*Women* Cases 569	Exercise, sport or walking	No yes	1.00 (ref) 0.67 (0.52, 0.86)	Never Smokers 1.00 (ref) w0.97 (0.62, 1.52)	Ever Smokers 1.00 (ref) 0.59 (0.42, 0.83)	Age, residence, education. Longer FUP of same case-control reported in Kubik et al., 2004
Kubik et al., 2008, Czech Republic, 1998-2006	*Women* Cases 587	Exercise, sport or walking >1 hour/ week	No yes		Never Smokers 1.00 (ref) 0.97 (0.62, 1.52) Ever Smokers 1.00 (ref) 0.64 (0.45, 0.90)	Squamous 0.71 (0.46, 1.11) Adenocarcinoma 0.59 (0.42, 0.84) Small Cell 0.61 (0.39, 0.97)	Age, residence, education, smoking when right Longer FUP of same case-control reported in Kubik et al., 2007
	Men Cases 587	Exercise, sport or walking >1 hour/ week	No yes		Never Smokers (ref) 0.75 (0.15, 3.66) Ever Smokers 1.00 (ref) 0.73 (0.37, 1.41)	Squamous 0.63 (0.30, 1.29) Adenocarcinoma 1.80 (0.51, 6.41) Small Cell 0.79 (0.27, 2.26)	

5

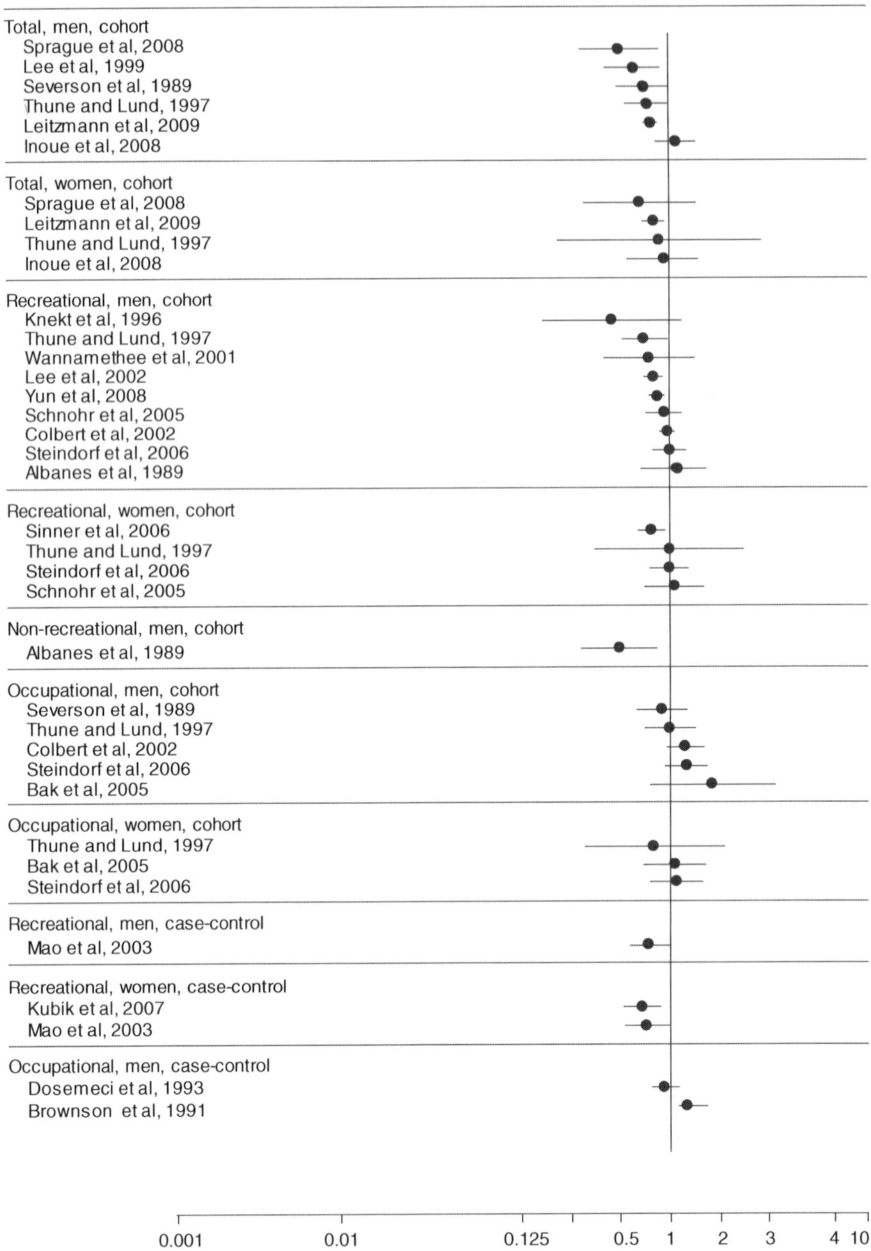

Fig. 5.2 Epidemiological studies of physical activity and lung cancer risk by type of physical activity and by gender. Relative risk (RR) for the lowest versus the highest level of physical activity and lung cancer risk by type of physical activity and gender. The RR of each study is represented by a circle, 95% Confidence Intervals (CIs) are represented by the horizontal lines. All studies except Knekt et al. have adjusted for smoking

activity (Bak et al. 2005; Colbert et al. 2002; Steindorf et al. 2006). Two early case control studies also reported statistically nonsignificant opposite results; Dosemeci et al. (Dosemeci et al. 1993) reported a non-significant decreased risk while Brownson et al. (Brownson et al. 1991) reported a statistically significant increased risk with increasing occupational activity.

5.2.2.2 Physical Activity, Smoking, and Lung Cancer Risk

Lung cancer is a multifactorial disease and smoking is thus far the most important carcino genic agent. Physical activity may interact with carcinogens in smoking and or/susceptibility genes and modify the association between smoking and lung cancer risk.

Among the eight studies (Kubik et al. 2008; Kubik et al. 2007; Kubik et al. 2004; Lee et al. 1999; Leitzmann et al. 2009; Mao et al. 2003; Sinner et al. 2006; Sprague et al. 2008) that stratified by smoking status (Fig. 5.3), Sprague et al. (Sprague et al. 2008) found a reduction in lung cancer risk with increasing total physical activity in both current and never/former smokers for both genders combined, although the risk reduction was somewhat stronger and statistically significant only in current smokers. Additionally, Leitzmann et al. (Leitzmann et al. 2009) found increased physical activity among both genders combined to be similarly related to decreased risk of total lung cancer among both current and former smokers, but unrelated to total lung cancer among never-smokers. Furthermore, the physical activity associated risk reduction for lung cancer found in a Canadian study was greater among smokers than nonsmokers (Mao et al. 2003). Thune and Lund (Thune and Lund 1997) stratified their analysis among male current smokers of over or above 15 cigarettes/day and found a statistically significant lung cancer risk reduction only among the heavy smokers, indicating a dose-dependent relationship. It has been suggested that the etiology of lung cancer among never-smokers is distinct from that among smokers (Leitzmann et al. 2009; Subramanian and Govindan 2007; Wakelee et al. 2007).

Cigarette smoking is associated with all histological types of lung cancer but the strength of the association varies by different histological subtypes of the disease: a stronger association is observed for squamous cell carcinoma and SCLC than for large cell carcinoma and adenocarcinoma (Khuder 2001). Given the differential effects smoking may have on histologic subtypes of lung carcinoma, smoking and physical activity may potentially have a different influence on the occurrence of each specific subtype of lung cancer. Only a few studies have investigated physical activity in relation to lung cancer by histological subtypes according to smoking status. Leitzmann et al. (Leitzmann et al. 2009) found an inverse relationship between increased physical activity and decreased lung cancer risk among current and former smokers for all histological subtypes (Leitzmann et al. 2009).

None of the studies that stratified their analyses by smoking status (Kubik et al. 2004; Leitzmann et al. 2009; Mao et al. 2003; Sinner et al. 2006; Sprague et al. 2008) found a significant inverse relationship between increased physical activity and decreased lung cancer risk among never-smokers. However, in a recent EPIC study (Rundle et al. 2010) recreational activity was observed to decrease lung cancer risk among ex-smokers (<10 years), and a non-significantly lower risk was observed among never-smokers compared to recreational inactive ex- or never-smokers, respectively. Furthermore, in the same study, the same intensity and amount of recreational physical activity was positively associated with glutathione (GSH)/hemoglobin levels, an important cofactor in detoxification of carcinogens of particular importance in the respiratory tract (Rundle et al.

5

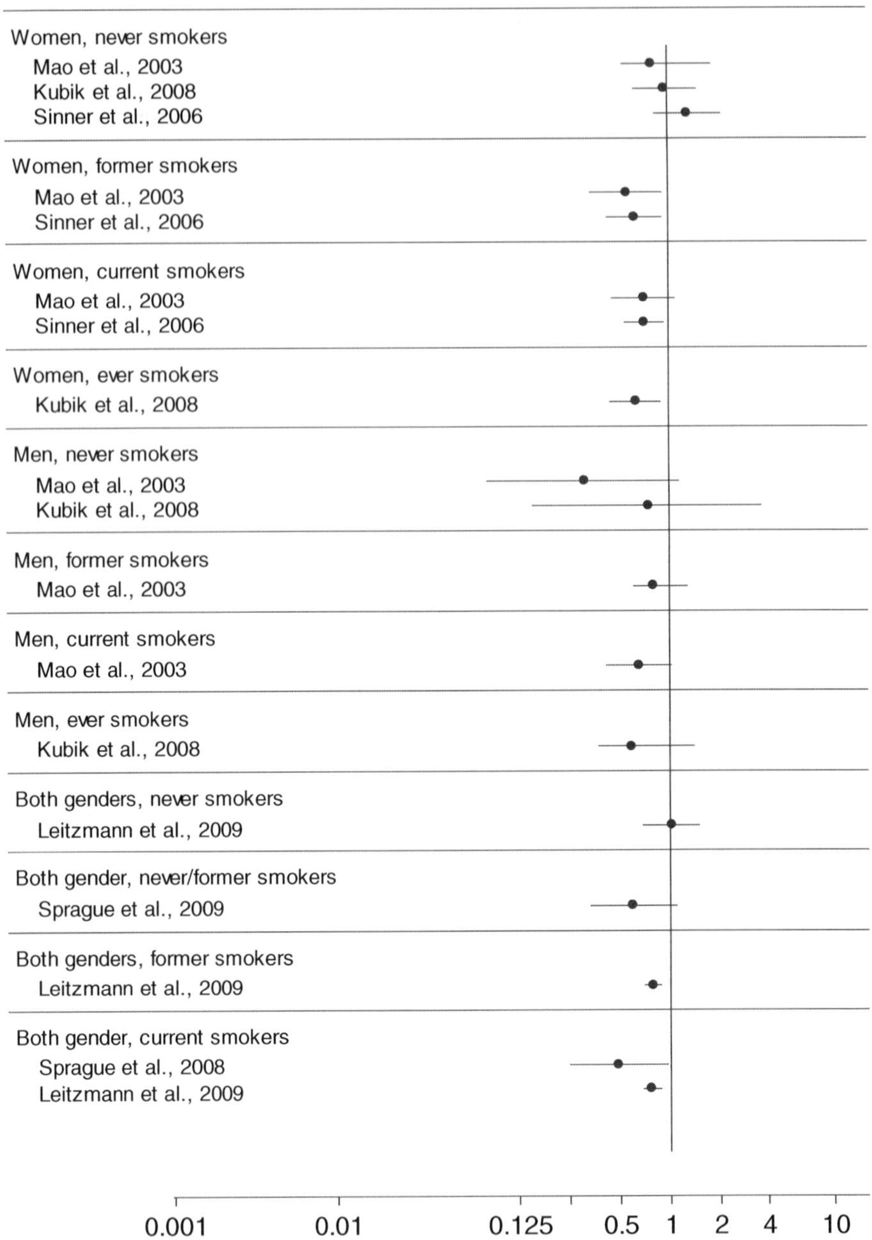

Fig. 5.3 Epidemiological studies of physical activity and lung cancer risk by smoking status and by gender. Relative risks (RR) for the lowest versus the highest level of physical activity and lung cancer risk by smoking status and gender. The RR of each study is represented by a circle, 95% Confidence Intervals (CIs) are represented by the horizontal lines

2010). These results point to important biological mechanisms and to associations among ex- and never-smokers. However, a relation between physical activity and lung cancer risk is also dependent on methodological factors such as the study design, sample size and consequent statistical power, exposure measurement, and possible misclassification. More studies are needed to clarify whether or not any association exists between physical activity and lung cancer among never-smokers.

5.2.2.3 Physical Activity and Histological Subtypes of Lung Cancer

The incidence rate patterns of the main histological subtypes of lung cancers – small cell (SCLC) and nonsmall cell (NSCLC) carcinoma (adenocarcinoma, squamous carcinoma and large cell carcinoma) – differ over time. Furthermore, the concept of differing mechanisms of lung carcinogenesis for the various histological subtypes supports a hypothesis that the etiology varies by tumor type; however it is still unclear whether or not the association between physical activity and lung cancer is different for the various histologic subtypes (Steindorf et al. 2006), and the research conducted in this field has yielded inconsistent results (Fig. 5.4). Thune and Lund found in a large Norwegian cohort that recreational physical activity had the strongest association with SCLC: the association was less marked for adenocarcinoma and no association was found for squamous cell carcinoma in men (Thune and Lund 1997). A Canadian study conducted by Mao and colleagues observed a greater risk reduction between recreational physical activity for squamous cell carcinoma in women and for SCLC in men (Mao et al. 2003). In a case control study of lifestyle and lung cancer associations by major histological subtypes, Kubik et al. found physical activity exercise in women to be inversely associated with the risk of both adenocarcinoma and SCLC, but not squamous cell cancer (Kubik et al. 2008). Leitzmann et al. reported in a recent large cohort study an inverse relation with physical activity that was apparent for all histologic subtypes of lung carcinomas (Leitzmann et al. 2009). Three other studies (Colbert et al. 2002; Sinner et al. 2006; Steindorf et al. 2006) reported nonsignificant inverse associations with physical activity that did not seem to vary by histologic subtype. These limited data underline the fact that more studies are warranted regarding the association between physical activity and subtypes of lung cancer.

5.2.2.4 Possible Effect Modifiers in Relation to Physical Activity and Lung Cancer

Studies suggest that there is substantial individual variation (inherited or acquired) in the susceptibility to respiratory carcinogens, pointing to possible effect modification between inhalation of carcinogens and the development of lung cancer. It is not clear if physical activity influences this association. Furthermore, age, gender, ethnicity, and body mass index (BMI) might be possible effect modifiers of the association between physical activity and lung cancer.

Earlier studies have indicated a stronger association for physical activity and lung cancer among younger participants (Alfano et al. 2004; Colbert et al. 2002). Alfano et al. suggested that the benefit of physical activity may not be great enough to counteract the carcinogenic effect of numerous years of cigarette smoking, which would likely be greater in older smoking patients (Alfano et al. 2004). It is not clear if age is an effect modifier among never-smokers, and the benefit of physical activity may vary by age and length of time period at exposure.

Far more men than women still die from lung cancer each year, but the gender gap in lung

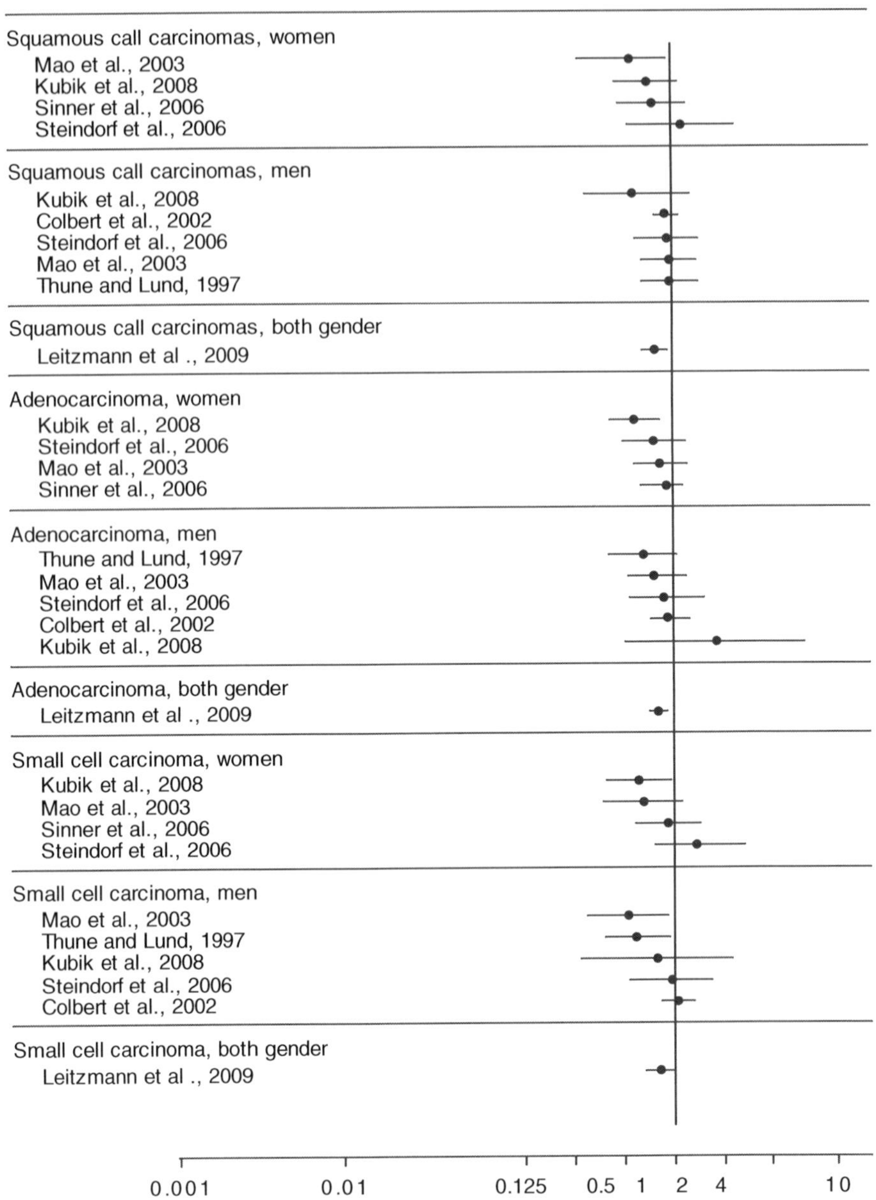

Fig. 5.4 Epidemiological studies of physical activity and lung cancer risk by histologic subtype and gender. Relative risks (RR) for the lowest versus the highest level of physical activity and lung cancer risk by histologic subtype and gender. The RR of each study is represented by a circle, 95% Confidence Interval (95% CIs) are represented by the horizontal lines. All studies have adjusted for smoking

cancer mortality is steadily narrowing and may eventually close (Jemal et al. 2003; Thun et al. 2006). This trend is most likely attributable to smoking patterns, with smoking prevalence having peaked approximately two decades earlier among men than women (Alberg et al. 2007; Thun et al. 2006). Thune and Lund (Thune and Lund 1997) found no effect of physical activity on lung cancer in women, only in men. Sprague et al. (Sprague et al. 2008) found that lung cancer risk declined with increasing total physical activity among both men and women, although the risk reduction was stronger and statistically significant only in men. As shown in this chapter, other studies (see Table 5.1 and Fig. 5.2) have found an association in both men and women, but the effect seems to be less clear for women than it is for men. These findings may be explained by the larger statistical power to detect any influence in certain studies because of, for example, the larger sample sizes of men versus women (Thune and Lund 1997).

Lung cancer incidence rates are similar among African-American and white women, while lung cancer occurrence is approximately 45% higher among African-American men than among white men (Alberg et al. 2007). Whether or not physical activity affects this association still remains unknown since no studies, to our knowledge, have examined effect modification by ethnicity or race.

Interestingly, a more profound risk reduction of lung cancer was observed among those with low and medium BMI compared to those with a high BMI in a Canadian study (Mao et al. 2003), while Leitzmann et al. (Leitzmann et al. 2009) found no difference in risk reduction with increasing physical activity among those with low, medium, and high BMI. More studies are needed in order to clarify whether or not body mass plays a role in modifying the effect of physical activity on lung cancer risk.

5.3 Hypothesized Biological Mechanisms Relating Physical Activity to Lung Cancer

Several plausible biological mechanisms have been hypothesized linking physical activity to reduced lung cancer risk. These mechanisms include increased pulmonary function reducing concentrations of carcinogenic agents in the lungs and shorter duration of agent–airway interaction, enhanced immune function, reduced inflammation, enhanced DNA repair capacity, and changes in growth factor levels (Fig. 5.5) (Lee et al. 1999; McTiernan 2008; Rundle 2005; Thune and Lund 1997). An understanding of these possible biological mechanisms is

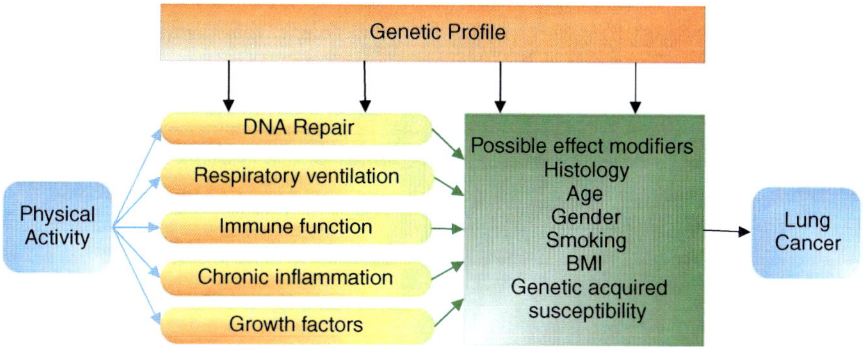

Fig. 5.5 Hypothesized biological mechanisms linking physical activity to lung cancer risk

5

needed to comprehend more completely how variation in physical activity can influence lung cancer risk.

Physical activity improves pulmonary function thereby improving pulmonary ventilation and perfusion (Cheng et al. 2003; Jakes et al. 2002; Sin et al. 2004). The improvement may reduce the amount of particle deposition and concentration of any carcinogenic agent in the airways and the duration of agent–air–particle interaction time (IARC 2002; Tockman et al. 1987). Interestingly, it has been found that reduced lung function is an important risk factor for lung cancer (Wasswa-Kintu et al. 2005), supporting a role for physical activity in preventing this lung disease.

Furthermore, regular physical activity enhances immune function (Fairey et al. 2005; Shephard and Shek 1995), which may also play a role in lung cancer etiology. Physical activity may improve the number or functional capacity of natural killer cells, protecting against carcinogenesis by recognizing and eliminating abnormal cells through acquired and/or innate immune system components (Jakobisiak et al. 2003; Rundle 2005; Wetmore and Ulrich 2006).

Additionally, the lung is an organ exposed to inflammation and infectious disease, which may increase susceptibility for malignant transformation (Engels 2008). Inflammation is a complex host response to a variety of injuries or insults, including microbial infections, chemical or particulate exposures (tobacco), and physical wounds (Engels 2008). Increased levels of proinflammatory factors, such as interleukin 6 (IL-6), C-reactive protein (CRP), and tumor necrosis factor-α (TNF-α) have been linked to increased cancer risk (Ballaz and Mulshine 2003). It is suggested that increasing levels of moderate intensity physical activity decreases inflammation markers, such as IL-6, CRP, and TNF-α, but not all studies are conclusive (Bruunsgaard 2005; Ford 2002; Kasapis and Thompson 2005; Sprague et al. 2008; Wetmore and Ulrich 2006).

Physical activity may protect against lung cancer risk by reversing DNA damage, or enhancing DNA repair capacity (Elosua et al. 2003). Inhaled carcinogens, such as benzo(a) pyrene in tobacco, radon, or asbestos can interact directly with the DNA of lung cells. Because the whole lung is exposed to inhaled carcinogens, several sites may accumulate different cancerous changes, leading to multiple cancers originating in different types of cells. High or moderate levels of physical activity may reduce the production of free radicals and carcinogenic metabolites produced by, for example, cigarette smoking (Asami et al. 1997; Rundle 2005). Because smoking plays such a major role in the etiology of lung cancer, residual confounding by this major risk factor remains a possibility in the pathway between physical activity and lung cancer.

Growth factors may also be reduced with increasing physical activity (Friedenreich and Orenstein 2002). Among the growth factors, insulin-like growth factors (IGFs) play a crucial role in regulating cell proliferation and differentiation (Pollak et al. 2004; Yu et al. 1999). IGFs are peptide hormones with a strong mitogenic effect on both normal and cancerous cells, including lung cancer cells (Jones and Clemmons 1995; Pollak et al. 2004). Higher IGF-1 levels have been associated with an increased risk of lung cancer in a case control study (Yu et al. 1999); however, other studies have observed no association between IGF-I and lung cancer risk (Ahn et al. 2006; London et al. 2002; Lukanova et al. 2001; Renehan et al. 2004).

Recent advances have occurred in understanding lung carcinogenesis, with the implementation of molecular epidemiological biomarker studies identifying the genetic profile of those most susceptible to disease (Reid et al. 2008). Susceptibility differences may be inherited or may be acquired through epigenetic mechanisms (Schwartz et al. 2007). A diverse range of genetic abnormalities are seen in lung cancer cells. Some may be markers of disease progression; others may have a direct role in lung cancer etiology by themselves or through gene–environment interactions. Common polymorphisms of certain genes may help explain why some smokers are more susceptible to lung cancer than others. In particular, glutathione S-transferase (GSTs), CYP1A1, and myeloperoxidase (MPO) have been extensively studied in relation to lung cancer (Schwartz et al. 2007). Additionally, individual variability in DNA repair genes, inflammation-related genes, and mutations have been studied as possible mechanisms that may be involved in lung cancer etiology (Schwartz et al. 2007). More recently, genome-wide associations studies (GWAS) have identified specific region on genes associated with lung cancer risk (Amos et al. 2008; Hung et al. 2008; Landi et al. 2009). However, to our knowledge, no studies today have elucidated the association of physical activity, susceptibility genes, and lung cancer risk, but susceptibility genes may interact and play an important role between physical activity and lung cancer.

In addition, effect modification by age, gender, BMI, and histological type of lung cancer are also possible. Hypothesized possible mechanisms and effect modifiers linking increased physical activity to reduced lung cancer are presented in Fig. 5.5.

5.4 Main Findings and Further Implications

This chapter focuses on a relatively new research area and the evidence is still inconclusive regarding whether or not physical activity influences lung cancer risk. When judging the evidence regarding the association between physical activity and lung cancer several methodological issues need to be considered. The observational epidemiological studies conducted thus far show an inverse graded dose–response association between physical activity and lung cancer risk and suggest that physical activity decreases lung cancer risk by 20–30% for women and 20–50% for men. These clear patterns have been observed across continents, time periods, and among both genders and support a true effect. Moreover, hypothesized plausible biological mechanisms exist, including improved pulmonary function, reduced concentrations of carcinogenic agents in the lungs, enhanced immune function, reduced inflammation, enhanced DNA repair capacity, changes in growth factor levels, and possible gene–physical activity interactions. Furthermore, recent studies identifying the genetic profile of those most susceptible to lung cancer support the fact that genetic factors may play a role linking physical activity to lung cancer. These associations might be explained by variation in susceptibility, indicating a gene–environment interaction and are supported by hypothesized biological mechanisms supporting the preventive role of physical activity on lung cancer risk. However, even if emerging evidence is available, the complex relationship between smoking, physical activity, and lung cancer risk has not been sufficiently investigated and needs further elucidation. Importantly, the variation in physical activity measurements used in the presented studies points to caution when interpreting the results. As well, the effect of physical activity on lung cancer risk may vary by smoking status, histological subtypes of lung cancer, gender, and body mass.

In conclusion, physical activity is a preventive measure influencing pulmonary and physical functioning throughout life that can be instituted to decrease the risk of several health problems, including possibly lung cancer. If physical activity is proven to protect against lung cancer in further research, it can be seen to provide an opportunity to reduce the incidence of this fatal cancer. However, so far the most important health strategy for lung cancer prevention has been to discourage smoking

5

initiation among adolescents, especially in the developing world, and among women, and to advocate for smoking cessation among tobacco users of any age.

Acknowledgment Aina Emaus was funded by the Norwegian Cancer Society (grant 05087) and Inger Thune was funded by The Research Council of Norway while working on this book chapter. The authors would like to express their appreciation for the helpful suggestions and discussions made by Jessica Clague and other colleagues at the Department of Etiology, City of Hope, CA, USA.

References

Ahn J, Weinstein SJ, Snyder K, Pollak MN, Virtamo J, Albanes D (2006) No association between serum insulin-like growth factor (IGF)-I, IGF-binding protein-3, and lung cancer risk. Cancer Epidemiol Biomarkers Prev 15:2010–2012

Albanes D, Blair A, Taylor PR (1989) Physical activity and risk of cancer in the NHANES I population. Am J Public Health 79:744–750

Alberg AJ, Ford JG, Samet JM (2007) Epidemiology of lung cancer: ACCP evidence-based clinical practice guidelines, 2nd edn. Chest 132: 29S–55S

Alfano CM, Klesges RC, Murray DM, Bowen DJ, McTiernan A, Vander Weg MW, Robinson LA, Cartmel B, Thornquist MD, Barnett M, Goodman GE, Omenn GS (2004) Physical activity in relation to all-site and lung cancer incidence and mortality in current and former smokers. Cancer Epidemiol Biomarkers Prev 13:2233–2241

American Cancer Society (2009) Cancer Facts & Figures 2009. American Cancer Society, Atlanta

Amos CI, Xu W, Spitz MR (1999) Is there a genetic basis for lung cancer susceptibility? Recent Results Cancer Res 151:3–12

Amos CI, Wu X, Broderick P, Gorlov IP, Gu J, Eisen T, Dong Q, Zhang Q, Gu X, Vijayakrishnan J, Sullivan K, Matakidou A, Wang Y, Mills G, Doheny K, Tsai YY, Chen WV, Shete S, Spitz MR, Houlston RS (2008) Genome-wide association scan of tag SNPs identifies a susceptibility locus for lung cancer at 15q25.1. Nat Genet 40:616–622

Asami S, Manabe H, Miyake J, Tsurudome Y, Hirano T, Yamaguchi R, Itoh H, Kasai H (1997) Cigarette smoking induces an increase in oxidative DNA damage, 8-hydroxydeoxyguanosine, in a central site of the human lung. Carcinogenesis 18:1763–1766

Bak H, Christensen J, Thomsen BL, Tjonneland A, Overvad K, Loft S, Raaschou-Nielsen O (2005) Physical activity and risk for lung cancer in a Danish cohort. Int J Cancer 116:439–444

Ballaz S, Mulshine JL (2003) The potential contributions of chronic inflammation to lung carcinogenesis. Clin Lung Cancer 5:46–62

Blair SN, Powell KE, Bazzarre TL, Early JL, Epstein LH, Green LW, Harris SS, Haskell WL, King AC, Koplan J et al. (1993) Physical inactivity. Workshop V. AHA Prevention Conference III. Behavior change and compliance: keys to improving cardiovascular health. Circulation 88:1402–1405

Bouchard C (2001) Physical activity and health: introduction to the dose-response symposium. Med Sci Sports Exerc 33:S347–S350

Brownson RC, Chang JC, Davis JR, Smith CA (1991) Physical activity on the job and cancer in Missouri. Am J Public Health 81:639–642

Bruske-Hohlfeld I (2009) Environmental and occupational risk factors for lung cancer. Methods Mol Biol 472:3–23

Bruunsgaard H (2005) Physical activity and modulation of systemic low-level inflammation. J Leukoc Biol 78:819–835

Cheng YJ, Macera CA, Addy CL, Sy FS, Wieland D, Blair SN (2003) Effects of physical activity on exercise tests and respiratory function. Br J Sports Med 37:521–528

Colbert LH, Hartman TJ, Tangrea JA, Pietinen P, Virtamo J, Taylor PR, Albanes D (2002) Physical activity and lung cancer risk in male smokers. Int J Cancer 98:770–773

DeVita VT, Lawrence TS, Rosenberg SA (2008) DeVita, Hellman, and Rosenberg's cancer: principles & practice of oncology. Philadelphia, PA

Dosemeci M, Hayes RB, Vetter R, Hoover RN, Tucker M, Engin K, Unsal M, Blair A (1993) Occupational physical activity, socioeconomic status, and risks of 15 cancer sites in Turkey. Cancer Cause Control 4:313–321

Elosua R, Molina L, Fito M, Arquer A, Sanchez-Quesada JL, Covas MI, Ordonez-Llanos J, Marrugat J (2003) Response of oxidative stress biomarkers to a 16-week aerobic physical activity program, and to acute physical activity, in healthy young men and women. Atherosclerosis 167:327–334

Engels EA (2008) Inflammation in the development of lung cancer: epidemiological evidence. Expert Rev Anticancer Ther 8:605–615

Fairey AS, Courneya KS, Field CJ, Bell GJ, Jones LW, Mackey JR (2005) Randomized controlled trial of exercise and blood immune function in postmenopausal breast cancer survivors. J Appl Physiol 98:1534–1540

Ferlay J, Autier P, Boniol M, Heanue M, Colombet M, Boyle P (2007) Estimates of the cancer incidence and mortality in Europe in 2006. Ann Oncol 18:581–592

Ford ES (2002) Does exercise reduce inflammation? Physical activity and C-reactive protein among U.S. adults. Epidemiology 13:561–568

Friedenreich CM, Orenstein MR (2002) Physical activity and cancer prevention: etiologic evidence and biological mechanisms. J Nutr 132:3456S–3464S

Hung RJ, McKay JD, Gaborieau V, Boffetta P, Hashibe M, Zaridze D, Mukeria A, Szeszenia-Dabrowska N, Lissowska J, Rudnai P, Fabianova E, Mates D, Bencko V, Foretova L, Janout V, Chen C, Goodman G, Field JK, Liloglou T, Xinarianos G, Cassidy A, McLaughlin J, Liu G, Narod S, Krokan HE, Skorpen F, Elvestad MB, Hveem K, Vatten L, Linseisen J, Clavel-Chapelon F, Vineis P, Bueno-de-Mesquita HB, Lund E, Martinez C, Bingham S, Rasmuson T, Hainaut P, Riboli E, Ahrens W, Benhamou S, Lagiou P, Trichopoulos D, Holcatova I, Merletti F, Kjaerheim K, Agudo A, Macfarlane G, Talamini R, Simonato L, Lowry R, Conway DI, Znaor A, Healy C, Zelenika D, Boland A, Delepine M, Foglio M, Lechner D, Matsuda F, Blanche H, Gut I, Heath S, Lathrop M, Brennan P (2008) A susceptibility locus for lung cancer maps to nicotinic acetylcholine receptor subunit genes on 15q25. Nature 452:633–637

IARC (2002) Weight control and physical activity. International Agency for Research on Cancer, Lyon

Inoue M, Yamamoto S, Kurahashi N, Iwasaki M, Sasazuki S, Tsugane S (2008) Daily total physical activity level and total cancer risk in men and women: results from a large-scale population-based cohort study in Japan. Am J Epidemiol 168:391–403

Jakes RW, Day NE, Patel B, Khaw KT, Oakes S, Luben R, Welch A, Bingham S, Wareham NJ (2002) Physical inactivity is associated with lower forced expiratory volume in 1 second: European prospective investigation into cancer-norfolk prospective population study. Am J Epidemiol 156:139–147

Jakobisiak M, Lasek W, Golab J (2003) Natural mechanisms protecting against cancer. Immunol Lett 90:103–122

Jemal A, Travis WD, Tarone RE, Travis L, Devesa SS (2003) Lung cancer rates convergence in young men and women in the United States: analysis by birth cohort and histologic type. Int J Cancer 105:101–107

Jemal A, Siegel R, Ward E, Hao Y, Xu J, Thun MJ (2009) Cancer statistics, 2009. CA Cancer J Clin 59:225–249

Jones JI, Clemmons DR (1995) Insulin-like growth factors and their binding proteins: biological actions. Endocr Rev 16:3–34

Kasapis C, Thompson PD (2005) The effects of physical activity on serum C-reactive protein and inflammatory markers: a systematic review. J Am Coll Cardiol 45:1563–1569

Khuder SA (2001) Effect of cigarette smoking on major histological types of lung cancer: a meta-analysis. Lung Cancer 31:139–148

Knekt P, Raitasalo R, Heliovaara M, Lehtinen V, Pukkala E, Teppo L, Maatela J, Aromaa A (1996) Elevated lung cancer risk among persons with depressed mood. Am J Epidemiol 144: 1096–1103

Knuth AG, Hallal PC (2009) Temporal trends in physical activity: a systematic review. J Phys Act Health 6:548–559

Kubik A, Zatloukal P, Tomasek L, Pauk N, Petruzelka L, Plesko I (2004) Lung cancer risk among nonsmoking women in relation to diet and physical activity. Neoplasma 51: 136–143

Kubik A, Zatloukal P, Tomasek L, Pauk N, Havel L, Dolezal J, Plesko I (2007) Interactions between smoking and other exposures associated with lung cancer risk in women: diet and physical activity. Neoplasma 54:83–88

Kubik A, Zatloukal P, Tomasek L, Dolezal J, Syllabova L, Kara J, Kopecky P, Plesko I (2008)

5

A case-control study of lifestyle and lung cancer associations by histological types. Neoplasma 55:192–199

Kubik AK, Zatloukal P, Tomasek L, Petruzelka L (2002) Lung cancer risk among Czech women: a case-control study. Prev Med 34:436–444

Landi MT, Chatterjee N, Yu K, Goldin LR, Goldstein AM, Rotunno M, Mirabello L, Jacobs K, Wheeler W, Yeager M, Bergen AW, Li Q, Consonni D, Pesatori AC, Wacholder S, Thun M, Diver R, Oken M, Virtamo J, Albanes D, Wang Z, Burdette L, Doheny KF, Pugh EW, Laurie C, Brennan P, Hung R, Gaborieau V, McKay JD, Lathrop M, McLaughlin J, Wang Y, Tsao MS, Spitz MR, Wang Y, Krokan H, Vatten L, Skorpen F, Arnesen E, Benhamou S, Bouchard C, Metsapalu A, Vooder T, Nelis M, Valk K, Field JK, Chen C, Goodman G, Sulem P, Thorleifsson G, Rafnar T, Eisen T, Sauter W, Rosenberger A, Bickeboller H, Risch A, Chang-Claude J, Wichmann HE, Stefansson K, Houlston R, Amos CI, Fraumeni JF Jr, Savage SA, Bertazzi PA, Tucker MA, Chanock S, Caporaso NE (2009) A genome-wide association study of lung cancer identifies a region of chromosome 5p15 associated with risk for adenocarcinoma. Am J Hum Genet 85:679–691

Lee IM, Sesso HD, Paffenbarger RS Jr (1999) Physical activity and risk of lung cancer. Int J Epidemiol 28:620–625

Lee SY, Kim MT, Jee SH, Im JS (2002) Does hypertension increase mortality risk from lung cancer? A prospective cohort study on smoking, hypertension and lung cancer risk among Korean men. J Hypertens 20:617–622

Leitzmann MF, Koebnick C, Abnet CC, Freedman ND, Park Y, Hollenbeck A, Ballard-Barbash R, Schatzkin A (2009) Prospective study of physical activity and lung cancer by histologic type in current, former, and never smokers. Am J Epidemiol 169:542–553

London SJ, Yuan JM, Travlos GS, Gao YT, Wilson RE, Ross RK, Yu MC (2002) Insulin-like growth factor I, IGF-binding protein 3, and lung cancer risk in a prospective study of men in China. J Natl Cancer Inst 94:749–754

Lukanova A, Toniolo P, Akhmedkhanov A, Biessy C, Haley NJ, Shore RE, Riboli E, Rinaldi S, Kaaks R (2001) A prospective study of insulin-like growth factor-I, IGF-binding proteins-1, -2 and -3 and lung cancer risk in women. Int J Cancer 92:888–892

Mao Y, Pan S, Wen SW, Johnson KC (2003) Physical activity and the risk of lung cancer in Canada. Am J Epidemiol 158:564–575

McTiernan A (2008) Mechanisms linking physical activity with cancer. Nat Rev Cancer 8:205–211

Olson JE, Yang P, Schmitz K, Vierkant RA, Cerhan JR, Sellers TA (2002) Differential association of body mass index and fat distribution with three major histologic types of lung cancer: evidence from a cohort of older women. Am J Epidemiol 156:606–615

Parkin DM, Whelan SL, Ferlay J, Teppo L, Thomas DM (2006) Cancer incidence in five continents, vol. VIII. I S P N 155. International Agency for Research on Cancer, Lyon, France

Pollak MN, Schernhammer ES, Hankinson SE (2004) Insulin-like growth factors and neoplasia. Nat Rev Cancer 4:505–518

Reid ME, Santella R, Ambrosone CB (2008) Molecular epidemiology to better predict lung cancer risk. Clin Lung Cancer 9:149–153

Renehan AG, Zwahlen M, Minder C, O'Dwyer ST, Shalet SM, Egger M (2004) Insulin-like growth factor (IGF)-I, IGF binding protein-3, and cancer risk: systematic review and meta-regression analysis. Lancet 363:1346–1353

Rundle A (2005) Molecular epidemiology of physical activity and cancer. Cancer Epidemiol Biomarkers Prev 14:227–236

Rundle A, Richie J, Steindorf K, Peluso M, Overvad K, Raaschou-Nielsen O, Clavel-Chapelon F, Linseisen JP, Boeing H, Trichopoulou A, Palli D, Krogh V, Tumino R, Panico S, Bueno-De-Mesquita HB, Peeters PH, Lund E, Gonzalez CA, Martinez C, Dorronsoro M, Barricarte A, Tormo MJ, Quiros J, Agudo A, Berglund G, Jarvholm B, Bingham S, Key TJ, Gormally E, Saracci R, Kaaks R, Riboli E, Vineis P (2010) Physical activity and lung cancer among non-smokers: a pilot molecular epidemiological study within EPIC. Biomarkers 15:20–30

Sano H, Marugame T (2006) International comparisons of cumulative risk of lung cancer, from cancer incidence in five continents, vol VIII. Jpn J Clin Oncol 36:334–335

Schnohr P, Gronbaek M, Petersen L, Hein HO, Sorensen TI (2005) Physical activity in leisure-time and risk of cancer: 14-year follow-up of 28, 000 Danish men and women. Scand J Public Health 33:244–249

Schwartz AG, Prysak GM, Bock CH, Cote ML (2007) The molecular epidemiology of lung cancer. Carcinogenesis 28:507–518

Sellers TA, Potter JD, Folsom AR (1991) Association of incident lung cancer with family history of female reproductive cancers: the Iowa Women's Health Study. Genet Epidemiol 8:199–208

Severson RK, Nomura AM, Grove JS, Stemmermann GN (1989) A prospective analysis of physical activity and cancer. Am J Epidemiol 130:522–529

Shephard RJ, Shek PN (1995) Cancer, immune function, and physical activity. Can J Appl Physiol 20:1–25

Sin DD, Jones RL, Mannino DM, Paul Man SF (2004) Forced expiratory volume in 1 second and physical activity in the general population. Am J Med 117:270–273

Sinner P, Folsom AR, Harnack L, Eberly LE, Schmitz KH (2006) The association of physical activity with lung cancer incidence in a cohort of older women: the Iowa Women's Health Study. Cancer Epidemiol Biomarkers Prev 15: 2359–2363

Sprague BL, Trentham-Dietz A, Klein BE, Klein R, Cruickshanks KJ, Lee KE, Hampton JM (2008) Physical activity, white blood cell count, and lung cancer risk in a prospective cohort study. Cancer Epidemiol Biomarkers Prev 17: 2714–2722

Steenland K, Nowlin S, Palu S (1995) Cancer incidence in the National Health and Nutrition Survey I. Follow-up data: diabetes, cholesterol, pulse and physical activity. Cancer Epidemiol Biomarkers Prev 4:807–811

Steindorf K, Friedenreich C, Linseisen J, Rohrmann S, Rundle A, Veglia F, Vineis P, Johnsen NF, Tjonneland A, Overvad K, Raaschou-Nielsen O, Clavel-Chapelon F, Boutron-Ruault MC, Schulz M, Boeing H, Trichopoulou A, Kalapothaki V, Koliva M, Krogh V, Palli D, Tumino R, Panico S, Monninkhof E, Peeters PH, Boshuizen HC, Bueno-de-Mesquita HB, Chirlaque MD, Agudo A, Larranaga N, Quiros JR, Martinez C, Barricarte A, Janzon L, Berglund G, Bingham S, Khaw KT, Key TJ, Norat T, Jenab M, Cust A, Riboli E (2006) Physical activity and lung cancer risk in the European Prospective Investigation into Cancer and Nutrition Cohort. Int J Cancer 119:2389–2397

Subramanian J, Govindan R (2007) Lung cancer in never smokers: a review. J Clin Oncol 25: 561–570

Tardon A, Lee WJ, Delgado-Rodriguez M, Dosemeci M, Albanes D, Hoover R, Blair A (2005) Leisure-time physical activity and lung cancer: a meta-analysis. Cancer Causes Control 16:389–397

Thun MJ, Henley SJ, Burns D, Jemal A, Shanks TG, Calle EE (2006) Lung cancer death rates in lifelong nonsmokers. J Natl Cancer Inst 98: 691–699

Thune I, Lund E (1997) The influence of physical activity on lung-cancer risk: a prospective study of 81, 516 men and women. Int J Cancer 70: 57–62

Tockman MS, Anthonisen NR, Wright EC, Donithan MG (1987) Airways obstruction and the risk for lung cancer. Ann Intern Med 106:512–518

Wakelee HA, Chang ET, Gomez SL, Keegan TH, Feskanich D, Clarke CA, Holmberg L, Yong LC, Kolonel LN, Gould MK, West DW (2007) Lung cancer incidence in never smokers. J Clin Oncol 25:472–478

Wannamethee SG, Shaper AG, Walker M (2001) Physical activity and risk of cancer in middle-aged men. Br J Cancer 85:1311–1316

Wasswa-Kintu S, Gan WQ, Man SF, Pare PD, Sin DD (2005) Relationship between reduced forced expiratory volume in one second and the risk of lung cancer: a systematic review and meta-analysis. Thorax 60:570–575

WCRF/AICR (2007) World Cancer Research Fund/American Institute for Cancer Research: food, nutrition, physical activity, and the prevention of cancer: a global perspective. AICR, Washington DC

Wetmore C, Ulrich CM (2006) Mechanisms associating physical activity with cancer incidence: exercise and immune function. CRC Press, Taylor & Francis

Yu H, Spitz MR, Mistry J, Gu J, Hong WK, Wu X (1999) Plasma levels of insulin-like growth factor-I and lung cancer risk: a case-control analysis. J Natl Cancer Inst 91:151–156

Yun YH, Lim MK, Won YJ, Park SM, Chang YJ, Oh SW, Shin SA (2008) Dietary preference, physical activity, and cancer risk in men: national health insurance corporation study. BMC Cancer 8:366

Physical Activity and Hematologic Cancer Prevention

6

Sai Yi Pan and Howard Morrison

Abstract This chapter presents the epidemio logic evidence on the association between physical activity and hematologic cancers and related hypothesized biologic mechanisms. Some preliminary indications of a protective role for physical activity for non-Hodgkin's lymphoma, leukemia, multiple myeloma, and Hodgkin's lymphoma exist, but the level of epidemiologic evidence is still insufficient to make any definitive conclusions regarding the nature of these associations. Several plausible biologic mechanisms underlying the possible associations between physical activity and hematologic cancers have been proposed, including enhancement of immune function, reduction in obesity, improvement of antioxidant defense systems, impact on metabolic hormones, and anti-inflammatory effects. Future studies should improve the estimation of physical activity by using more reliable, valid, and comprehensive measurement tools, assessing all components of physical activity (type, intensity, and time period), and conducting intervention studies to evaluate the effect of physical activity on various biomarkers of cancer in order to provide further insight into plausible biologic mechanisms underlying the possible association between physical activity and hematologic cancers.

S.Y. Pan (✉) and H. Morrison
Centre for Chronic Disease Prevention and Control, Public Health Agency of Canada, 785 Carling Avenue, Locator: 6807B Ottawa, Ontario, K1A 0K9, Canada
e-mail: sai.yi.pan@phac-aspc.gc.ca; howard.morrison@phac-aspc.gc.ca

6.1 Introduction

Hematologic cancers are cancers of the blood, bone marrow, and lymphatic tissues, and include leukemia, Hodgkin's lymphoma (HL), non-Hodgkin's lymphoma (NHL), and myeloma. Leukemia is divided into lymphocytic leukemia and myelogenous leukemia (also known as myeloid or myelocytic leukemia), and may be either chronic or acute (Bhatia and Robison 1999). According to the World Health Organization classification of lymphomas, which was based on the Revised European–American Lymphoma classification, HL (also called Hodgkin's disease) includes two main types: nodular lymphocyte predominant and classic HL (the latter is further divided into four histologically and clinically defined subtypes: nodular sclerosis, mixed cellularity, lymphocyte rich, and lymphocyte depleted) (Harris et al. 2000). NHL is a heterogeneous

K.S. Courneya and C.M. Friedenreich (eds.), *Physical Activity and Cancer*, Recent Results in Cancer Research 186, DOI: 10.1007/978-3-642-04231-7_6,

6

group of malignancies and classified into dozens of distinct histologic entities with the most common types being diffuse large B-cell lymphoma and follicular lymphoma (Harris et al. 1994, 1999, 2000; Alexander et al. 2007a). Multiple myeloma (MM) is a cancer of plasma cells that is characterized by skeletal destruction, renal failure, anemia, and hypercalcemia (Sirohi and Powles 2006; Alexander et al. 2007b). MM is closely related to monoclonal gammopathy of unknown significance (MGUS) and is sometimes preceded by MGUS, a condition common in older populations. MM develops from MGUS at the rate of about 1% per year (Sirohi and Powles 2006).

6.1.1 Epidemiology

According to global cancer statistics, in 2002, 6.9% of all cancer cases and 7.1% of all cancer deaths were cases with, and deaths from, hematologic cancer (including leukemia, NHL, HL, and MM) (Parkin et al. 2005). Worldwide, leukemia represented 2.8% of all cancer cases and 3.3% of all cancer deaths in 2002; the age-standardized incidence rates were 5.9 per 100,000 for men and 4.1 for women, and the age-standardized mortality rates were 4.3 and 3.1 per 100,000 for men and women; the incidence was lowest in sub-Saharan Africa and highest in North America, Australia, and New Zealand (Parkin et al. 2005). Among children and teens less than 20 years old, leukemia is the most common cancer and the leading cause of cancer death (U.S. Cancer Statistics Working Group 2009; Canadian Cancer Society 2009; Lightfoot 2005). Chronic lymphocytic leukemia (CLL) accounts for 30% of all leukemia and is the most common form of leukemia among adults in the developed countries while it is most often diagnosed over age 55 and almost never affects children (Kalil and Cheson 1999); however, acute lymphocytic leukemia (ALL) represents over 80% of all childhood leukemia and also affects adults (Lightfoot 2005). Chronic myeloid leukemia (CML) mainly affects adults and its incidence increases with age and is higher in men than in women (Rohrbacher and Hasford 2009). Acute myeloid leukemia (AML) occurs in both adults and children, accounting for approximately 25% of all leukemia in adults in the Western world and 15–20% of all leukemia cases in children aged ≤15 years (Deschler and Lubbert 2006).

NHL accounted for 2.8% of all cancer cases and 2.6% of cancer deaths in 2002 worldwide, with world incidence rates of 6.1 and 3.9 per 100,000 for men and women, respectively, and mortality rates of 3.5 and 2.3 for men and women (Parkin et al. 2005). The higher incidence in men than in women is apparent throughout all age groups. NHL incidence is higher in whites than in blacks, and in Northern America, Australia, and Western Europe than in Asia, Eastern Europe, and Africa (Muller et al. 2005; Curado et al. 2007; Ferlay et al. 2010). Higher rates of follicular lymphoma have been observed in Western nations than elsewhere, as have aggressive NHL, T-cell lymphomas, and extranodal NHL in Asians, endemic Burkitt's lymphoma in Africa, and intestinal extranodal NHL in the Middle East (Muller et al. 2005). The incidence and mortality of NHL have steadily increased in many countries of the world, but have stabilized in recent years (Alexander et al. 2007a; Muller et al. 2005). This increase has been observed in both men and women, white and black people, younger and older persons, and is more evident for aggressive NHL among older persons (Muller et al. 2005).

HL is a rare malignancy with a worldwide incidence rate of 1.2 per 100,000 for men and 0.8 for women, and a death rate of 0.4 per 100,000 (Parkin et al. 2005). While North America and Europe have the highest incidence rates of 2–3 per 100,000 (Caporaso et al. 2009) with a similar death rate of 0.4 per

100,000 (Horner et al. 2009), HL is rare in Asia (Curado et al. 2007). Data from the USA showed that the HL incidence rate was highest among whites, followed by African-Americans and Hispanics, and lowest among people of Asian descent (Caporaso et al. 2009). HL exhibited a bimodal age-incidence shape with a first peak in the third decade and a second peak after the age of 50 in industrialized countries, whereas HL occurs mainly in children and in the elderly in developing countries (Caporaso et al. 2009; Parkin et al. 2005).

MM accounted for about 0.8% of all cancer diagnoses and 0.9% of cancer deaths in 2002 worldwide (Parkin et al. 2005), while it accounted for approximately 1.3% of all cancers diagnosed in Canada (Canadian Cancer Society 2009) and 1.2% in the United States (U.S. Cancer Statistics Working Group, 2009). In 2002, the worldwide age-standardized incidence rates were 1.7 and 1.2 per 100,000 population for men and women, respectively (Parkin et al. 2005). Incidence rates were higher in America, Europe, and Oceania than in Asia, and highest among African-Americans (Curado et al. 2007). The incidence of MM has increased slightly in most parts of the world since 1975 and improved case ascertainment might be one of the reasons for this increase (Bray et al. 2001; Morgan et al. 2002). MM is rarely diagnosed before the age of 40, with incidence increasing rapidly after that age (Alexander et al. 2007b).

6.1.2 Etiology and Risk Factors

The etiologies of these hematopoietic cancers are largely unknown. Family history, obesity, genetic susceptibility, infection, exposure to ionizing radiation, hair dyes, chemicals such as benzene, insecticides, herbicides, and animal rearing, and chemicals used in the rubber industry are believed to be the putative risk factors for leukemia (Lightfoot 2005; Bhatia and Robison 1999; Larsson and Wolk 2008). Suspected risk factors for NHL include immunosuppression; infections of human T-cell lymphotropic virus (type I and II), Epstein-Barr Virus, *Helicobacter pylori*, hepatitis C, and simian virus 40; ultraviolet radiation; chemicals and agricultural exposure, hair dyes; blood transfusions (Fisher and Fisher 2004; Alexander et al. 2007a); and obesity (Larsson and Wolk 2007b). Epstein-Barr virus infection has long been considered as the etiologic agent for HL; autoimmune diseases or conditions, organ or bone marrow transplants, and genetic factors have also been suggested to be associated with an increased HL risk (Caporaso et al. 2009). Both environmental and genetic factors may play a role in the development of MM. Age is the most significant risk factor for developing myeloma, with people under 40 rarely developing the disease. Chronic immune stimulation, autoimmune disorders, MGUS, ionizing radiation, agricultural exposure to pesticides or herbicides, long-term use of hair dyes, and obesity have been suggested to be associated with MM (Alexander et al. 2007b; Larsson and Wolk 2007a).

Because the etiologies of these cancers are poorly understood, identification of modifiable risk factors for these diseases is particularly important for the purpose of prevention and control. There is convincing evidence to support a role for physical activity in preventing cancers of the colon and breast, whereas physical activity likely reduces the risk of cancers of the endometrium, lung, and prostate (Pan and Desmeules 2009). Obesity is suggested to be a risk factor for NHL, leukemia, and MM, and immune deficiency is also considered to be associated with NHL and HL. While physical activity has been hypothesized to reduce obesity and improve immune function, it may decrease the risk of these cancers.

This review aims to provide: (1) a review of the literature on the epidemiologic evidence for the association between physical activity and hematologic cancers; and (2) an overview of the

6

hypothesized biologic mechanisms operative in the associations.

6.2 Epidemiologic Studies on Physical Activity and Hematologic Cancers

6.2.1 Non-Hodgkin's Lymphoma (NHL)

There have been four cohort studies (Lu et al. 2009; Cerhan et al. 2002; Paffenbarger et al. 1987, 1992) and four case-control studies (Pan et al. 2005; Cerhan et al. 2005; Zahm et al. 1999; Brownson et al. 1991) published that assessed the association between physical activity (PA) and NHL risk. A summary of these studies is provided in Table 6.1.

The largest cohort study (Lu et al. 2009) found no evidence of an association of NHL risk with long-term recreational PA or activity in the past 3 years or activity during early adulthood (prior to age 25 years), overall and by histologic subtype. The Iowa Women's Health Study (Cerhan et al. 2002) also observed no association for NHL overall, or diffuse or small lymphocytic lymphoma, although there was a suggestion of nonsignificant inverse association for follicular subtype. In addition, there were suggestive nonsignificant effects of sports or leisure-time physical activity on NHL risk in two other cohort studies (Paffenbarger et al. 1987, 1992); however, these two studies had relatively small numbers of cases, with one as a mortality study (Paffenbarger et al. 1987).

Of the four relatively large case-control studies, three (Cerhan et al. 2005; Zahm et al. 1999; Brownson et al. 1991) assessed the impact of occupational PA on the risk of NHL and found no association. Two population-based studies examined the effect of recreational PA. One (Pan et al. 2005) observed various degrees of reduction in NHL risk related to recreational PA for both men and women, and for all four histologic subtypes of NHL, with a larger effect for follicular, small lymphocytic types and a smaller effect for the diffuse type. The other study (Cerhan et al. 2005) suggested that nonoccupational PA was inversely but weakly associated with risks of all NHL and of diffuse and follicular NHL, with a slightly stronger inverse association for vigorous than for moderate leisure-time PA.

Overall, although there is a suggestive protective role of recreational PA against NHL, study results are inconsistent, and there is insufficient evidence for a firm conclusion on the relationship between PA and NHL.

6.2.2 Leukemia

Three cohort studies (Cerhan et al. 2002; Paffenbarger et al. 1987, 1992) and two case-control studies (Brownson et al. 1991; Kasim et al. 2009) have been conducted on the association between leukemia and physical activity (Table 6.2). All three cohort studies had a small number of cases: 63 cases of B-cell chronic lymphocytic leukemia (Cerhan et al. 2002), 81 cases of leukemia (Paffenbarger et al. 1992), and 24 deaths of leukemia (Paffenbarger et al. 1987), respectively, and all cohort studies demonstrated no association between physical activity and leukemia risk.

Of the two case-control studies, one assessed occupational physical activity by using occupational title as an index of physical activity and used cancer patients other than leukemia as the control group (Brownson et al. 1991). No effect of occupational physical activity on leukemia risk was found in this study. Another case-control study on recreational physical activity and the risk of adult leukemia (Kasim et al. 2009) observed a 25% reduction in leukemia risk

Table 6.1 Studies of physical activity and the risk of non-Hodgkin's lymphoma

Author, date, study location	Study dates	Study population	No. of cases	Physical activity assessment	RR or OR (95% CI)	Trend	Adjustment for confounding
Cohort studies							
Lu et al. 2009, USA	1995–2007	The California Teachers Study. 121,216 women aged 22–84 years	574 all B-cell NHL 155 diffuse large 121 follicular 124 CLL/SLL	Strenuous & moderate recreational PA (long-term from high school to age 54 yrs or age at cohort entry and recent in the past 3 yrs before cohort entry	≥4 versus ≤0.5 h week^{-1} year^{-1}: *Long-term PA*: All: 1.00 (0.78–1.29) Diffuse large: 0.97 (0.60–1.55) Follicular: 1.29 (0.69–2.41) CLL/SLL: 0.94 (0.55–1.60) Recent PA (the past 3 years): All: 1.11 (0.86–1.44) Diffuse large: 1.00 (0.62–1.62) Follicular: 1.01 (0.57–1.79) CLL/SLL: 1.50 (0.86–2.63)	 0.27 0.46 0.43 0.92 0.63 0.98 0.58 0.31	 Age at menarche, height, weight at cohort entry Age at menarche, height, weight at cohort entry, long-term PA
Cerhan et al. 2002, USA	1986–1998	The Iowa Women's Health Study 37,931 women aged 55–69 years	261 total 137 diffuse 58 follicular 32 SLL	Frequency of moderate and vigorous recreational PA at baseline	High versus low PA index: All: 0.83 (0.59–1.11) Diffuse: 1.00 (0.63–1.43) Follicular: 0.55 (0.28–1.11) SLL: 0.91 (0.45–1.67)		Age
Paffenbarger et al. 1992, USA	1916–1978	56,683 Harvard and University of Pennsylvania Alumni M: 51977 W: 4706	86	Hours in sports play per week during early college	≥5 versus <5 h/week: 0.67 ($p = 0.134$)		Age and sex
Paffenbarger et al. 1987, USA	1962 or 1966–1978	16,936 male Harvard alumni, aged 35–74 years	death: 34	Energy expenditure (EE) (kcal/week), leisure time PA	EE >2,000 versus <500: Mortality: 0.72 (= 1.3/1.8)	0.45	Age, cigarette smoking, BMI

(*continued*)

6

Table 6.1 (continued)

Author, date, study location	Study dates	Study population	No. of cases	Physical activity assessment	RR or OR (95% CI)	Trend	Adjustment for confounding
Case-control studies:							
Pan et al. 2005, Canada	1994–1997	Adults aged 20–76 years. Population-based cancer registry data	1,030 cases 419 diffuse 242 follicular 100 SLL 269 others 3,106 controls	Recreational PA 2 years ago, MET-hours/week	Highest versus lowest quartile: Men: 0.79 (0.59–1.05) Women: 0.59 (0.42–0.81) Diffuse: 0.84 (0.62–1.13) Follicular: 0.64 (0.42–0.97) SLL: 0.74 (0.41–1.33) Others: 0.64 (0.45–0.92)	0.024 0.0002 0.12 0.042 0.27 0.008	Age, province, sex, education, smoking pack-years, alcohol drinking, chemical exposure, BMI, calorie intake
Cerhan et al. 2005, USA	1998–2000	Adults aged 20–74 years Population based cancer registry data (SEER)	1,321 cases 423 diffuse 317 follicular 79 T-cell 502 others 1,057 controls	PA 1 year ago: Categorized occupational activity and nonoccupational PA (vigorous housework plus vigorous & moderate leisure-time PA (MET-min/week)	Highest versus lowest index: Occupational: 0.98 (0.55–1.74) Nonoccupational (MET-min/week): Overall: 0.68 (0.43–1.08) Diffuse: 0.53 (0.29–0.99) Follicular: 0.79 (0.40–1.56) Vigorous leisure-time PA (min/day) Overall: 0.68 (0.47–0.99) Diffuse: 0.51 (0.30–0.88) Follicular: 0.82 (0.46–1.45)	 0.04 0.08 0.5 0.02 0.005 0.3	Age
Zahm et al. 1999, USA	Nebraska: 1983–1986 Kansas: 1976–1982 Minnesota: 1980–1982	Men and women ≥21 years. Population-based.	1,177 cases (M-993, W-184) 3,625 controls (M-2918, W-707)	EE and sitting time of usual occupation EE and sitting time of lifetime occupational	High versus sedentary: EE: M: 1.0 (0.7–1.3) W: 1.7 (0.2–11.5) Sitting time: M: 1.0 (0.8–1.3) W: 1.2 (0.7–2.3)	 0.46 0.32 0.43 0.31	Age, state of residence

	Iowa: 1981–1983			cumulative and average level of	Cumulative: EE: 1.0 (0.7–1.4)	0.41	
				PA among men in Iowa & Minnesota	Sitting time: 1.2 (0.9–1.6) Average: EE: 1.1 (0.7–1.7) Sitting time: 1.0 (0.7–1.4)	0.19 0.28 0.41	
Brownson et al. 1991, USA	1984–1989	White men ≥20 years. Cancer registry data.	536 cases 16.611 other cancer patients as controls	Occupational titles. High, moderate & low activity: PA is required ≥80, 20–80 and ≤20% of the work time	Moderate versus high: 1.0 (0.8–1.4) Low versus high: 1.2 (0.8–1.8)	0.23	Age, smoking

SLL small lymphocytic lymphoma; *CLL* chronic lymphocytic leukemia; *EE* energy expenditure; *M* men; *W* women

Table 6.2 Studies of physical activity and the risk of leukemia

Author, date, study location	Study dates	Study population	No. of cases	Physical activity assessment	RR or OR (95% CI)	Trend	Adjustment for confounding
Cohort studies							
Cerhan et al. 2002, USA	1986–1998	The Iowa Women's Health Study. 37,931 women aged 55–69 years	63 B-cell chronic lymphocytic leukemia	Frequency of moderate and vigorous recreational PA	Low versus high PA index 1.1 (0.6–2.2)		Age
Paffenbarger et al. 1992, USA	1916–1978	56,683 Harvard and University of Pennsylvania Alumni M: 51977 W: 4706	81	Hours in sports play per week	≥5 h versus < 5 0.84 ($p = 0.588$)		Age and sex
Paffenbarger et al. 1987, USA	1962 or 1966–1978	16,936 male Harvard alumni, aged 35–74 years	death: 24	Energy expenditure (EE) (kcal/week) (leisure time)	EE >2,000 versus <500: mortality: 0.83 (= 1.5/1.8)	0.99	Age, cigarette smoking, body mass index
Case-control studies							
Kasim et al. 2009, Canada	1994–1997	Adults aged 20–74 years. Population-based cancer registry data	653 cases 179 AML 27 ALL 96 CML 254 CLL	Moderate & vigorous Recreational PA 2 years ago, MET-hours/week	Highest versus lowest quartile: *Total PA:* W: 0.97 (0.66–1.42)	0.50	Age group, occupational exposure to benzene and ionizing, BMI, passive smoking, smoking pack-years, residence, vegetable and fruit consumption

			55 HCL 3,106 controls		M: 1.31 (0.93–1.85)	0.16	
					W + M: 1.17 (0.91–1.51)	0.23	
					Vigorous PA:		
					W: 0.82 (0.52–1.29)	0.48	
					M: 0.64 (0.41–0.95)	0.99	
					W + M:0.75 (0.57–0.99)	0.88	
					AML: 0.82 (0.46–1.47)	0.74	
					ALL: 0.52 (0.12–2.43)	0.81	
					CML: 1.27 (0.61–2.62)	0.1	
					CLL: 0.75 (0.49–1.20)	0.16	
					HCL: 0.60 (0.22–1.63)	0.35	
Brownson et al. 1991, USA	1984–1989	White men ≥20 years in Missouri. Cancer registry data	438 cases, 16,709 other cancer patients as controls	Occupational titles. High, moderate & low activity: PA is required ≥80, 20–80 and ≤20% of the work time	Moderate versus high: 1.0 (0.8–1.3) Low versus high: 1.1 (0.7–1.7)	0.47	Age, smoking

AML acute myeloid leukemia; *ALL* acute lymphoid leukemia; *CML* chronic myeloid leukemia; *CLL* chronic lymphoid leukemia; *HCL* hairy cell leukemia
MET metabolic equivalent; *W* women; *M* men

among people who reported more than 11.8 MET-h per week of vigorous physical activity, and this association was stronger in men than in women. This study also examined the association by leukemia subtype and suggested some degrees of risk reduction associated with higher levels of vigorous physical activity for each of the five histological subtypes assessed (except chronic myeloid leukemia) although the number of cases for each subtype was small and the associations were nonsignificant.

6.2.3 Multiple Myeloma and Hodgkin's Lymphoma

Four cohort studies have been published that examined the role of physical activity on the risk of multiple myeloma and HL, two studies for each site (Table 6.3). The study by Birmann et al. (2007) analyzed data from the Nurses' Health Study cohort and the Health Professionals Follow-up Study cohort separately and on both cohorts combined. This study did not find a significant association between long-term moderate or vigorous recreational physical activity and MM risk although there was a suggestion of an inverse association among women. In the Japanese study (Khan et al. 2006), people walking less than 30 min per day had a significantly higher risk of dying from MM (RR = 1.99 with 95% CI: 1.16–3.39) compared with those walking more than 1 h per day.

For HL, the only two cohort studies (Paffenbarger et al. 1987, 1992), both with a small number of cases or deaths, observed no relations between physical activity measured as hours of sports or energy expenditure of leisure-time activity and the risk of HL. In addition, one cohort study examined the impact of recreational physical activity on the risk of lymphatic/hematopoietic cancers on British men (Wannamethee et al. 2001). This study had only 61 cases of lymphatic/hematopoietic cancers all combined, and did not assess the risk associated with each specific type of hematologic cancer separately. These investigators found a risk reduction for lymphatic/hematopoietic cancers associated with sporting activity, although the risk decrease was not statistically significant.

In summary, although observational epidemiologic studies have provided some preliminary indications of an etiologic role for physical activity for these hematologic cancers, the level of evidence is still too limited to make any definitive assessments regarding causal associations, and thus the role of physical activity is classified as insufficient for NHL, leukemia, MM, and HL (Fig. 6.1).

6.3 Main Hypothesized Biologic Mechanisms

The underlying biologic mechanisms for the possible association between physical activity and hematologic cancers have not been established. Several plausible mechanisms are presented here (Fig. 6.2).

6.3.1 Enhancement of Immune System

Physical activity has the potential to influence cancer development by enhancing antitumor immune defenses (Westerlind 2003; McTiernan 2008; Shephard and Shek 1995). Although too much exercise can suppress immune function (Malm et al. 2005), moderate habitual physical activity may enhance immune function by increasing the number and activity of macrophages, natural killer cells, lymphokine-activated killer cells, and regulating cytokines (Woods 2005; Rogers et al. 2008; Woods et al. 1999; Nieman and Pedersen 1999), thus enhancing immune surveillance and killing of abnormal cells. Experimental studies have

Table 6.3 Studies of physical activity and the risk of Hodgkin's lymphoma, multiple myeloma, and lymphatic/hematopoietic cancer

Author, date, study location	Study dates	Study population	No. of cases	Physical activity assessment	RR or OR (95% CI)	Trend	Adjustment for confounding
Cohort studies							
Hodgkin's lymphoma							
Paffenbarger et al. 1992, USA	1916–1978	56,683 Harvard and University of Pennsylvania Alumni M: 51,977 W: 4,706	52	Hours in sports play per week	≥5 h versus <5 0.73 (p = 0.336)		Age and sex
Paffenbarger et al. 1987, USA	1962 or 1966–1978	16,936 male Harvard alumni, aged 35–74 years	death:10	Energy expenditure (EE) (kcal/week) (leisure-time PA)	EE >2,000 versus <500: mortality: 0.33 (0.3/0.9)	0.12	Age, cigarette smoking, body mass index
Multiple myeloma							
Birmann et al. 2007, USA	W: 1980–2002 M: 1986–2002	The Nurse's Health Study and The Health Professional Follow-up Study: 89663 nurses and 46,960 male health professional	215 cases W: 129 M: 86	Cumulative average hours/week of recreational PA	≥7 versus <2 h/week: W: 0.5 (0.2–1.4) M: 0.8 (0.5–1.5) W+M: 0.7 (0.5–1.1)	 0.14 0.78 0.20	Age, study, cohort, BMI
Khan et al. 2006, Japan	1988–2003	The Japan Collaborative Cohort Study: 46,157 men and 63,541 women aged 40–79 years	98 deaths W: 49 M: 49	Walking minutes/day	≤0.5 versus ≥1 h/day: M: 2.25 (1.08–4.67) W: 1.73 (0.79–3.79) M + W: 1.99 (1.16–3.39)	 0.032 0.178 0.01	Age, sex

(*continued*)

Table 6.3 (continued)

Author, date, study location	Study dates	Study population	No. of cases	Physical activity assessment	RR or OR (95% CI)	Trend	Adjustment for confounding
Lymphatic/haematopoietic cancer							
Wannamethee et al., UK	1978–1980, 1980–1997	7,588 British men aged 40–59 years	61 cases	PA index based on frequency & intensity of PA: regular walking/cycling, recreational activity, sporting (vigorous) activity	Moderate-vigorous versus non/occasional: 0.73 (0.33–1.63) Vigorous versus non/occasional: 0.47 (0.11–1.96) Sporting activity > per month versus no: 0.59 (0.30–1.16) Regular walking >60 versus <20 min/day: 1.47 (0.52–4.15)	0.21	Age, cigarette smoking, BMI, alcohol intake, social class

M men; *W* women

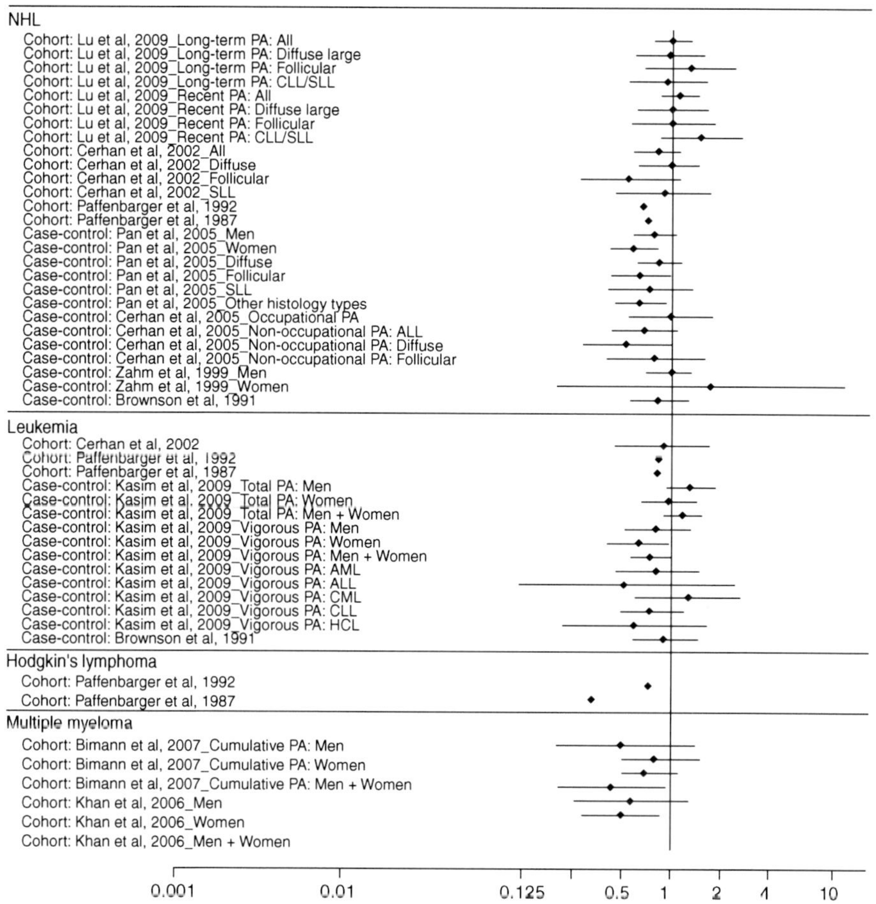

Fig. 6.1 Epidemiologic studies of physical activity and hematologic cancer type. Relative risks and 95% confidence intervals indicated with *circular* dots and *horizontal lines*

demonstrated greater activity of natural killer cells and of lymphokine-activated killer cells in trained or physically active mice, resulting in greater clearance of tumor cells and lower incidence of tumors (Rogers et al. 2008; MacNeil and Hoffman-Goetz 1993; Hoffman-Goetz et al. 1994; Woods and Davis 1994). Studies in humans have suggested that moderate exercise training has been associated with increases in natural killer cell activity or cell count (Hoffman-Goetz 1998; Rhind et al. 1994, 1996; Nieman et al. 1990), alterations in lymphocyte subpopulations (LaPerriere et al. 1994; Host et al. 1995), changes in interleukin-2 production and interleukin-2 receptor expression (Rhind et al. 1994, 1996), and elevation in immunoglobulin levels (Nehlsen-Cannarella et al. 1991). Long-term, moderate physical activity in geriatric populations seems to reduce infectious disease risk, increase rates of vaccine efficacy, and improve both physical and psychosocial aspects of daily living through its enhancement on immune response including T-cell phenotype and proliferation,

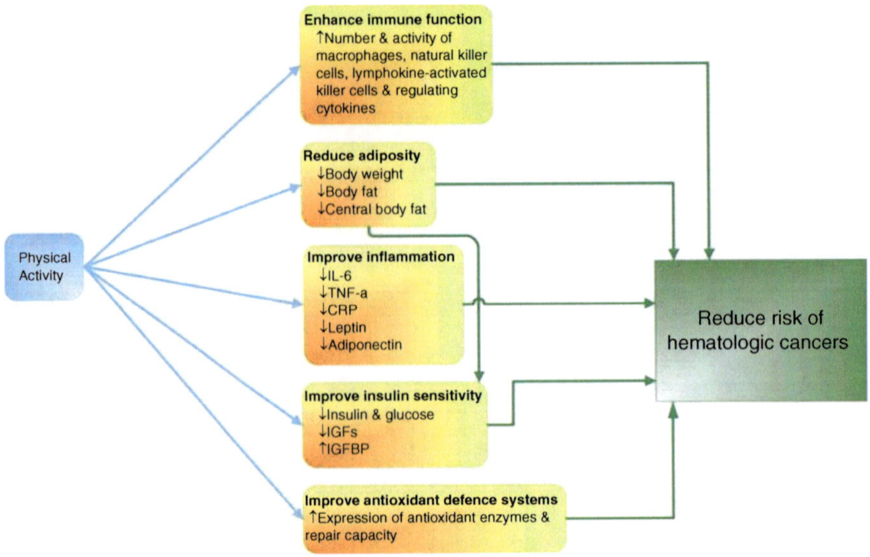

Fig. 6.2 Hypothesized biologic mechanisms involved in the etiology of physical activity and hematologic cancers

antibody response to vaccination, and cytokine production (Senchina and Kohut 2007). Immunosenescence (decreased immune function with aging) has been shown to be associated with a dramatic reduction in responsiveness and functional deregulation which may, in part, contribute to the increased incidence of cancer (Malaguarnera et al. 2009).

Because immunodeficiency is a risk factor for NHL and HL, physical activity-related improvement in immune function may play a role in the protective effect of physical activity against developing NHL and HL. Studies demonstrated that immunotherapy with immune splenocytes caused regression and cure of mouse lymphoma (Mule et al. 1985). Immunotherapy with anti-CD antibodies has also shown convincing efficacy on treating NHL patients (Otte et al. 2009). In addition, dendritic cell-based immunotherapy for the treatment of hematologic malignancies has already shown promising results (Buchler et al. 2003; Van et al. 2008; Radford et al. 2005).

6.3.2 Maintenance of Energy Balance

Obesity has been associated with significant metabolic abnormalities, including insulin resistance, hyperinsulinemia, hypertriglyceridemia, and increase in insulin-like growth factors (IGFs) (Kaaks and Lukanova 2001, 2002). It is also hypothesized that obesity has been associated with increased endogenous production of reactive oxygen species leading to DNA damage, impaired immune function by leptin and other factors, and increased inflammatory response (Calle and Kaaks 2004; Fair and Montgomery 2009; Marti et al. 2001; Bastard et al. 2006; Skibola et al. 2004). Obesity has been suggested to be a risk factor for hematologic cancers (Larsson and Wolk, 2007a, b; , 2008; Lu et al. 2009; Lim et al. 2007; Reeves et al. 2007; Maskarinec et al. 2008; Birmann et al. 2007), while physical activity increases energy expenditure and reduces body weight, body fat, or changes body composition (McTiernan et al.

2007; Irwin et al. 2003), and thus may decrease the risks of hematologic cancers. The greater reduction in NHL risk associated with physical activity among obese men observed in one case-control study supports a possible role of physical activity in affecting NHL risk for men through its influence on obesity (Pan et al. 2005).

6.3.3 Improvement of Antioxidant Defense Systems

Exercise increases oxygen uptake and the production of oxygen free radicals but also improves antioxidant enzyme repair capacity (Gomez-Cabrera et al. 2008; Ji 2008). Excessive free radicals have been shown to induce cell mutagenesis and tumor cell proliferation of hematopoietic cells (Lyu et al. 2008; Sallmyr et al. 2008; Valko et al. 2006; Hurt et al. 2007; Kuku et al. 2005).

Exercise could be beneficial or harmful, depending on the intensity and duration of exercise, and nutritional status. Heavy exercise could cause excessive increase of free radicals and disturbance of intracellular prooxidant–antioxidant homeostasis (i.e., overwhelm cellular antioxidant defenses), and thus damage to biomolecules may occur (Vina et al. 2000; Sachdev and Davies 2008; Chevion et al. 2003; Poulsen et al. 1996; Sastre et al. 1992). However, moderate intensity exercises exert low oxidative stress without oxidative damage impulses in normally nourished subjects (Apor and Radi 2006). When exercise is performed in moderation (in terms of intensity or duration), muscle antioxidant defense systems are upregulated as an adaptive response to exercise, and the expression of antioxidant enzymes is increased (Gomez-Cabrera et al. 2008; Ji 2008; Morton et al. 2009).

Aging is associated with increased free radical generation in the skeletal muscle and decreased antioxidant defense and repair capacity (Kretzschmar and Muller 1993; Ji 2001). This age-related change can be partly compensated by moderate exercise (Asha 2009; Kretzschmar and Muller 1993). Thus, older populations could experience significant benefit from regular exercise through an exercise-induced adaptation in cellular antioxidant defense systems that is necessary to deal with the daily production of reactive oxygen species (Goto et al. 2007).

6.3.4 Impact on Metabolic Hormones

Another hypothesized mechanism is the exercise-related improvement in insulin sensitivity, and reduction in levels of insulin and IGFs (McTiernan 2008). Increasing evidence has shown that insulin and IGFs are growth factors for tumor formation by enhancing DNA synthesis, resulting in tumor cell proliferation, inhibition of apoptosis, and an altered sex hormone milieu (Gupta et al. 2002; Khandwala et al. 2000). Studies also demonstrated that insulin receptors and IGF receptors are expressed in human neoplastic hematopoietic cells (Khandwala et al. 2000; Vetter et al. 1986; Frasca et al. 2008). IGF-1 has been shown to have both an antiapoptotic and a proliferative effect on MM cells and can induce migration, and thus may play a role in MM development (Menu et al. 2009; Jernberg-Wiklund and Nilsson 2007; Ge and Rudikoff 2000; Qiang et al. 2004). In studies of IGF effects on tumor growth, IGF had stimulatory effects and mitogenic effects on cell lines of Burkitt type, HL, acute lymphoblastic leukemia, and acute myeloblastic leukemia (Khandwala et al. 2000).

Physical activity can improve insulin sensitivity (Mayer-Davis et al. 1998; Borghouts and Keizer 2000; Hawley and Lessard 2008) and decrease insulin concentrations (Irwin et al. 2009, 2000; Fairey et al. 2003; Pischon et al. 2003) by enhancing glucose uptake and

6

insulin sensitivity in skeletal muscles and by avoiding excessive weight gain (Dossus and Kaaks 2008; McTiernan 2008). Chronic exercise has been reported to be associated with decreased levels of IGF-1 (Schmitz et al. 2002; Irwin et al. 2009; Fairey et al. 2003; Eliakim et al. 1998; Nguyen et al. 1998) and increased levels of IGF binding protein (IGFBP) (Fairey et al. 2003; Eliakim et al. 1998; Nguyen et al. 1998). However, the independent effect of physical activity on the IGF system (such as IGF-1 and IGFBP-3) is less clear and the evidence from research is mixed (Voskuil et al. 2001; Dossus and Kaaks 2008; Chang et al. 2002; Schmitz et al. 2002; Friedenreich and Orenstein 2002; Allen et al. 2003). Physical activity may indirectly influence the IGF system through its effect on body composition and insulin sensitivity.

6.3.5 Anti-inflammatory Effects

Increased circulation levels of proinflammatory factors such as C-reactive protein (CRP), interleukin (IL-6), tumor necrosis factor-α (TNF-α), and decreased anti-inflammatory factors (such as adiponectin) have been shown to be associated with increased cancer risk (Il'yasova et al. 2005; Allin et al. 2009), including lymphoma, leukemia, and MM (Mischke et al. 2007; Nilsson et al. 1992; Sugiyama et al. 1996; Klein et al. 2003; Petridou et al. 2006, 2009; Avcu et al. 2006; Yokota et al. 2000; Reseland et al. 2009; Dalamaga et al. 2009). For example, CRP has been demonstrated to be a prognostic factor affecting the survival of patients with MM (Offidani et al. 2008; Tao et al. 2007). It has also been shown that CRP enhanced myeloma cell proliferation under stressed conditions and protected myeloma cells from chemotherapy drug-induced apoptosis in vitro and in vivo, as well as enhanced myeloma cell secretion of IL-6 and synergized with IL-6 to protect myeloma cells from chemotherapy drug-induced apoptosis (Yang et al. 2007). IL-6 is suggested as a growth and survival factor in MM via activation of extracellular signal-regulated kinase and the phosphatidylinositol 3-kinase signaling cascade (Hsu et al. 2004; Lauta 2003).

Observational studies have observed that adiposity, specifically percentage of body fat, is positively associated with inflammatory markers (IL-6, TNF-α, and CRP), while regular exercise improves inflammation in terms of both inflammatory markers (such as CRP, TNF-alpha, IL-6, and leptin) and anti-inflammatory factors (adiponectin) (Puglisi and Fernandez 2008; Woods et al. 2009; Forsythe et al. 2008; Mathur and Pedersen 2008; Pischon et al. 2003; Moldoveanu et al. 2001). Body fat reduction resulting from exercise may partially account for the association between physical activity and its anti-inflammatory effect; however, some studies also report that physical activity has an anti-inflammatory effect independent of adiposity (Woods et al. 2009; Thomas and Williams 2008; Pischon et al. 2003). It is suggested that regular exercise induces suppression of TNF-α and thereby offers protection against TNF-α-induced insulin resistance (Pedersen and Bruunsgaard 2003; Pedersen 2006).

It is likely that multiple mechanisms may be operative for the possible association between physical activity and hematologic cancers, some of which are interrelated. However, the evidence for these mechanisms is still limited and much more experimental research in animal models and in human intervention studies is needed to provide further information on the biologic mechanisms underlying the possible effect of physical activity on hematologic cancers.

6.4 Conclusion and Future Directions

In summary, the epidemiologic evidence for the association with physical activity is classified as *insufficient* for NHL, leukemia, MM, and HL. Several plausible biologic mechanisms underlying the possible associations between physical activity and hematologic cancers are hypothesized, including enhancement of immune function, maintenance of energy balance, improvement of the antioxidant defense system, impact on metabolic hormones, and anti-inflammatory effects.

Research on the relations between physical activity and hematologic cancers is scarce, and more studies are needed that take into consideration the following methodologic issues in order to improve understanding in this area. First of all, reliable, valid, and comprehensive measures of physical activity are needed that include a combination of self-report methods along with objective measures such as pedometers, accelerometers, and heart-rate monitors in order to assess more accurately the type and dose (frequency, duration, and intensity) of activity required for a risk reduction (Tudor-Locke et al. 2002; Le Masurier and Tudor-Locke 2003; Corder et al. 2007; Michaud et al. 2002; Janz 2006; Freedson and Miller 2000; Howe et al. 2009; Hasson et al. 2009; Pober et al. 2006; Janz 2006; Metallinos-Katsaras et al. 2007).

To facilitate comparisons across studies, all dimensions or components of physical activity should be measured and assessed, including type (recreational, occupational, transportation, and household physical activity), dose, and time in life when physical activity is performed.

Secondly, NHL and leukemia are heterogeneous groups of malignancies that may significantly vary in their causes. The effect of physical activity may differ by histologic subtype of NHL and leukemia. Future studies should examine the impact of physical activity on these cancers by histologic subtype. These future studies should also consider effect modification by other risk factors for these cancers.

Finally, intervention studies, especially randomized controlled trials, are warranted to evaluate the effect of physical activity on various hypothesized biomarkers of cancer, including insulin-related hormones, and biomarkers of immune function, inflammation, and oxidative stress (Rundle 2005; McTiernan 2008). These studies would shed light on the underlying biological mechanisms linking physical activity and hematologic cancers.

References

Alexander DD, Mink PJ, Adami HO, Chang ET, Cole P, Mandel JS, Trichopoulos D (2007a) The non-Hodgkin lymphomas: a review of the epidemiologic literature. Int J Cancer 120(Suppl 12): 1–39

Alexander DD, Mink PJ, Adami HO, Cole P, Mandel JS, Oken MM, Trichopoulos D (2007b) Multiple myeloma: a review of the epidemiologic literature. Int J Cancer 120(Suppl 12):40–61

Allen NE, Appleby PN, Kaaks R, Rinaldi S, Davey GK, Key TJ (2003) Lifestyle determinants of serum insulin-like growth-factor-I (IGF-I), C-peptide and hormone binding protein levels in British women. Cancer Causes Control 14: 65–74

Allin KH, Bojesen SE, Nordestgaard BG (2009) Baseline C-reactive protein is associated with incident cancer and survival in patients with cancer. J Clin Oncol 27:2217–2224

Apor P, Radi A (2006) Physical exercise, oxidative stress and damage. Orv Hetil 147:1025–1031

Asha DS (2009) Aging brain: prevention of oxidative stress by vitamin E and exercise. Sci World J 9:366–372

6

Avcu F, Ural AU, Yilmaz MI, Bingol N, Nevruz O, Caglar K (2006) Association of plasma adiponectin concentrations with chronic lymphocytic leukemia and myeloproliferative diseases. Int J Hematol 83:254–258

Bastard JP, Maachi M, Lagathu C, Kim MJ, Caron M, Vidal H, Capeau J, Feve B (2006) Recent advances in the relationship between obesity, inflammation, and insulin resistance. Eur Cytokine Netw 17:4–12

Bhatia S, Robison LL (1999) Epidemiology of leukemia and lymphoma. Curr Opin Hematol 6:201

Birmann BM, Giovannucci E, Rosner B, Anderson KC, Colditz GA (2007) Body mass index, physical activity, and risk of multiple myeloma. Cancer Epidemiol Biomark Prev 16:1474–1478

Borghouts LB, Keizer HA (2000) Exercise and insulin sensitivity: a review. Int J Sports Med 21:1–12

Bray I, Brennan P, Boffetta P (2001) Recent trends and future projections of lymphoid neoplasms–a Bayesian age-period-cohort analysis. Cancer Causes Control 12:813–820

Brownson RC, Chang JC, Davis JR, Smith CA (1991) Physical activity on the job and cancer in Missouri. Am J Public Health 81:639–642

Buchler T, Michalek J, Kovarova L, Musilova R, Hajek R (2003) Dendritic cell-based immunotherapy for the treatment of hematological malignancies. Hematology 8:97–104

Calle EE, Kaaks R (2004) Overweight, obesity and cancer: epidemiological evidence and proposed mechanisms. Nat Rev Cancer 4:579–591

Canadian Cancer Society (2009) Canadian cancer statistics 2009. Canadian Cancer Society, Toronto, Canada

Caporaso NE, Goldin LR, Anderson WF, Landgren O (2009) Current insight on trends, causes, and mechanisms of Hodgkin's lymphoma. Cancer J 15:117–123

Cerhan JR, Janney CA, Vachon CM, Habermann TM, Kay NE, Potter JD, Sellers TA, Folsom AR (2002) Anthropometric characteristics, physical activity, and risk of non-Hodgkin's lymphoma subtypes and B-cell chronic lymphocytic leukemia: a prospective study. Am J Epidemiol 156:527–535

Cerhan JR, Bernstein L, Severson RK, Davis S, Colt JS, Blair A, Hartge P (2005) Anthropometrics, physical activity, related medical conditions, and the risk of non-hodgkin lymphoma. Cancer Causes Control 16:1203–1214

Chang S, Wu X, Yu H, Spitz MR (2002) Plasma concentrations of insulin-like growth factors among healthy adult men and postmenopausal women: associations with body composition, lifestyle, and reproductive factors. Cancer Epidemiol Biomark Prev 11:758–766

Chevion S, Moran DS, Heled Y, Shani Y, Regev G, Abbou B, Berenshtein E, Stadtman ER, Epstein Y (2003) Plasma antioxidant status and cell injury after severe physical exercise. Proc Natl Acad Sci USA 100:5119–5123

Corder K, Brage S, Ekelund U (2007) Accelerometers and pedometers: methodology and clinical application. Curr Opin Clin Nutr Metab Care 10:597–603

Curado MP, Edwards B, Shin HR, Storm H, Ferlay J, Heanue M, Boyle P (2007) Cancer incidence in five continents, vol IX, IARC Scientific Publication No. 160. IARC, Lyon

Dalamaga M, Karmaniolas K, Panagiotou A, Hsi A, Chamberland J, Dimas C, Lekka A, Mantzoros CS (2009) Low circulating adiponectin and resistin, but not leptin, levels are associated with multiple myeloma risk: a case-control study. Cancer Causes Control 20:193–199

Deschler B, Lubbert M (2006) Acute myeloid leukemia: epidemiology and etiology. Cancer 107:2099–2107

Dossus L, Kaaks R (2008) Nutrition, metabolic factors and cancer risk. Best Pract Res Clin Endocrinol Metab 22:551–571

Eliakim A, Brasel JA, Mohan S, Wong WL, Cooper DM (1998) Increased physical activity and the growth hormone-IGF-I axis in adolescent males. Am J Physiol 275:R308–R314

Fair AM, Montgomery K (2009) Energy balance, physical activity, and cancer risk. Methods Mol Biol 472:57–88

Fairey AS, Courneya KS, Field CJ, Bell GJ, Jones LW, Mackey JR (2003) Effects of exercise training on fasting insulin, insulin resistance, insulin-like growth factors, and insulin-like growth factor binding proteins in postmenopausal breast cancer survivors: a randomized controlled trial. Cancer Epidemiol Biomark Prev 12:721–727

Ferlay J, Parkin DM, Steliarova-Foucher E (2010) Estimates of cancer incidence and mortality in Europe in 2008. Eur J Cancer 46:765–781

Fisher SG, Fisher RI (2004) The epidemiology of non-Hodgkin's lymphoma. Oncogene 23: 6524–6534

Forsythe LK, Wallace JM, Livingstone MB (2008) Obesity and inflammation: the effects of weight loss. Nutr Res Rev 21:117–133

Frasca F, Pandini G, Sciacca L, Pezzino V, Squatrito S, Belfiore A, Vigneri R (2008) The role of insulin receptors and IGF-I receptors in cancer and other diseases. Arch Physiol Biochem 114: 23–37

Freedson PS, Miller K (2000) Objective monitoring of physical activity using motion sensors and heart rate. Res Q Exerc Sport 71: S21–S29

Friedenreich CM, Orenstein MR (2002) Physical activity and cancer prevention: etiologic evidence and biological mechanisms. J Nutr 132: 3456S–3464S

Ge NL, Rudikoff S (2000) Insulin-like growth factor I is a dual effector of multiple myeloma cell growth. Blood 96:2856–2861

Gomez-Cabrera MC, Domenech E, Vina J (2008) Moderate exercise is an antioxidant: upregulation of antioxidant genes by training. Free Radic Biol Med 44:126–131

Goto S, Naito H, Kaneko T, Chung HY, Radak Z (2007) Hormetic effects of regular exercise in aging: correlation with oxidative stress. Appl Physiol Nutr Metab 32:948–953

Gupta K, Krishnaswamy G, Karnad A, Peiris AN (2002) Insulin: a novel factor in carcinogenesis. Am J Med Sci 323:140–145

Harris NL, Jaffe ES, Stein H, Banks PM, Chan JK, Cleary ML, Delsol G, De Wolf-Peeters C, Falini B, Gatter KC (1994) A revised European-American classification of lymphoid neoplasms: a proposal from the international lymphoma study group. Blood 84:1361–1392

Harris NL, Jaffe ES, Diebold J, Flandrin G, Muller-Hermelink HK, Vardiman J, Lister TA, Bloomfield CD (1999) World Health Organization classification of neoplastic diseases of the hematopoietic and lymphoid tissues: report of the Clinical Advisory Committee meeting-Airlie House, Virginia, November 1997. J Clin Oncol 17:3835–3849

Harris NL, Jaffe ES, Diebold J, Flandrin G, Muller-Hermelink HK, Vardiman J (2000) Lymphoma classification – from controversy to consensus: the R.E.A.L. and WHO classification of lymphoid neoplasms. Ann Oncol 11(Suppl 1): 3–10

Hasson RE, Haller J, Pober DM, Staudenmayer J, Freedson PS (2009) Validity of the Omron HJ-112 pedometer during treadmill walking. Med Sci Sports Exerc 41:805–809

Hawley JA, Lessard SJ (2008) Exercise training-induced improvements in insulin action. Acta Physiol (Oxf) 192:127–135

Hoffman-Goetz L (1998) Influence of physical activity and exercise on innate immunity. Nutr Rev 56:S126–S130

Hoffman-Goetz L, May KM, Arumugam Y (1994) Exercise training and mouse mammary tumour metastasis. Anticancer Res 14:2627–2631

Horner MJ, Ries LAG, Krapcho M, Neyman N, Aminou R, Howlader N, Altekruse SF, Feuer EJ, Huang L, Mariotto A, Miller BA, Lewis DR, Eisner MP, Stinchcomb DG, Edwards BK (eds) (2009) SEER Cancer statistics review, 1975–2006. National Cancer Institute, Bethesda, MD. http://seer.cancer.gov/csr/1975_2006/

Host CR, Norton KI, Olds TS, Lowe EL, Mulligan SP (1995) The effects of altered exercise distribution on lymphocyte subpopulations. Eur J Appl Physiol Occup Physiol 72:157–164

Howe CA, Staudenmayer JW, Freedson PS (2009) Accelerometer prediction of energy expenditure: vector magnitude versus vertical axis. Med Sci Sports Exerc 41:2199–2206

Hsu JH, Shi Y, Frost P, Yan H, Hoang B, Sharma S, Gera J, Lichtenstein A (2004) Interleukin-6 activates phosphoinositol-3′ kinase in multiple myeloma tumor cells by signaling through RAS-dependent and, separately, through p85-dependent pathways. Oncogene 23:3368–3375

Hurt EM, Thomas SB, Peng B, Farrar WL (2007) Integrated molecular profiling of SOD2 expression in multiple myeloma. Blood 109: 3953–3962

Il'yasova D, Colbert LH, Harris TB, Newman AB, Bauer DC, Satterfield S, Kritchevsky SB (2005) Circulating levels of inflammatory markers and cancer risk in the health aging and body composition cohort. Cancer Epidemiol Biomark Prev 14:2413–2418

Irwin ML, Mayer-Davis EJ, Addy CL, Pate RR, Durstine JL, Stolarczyk LM, Ainsworth BE (2000) Moderate-intensity physical activity and fasting insulin levels in women: the cross-cultural activity participation study. Diab Care 23:449–454

6

Irwin ML, Yasui Y, Ulrich CM, Bowen D, Rudolph RE, Schwartz RS, Yukawa M, Aiello E, Potter JD, McTiernan A (2003) Effect of exercise on total and intra-abdominal body fat in postmenopausal women: a randomized controlled trial. JAMA 289:323–330

Irwin ML, Varma K, Varez-Reeves M, Cadmus L, Wiley A, Chung GG, DiPietro L, Mayne ST, Yu H (2009) Randomized controlled trial of aerobic exercise on insulin and insulin-like growth factors in breast cancer survivors: the Yale exercise and survivorship study. Cancer Epidemiol Biomark Prev 18:306–313

Janz KF (2006) Physical activity in epidemiology: moving from questionnaire to objective measurement. Br J Sports Med 40:191–192

Jernberg-Wiklund H, Nilsson K (2007) Control of apoptosis in human multiple myeloma by insulin-like growth factor I (IGF-I). Adv Cancer Res 97:139–165

Ji LL (2001) Exercise at old age: does it increase or alleviate oxidative stress? Ann NY Acad Sci 928:236–247

Ji LL (2008) Modulation of skeletal muscle antioxidant defense by exercise: Role of redox signaling. Free Radic Biol Med 44:142–152

Kaaks R, Lukanova A (2001) Energy balance and cancer: the role of insulin and insulin-like growth factor-I. Proc Nutr Soc 60:91–106

Kaaks R, Lukanova A (2002) Effects of weight control and physical activity in cancer prevention: role of endogenous hormone metabolism. Ann NY Acad Sci 963:268–281

Kalil N, Cheson BD (1999) Chronic lymphocytic leukemia. Oncologist 4:352–369

Kasim K, Johnson KC, Levallois P, Abdous B, Auger P (2009) Recreational physical activity and the risk of adult leukemia in Canada. Cancer Causes Control 20(8):1377–1386

Khan MM, Mori M, Sakauchi F, Matsuo K, Ozasa K, Tamakoshi A (2006) Risk factors for multiple myeloma: evidence from the Japan Collaborative Cohort (JACC) study. Asian Pac J Cancer Prev 7:575–581

Khandwala HM, McCutcheon IE, Flyvbjerg A, Friend KE (2000) The effects of insulin-like growth factors on tumorigenesis and neoplastic growth. Endocr Rev 21:215–244

Klein B, Tarte K, Jourdan M, Mathouk K, Moreaux J, Jourdan E, Legouffe E, De VJ, Rossi JF (2003) Survival and proliferation factors of normal and malignant plasma cells. Int J Hematol 78: 106–113

Kretzschmar M, Muller D (1993) Aging, training and exercise. A review of effects on plasma glutathione and lipid peroxides. Sports Med 15: 196–209

Kuku I, Aydogdu I, Bayraktar N, Kaya E, Akyol O, Erkurt MA (2005) Oxidant/antioxidant parameters and their relationship with medical treatment in multiple myeloma. Cell Biochem Funct 23:47–50

LaPerriere A, Antoni MH, Ironson G, Perry A, McCabe P, Klimas N, Helder L, Schneiderman N, Fletcher MA (1994) Effects of aerobic exercise training on lymphocyte subpopulations. Int J Sports Med 15(Suppl 3):S127–S130

Larsson SC, Wolk A (2007a) Body mass index and risk of multiple myeloma: a meta-analysis. Int J Cancer 121:2512–2516

Larsson SC, Wolk A (2007b) Obesity and risk of non-Hodgkin's lymphoma: a meta-analysis. Int J Cancer 121:1564–1570

Larsson SC, Wolk A (2008) Overweight and obesity and incidence of leukemia: a meta-analysis of cohort studies. Int J Cancer 122:1418–1421

Lauta VM (2003) A review of the cytokine network in multiple myeloma: diagnostic, prognostic, and therapeutic implications. Cancer 97: 2440–2452

Le Masurier GC, Tudor-Locke C (2003) Comparison of pedometer and accelerometer accuracy under controlled conditions. Med Sci Sports Exerc 35:867–871

Lightfoot T (2005) Aetiology of childhood leukemia. Bioelectromagnetics Suppl 7:S5–S11

Lim U, Morton LM, Subar AF, Baris D, Stolzenberg-Solomon R, Leitzmann M, Kipnis V, Mouw T, Carroll L, Schatzkin A, Hartge P (2007) Alcohol, smoking, and body size in relation to incident Hodgkin's and non-Hodgkin's lymphoma risk. Am J Epidemiol 166: 697–708

Lu Y, Prescott J, Sullivan-Halley J, Henderson KD, Ma H, Chang ET, Clarke CA, Horn-Ross PL, Ursin G, Bernstein L (2009) Body size, recreational physical activity, and b-cell non-hodgkin lymphoma risk among women in the California teachers study. Am J Epidemiol 170(10): 1231–1240

Lyu BN, Ismailov SB, Ismailov B, Lyu MB (2008) Mitochondrial concept of leukemogenesis: key role of oxygen-peroxide effects. Theor Biol Med Model 5:23

MacNeil B, Hoffman-Goetz L (1993) Chronic exercise enhances in vivo and in vitro cytotoxic mechanisms of natural immunity in mice. J Appl Physiol 74:388–395

Malaguarnera L, Cristaldi E, Malaguarnera M (2009) The role of immunity in elderly cancer. Crit Rev Oncol Hematol 74:40–60

Malm C, Celsing F, Friman G (2005) Immune defense is both stimulated and inhibited by physical activity. Lakartidningen 102:867–868, 870, 873

Marti A, Marcos A, Martinez JA (2001) Obesity and immune function relationships. Obes Rev 2:131–140

Maskarinec G, Erber E, Gill J, Cozen W, Kolonel LN (2008) Overweight and obesity at different times in life as risk factors for non-Hodgkin's lymphoma: the multiethnic cohort. Cancer Epidemiol Biomark Prev 17:196–203

Mathur N, Pedersen BK (2008) Exercise as a mean to control low-grade systemic inflammation. Mediators Inflamm 2008:109502

Mayer-Davis EJ, D'Agostino R Jr, Karter AJ, Haffner SM, Rewers MJ, Saad M, Bergman RN (1998) Intensity and amount of physical activity in relation to insulin sensitivity: the insulin resistance atherosclerosis study. JAMA 279: 669–674

McTiernan A (2008) Mechanisms linking physical activity with cancer. Nat Rev Cancer 8:205–211

McTiernan A, Sorensen B, Irwin ML, Morgan A, Yasui Y, Rudolph RE, Surawicz C, Lampe JW, Lampe PD, Ayub K, Potter JD (2007) Exercise effect on weight and body fat in men and women. Obesity (Silver Spring) 15:1496–1512

Menu E, Van VE, Van CB, Vanderkerken K (2009) The role of the insulin-like growth factor 1 receptor axis in multiple myeloma. Arch Physiol Biochem 115:49–57

Metallinos-Katsaras ES, Freedson PS, Fulton JE, Sherry B (2007) The association between an objective measure of physical activity and weight status in preschoolers. Obesity (Silver Spring) 15:686–694

Michaud PA, Cauderay M, Narring F, Schutz Y (2002) Assessment of physical activity with a pedometer and its relationship with VO2max among adolescents in Switzerland. Soz Praventivmed 47:107–115

Mischke R, Waterston M, Eckersall PD (2007) Changes in C-reactive protein and haptoglobin in dogs with lymphatic neoplasia. Vet J 174:188–192

Moldoveanu AI, Shephard RJ, Shek PN (2001) The cytokine response to physical activity and training. Sports Med 31:115–144

Morgan GJ, Davies FE, Linet M (2002) Myeloma aetiology and epidemiology. Biomed Pharmacother 56:223–234

Morton JP, Kayani AC, McArdle A, Drust B (2009) The exercise-induced stress response of skeletal muscle, with specific emphasis on humans. Sports Med 39:643–662

Mule JJ, Rosenstein M, Shu S, Rosenberg SA (1985) Eradication of a disseminated syngeneic mouse lymphoma by systemic adoptive transfer of immune lymphocytes and its dependence upon a host component(s). Cancer Res 45:526–531

Muller AM, Ihorst G, Mertelsmann R, Engelhardt M (2005) Epidemiology of non-Hodgkin's lymphoma (NHL): trends, geographic distribution, and etiology. Ann Hematol 84:1–12

Nehlsen-Cannarella SL, Nieman DC, Balk-Lamberton AJ, Markoff PA, Chritton DB, Gusewitch G, Lee JW (1991) The effects of moderate exercise training on immune response. Med Sci Sports Exerc 23:64–70

Nguyen UN, Mougin F, Simon-Rigaud ML, Rouillon JD, Marguet P, Regnard J (1998) Influence of exercise duration on serum insulin-like growth factor and its binding proteins in athletes. Eur J Appl Physiol Occup Physiol 78: 533–537

Nieman DC, Pedersen BK (1999) Exercise and immune function. Recent developments. Sports Med 27:73–80

Nieman DC, Nehlsen-Cannarella SL, Markoff PA, Balk-Lamberton AJ, Yang H, Chritton DB, Lee JW, Arabatzis K (1990) The effects of moderate exercise training on natural killer cells and acute upper respiratory tract infections. Int J Sports Med 11:467–473

Nilsson K, Larsson LG, Soderberg O, Schena M, Gottardi D, Caligaris-Cappio F, Carlsson M (1992) On the role of endogenously produced TNF-alpha and IL-6 as regulators of growth and differentiation of B-type chronic lymphocytic leukemia cells in vitro. Curr Top Microbiol Immunol 182:271–277

Offidani M, Corvatta L, Polloni C, Piersantelli MN, Galieni P, Visani G, Alesiani F, Catarini

6

M, Brunori M, Burattini M, Centurioni R, Ferranti M, Giuliodori L, Candela M, Mele A, Marconi M, Leoni P (2008) Serum C-reactive protein at diagnosis and response to therapy is the most powerful factor predicting outcome of multiple myeloma treated with thalidomide/anthracycline-based therapy. Clin Lymphoma Myeloma 8:294–299

Otte A, de WC Van, Dierckx RA (2009) Radiolabeled immunotherapy in non-Hodgkin's lymphoma treatment: the next step. Nucl Med Commun 30:5–15

Paffenbarger RS Jr, Hyde RT, Wing AL (1987) Physical activity and incidence of cancer in diverse populations: a preliminary report. Am J Clin Nutr 45:312–317

Paffenbarger RS Jr, Lee IM, Wing AL (1992) The influence of physical activity on the incidence of site-specific cancers in college alumni. Adv Exp Med Biol 322:7–15

Pan SY, Desmeules M (2009) Energy intake, physical activity, energy balance, and cancer: epidemiologic evidence. Methods Mol Biol 472:191–215

Pan SY, Mao Y, Ugnat AM (2005) Physical activity, obesity, energy intake, and the risk of non-Hodgkin's lymphoma: a population-based case-control study. Am J Epidemiol 162:1162–1173

Parkin DM, Bray F, Ferlay J, Pisani P (2005) Global cancer statistics, 2002. CA Cancer J Clin 55:74–108

Pedersen BK (2006) The anti-inflammatory effect of exercise: its role in diabetes and cardiovascular disease control. Essays Biochem 42:105–117

Pedersen BK, Bruunsgaard H (2003) Possible beneficial role of exercise in modulating low-grade inflammation in the elderly. Scand J Med Sci Sports 13:56–62

Petridou E, Mantzoros CS, Dessypris N, Dikalioti SK, Trichopoulos D (2006) Adiponectin in relation to childhood myeloblastic leukaemia. Br J Cancer 94:156–160

Petridou ET, Sergentanis TN, Dessypris N, Vlachantoni IT, Tseleni-Balafouta S, Pourtsidis A, Moschovi M, Polychronopoulou S, Thanasiadou-Piperopoulou F, Kalmanti M, Mantzoros CS (2009) Serum adiponectin as a predictor of childhood non-Hodgkin's lymphoma: a nationwide case-control study. J Clin Oncol 27(30):5049–5055

Pischon T, Hankinson SE, Hotamisligil GS, Rifai N, Rimm EB (2003) Leisure-time physical activity and reduced plasma levels of obesity-related inflammatory markers. Obes Res 11:1055–1064

Pober DM, Staudenmayer J, Raphael C, Freedson PS (2006) Development of novel techniques to classify physical activity mode using accelerometers. Med Sci Sports Exerc 38:1626–1634

Poulsen HE, Loft S, Vistisen K (1996) Extreme exercise and oxidative DNA modification. J Sports Sci 14:343–346

Puglisi MJ, Fernandez ML (2008) Modulation of C-reactive protein, tumor necrosis factor-alpha, and adiponectin by diet, exercise, and weight loss. J Nutr 138:2293–2296

Qiang YW, Yao L, Tosato G, Rudikoff S (2004) Insulin-like growth factor I induces migration and invasion of human multiple myeloma cells. Blood 103:301–308

Radford KJ, Vari F, Hart DN (2005) Vaccine strategies to treat lymphoproliferative disorders. Pathology 37:534–550

Reeves GK, Pirie K, Beral V, Green J, Spencer E, Bull D (2007) Cancer incidence and mortality in relation to body mass index in the million women study: cohort study. BMJ 335:1134

Reseland JE, Reppe S, Olstad OK, Hjorth-Hansen H, Brenne AT, Syversen U, Waage A, Iversen PO (2009) Abnormal adipokine levels and leptin-induced changes in gene expression profiles in multiple myeloma. Eur J Haematol 83: 460–470

Rhind SG, Shek PN, Shinkai S, Shephard RJ (1994) Differential expression of interleukin-2 receptor alpha and beta chains in relation to natural killer cell subsets and aerobic fitness. Int J Sports Med 15:311–318

Rhind SG, Shek PN, Shinkai S, Shephard RJ (1996) Effects of moderate endurance exercise and training on in vitro lymphocyte proliferation, interleukin-2 (IL-2) production, and IL-2 receptor expression. Eur J Appl Physiol Occup Physiol 74:348–360

Rogers CJ, Berrigan D, Zaharoff DA, Hance KW, Patel AC, Perkins SN, Schlom J, Greiner JW, Hursting SD (2008) Energy restriction and exercise differentially enhance components of systemic and mucosal immunity in mice. J Nutr 138:115–122

Rohrbacher M, Hasford J (2009) Epidemiology of chronic myeloid leukaemia (CML). Best Pract Res Clin Haematol 22:295–302

Rundle A (2005) Molecular epidemiology of physical activity and cancer. Cancer Epidemiol Biomark Prev 14:227–236

Sachdev S, Davies KJ (2008) Production, detection, and adaptive responses to free radicals in exercise. Free Radic Biol Med 44:215–223

Sallmyr A, Fan J, Rassool FV (2008) Genomic instability in myeloid malignancies: increased reactive oxygen species (ROS), DNA double strand breaks (DSBs) and error-prone repair. Cancer Lett 270:1–9

Sastre J, Asensi M, Gasco E, Pallardo FV, Ferrero JA, Furukawa T, Vina J (1992) Exhaustive physical exercise causes oxidation of glutathione status in blood: prevention by antioxidant administration. Am J Physiol 263:R992–R995

Schmitz KH, Ahmed RL, Yee D (2002) Effects of a 9-month strength training intervention on insulin, insulin-like growth factor (IGF)-I, IGF-binding protein (IGFBP)-1, and IGFBP-3 in 30–50-year-old women. Cancer Epidemiol Biomark Prev 11:1597–1604

Senchina DS, Kohut ML (2007) Immunological outcomes of exercise in older adults. Clin Interv Aging 2:3–16

Shephard RJ, Shek PN (1995) Cancer, immune function, and physical activity. Can J Appl Physiol 20:1–25

Sirohi B, Powles R (2006) Epidemiology and outcomes research for MGUS, myeloma and amyloidosis. Eur J Cancer 42:1671–1683

Skibola CF, Holly EA, Forrest MS, Hubbard A, Bracci PM, Skibola DR, Hegedus C, Smith MT (2004) Body mass index, leptin and leptin receptor polymorphisms, and non-hodgkin lymphoma. Cancer Epidemiol Biomark Prev 13:779–786

Sugiyama H, Inoue K, Ogawa H, Yamagami T, Soma T, Miyake S, Hirata M, Kishimoto T (1996) The expression of IL-6 and its related genes in acute leukemia. Leuk Lymphoma 21: 49–52

Tao ZF, Fu WJ, Yuan ZG, Wang DX, Chen YB, Hou J (2007) Prognostic factors and staging systems of multiple myeloma. Chin Med J (Engl) 120:1655–1658

Thomas NE, Williams DR (2008) Inflammatory factors, physical activity, and physical fitness in young people. Scand J Med Sci Sports 18: 543–556

Tudor-Locke C, Williams JE, Reis JP, Pluto D (2002) Utility of pedometers for assessing physical activity: convergent validity. Sports Med 32:795–808

U.S. Cancer Statistics Working Group (2009) United States Cancer Statistics: 1999–2005 Incidence and Mortality Web-based Report. Department of Health and Human Services, Centers for Disease Control and Prevention, and National Cancer Institute, Atlanta, GA. Ref Type: Report

Valko M, Rhodes CJ, Moncol J, Izakovic M, Mazur M (2006) Free radicals, metals and antioxidants in oxidative stress-induced cancer. Chem Biol Interact 160:1–40

Van de Velde ALR, Berneman ZN, Van Tendeloo VF (2008) Immunotherapy of hematological malignancies using dendritic cells. Bull Cancer 95:320–326

Vetter U, Schlickenrieder JH, Zapf J, Hartmann W, Heit W, Hitzler H, Byrne P, Gaedicke G, Heinze E, Teller WM (1986) Human leukemic cells: receptor binding and biological effects of insulin and insulin-like growth factors. Leuk Res 10: 1201–1207

Vina J, Gomez-Cabrera MC, Lloret A, Marquez R, Minana JB, Pallardo FV, Sastre J (2000) Free radicals in exhaustive physical exercise: mechanism of production, and protection by antioxidants. IUBMB Life 50:271–277

Voskuil DW, Bueno de Mesquita HB, Kaaks R, van Noord PA, Rinaldi S, Riboli E, Grobbee DE, Peeters PH (2001) Determinants of circulating insulin-like growth factor (IGF)-I and IGF binding proteins 1–3 in premenopausal women: physical activity and anthropometry (Netherlands). Cancer Causes Control 12: 951–958

Wannamethee SG, Shaper AG, Walker M (2001) Physical activity and risk of cancer in middle-aged men. Br J Cancer 85:1311–1316

Westerlind KC (2003) Physical activity and cancer prevention – mechanisms. Med Sci Sports Exerc 35:1834–1840

Woods JA (2005) Physical activity, exercise, and immune function. Brain Behav Immun 19: 369–370

Woods JA, Davis JM (1994) Exercise, monocyte/macrophage function, and cancer. Med Sci Sports Exerc 26:147–156

Woods JA, Davis JM, Smith JA, Nieman DC (1999) Exercise and cellular innate immune function. Med Sci Sports Exerc 31:57–66

Woods JA, Vieira VJ, Keylock KT (2009) Exercise, inflammation, and innate immunity. Immunol Allergy Clin North Am 29:381–393

6

Yang J, Wezeman M, Zhang X, Lin P, Wang M, Qian J, Wan B, Kwak LW, Yu L, Yi Q (2007) Human C-reactive protein binds activating Fcgamma receptors and protects myeloma tumor cells from apoptosis. Cancer Cell 12: 252–265

Yokota T, Oritani K, Takahashi I, Ishikawa J, Matsuyama A, Ouchi N, Kihara S, Funahashi T, Tenner AJ, Tomiyama Y, Matsuzawa Y (2000) Adiponectin, a new member of the family of soluble defense collagens, negatively regulates the growth of myelomonocytic progenitors and the functions of macrophages. Blood 96: 1723–1732

Zahm SH, Hoffman-Goetz L, Dosemeci M, Cantor KP, Blair A (1999) Occupational physical activity and non-Hodgkin's lymphoma. Med Sci Sports Exerc 31:566–571

Physical Activity and Gynecologic Cancer Prevention 7

Anne E. Cust

Abstract This chapter reviews the findings from epidemiologic studies of the associations of physical activity with gynecologic cancers, including those of the endometrium, ovaries, and cervix, and the biologic mechanisms mediating the associations. The epidemiologic evidence to date suggests that physical activity probably protects against endometrial cancer, with a risk reduction of about 20–30% for those with the highest levels of physical activity compared to those with the lowest levels, and that light to moderate physical activity including housework, gardening, or walking for transportation may reduce risk. The role of physical activity in ovarian cancer development remains uncertain, as findings from these studies have been inconsistent with about half the studies suggesting physical activity modestly decreases risk and about half the studies suggesting no association. A recent meta-analysis of studies examining recreational physical activity with ovarian cancer risk estimated a 20% reduced risk for the most active versus least active women. There is mounting evidence that sedentary behaviors such as sitting time probably increase risk of endometrial and ovarian cancers. Overall, there is insufficient evidence to draw a conclusion on a possible role of physical activity in the development of cervical cancer, although a modest influence on risk is possible through effects on sex steroid hormones and immune function. The biologic evidence provides strong support for a protective role of physical activity on cancer of the endometrium, and moderate support for cancer of the ovaries, as these cancers have a strong hormonal etiology. The more established biologic mechanisms that are supported by epidemiologic and experimental data involve endogenous sex hormone levels, insulin-mediated pathways, and maintenance of energy balance.

In this chapter, we will discuss the evidence for an association of physical activity with gynecologic cancers including those of the endometrium, ovaries, and cervix. Cancers of the endometrium and ovaries have a strong hormonal etiology (Risch 1998; Kaaks et al. 2002; Lukanova and Kaaks 2005), and physical activity has been postulated as a potential modifiable risk factor for prevention of these cancers because it can influence circulating hormone levels, energy balance, and insulin-mediated pathways that are thought to be important

A.E. Cust
Centre for Molecular, Environmental, Genetic and Analytic Epidemiology, School of Population Health, The University of Melbourne,
Level 1, 723 Swanston Street, VIC 3010, Australia
e-mail: aecust@unimelb.edu.au

K.S. Courneya and C.M. Friedenreich (eds.), *Physical Activity and Cancer*,
Recent Results in Cancer Research 186, DOI: 10.1007/978-3-642-04231-7_7,

7

mediators underlying the associations. Few studies have evaluated the association of physical activity with cervical cancer because the main causal factor is infection with certain types of human papillomavirus (HPV), although other hormonal and immune factors are also thought to play a role (Smith et al. 2003; Waggoner 2003). We review the findings from epidemiologic studies that have examined the associations of physical activity with gynecologic cancers, and the biologic mechanisms that might mediate the associations.

7.1 Endometrial Cancer

The endometrium is the lining of the uterus, and is made up of several layers of cells, blood vessels, tissue, and glands. An estimated 200,000 women are diagnosed each year with endometrial cancer worldwide, and approximately 50,000 women die from the disease (Ferlay et al. 2004). Incidence rates vary considerably across countries. Overall, the age-standardized rates in more developed regions are 4.5 times higher than in less developed regions (13.6 versus 3.0 per 100,000 person-years), but the difference is up to tenfold between the USA and parts of Africa and Asia (Ferlay et al. 2004). The median age of diagnosis of endometrial cancer in Western populations is approximately 63 years (Rose 1996). The age-specific incidence rates increase markedly around the time of menopause and usually peak at age 65–75 years. Seventy-five percent of cases occur in postmenopausal women, and 25% in premenopausal women (Rose 1996). The overall 5-year survival rates for endometrial cancer are around 80%, although the prognosis depends on the histological type and grade, and surgical stage of the tumor (Pecorelli et al. 1999; Mota and De Oliveira 2003; Amant et al. 2005).

7.1.1 Overall Findings

Lifestyle factors are strongly implicated in the etiology of endometrial cancer (Kaaks et al. 2002; Amant et al. 2005), and there is some epidemiologic evidence that physical activity may play a preventive role (Friedenreich 2001; Thune and Furberg 2001; International Agency for Research on Cancer (IARC) World Health Organization (WHO) 2002; Cust et al. 2007b; Voskuil et al. 2007). In 2002, the International Agency for Research on Cancer concluded, based on a review of ten studies, that regular physical activity possibly reduces risk of endometrial cancer (International Agency for Research on Cancer (IARC) World Health Organization (WHO) 2002). There was no consistent dose-response relation and the risk estimates varied somewhat across the studies. There was also insufficient information about how different physical activity domains (occupational, recreational, household, transport), characteristics (frequency, intensity, duration), and distributions throughout life might influence endometrial cancer risk (Friedenreich 2001; Thune and Furberg 2001; International Agency for Research on Cancer (IARC) World Health Organization (WHO) 2002). To date, 26 studies have examined the association between physical activity, as a primary exposure variable, and endometrial cancer, using a diverse range of study designs, study populations, and physical activity assessment methods (Dosemeci et al. 1993; Levi et al. 1993; Pukkala et al. 1993; Shu et al. 1993; Sturgeon et al. 1993; Zheng et al. 1993; Hirose et al. 1996; Kalandidi et al. 1996; Goodman et al. 1997; Olson et al. 1997; Moradi et al. 1998, 2000; Terry et al. 1999; Salazar-Martinez et al. 2000; Littman et al. 2001; Colbert et al. 2003; Furberg and Thune 2003; Schouten et al. 2004; Matthews et al. 2005; Friberg et al. 2006; Friedenreich et al. 2007; Patel et al. 2008; Conroy et al. 2009; Gierach et al. 2009; Tavani et al. 2009; Friedenreich et al. 2010).

Recent reviews of the literature have concluded that physical activity probably protects against endometrial cancer, independently of body fatness (Cust et al. 2007b; Voskuil et al. 2007; World Cancer Research Fund & American Institute for Cancer Research 2007). A systematic review by Voskuil and colleagues (Voskuil et al. 2007) included seven cohort and 13 case-control studies that assessed either total, recreational or occupational physical activities. The studies consistently showed that physical activity was associated with a decreased risk of endometrial cancer; however, the magnitude of risk reduction varied considerably across studies. A 'best evidence' synthesis showed that the majority (80%) of ten high-quality studies found risk reductions of greater than 20% (Voskuil et al. 2007). Pooling of seven high-quality cohort studies that measured total, recreational, or occupational activity showed a significantly decreased risk of endometrial cancer (summary odds ratio (OR) 0.77; 95% CI 0.70–0.85) for the most active women compared to the least active (Voskuil et al. 2007). The review by Cust and colleagues (Cust et al. 2007b) did not pool results from the different studies due to the heterogeneity in methods across studies used for measuring physical activity; however, they noted that 14 of the 18 studies included in their review found a 'convincing' or 'possible' inverse association between physical activity and endometrial cancer risk, with an average risk reduction of around 30%.

Of 20 studies that examined whether or not a dose-response relation was present between increasing frequency, duration, intensity or METs of physical activity, and risk of endometrial cancer, about half observed a statistically significant dose-response relation (Levi et al. 1993; Moradi et al. 1998, 2000; Terry et al. 1999; Salazar-Martinez et al. 2000; Schouten et al. 2004; Matthews et al. 2005; Gierach et al. 2009) or borderline-significant association (Furberg and Thune 2003; Patel et al. 2008), and half the studies observed no clear dose-response relation (Dosemeci et al. 1993; Goodman et al. 1997; Olson et al. 1997; Littman et al. 2001; Colbert et al. 2003; Friberg et al. 2006; Friedenreich et al. 2007; Conroy et al. 2009; Tavani et al. 2009; Friedenreich et al. 2010). In some studies, a dose-response relation was only observed for certain domains or types of activity. Matthews et al. (2005) observed a dose-response for exercise and lifestyle activity but not for occupational activity; Levi et al. (1993) observed a dose-response for housework, sports, and occupational activity but not for climbing stairs or walking; Schouten et al. (2004) found a dose-response for nonoccupational activity and walking for transport but not for sports or household activity separately; and Friedenreich et al. (2010) noted a dose-response association for recreational activity but not for other activity domains or after adjustment for body mass index (BMI). Littman et al. (2001) did not observe a dose-response relation except for increasing duration of low intensity activities.

The reviews also assessed the methodological quality of the studies. Cust et al. (2007b) reported that prospective cohort studies and population-based case-control studies had better assessment of physical activity, and that the quality of physical activity measures improved over time; however, the quality of physical activity assessment methods did not appear to be related to the observed strength of association or the presence of a dose-response relation between physical activity level and endometrial cancer risk. They noted that case-control studies were more likely than cohort studies to have 'convincing' findings, which could have been influenced by recall bias. The second expert report by the World Cancer Research Fund & American Institute for Cancer Research (2007) also reported that most of the evidence for a protective effect was from case-control studies. Voskuil et al. (2007) noted that case-control studies with relatively unfavorable quality scores reported more divergent risk estimates than studies with higher quality scores.

7.1.2 Domain of Physical Activity

Although there was a large variation in the relative risk estimates, most studies showed an inverse association between physical activity and endometrial cancer risk, with an average reduction of about 30% (Fig. 7.1). A few studies used a summary measure of total physical activity, derived from activity across occupational, household, and recreational domains, and these studies showed relative risk reductions in the range of 8–63%. Most studies measured occupational activity or recreational activity, but fewer studies evaluated household or transport activity. Recently, there has been particular interest in the association of sedentary behaviors, such as sitting time, with cancer risk because these behaviors may be easier to recall than periods of activity (Clark et al. 2008). There were no clear differences in the associations of physical activity in different domains, although it appeared that the relative risk estimates were slightly stronger for total, household, and transport physical activity. This is consistent with the hypothesis that overall energy expenditure, and in particular daily lifestyle-related activities contributing to nonexercise activity thermogenesis (Levine 2004; Ravussin 2005), may be the most important dimension of physical activity assessment. Most of the studies that examined nonoccupational activity controlled reasonably well for potential confounders (such as age, adiposity, reproductive and menstrual factors, and use of exogenous hormones), so it is unlikely that a lack of adjustment of confounders could directly explain the differences in the relative risk estimates among the nonoccupational activity domains.

7.1.3 Intensity, Duration and Frequency of Exposure

Most studies have evaluated some aspect of intensity, duration, and frequency of activity, although few studies measured all of these aspects (Littman et al. 2001; Friedenreich et al. 2007, 2010). With respect to intensity, several studies suggested a 30–40% reduced risk for higher versus lower levels of vigorous activity (Olson et al. 1997; Littman et al. 2001; Conroy et al. 2009; Gierach et al. 2009), whereas other studies observed no association (Colbert et al. 2003; Friedenreich et al. 2007, 2010). Several studies (Terry et al. 1999; Littman et al. 2001; Colbert et al. 2003; Schouten et al. 2004; Matthews et al. 2005; Patel et al. 2008; Friedenreich et al. 2010) demonstrated risk reductions of about 20–50% for light-moderate physical activities, such as walking, gardening, daily household activities, and active transportation. Friedenreich and colleagues observed a 32% reduced risk for the highest versus lowest quartile (corresponding to >21.6 versus ≤11.1 h per week per year) of lifetime total light physical activity, but no association with moderate or vigorous activities (Friedenreich et al. 2010). Colbert et al. (2003) reported a reduced risk with moderate physical activity but only after several years of exposure. Studies that have assessed the role of inactivity, such as sitting time, found increased risk for those sitting for more than about 5 h a day (Friberg et al. 2006; Patel et al. 2008; Gierach et al. 2009). Friedenreich et al. reported an 11% increased risk for every 5 h per week per year of sedentary occupational activity (Friedenreich et al. 2010).

For duration of physical activity, Schouten et al. (2004) found that increasing the duration of nonoccupational physical activities (combining walking and/or cycling for transportation or recreation, gardening and odd jobs, sports or exercise) was significantly associated with reduced risk, with 1 h or more per day (versus <30 min per day) required to reduce risk by 40–50%. Transportation physical activity for 1 h or more per day versus <10 min per day was associated with a 50% reduced risk (Schouten et al. 2004). Matthews and colleagues (2005) reported that walking for transport for at least 1 h a day, or 4 or more h of daily household activities, was associated with a

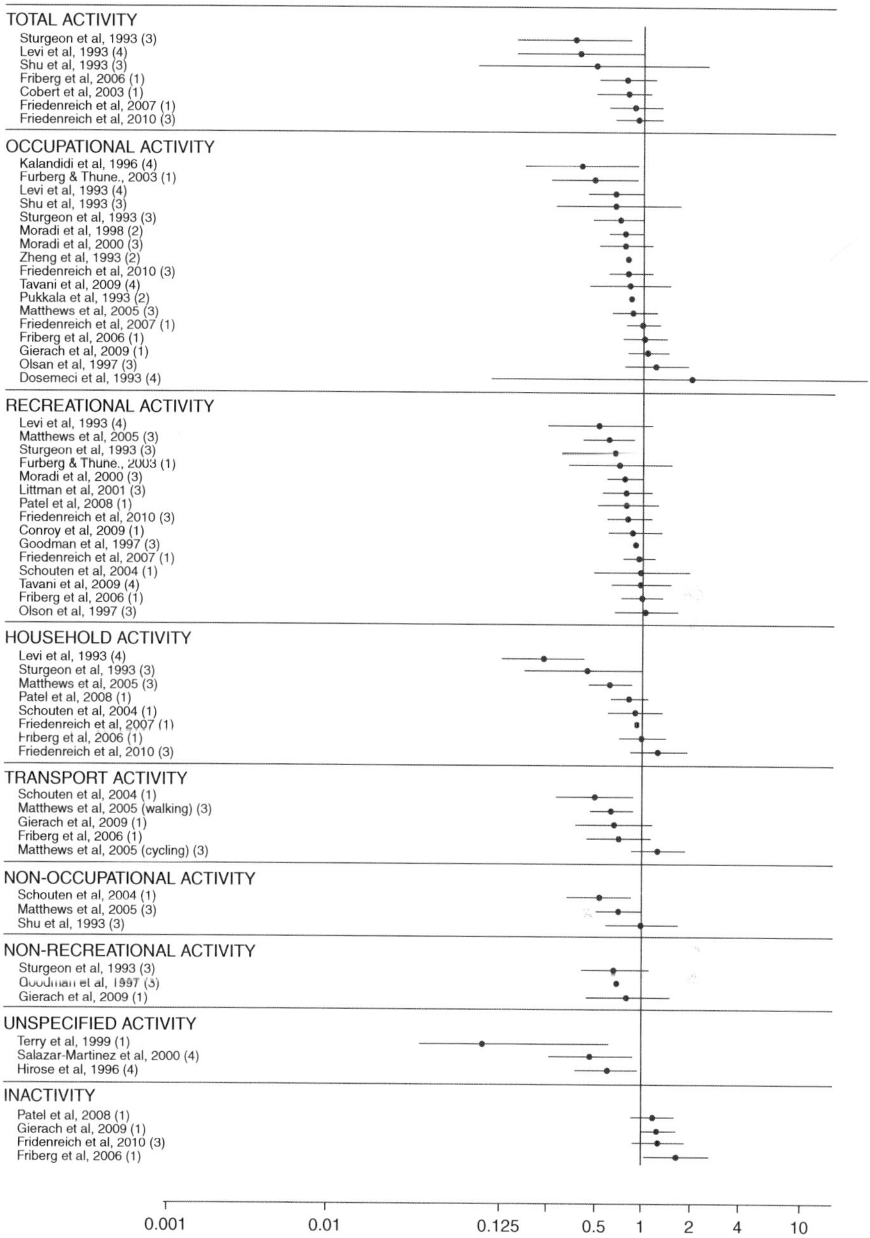

Fig. 7.1 Epidemiologic studies of physical activity and endometrial cancer. Relative risk estimates for endometrial cancer by different domains of physical activity for published studies. The risk estimates are adjusted for confounders where published and are presented for the most active category compared to the least active (reference) category, except for 'Inactivity', which compares the most inactive to least inactive category. Solid squares = relative risk (RR), odds ratio (OR), or standardized incidence ratio (SIR) as reported in the studies. The area of the square reflects the statistical weight (inverse of the variance) of the study. Horizontal bars = 95% confidence intervals (CIs). Some studies did not report CIs; these studies are shown without horizontal bars and 'N/A' is displayed. The numbers in brackets refer to the study design: (1) = prospective cohort, (2) = historical cohort, (3) = population-based case-control study, (4) = hospital-based case-control study

30–40% reduction in risk compared with sedentary women. Moradi et al. (2000) observed a protective effect with about 2 h of recreational activity per week. Friberg et al. (2006) reported that recreational inactivity such as watching TV or sitting for 5 or more h daily versus <5 h was associated with a statistically significantly 66% increased risk of endometrial cancer and that walking or bicycling at least 1 h daily versus <1 h was associated with a 30% nonsignificant decreased risk.

Some studies combined the characteristics of exposure into metabolic equivalent (MET)-hours (Ainsworth et al. 2000). Matthews et al. (2005) observed that women participating in at least 10 MET-h per day of combined lifestyle and other non-occupational activities had a 30% reduced risk compared to women with less than 7 MET-h per day. In the study by Salazar-Martinez and colleagues (2000), women in the top two tertiles of physical activity, corresponding to 30 or more MET-h per week, had a 50% lower risk compared to women doing less than 30 MET-h per week of activity.

7.1.4 Age Period

There is limited information about which age periods physical activity might have the most impact on in reducing endometrial cancer risk, because the majority of studies have measured only recent or usual physical activity. Of those that have measured activity in one or more longer periods in adulthood or adolescence (Dosemeci et al. 1993; Levi et al. 1993; Pukkala et al. 1993; Shu et al. 1993; Sturgeon et al. 1993; Goodman et al. 1997; Olson et al. 1997; Moradi et al. 1998, 2000; Matthews et al. 2005; Tavani et al. 2009; Friedenreich et al. 2010) the evidence generally indicates that recent activity and lifetime activity might be more important than activity in the distant past, but there are no clear patterns for any particular age or biologically relevant periods in life.

Matthews et al. (2005) observed that recalled exercise and lifestyle activities in adolescence and adulthood were generally each associated with a reduced risk of endometrial cancer, but there appeared to be a stronger effect for lifetime exercisers. Moradi et al. (2000) observed a 20–30% reduced risk associated with highly active recreational behavior compared to sedentary behavior in recent years and in early adulthood, which was stronger if the recreational activity was sustained over both of these adult periods; however, adolescent recreational physical activity level was not associated with risk. Olson et al. (1997) found that physical activity was generally not associated with risk assessed at four different life periods ranging from age 16 to late adulthood. Similarly, Shu et al. (1993) did not observe any relation during 4 different decades in adulthood, and nor did Friedenreich et al. (2010) when they examined biologically relevant life periods.

The two studies by Moradi et al. (1998, 2000) suggest that the effect of occupational activity on endometrial cancer risk was largely attributable to recent activity rather than past activity levels. Levi et al. (1993) reported an inverse association between total physical level and risk at all ages, but that was stronger at ages 55 years and older. Similarly, Sturgeon et al. (1993) observed that high levels of recent physical activity were generally associated with greater risk reductions than high levels of lifetime physical activity. Colbert et al. (2003) suggested that at least 8 years of sustained moderate physical activity may be necessary to reduce risk. Patel et al. (2008) prospectively measured exercise at two time-points 10 years apart and found that compared to participants who were inactive at both periods, those who were consistently active or active in only one of the periods had similar risk reductions.

7.1.5 Population Subgroups

Risk information for different subgroups is important for identifying women at high risk of developing cancer who could benefit from increased surveillance, screening, or interventions, as well as for providing clues regarding the biologic mechanisms underlying associations with risk. There has been no consistent evidence that the association of physical activity with endometrial cancer risk might differ for different population subgroups. Several studies reported a stronger effect of physical activity in women with a high BMI (Levi et al. 1993; Sturgeon et al. 1993; Furberg and Thune 2003; Patel et al. 2008) or high caloric intake (Levi et al. 1993); however, conversely, one study found a stronger effect in women with a lower BMI (Moradi et al. 2000), and other studies found no effect modification by BMI (Friberg et al. 2006; Friedenreich et al. 2007, 2010). There were also suggestions of a stronger benefit of physical activity among women who had never smoked (Moradi et al. 2000) or who had never used oral contraceptives (Schouten et al. 2004; Friedenreich et al. 2007) or hormone replacement therapy (Friedenreich et al. 2007).

There was no strong evidence for effect modification by menopausal status (Sturgeon et al. 1993; Colbert et al. 2003; Matthews et al. 2005; Friedenreich et al. 2010) or age (Levi et al. 1993; Moradi et al. 1998; Furberg and Thune 2003), as the observed effect modification was not statistically significant in any study. Friedenreich et al. (2007) observed a somewhat stronger protective association among premenopausal women than among postmenopausal women, which was most apparent for household and recreational activities. Matthews et al. (2005) reported a slightly stronger association of household and walking activities, but not total lifestyle activity, in premenopausal women. Some studies observed an apparently stronger association in older (>50 years) than in younger women for total (Levi et al. 1993), recreational, (Furberg and Thune 2003) or occupational activity (Moradi et al. 1998); although Furberg et al. (Furberg and Thune 2003) suggested a stronger association of occupational activity in women younger than 50 years.

7.1.6 Conclusions

The epidemiologic evidence from the studies to date suggest that physical activity probably protects against endometrial cancer, with a risk reduction of about 20–30% for those with the highest levels of physical activity compared to those with the lowest levels. Given that measurement of physical activity is difficult because of its complex and varied characteristics, errors in measurement are expected to lead to nondifferential misclassification of exposure and underestimation of the relative risk (Willett 1989; Armstrong et al. 1992; International Agency for Research on Cancer (IARC) World Health Organization (WHO) 2002). Thus, the 'true' risk reduction could be greater than the average 20–30% observed in the studies conducted to date.

The main gaps in the literature include a lack of a consistent dose-response relation, imprecise risk estimates, and insufficient information about how different physical activity domains, characteristics (frequency, intensity, duration), and distributions throughout life might influence endometrial cancer risk. A major methodological limitation that has hindered progress in determining the precise nature of the association between physical activity and cancer risk is the heterogeneous and relatively crude methods used to measure physical activity across studies, although this limitation is common to the majority of studies on physical activity.

The available evidence suggests that light and moderate physical activity, including housework, gardening, or walking for transportation, may reduce risk, and that sitting time may increase risk. The effect of light- and moderate-intensity activities is of significant public health importance because such activities comprise the majority of women's daily energy expenditure (Ainsworth 2000) and are easier to adopt and maintain participation in compared to vigorous activities (Pate et al. 1995). Currently, public health guidelines recommend that adults perform moderate-intensity physical activity for a minimum of 30 min 5 days each week to maintain good health (National Center for Chronic Disease Prevention and Health Promotion; Centers for Disease Control and Prevention 1996; Australian Government Department of Health and Ageing 2005; Haskell et al. 2007) and 60 min each day for cancer risk reduction (World Cancer Research Fund & American Institute for Cancer Research 2007). Although imprecise, some of the studies conducted to date suggest that about 1 h per day of light to moderate-intensity activity may confer a reduction in endometrial cancer risk.

7.2 Ovarian Cancer

Ovarian cancer is the sixth most common incident cancer and cause of cancer deaths in women in developed countries (Ferlay et al. 2004). The prognosis upon diagnosis is relatively poor because clinical presentation of the disease often occurs at an advanced stage (Cannistra 2004). Thus, it is particularly important to identify potentially modifiable risk factors for prevention of ovarian cancer. Although the causes of ovarian cancer are not fully understood, hormonal factors are known to play a role. Use of oral contraceptives confers long-term protection against ovarian cancer (Beral et al. 2008), whereas nulliparity (Kristensen and Trope 1997), overweight (Olsen et al. 2007b; Schouten et al. 2008; Lahmann et al. 2009a) and incessant ovulation (Purdie et al. 2003) increase risk. Physical activity has been proposed as a possible protective factor particularly by affecting levels of endogenous hormones as well as through other mechanisms.

7.2.1 Overall Findings

To date, 21 studies have examined the association between physical activity and ovarian cancer risk, including nine prospective cohort studies (Bertone et al. 2001; Anderson et al. 2004; Hannan et al. 2004; Schnohr et al. 2005; Biesma et al. 2006; Patel et al. 2006; Weiderpass et al. 2006; Lahmann et al. 2009b; Leitzmann et al. 2009), two historical cohort studies (Pukkala et al. 1993; Zheng et al. 1993), seven population-based case-control studies (Cottreau et al. 2000; Bertone et al. 2002; Riman et al. 2004; Pan et al. 2005; Olsen et al. 2007a; Carnide et al. 2009; Rossing et al. 2010), and three hospital-based case-control studies (Dosemeci et al. 1993; Tavani et al. 2001; Zhang et al. 2003).

Despite more than 20 published studies on this topic, the role of physical activity in ovarian cancer development remains uncertain because the findings from these studies have been inconsistent. About half of the studies have indicated a decreased risk with increasing physical activity (Cottreau et al. 2000; Tavani et al. 2001; Zhang et al. 2003; Riman et al. 2004; Pan et al. 2005; Schnohr et al. 2005; Biesma et al. 2006; Carnide et al. 2009; Rossing et al. 2010), half observed no association (Dosemeci et al. 1993; Pukkala et al. 1993; Zheng et al. 1993; Bertone et al. 2001, 2002; Hannan et al. 2004; Patel et al. 2006; Weiderpass et al. 2006; Olsen et al. 2007a; Lahmann et al. 2009b; Leitzmann et al. 2009), and one reported an increased risk (Anderson et al. 2004). In addition, of studies that observed an inverse association of physical activity with risk, a dose-response relation was not always observed for all types of activity. Tavani et al. (2001) found a dose–response only for occupational activity but not for recreational activity. Rossing and colleagues (2010) observed a statistically significant trend of decreasing risk with increasing duration of high-intensity recreational activity; however, no trend was observed for either duration of total recreational physical activity, low-intensity or moderate-intensity activity, or MET-hours per week of recreational activity.

The 2007 second expert report by the World Cancer Research Fund & American Institute for

Cancer Research (2007) examined the role of physical activity on ovarian cancer risk but found that the data were inadequate to draw a conclusion. A recent meta-analysis of six case-control studies and six cohort studies that assessed the association of recreational physical activity with ovarian cancer risk reported a pooled relative risk of 0.81 (95% CI 0.72–0.92) for the most active versus the least active women (Olsen et al. 2007a). The risk estimates were similar for cohort studies (relative risk (RR) = 0.81) and case-control studies (RR = 0.79), although the 95% confidence intervals for the cohort studies pooled estimate included the null (95% CI 0.57–1.17). Heterogeneity was present among the cohort studies, which was attributed to one study that observed an increased risk with higher levels of physical activity (Anderson et al. 2004).

7.2.2 Domain of Physical Activity

Most studies assessed recreational activity, but a few examined the other domains of physical activity (Fig. 7.2). A meta-analysis of six case-control studies and six cohort studies estimated a statistically significant 19% relative risk reduction of ovarian cancer for the highest versus lowest levels of recreational physical activity (Olsen et al. 2007a). Olsen and colleagues also reviewed studies assessing occupational activity but found no consistency in results, with about half the studies observing a modest inverse association of physical activity with ovarian cancer risk, and half the studies reporting no association with risk (Olsen et al. 2007a). Lahmann et al. (2009b) observed no association with physical activity and this was consistent for occupational, recreational, household, and total physical activity level. Pan et al. (2005) observed risk reductions for both recreational and occupational physical activity. Biesma and colleagues (Biesma et al. 2006) noted a weak, inverse association with nonoccupational physical activity; when they examined the different types of activities, the inverse association was stronger (35% relative risk reduction) for women who spent more than 2 h per week on recreational biking and walking compared to women who did not do these activities, and there was no association with gardening or sports activities.

7.2.3 Intensity, Duration and Frequency of Exposure

With regard to intensity of physical activity, Patel et al. (2006) observed no association of light, moderate, or vigorous recreational physical activity with risk, but they did observe a positive association with increasing sitting time; 3–5 h of sitting per day were associated with a 21% increased risk, and 6 or more h per day of sitting was associated with a 55% increased risk. Similarly, Zhang et al. (2004) also found that sedentary behaviors, including sitting at work, sitting while watching television, and total sitting duration were associated with an increased risk. One small study suggested an inverse association of occupational sitting time with risk, but the confidence intervals were very wide (OR 0.4, 95% CI 0.1–1.9) (Dosemeci et al. 1993).

Findings from several studies suggest that vigorous-intensity physical activity might increase ovarian cancer risk. Anderson et al. (2004) was the only study that found a statistically significant increased risk with higher levels of recreational physical activity, and they noted that the association was particularly strong for frequency of vigorous physical activity, where the risk was approximately doubled for activity more than four times per week versus rarely or never. Bertone et al. (2001) also found the possibility of a modest increase in risk with frequent vigorous activity. Carnide et al. (2009) reported an increased risk associated with strenuous recreational activity up to two times per week during adolescence and early adulthood, but observed a decreased risk for recent moderate or strenuous

7

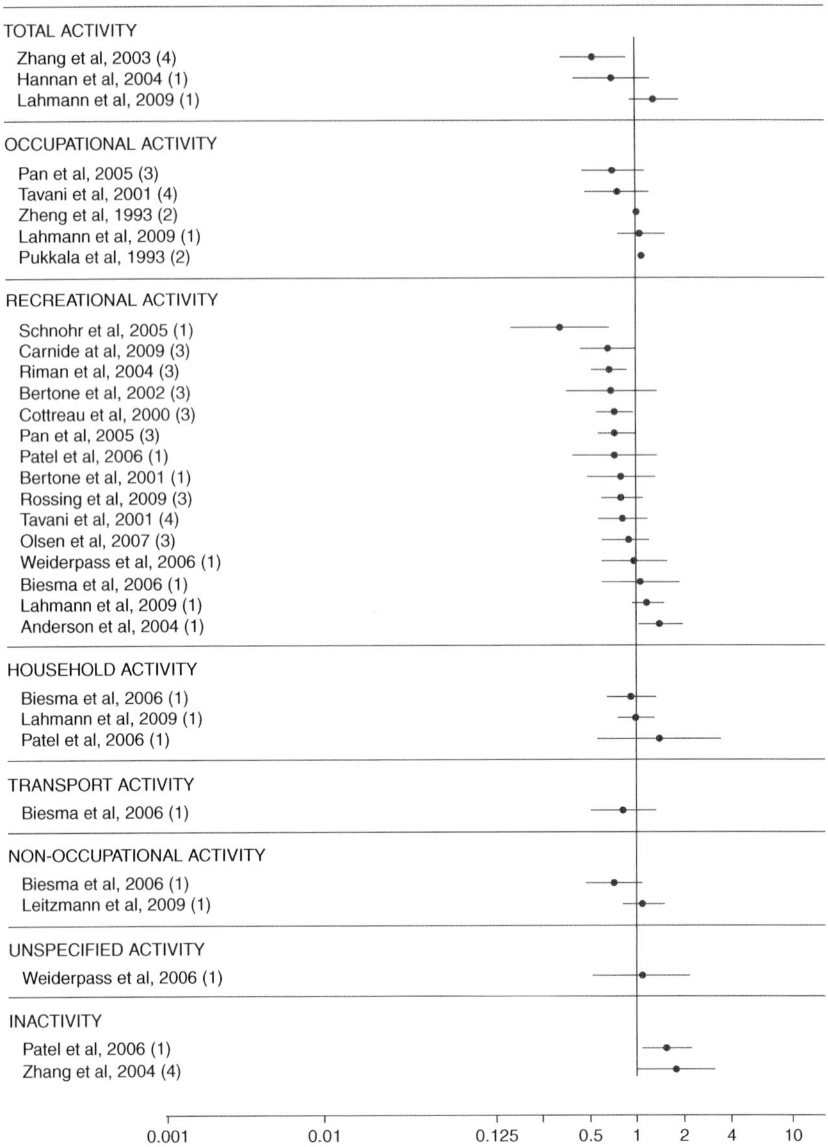

Fig. 7.2 Epidemiologic studies of physical activity and ovarian cancer. Relative risk estimates for ovarian cancer by different domains of physical activity for published studies. The risk estimates are adjusted for confounders where published and are presented for the most active category compared to the least active (reference) category, except for 'Inactivity', which compares the most inactive to least inactive category. The risk estimate from the study by Dosemeci et al. (1993) is not included in the figure due to the very wide confidence intervals (OR 0.26, 95% CI 0.001–10.0). Solid squares = relative risk (RR), odds ratio (OR), or standardized incidence ratio (SIR) as reported in the studies. The area of the square reflects the statistical weight (inverse of the variance) of the study. Horizontal bars = 95% confidence intervals (CIs). Some studies did not report CIs; these studies are shown without horizontal bars and 'N/A' is displayed. The numbers in brackets refer to the study design: (1) = prospective cohort, (2) = historical cohort, (3) = population-based case-control study, (4) = hospital-based case-control study

activity up to two times per week; however, no dose-response relation was observed. When moderate and strenuous recreational activity was combined, there was an inverse association between frequency of recent activity and ovarian cancer risk (Carnide et al. 2009). Leitzmann and colleagues (2009) observed a statistically non-significant increased risk of serous cancer and a decreased risk of non-serous cancer among women who engaged in vigorous activity. The authors hypothesized that the positive relation between physical activity and ovarian cancer could be attributable to detection bias if more vigorously active women tended to be more symptomatic (Leitzmann et al. 2009). Two studies (Pan et al. 2005; Biesma et al. 2006) observed decreasing risk with increasing levels of moderate recreational physical activity but no association with vigorous physical activity. Similarly, Pan et al. (2005) observed statistically significant risk reductions for moderate occupational physical activity compared to those who worked in sedentary occupations, but weaker risk reductions for strenuous occupational activity.

Conversely, other studies have observed a decreased risk of ovarian cancer with increasing vigorous activity (Zhang et al. 2003; Schnohr et al. 2005; Rossing et al. 2010). Rossing and colleagues (2010) observed a 40% reduced risk of invasive ovarian cancer for women who reported more than 1.5 h per week of high intensity recreational activity compared to inactive women; however, no association with risk was observed for a measure of MET-hours per week of moderate- and high-intensity activity combined. Several studies did not observe any differences between moderate and vigorous activity and risk of ovarian cancer (Bertone et al. 2002; Zhang et al. 2003; Hannan et al. 2004; Olsen et al. 2007a).

7.2.4 Age Period

Most studies that measured physical activity at different age periods reported consistent findings for the associations during childhood, adolescence, and various stages of adulthood, including consistent risk reductions (Cottreau et al. 2000; Tavani et al. 2001; Riman et al. 2004; Pan et al. 2005; Rossing et al. 2010) or consistent null associations (Bertone et al. 2002; Patel et al. 2006; Weiderpass et al. 2006; Olsen et al. 2007a). Conversely, the findings by Carnide et al. (2009) suggested that strenuous recreational activity early in life might increase risk of ovarian cancer, whereas more recent recreational activity may reduce risk.

7.2.5 Population Subgroups

Most studies did not find evidence for effect modification of the association between physical activity and ovarian cancer risk by BMI, menopausal status, hormone use, parity, smoking status, family history, or for different histological subtypes, although most of the studies had limited ability to detect associations with risk for different population subgroups due to relatively small sample sizes. Pan et al. (2005) observed similar risk reductions for pre- and postmenopausal women, but a slightly stronger protective effect for overweight and obese women. An analysis of the Nurses' Health Study cohort (Bertone et al. 2001) showed a modest increased risk of ovarian cancer for women who frequently engaged in vigorous activity compared with inactive women that was stronger in leaner women (BMI < 25 kg/m^2), but the interaction was not statistically significant. One large population-based case-control study (Olsen et al. 2007a) found no effect modification by menopausal status or BMI.

Associations of physical activity with ovarian cancer might differ according to the specific histological subtype, because each subtype has distinct clinical and morphological features and potentially different etiologies (Chen et al. 2003; Kurian et al. 2005). However, findings

7

for specific histological subtypes have been inconsistent across studies. Pan et al. (2005) observed that for moderate recreational physical activity, increasing activity level was associated with a statistically significant trend of decreasing risk of serous, endometrioid, and other types of ovarian tumors, but no significant association with mucinous tumors. For vigorous activity, no association was observed for serous and endometrioid tumors, but there was a suggestion of an increased risk for mucinous and other types of tumors (Pan et al. 2005). Findings from two other studies also indicated that physical activity might offer no protection against mucinous tumors (Riman et al. 2004; Olsen et al. 2007a).

Rossing and colleagues (2010) observed an inverse association of vigorous physical activity with risk of invasive but not borderline epithelial ovarian tumors. They also noted important differences for invasive tumors according to histological subtype; relative to inactive women, the risk of serous invasive cancer was reduced for women who reported any recreational physical activity; however, in contrast, risk of endometrioid/clear cell tumors was positively associated with physical activity and this was consistent across different age-periods (Rossing et al. 2010). No dose-response trend was apparent for the inverse association with serous invasive cancer, as 30 min per day and 3 h per day of activity were associated with the same risk reductions. However, there was a dose–response for the positive association with endometrioid/clear cell tumors; with risk more than doubled for women reporting more than 3 h per week of recreational activity (Rossing et al. 2010). Conversely, Leitzmann et al. (2009) noted an increased risk of serous cancer and a decreased risk of nonserous cancer among women who engaged in vigorous activity, although neither association was statistically significant. Olsen et al. (2007a) reported a nonsignificant reduced risk of invasive endometrioid tumors with moderate levels of physical activity.

In the prospective Nurses Health Study, Hecht and colleagues (2009) examined whether or not the association of physical activity with ovarian cancer risk might differ according to the estrogen receptor or progesterone receptor status of the tumor, but they found no association with risk for all receptor expression subgroups.

7.2.6 Conclusions

Despite more than 20 published studies on this topic, the role of physical activity in ovarian cancer development remains uncertain, as findings from these studies have been inconsistent. About half of the studies suggest a decreased risk of ovarian cancer with increasing physical activity, and about half the studies suggest no association. In addition, some studies reported a positive association of vigorous levels of physical activity with risk. Several plausible biologic mechanisms have been postulated to support a protective effect of physical activity on ovarian cancer risk, although there is also some biologic plausibility for vigorous activity increasing risk. Some recent studies have also evaluated the role of sedentary behaviors such as sitting time, which, similar to endometrial cancer, does appear to increase ovarian cancer risk. The public health implications of a positive association of inactivity with risk are substantial, given the long duration that most people spend sitting each day.

Inconsistencies in results across studies may be attributable to variation in physical activity measurement between studies, study designs, study populations, or bias. Any protective effect of physical activity on ovarian cancer risk is likely to be modest, and thus may be difficult to detect using questionnaire measurement because of misclassification of physical activity levels. Most studies also had limited numbers of cases and so they suffered a lack of power to detect modest associations, and were thus unable to exclude chance as an explanation of findings. Conducting a meta-analysis is one way of overcoming the lack of power in individual studies, and a recent meta-analysis of studies examining recreational physical activity with ovarian cancer risk estimated a 20% reduction in risk for the most active versus least active women (Olsen et al. 2007a). There is limited evidence concerning the role of other types of activity, including total, occupational, household, or transport activity. There was some indication that associations might differ according to the histological subtype of the tumor, but studies with larger sample sizes or more detailed physical activity measures are required to investigate these associations more fully.

7.3 Cervical Cancer

Cancer of the cervix is the second most frequent cancer in women worldwide, although incidence and mortality are decreasing in developed countries due to the success of cervical cancer screening and the recent development of the HPV vaccine (Mathew and George 2009). In 2002, around half a million new cases per year were recorded, accounting for around 10% of all new cancers in women (Ferlay et al. 2004; Parkin et al. 2005). Cervical cancer is much more common in developing countries, where 83% of cases occur, largely because screening is not at optimum levels (Parkin et al. 2005). It is the third most common cause of cancer death in women, with 5-year survival rates around 40% in developing countries and 60% in developed countries (Parkin et al. 2005; World Cancer Research Fund & American Institute for Cancer Research 2007).

It is firmly established that the major causal factor for cervical cancer is infection with specific oncogenic subtypes of HPV (Waggoner 2003; Parkin et al. 2005). However, although HPV is recognized as a necessary agent for cervical carcinogenesis, it is by itself not a sufficient cause of cervical cancer, as only a minority of women who are infected by HPV develop cervical intraepithelial neoplasia (CIN) and progression of the lesions to invasive cervical cancer (World Cancer Research Fund & American Institute for Cancer Research 2007). Other cofactors that are believed to modify the risk of cervical cancer for women infected with HPV include parity, cigarette smoking, endogenous and exogenous hormones including long-term use of oral contraceptives, co-infection with other sexually transmitted infections, diet, as well as individual susceptibility, immune status, and viral characteristics (Stuver and Adami 2002; Moodley et al. 2003; Smith et al. 2003; Waggoner 2003; Parkin et al. 2005; Delvenne et al. 2007; Steben and Duarte-Franco 2007; World Cancer Research Fund & American Institute for Cancer Research 2007).

Physical activity is not considered to play an important role in modifying risk of cervical cancer, although a modest role of physical activity in influencing risk is plausible because a general nutritional status may affect a woman's vulnerability to infection, and because hormonal and immune factors can modify risk (Stuver and Adami 2002; Smith et al. 2003; Waggoner 2003; World Cancer Research Fund & American Institute for Cancer Research 2007).

7.3.1 Overall Findings and Conclusions

Three studies have evaluated the association of physical activity with cervical cancer (Fig. 7.3). In the prospective National Health and Nutrition Examination Survey (NHANES I) cohort, women who reported their nonrecreational activity as 'quite inactive' had a statistically significant fivefold increased risk compared to those who were 'very active', although the confidence intervals were wide (95% CI = 1.4–14.5)

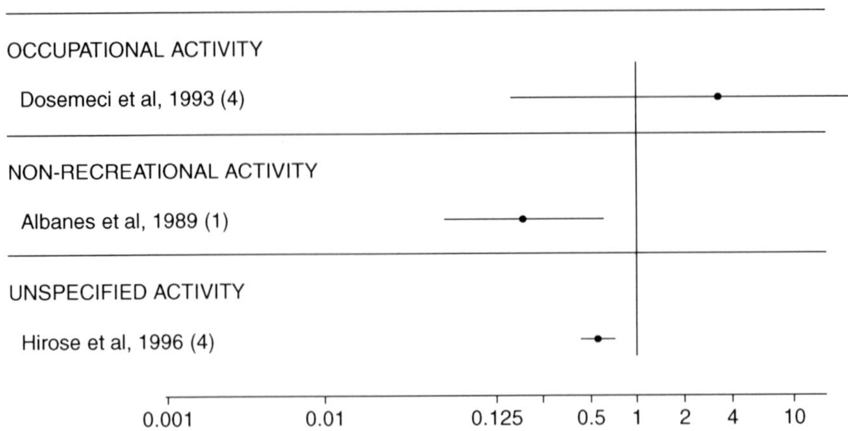

Fig. 7.3 Epidemiologic studies of physical activity and cervical cancer. Relative risk estimates for cervical cancer by different domains of physical activity for published studies. The risk estimates are adjusted for confounders where published and are presented for the most active category compared to the least active (reference) category. Solid squares = relative risk (RR), odds ratio (OR), or standardized incidence ratio (SIR) as reported in the studies. Horizontal bars = 95% confidence intervals. The numbers in brackets refer to the study design: (1) = prospective cohort, (4) = hospital-based case-control study

(Albanes et al. 1989). Conversely, in the NHANES study, recreational exercise was not related to risk although the risk estimate was not provided (Albanes et al. 1989). A hospital-based case-control study from Japan (Hirose et al. 1996) observed a protective association of physical exercise with risk of cervical cancer (OR 0.56, 95% CI 0.44–0.72), adjusted only for age and year of first hospital visit. Conversely, a small hospital-based case control study (Dosemeci et al. 1993) reported a nonsignificant increased risk of cervical cancer with increased occupational activity although the confidence intervals were very wide. Occupational activity was classified using occupational job titles and risk estimates were adjusted for age, smoking, and socioeconomic status (Dosemeci et al. 1993).

A major limitation of the published studies to date is the inability to control for HPV status or sexual behavior, because none of the studies were specifically designed to examine the relation between physical activity and risk of cervical cancer. Overall, there is insufficient evidence to draw a conclusion on a possible role of physical activity in the development of cervical cancer.

7.4 Biologic Mechanisms

Understanding the biologic mechanisms that might underlie associations between physical activity and cancer incidence is important because it can (a) support the epidemiologic evidence, (b) inform the design and implementation of physical activity interventions at the population and individual level to reduce cancer risk, and (c) give new clues to cancer biology that could help design new cancer treatments or prevention strategies (McTiernan 2008). There are several biologic mechanisms that might mediate a protective effect of higher levels of physical activity on risk of gynecologic cancers. They include direct and indirect effects of physical activity on endogenous sex hormone levels, body weight and fatness, insulin-mediated pathways, inflammation, and immune function (Fig. 7.4).

7.4.1 Sex Hormone Levels

Modification of endogenous sex hormone levels is the major hypothesized biologic mechanism mediating a possible association between physical activity and cancers of the endometrium and ovaries (Kaaks et al. 2002; Lukanova and Kaaks 2005). Physical activity could influence ovarian and endometrial cancer risk through its effects on sex hormone levels and menstrual function by influencing the balance of circulating estrogens, progesterone, and androgens (McTiernan 2008). Hormonal pathways are also considered to be important in cervical cancer carcinogenesis, because pregnancy and long-term use of oral contraceptives are associated with risk (Moodley et al. 2003; Smith et al. 2003; Delvenne et al. 2007).

Prolonged exposure to estrogens that are insufficiently counterbalanced by progesterone is a major etiologic determinant of endometrial cancer – known as the 'unopposed estrogens hypothesis' (Key and Pike 1988; Kaaks et al. 2002). In postmenopausal women, estrogen levels appear to be the main determinant of endometrial cancer risk, whereas among premenopausal women, progesterone deficiency is the main risk factor (Key and Pike 1988; Kaaks et al. 2002). For ovarian cancer, risk is increased when levels of androgens and estrogens are elevated and levels of progesterone decreased, which results in proliferative and anti-apoptotic effects on ovarian epithelial tissue (Risch 1998; Lukanova and Kaaks 2005; Olsen et al. 2008).

For cervical cancer, there is evidence suggesting that sex steroid hormones can influence the tumorigenic effect of HPV on cervical tissue (Stuver and Adami 2002; Moodley et al. 2003; Delvenne et al. 2007). Sex steroid hormones could facilitate cervical carcinogenesis by different mechanisms, including the induction of

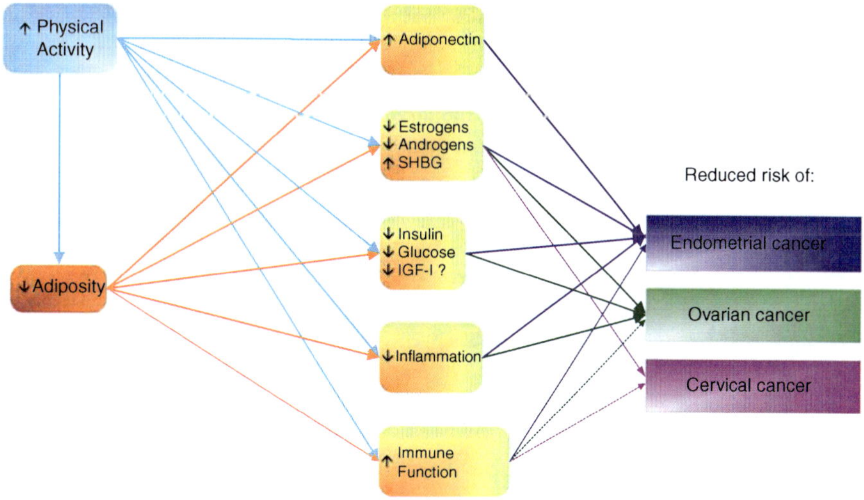

Fig. 7.4 Hypothesized biologic model mediating possible associations between physical activity and risk of endometrial, ovarian, and cervical cancers. Dotted lines indicate limited evidence for pathway

7

squamous metaplasia, interactions between sex steroid hormones and HPV gene expression, and alterations of the local immune microenvironment (Delvenne et al. 2007). Sex steroid hormones could stimulate or suppress transcription of various genes by binding to specific DNA sequences within transcriptional regulatory regions on the HPV DNA (Stuver and Adami 2002; Moodley et al. 2003; Delvenne et al. 2007). They could also affect the immune response to HPV by altering the local immune microenvironment and also by acting on cytokine production (Stuver and Adami 2002; Delvenne et al. 2007). In addition, the mitogenic activity of estrogens may be amplified by viral oncoproteins (Delvenne et al. 2007).

Several observational studies have shown physical activity to be inversely associated with total and bioavailable estrogen levels (Nelson et al. 1988; Cauley et al. 1989; Verkasalo et al. 2001). One study observed a nonlinear U-shaped relation between recreational physical activity and sex hormone levels in postmenopausal women (Bertone-Johnson et al. 2009). Stronger evidence comes from intervention studies (McTiernan et al. 2004a, b; McTiernan 2008), where regular, moderate physical activity over 12 months resulted in lower serum levels of estrogens and androgens, which was only partly explained by decreased fat mass.

Participation in regular moderate- to vigorous-intensity sports has been associated with menstrual cycle irregularities including delayed onset of menarche, increased incidence of oligomenorrhea and secondary amenorrhea (irregular or absent menstrual periods), abnormal luteal function, loss of the surge in luteinizing hormone, and a longer menstrual cycle length (Dale et al. 1979; Frisch et al. 1980; Warren 1980; Frisch et al. 1981; Bullen et al. 1985; Bernstein et al. 1987; Broocks et al. 1990; De Souza et al. 1998; De Souza 2003): factors that are generally associated with decreased risk of endometrial and ovarian cancers (Key and Pike 1988; Risch 1998; Kaaks et al. 2002; Lukanova and Kaaks 2005; Olsen et al. 2008). However, not all studies have observed disruption to menstrual function in response to moderate-intensity physical activity (Bonen 1992; Rogol et al. 1992; McTiernan 2008). It has been proposed that physical activity might only influence menstrual dysfunction when energy intake is insufficient to meet energy demands (Loucks 2003), or that suppression of ovulation might only occur with extreme activity levels (Bertone et al. 2001).

The delayed onset of menarche and menstrual cycle irregularities could have a protective effect on endometrial and ovarian cancer risk by decreasing the cumulative number of ovulatory cycles and subsequent diminution of lifetime exposure to endogenous estrogen (Dale et al. 1979; Broocks et al. 1990). On the other hand, these menstrual cycle irregularities are also characterized by lower peak (luteal phase) and average progesterone levels that lead to increased proliferation and mitotic activity in the endometrium and ovaries (Henderson et al. 1983; Key and Pike 1988; Risch 1998; Kaaks et al. 2002; Lukanova and Kaaks 2005). Thus, high-intensity activity might increase endometrial or ovarian cancer risk by lowering progesterone levels. Vigorous activity could also plausibly increase risk of ovarian cancer by increasing gonadotropins via hypothalamic feedback in response to lower estrogen levels (Gertig and Hunter 2002).

7.4.2 Adiposity

Obesity is a major established risk factor for endometrial cancer (Kaaks et al. 2002), and excess weight alone is estimated to cause around half of all endometrial cancer cases in Europe and the USA (2002; Calle and Kaaks 2004). Recent meta-analyses also demonstrate that obesity is associated with an estimated 30% increased risk of ovarian cancer when compared to normal weight (Olsen et al. 2007b; Schouten et al. 2008; Lahmann et al. 2009a). Thus, physical activity could protect against endometrial and ovarian cancers by maintaining energy balance and reducing excess adipose tissue. Low- and moderate-intensity physical activities are thought to be particularly important for maintaining energy balance and preventing weight gain because they are the main determinants of overall physical activity energy expenditure (King and Tribble 1991; Levine 2004, 2005, 2006; Ravussin 2005).

In postmenopausal women, in whom ovarian production of both estrogen and progesterone has ceased, the primary source of estrogens is from the conversion of androgens to estrogens within adipose tissue (Forney et al. 1981; Key and Pike 1988; Kaaks et al. 2002; Calle and Kaaks 2004; Lukanova and Kaaks 2005; Rinaldi et al. 2006). Therefore, in postmenopausal women, the degree of overweight or obesity directly influences the levels of total and bioavailable estrogens (Forney et al. 1981; Kaaks et al. 2002). In premenopausal women, obesity is associated with chronic anovulation, reduced luteal phase progesterone levels, and irregular menstrual periods (Key and Pike 1988; Key et al. 2001; Kaaks et al. 2002). In premenopausal women, adiposity has also been shown to be inversely associated with plasma concentrations of progesterone and sex hormone binding globulin (SHBG), and is positively associated with free testosterone (Kaaks et al. 2005; Tworoger et al. 2006; Rinaldi et al. 2007). Excess weight is also associated with both early menarche and delayed menopause (Sherman et al. 1981; Frisch et al. 1987), conditions that reflect prolonged cumulative exposure to unopposed estrogens and that are associated with increased endometrial and ovarian cancer risk (Key and Pike 1988; World Cancer Research Fund & American Institute for Cancer Research 2007). In addition, increased adiposity is linked to insulin resistance, hyperinsulinemia and hyperglycemia, inflammation and immune function; these pathways are discussed in more detail in the next section.

7.4.3 Insulin-Mediated Pathways

Insulin resistance and the insulin-like growth factor (IGF)-I pathway are implicated in the etiology of endometrial cancer (Kaaks and Lukanova 2001, 2002; Kaaks et al. 2002; Calle and Kaaks 2004; Lukanova et al. 2004; Cust et al. 2007a, d) and, to a lesser extent, ovarian cancer (Lukanova et al. 2002; Lukanova and Kaaks 2005; Peeters et al. 2007; Olsen et al. 2008). Physical activity could reduce risk of endometrial and ovarian cancers by enhancing insulin sensitivity, lowering insulin and glucose levels, and modifying the insulin-like growth factor (IGF) axis, independently of changes to body weight or body composition (McTiernan 2008).

Moderate- and vigorous-intensity activities have been associated with acute and prolonged improvements in glycemic control and insulin sensitivity (Mayer-Davis et al. 1998; Borghouts and Keizer 2000; Ross et al. 2000; Boule et al. 2001; Duncan et al. 2003; Ross et al. 2004; Frank et al. 2005), lower circulating insulin levels (Feskens et al. 1994; Irwin et al. 2000; Allen et al. 2003; Pischon et al. 2003), increased levels of SHBG (Hamalainen et al. 1987; van Gils et al. 2009) and IGFBP-1 (Rajaram et al. 1997; Kaaks and Lukanova 2001; Allen et al. 2003), and a reduced prevalence of metabolic syndrome (Irwin et al. 2002). Light-intensity physical activity and time spent in sedentary behaviors may also be important determinants of insulin sensitivity, as one study using objectively measured physical activity showed that blood glucose levels were inversely associated with light-intensity physical activity and positively associated with sedentary time (Healy et al. 2007).

There are several direct and indirect mechanisms by which insulin and IGF-I could influence endometrial and ovarian cancer risk (Kaaks and Lukanova 2001; Lukanova et al. 2002; Cust et al. 2007a; Peeters et al. 2007). Insulin can act directly as a mitogenic and anti-apoptotic

7

growth factor, and could increase total and bioavailable levels of estrogens and androgens by downregulating hepatic production of SHBG and upregulating ovarian sex steroid production. In addition, chronic high insulin levels can, in susceptible women, exacerbate ovarian hyperandrogenism and lead to increased frequency of anovulatory menstrual cycles and progesterone deficiency.

Observational studies have linked high IGF-I levels with ovarian cancer especially in premenopausal women (Lukanova et al. 2002; Peeters et al. 2007), and IGF-I levels in endometrial tissue is hypothesized to play a role in endometrial cancer development (Kaaks and Lukanova 2001; Kaaks et al. 2002). Insulin can increase the bioactivity of IGF-I in plasma and the local tissue by inhibiting the synthesis of binding proteins IGFBP-1 and IGFBP-2. One randomized clinical trial, however, showed no direct effect of a one-year moderate-intensity physical activity intervention on IGF-I and its main binding protein IGFBP-3 (McTiernan et al. 2005). The biologic mechanisms linking insulin and IGF-I with endometrial and ovarian cancer risk may differ considerably according to menopausal status (Kaaks and Lukanova 2001, 2002; Kaaks et al. 2002; Lukanova et al. 2002, 2003; Lukanova and Kaaks 2005; Peeters et al. 2007; Rinaldi et al. 2007).

7.4.4 Inflammation

There is some evidence that inflammation plays an etiologic role in endometrial (Modugno et al. 2005) and ovarian (Ness and Cottreau 1999) carcinogenesis. Physical activity could thus influence endometrial and ovarian cancer risk by affecting the balance of pro- and anti-inflammatory cytokines in the systemic circulation and local tissue (Ness and Cottreau 1999; Moldoveanu et al. 2001; Pischon et al. 2003; McTiernan 2008).

For endometrial cancer, many of the established risk factors including obesity, insulin resistance, polycystic ovarian syndrome, and diabetes (Kaaks et al. 2002) are associated with a state of chronic low-level systemic inflammation and increased proinflammatory cytokine production, especially of interleukin (IL)-1, IL-6 and tumor necrosis factor (TNF)-α (Modugno et al. 2005). Lower levels of adiponectin, an anti-inflammatory factor, are also associated with increased endometrial cancer risk (Cust et al. 2007c; McTiernan 2008). A proinflammatory milieu could increase endometrial cancer risk through increased estrogen production (Purohit et al. 2002), or alternatively through activation of nuclear factor-κB (NF-κB) and increased expression of cyclooxygenase (COX)-2 (an inflammatory enzyme) and prostaglandin E_2 (PGE_2) in endometrial tissue, which can initiate and promote endometrial tumor development (Modugno et al. 2005).

For ovarian cancer, incessant ovulation is associated with inflammation at the level of both the epithelium and the follicle, and other risk factors such as asbestos and talc exposure, endometriosis, and pelvic inflammatory disease also cause local pelvic inflammation (Ness and Cottreau 1999). Inflammation induces cell damage, oxidative stress, and elevations of cytokines and prostaglandins, all of which may be mutagenic to ovarian tissue (Ness and Cottreau 1999). It has been proposed that inflammation might be more strongly associated with the risk of cancer death than cancer incidence (Il'yasova et al. 2005).

Physical activity could increase circulating levels of anti-inflammatory cytokines, including IL-1rα, IL-4, and IL-10, which attenuate inflammation by restricting the production and activity of inflammatory cytokines (Moldoveanu et al. 2001; McTiernan 2008). Cross-sectional studies and some intervention studies support an association between chronic physical activity and lower levels of inflammatory markers such as C-reactive protein, IL-6, serum amyloid A, and TNF-α (Kasapis and Thompson 2005; McTiernan 2008). A reduction in body fat mass could partially explain the inverse association between physical activity level and plasma levels of inflammatory cytokines (Pischon et al. 2003; Campbell and McTiernan 2007; McTiernan 2008). The modulation of cytokine levels may be related to the type, intensity, and duration of exercise (Pedersen et al. 1998; Moldoveanu et al. 2001).

7.4.5 Immune Function

Innate and acquired components of the immune system (such as natural killer cells, macrophages, neutrophils, eosinophils, antibodies, and T cytotoxic cells) are implicated in the carcinogenic process by eliminating carcinogens and tumor cells and repairing DNA damage (Jakobisiak et al. 2003; McTiernan 2008). Physical activity is generally associated with improved immune function and an anti-inflammatory response (Shephard and Shek 1998; Moldoveanu et al. 2001), and has been proposed to decrease cancer risk by enhancing the immune system and reducing oxidative stress. This biologic mechanism might be important in the etiology of cervical cancer because oxidative stress and inflammatory immune responses are thought to be implicated in cervical carcinogenesis (Giuliano 2003; World Cancer Research Fund & American Institute for Cancer Research 2007). Physical activity might also improve immune function via reduced adiposity (Marti et al. 2001).

However, there is limited epidemiologic evidence to support a role of immune factors in reducing cancer risk. Although cross-sectional studies suggest that moderate physical activity is associated with enhanced resting immune function (Lee 1995; Nieman 1997; McTiernan 2008), a 12-month randomized controlled trial showed no effect of aerobic exercise on in vitro immune function in postmenopausal women (Campbell et al. 2008). The biologic mechanisms could depend on the intensity and duration of the physical activity, as there is some evidence that moderate activity results in enhanced immune function, whereas intense, vigorous exercise could actually induce immuno-suppression and an inflammatory response (Nieman 1997; Nehlsen-Cannarella 1998; Pedersen et al. 1998; Shephard and Shek 1998; Moldoveanu et al. 2001; McTiernan 2008). Similarly, effects of physical activity on antioxidant enzyme repair capacity and oxygen free radicals might also depend on the intensity of activity (Robertson et al. 1991; Dreher and Junod 1996; Miyazaki et al. 2001). Changes seen in immune function with physical activity also tend to be transient in nature (Lee 1995; Nieman 1997).

7.4.6 Metabolic and Cellular Pathways

Cellular pathways could also be activated by physical activity. Exercise can activate 5′-AMP-activated protein kinase (AMPK), a signaling molecule that has a major role in cellular lipid and protein metabolism (Luo et al. 2005). AMPK exerts direct effects on specific enzymes and transcriptional regulators to inhibit the development of insulin resistance and the growth and/or survival of cancer cells (Luo et al. 2005; Kelesidis et al. 2006). The AMPK pathway may be important in obesity-related cancers such as endometrial and ovarian cancers (Luo et al. 2005; Kelesidis et al. 2006).

Some observational studies have proposed that physical activity may decrease the risk of estrogen-related cancers by increasing the metabolism of estrogens to less potent forms, by favoring the 2-hydroxylation pathway rather than the more estrogenic and possibly genotoxic 16α-hydroxylation or 4-hydroxylation pathways (Shephard and Shek 1998; Matthews et al.

7

2004; Bentz et al. 2005; Modugno et al. 2005). The 2-hydroxyestradiol metabolite appears to inhibit tumor growth, induce apoptosis, and inhibit the production and action of cytokines IL-6 and TNF-α, whereas both the 16α-hydroxylation and 4-hydroxylation metabolites are potent estrogens with uterine activity (Modugno et al. 2005). However, findings from other observational (Campbell et al. 2005) and intervention studies (Atkinson et al. 2004) do not support this hypothesis.

7.4.7 Biologic Mechanisms – Conclusions

Of the gynecological cancers, the biologic evidence provides strong support for a protective role of physical activity on cancer of the endometrium, and moderate support for cancer of the ovaries, as these cancers have a strong hormonal etiology (Risch 1998; Kaaks et al. 2002; Lukanova and Kaaks 2005). The more established biologic mechanisms that are supported by epidemiologic and experimental data involve endogenous sex hormone levels, insulin-mediated pathways, and maintenance of energy balance. For cervical cancer, for which the major causal factor is HPV infection, it is possible that physical activity could influence risk through effects on sex steroid hormones and immune function.

Acknowledgment Anne Cust is the recipient of a National Health and Medical Research Council public health postdoctoral fellowship #520018

References

Ainsworth BE (2000) Issues in the assessment of physical activity in women. Res Q Exerc Sport 71:S37–S42

Ainsworth BE, Haskell WL, Whitt MC et al (2000) Compendium of physical activities: an update of activity codes and MET intensities. Med Sci Sports Exerc 32:S498–S504

Albanes D, Blair A, Taylor PR (1989) Physical activity and risk of cancer in the NHANES I population. Am J Public Health 79:744–750

Allen NE, Appleby PN, Kaaks R et al (2003) Lifestyle determinants of serum insulin-like growth-factor-I (IGF-I), C-peptide and hormone binding protein levels in British women. Cancer Causes Control 14:65–74

Amant F, Moerman P, Neven P et al (2005) Endometrial cancer. Lancet 366:491–505

Anderson JP, Ross JA, Folsom AR (2004) Anthropometric variables, physical activity, and incidence of ovarian cancer: The Iowa women's health study. Cancer 100:1515–1521

Armstrong BK, White E, Saracci R (1992) Principles of exposure measurement in epidemiology. Oxford University Press, Oxford, NY

Atkinson C, Lampe JW, Tworoger SS et al (2004) Effects of a moderate intensity exercise intervention on estrogen metabolism in postmenopausal women. Cancer Epidemiol Biomark Prev 13:868–874

Australian Government Department of Health and Ageing (2005) National physical activity guidelines for adults. Australian Government Department of Health and Ageing, Canberra

Bentz AT, Schneider CM, Westerlind KC (2005) The relationship between physical activity and 2-hydroxyestrone, 16alpha-hydroxyestrone, and the 2/16 ratio in premenopausal women (United States). Cancer Causes Control 16:455–461

Beral V, Doll R, Hermon C et al (2008) Ovarian cancer and oral contraceptives: collaborative reanalysis of data from 45 epidemiological studies including 23,257 women with ovarian cancer and 87,303 controls. Lancet 371:303–314

Bernstein L, Ross RK, Lobo RA et al (1987) The effects of moderate physical activity on menstrual cycle patterns in adolescence: implications for breast cancer prevention. Br J Cancer 55: 681–685

Bertone-Johnson ER, Tworoger SS, Hankinson SE (2009) Recreational physical activity and steroid hormone levels in postmenopausal women. Am J Epidemiol 170:1095–1104

Bertone ER, Willett WC, Rosner BA et al (2001) Prospective study of recreational physical activity and ovarian cancer. J Natl Cancer Inst 93: 942–948

Bertone ER, Newcomb PA, Willett WC et al (2002) Recreational physical activity and ovarian cancer in a population-based case-control study. Int J Cancer 99:431–436

Biesma RG, Schouten LJ, Dirx MJ et al (2006) Physical activity and risk of ovarian cancer: results from the Netherlands Cohort Study (The Netherlands). Cancer Causes Control 17: 109–115

Bonen A (1992) Recreational exercise does not impair menstrual cycles: a prospective study. Int J Sports Med 13:110–120

Borghouts LB, Keizer HA (2000) Exercise and insulin sensitivity: a review. Int J Sports Med 21: 1–12

Boule NG, Haddad E, Kenny GP et al (2001) Effects of exercise on glycemic control and body mass in type 2 diabetes mellitus: a meta-analysis of controlled clinical trials. JAMA 286:1218–1227

Broocks A, Pirke KM, Schweiger U et al (1990) Cyclic ovarian function in recreational athletes. J Appl Physiol 68:2083–2086

Bullen BA, Skrinar GS, Beitins IZ et al (1985) Induction of menstrual disorders by strenuous exercise in untrained women. N Engl J Med 312: 1349–1353

Calle EE, Kaaks R (2004) Overweight, obesity and cancer: epidemiological evidence and proposed mechanisms. Nat Rev Cancer 4:579–591

Campbell KL, Westerlind KC, Harber VJ et al (2005) Associations between aerobic fitness and estrogen metabolites in premenopausal women. Med Sci Sports Exerc 37:585–592

Campbell KL, McTiernan A (2007) Exercise and biomarkers for cancer prevention studies. J Nutr 137:161S–169S

Campbell PT, Wener MH, Sorensen B et al (2008) Effect of exercise on in vitro immune function: a 12-month randomized, controlled trial among postmenopausal women. J Appl Physiol 104: 1648–1655

Cannistra SA (2004) Cancer of the ovary. N Engl J Med 351:2519–2529

Carnide N, Kreiger N, Cotterchio M (2009) Association between frequency and intensity of recreational physical activity and epithelial ovarian cancer risk by age period. Eur J Cancer Prev 18:322–330

Cauley JA, Gutai JP, Kuller LH et al (1989) The epidemiology of serum sex hormones in postmenopausal women. Am J Epidemiol 129:1120–1131

Chen VW, Ruiz B, Killeen JL et al (2003) Pathology and classification of ovarian tumors. Cancer 97:2631–2642

Clark BK, Sugiyama T, Healy GN et al (2008) Validity and reliability of measures of television viewing time and other non-occupational sedentary behaviour of adults: a review. Obes Rev Jul 8

Colbert LH, Lacey JV Jr, Schairer C et al (2003) Physical activity and risk of endometrial cancer in a prospective cohort study (United States). Cancer Causes Control 14:559–567

Conroy MB, Sattelmair JR, Cook NR et al (2009) Physical activity, adiposity, and risk of endometrial cancer. Cancer Causes Control 20: 1107–1115

Cottreau CM, Ness RB, Kriska AM (2000) Physical activity and reduced risk of ovarian cancer. Obstet Gynecol 96:609–614

Cust AE, Allen NE, Rinaldi S et al (2007a) Serum levels of C-peptide, IGFBP-1 and IGFBP-2 and endometrial cancer risk; Results from the European prospective investigation into cancer and nutrition. Int J Cancer 120:2656–2664

Cust AE, Armstrong BK, Friedenreich CM et al (2007b) Physical activity and endometrial cancer risk: a review of the current evidence, biologic mechanisms and the quality of physical activity assessment methods. Cancer Causes Control 18:243–258

Cust AE, Kaaks R, Friedenreich C et al (2007c) Plasma adiponectin levels and endometrial cancer risk in pre- and postmenopausal women. J Clin Endocrinol Metab 92:255–263

Cust AE, Kaaks R, Friedenreich C et al (2007d) Metabolic syndrome, plasma lipid, lipoprotein and glucose levels, and endometrial cancer risk in the European Prospective Investigation into Cancer and Nutrition (EPIC). Endocr Relat Cancer 14:755–767

Dale E, Gerlach DH, Wilhite AL (1979) Menstrual dysfunction in distance runners. Obstet Gynecol 54:47–53

De Souza MJ, Miller BE, Loucks AB et al (1998) High frequency of luteal phase deficiency and anovulation in recreational women runners: blunted elevation in follicle-stimulating hormone observed during luteal-follicular transition. J Clin Endocrinol Metab 83:4220–4232

De Souza MJ (2003) Menstrual disturbances in athletes: a focus on luteal phase defects. Med Sci Sports Exerc 35:1553–1563

7

Delvenne P, Herman L, Kholod N et al (2007) Role of hormone cofactors in the human papillomavirus-induced carcinogenesis of the uterine cervix. Mol Cell Endocrinol 264:1–5

Dosemeci M, Hayes RB, Vetter R et al (1993) Occupational physical activity, socioeconomic status, and risks of 15 cancer sites in Turkey. Cancer Causes Control 4:313–321

Dreher D, Junod AF (1996) Role of oxygen free radicals in cancer development. Eur J Cancer 32A:30–38

Duncan GE, Perri MG, Theriaque DW et al (2003) Exercise training, without weight loss, increases insulin sensitivity and postheparin plasma lipase activity in previously sedentary adults. Diab Care 26:557–562

Ferlay J, Bray F, Pisani P et al (2004). GLOBOCAN 2002: Cancer incidence, mortality and prevalence worldwide. IARC CancerBase No. 5. version 2.0. IARC Press, Lyon. http://www-dep.iarc.fr/

Feskens EJ, Loeber JG, Kromhout D (1994) Diet and physical activity as determinants of hyperinsulinemia: the Zutphen Elderly Study. Am J Epidemiol 140:350–360

Forney JP, Milewich L, Chen GT et al (1981) Aromatization of androstenedione to estrone by human adipose tissue in vitro. Correlation with adipose tissue mass, age, and endometrial neoplasia. J Clin Endocrinol Metab 53:192–199

Frank LL, Sorensen BE, Yasui Y et al (2005) Effects of exercise on metabolic risk variables in overweight postmenopausal women: a randomized clinical trial. Obes Res 13:615–625

Friberg E, Mantzoros CS, Wolk A (2006) Physical activity and risk of endometrial cancer: a population-based prospective cohort study. Cancer Epidemiol Biomark Prev 15:2136–2140

Friedenreich CM (2001) Physical activity and cancer prevention: from observational to intervention research. Cancer Epidemiol Biomark Prev 10:287–301

Friedenreich CM, Cust A, Lahmann PH et al (2007) Physical activity and risk of endometrial cancer: The European prospective investigation into cancer and nutrition. Int J Cancer 121: 347–355

Friedenreich CM, Cook LS, Magliocco AM et al (2010) Case-control study of lifetime total physical activity and endometrial cancer risk. Cancer Causes Control Mar 25; epub ahead of print

Frisch RE, Wyshak G, Vincent L (1980) Delayed menarche and amenorrhea in ballet dancers. N Engl J Med 303:17–19

Frisch RE, Gotz-Welbergen AV, McArthur JW et al (1981) Delayed menarche and amenorrhea of college athletes in relation to age of onset of training. JAMA 246:1559–1563

Frisch RE, Wyshak G, Albright NL et al (1987) Lower lifetime occurrence of breast cancer and cancers of the reproductive system among former college athletes. Am J Clin Nutr 45: 328–335

Furberg AS, Thune I (2003) Metabolic abnormalities (hypertension, hyperglycemia and overweight), lifestyle (high energy intake and physical inactivity) and endometrial cancer risk in a Norwegian cohort. Int J Cancer 104: 669–676

Gertig D, Hunter D (2002) Ovarian Cancer. In: Adami HO, Hunter D, Trichopoulos D (eds) Textbook of cancer epidemiology. Oxford University Press, Oxford, pp 378–399

Gierach GL, Chang SC, Brinton LA et al (2009) Physical activity, sedentary behavior, and endometrial cancer risk in the NIH-AARP diet and health study. Int J Cancer 124:2139–2147

Giuliano A (2003) Cervical carcinogenesis: the role of co-factors and generation of reactive oxygen species. Salud Pública Méx 45(Suppl 3): S354–S360

Goodman MT, Hankin JH, Wilkens LR et al (1997) Diet, body size, physical activity, and the risk of endometrial cancer. Cancer Res 57:5077–5085

Hamalainen E, Tikkanen H, Harkonen M et al (1987) Serum lipoproteins, sex hormones and sex hormone binding globulin in middle-aged men of different physical fitness and risk of coronary heart disease. Atherosclerosis 67: 155–162

Hannan LM, Leitzmann MF, Lacey JV Jr et al (2004) Physical activity and risk of ovarian cancer: a prospective cohort study in the United States. Cancer Epidemiol Biomark Prev 13: 765–770

Haskell WL, Lee IM, Pate RR et al (2007) Physical activity and public health: updated recommendation for adults from the American college of sports medicine and the American heart association. Circulation 116:1081–1093

Healy GN, Dunstan DW, Salmon J et al (2007) Objectively measured light-intensity physical activity is independently associated with 2-hr plasma glucose. Diab Care 30:1384–1389

Hecht JL, Kotsopoulos J, Hankinson SE et al (2009) Relationship between epidemiologic risk factors and hormone receptor expression in ovarian cancer: results from the nurses' health study. Cancer Epidemiol Biomark Prev 18:1624–1630

Henderson BE, Casagrande JT, Pike MC et al (1983) The epidemiology of endometrial cancer in young women. Br J Cancer 47:749–756

Hirose K, Tajima K, Hamajima N et al (1996) Subsite (cervix/endometrium)-specific risk and protective factors in uterus cancer. Jpn J Cancer Res 87:1001–1009

Il'yasova D, Colbert LH, Harris TB et al (2005) Circulating levels of inflammatory markers and cancer risk in the health aging and body composition cohort. Cancer Epidemiol Biomark Prev 14:2413–2418

International Agency for Research on Cancer (IARC), World Health Organization (WHO) (2002) Weight control and physical activity. IARC Handbook for cancer prevention, vol 6. IARC Press, Lyon, France

Irwin ML, Mayer-Davis EJ, Addy CL et al (2000) Moderate-intensity physical activity and fasting insulin levels in women: the cross-cultural activity participation study. Diab Care 23:449–454

Irwin ML, Ainsworth BE, Mayer-Davis EJ et al (2002) Physical activity and the metabolic syndrome in a tri-ethnic sample of women. Obes Res 10:1030–1037

Jakobisiak M, Lasek W, Golab J (2003) Natural mechanisms protecting against cancer. Immunol Lett 90:103–122

Kaaks R, Lukanova A (2001) Energy balance and cancer: the role of insulin and insulin-like growth factor-I. Proc Nutr Soc 60:91–106

Kaaks R, Lukanova A (2002) Effects of weight control and physical activity in cancer prevention: role of endogenous hormone metabolism. Ann NY Acad Sci 963:268–281

Kaaks R, Lukanova A, Kurzer MS (2002) Obesity, endogenous hormones, and endometrial cancer risk: a synthetic review. Cancer Epidemiol Biomark Prev 11:1531–1543

Kaaks R, Berrino F, Key T et al (2005) Serum sex steroids in premenopausal women and breast cancer risk within the European Prospective Investigation into Cancer and Nutrition (EPIC). J Natl Cancer Inst 97:755–765

Kalandidi A, Tzonou A, Lipworth L et al (1996) A case-control study of endometrial cancer in relation to reproductive, somatometric, and life-style variables. Oncology 53:354–359

Kasapis C, Thompson PD (2005) The effects of physical activity on serum C-reactive protein and inflammatory markers: a systematic review. J Am Coll Cardiol 45:1563–1569

Kelesidis I, Kelesidis T, Mantzoros CS (2006) Adiponectin and cancer: a systematic review. Br J Cancer 94:1221–1225

Key TJ, Pike MC (1988) The dose-effect relationship between 'unopposed' oestrogens and endometrial mitotic rate: its central role in explaining and predicting endometrial cancer risk. Br J Cancer 57:205–212

Key TJ, Allen NE, Verkasalo PK et al (2001) Energy balance and cancer: the role of sex hormones. Proc Nutr Soc 60:81–89

King AC, Tribble DL (1991) The role of exercise in weight regulation in nonathletes. Sports Med 11:331–349

Kristensen GB, Trope C (1997) Epithelial ovarian carcinoma. Lancet 349:113–117

Kurian AW, Balise RR, McGuire V et al (2005) Histologic types of epithelial ovarian cancer: have they different risk factors? Gynecol Oncol 96:520–530

Lahmann PH, Cust AE, Friedenreich CM et al (2009a) Anthropometric measures and epithelial ovarian cancer risk in the Europeaneuropean prospective investigation into cancer and nutrition. Int J Cancer 126: 2404–2415

Lahmann PH, Friedenreich C, Schulz M et al (2009b) Physical activity and ovarian cancer risk: the European prospective investigation into cancer and nutrition. Cancer Epidemiol Biomark Prev 18:351–354

Lee IM (1995) Exercise and physical health: cancer and immune function. Res Q Exerc Sport 66:286–291

Leitzmann MF, Koebnick C, Moore SC et al (2009) Prospective study of physical activity and the risk of ovarian cancer. Cancer Causes Control 20:765–773

Levi F, La Vecchia C, Negri E et al (1993) Selected physical activities and the risk of endometrial cancer. Br J Cancer 67:846–851

Levine JA (2004) Non-exercise activity thermogenesis (NEAT). Nutr Rev 62:S82–S97

Levine JA, Lanningham-Foster LM, McCrady SK et al (2005) Interindividual variation in posture

7

allocation: possible role in human obesity. Science 307:584–586

Levine JA, Vander Weg MW, Hill JO et al (2006) Non-exercise activity thermogenesis: the crouching tiger hidden dragon of societal weight gain. Arterioscler Thromb Vasc Biol 26:729–736

Littman AJ, Voigt LF, Beresford SA et al (2001) Recreational physical activity and endometrial cancer risk. Am J Epidemiol 154:924–933

Loucks AB (2003) Energy availability, not body fatness, regulates reproductive function in women. Exerc Sport Sci Rev 31:144–148

Lukanova A, Lundin E, Toniolo P et al (2002) Circulating levels of insulin-like growth factor-I and risk of ovarian cancer. Int J Cancer 101: 549–554

Lukanova A, Lundin E, Akhmedkhanov A et al (2003) Circulating levels of sex steroid hormones and risk of ovarian cancer. Int J Cancer 104:636–642

Lukanova A, Zeleniuch-Jacquotte A, Lundin E et al (2004) Prediagnostic levels of C-peptide, IGF-I, IGFBP -1, -2 and -3 and risk of endometrial cancer. Int J Cancer 108:262–268

Lukanova A, Kaaks R (2005) Endogenous hormones and ovarian cancer: epidemiology and current hypotheses. Cancer Epidemiol Biomark Prev 14:98–107

Luo Z, Saha AK, Xiang X et al (2005) AMPK, the metabolic syndrome and cancer. Trends Pharmacol Sci 26:69–76

Marti A, Marcos A, Martinez JA (2001) Obesity and immune function relationships. Obes Rev 2:131–140

Mathew A, George PS (2009) Trends in incidence and mortality rates of squamous cell carcinoma and adenocarcinoma of cervix – worldwide. Asian Pac J Cancer Prev 10:645–650

Matthews CE, Fowke JH, Dai Q et al (2004) Physical activity, body size, and estrogen metabolism in women. Cancer Causes Control 15:473–481

Matthews CE, Xu WH, Zheng W et al (2005) Physical activity and risk of endometrial cancer: a report from the Shanghai endometrial cancer study. Cancer Epidemiol Biomark Prev 14: 779–785

Mayer-Davis EJ, D'Agostino R Jr, Karter AJ et al (1998) Intensity and amount of physical activity in relation to insulin sensitivity: the insulin resistance atherosclerosis study. JAMA 279: 669–674

McTiernan A, Tworoger SS, Rajan KB et al (2004a) Effect of exercise on serum androgens in postmenopausal women: a 12-month randomized clinical trial. Cancer Epidemiol Biomark Prev 13:1099–1105

McTiernan A, Tworoger SS, Ulrich CM et al (2004b) Effect of exercise on serum estrogens in postmenopausal women: a 12-month randomized clinical trial. Cancer Res 64:2923–2928

McTiernan A, Sorensen B, Yasui Y et al (2005) No effect of exercise on insulin-like growth factor 1 and insulin-like growth factor binding protein 3 in postmenopausal women: a 12-month randomized clinical trial. Cancer Epidemiol Biomark Prev 14:1020–1021

McTiernan A (2008) Mechanisms linking physical activity with cancer. Nat Rev Cancer 8:205–211

Miyazaki H, Oh-ishi S, Ookawara T et al (2001) Strenuous endurance training in humans reduces oxidative stress following exhausting exercise. Eur J Appl Physiol 84:1–6

Modugno F, Ness RB, Chen C et al (2005) Inflammation and endometrial cancer: a hypothesis. Cancer Epidemiol Biomark Prev 14: 2840–2847

Moldoveanu AI, Shephard RJ, Shek PN (2001) The cytokine response to physical activity and training. Sports Med 31:115–144

Moodley M, Moodley J, Chetty R et al (2003) The role of steroid contraceptive hormones in the pathogenesis of invasive cervical cancer: a review. Int J Gynecol Cancer 13:103–110

Moradi T, Nyren O, Bergstrom R et al (1998) Risk for endometrial cancer in relation to occupational physical activity: a nationwide cohort study in Sweden. Int J Cancer 76:665–670

Moradi T, Weiderpass E, Signorello LB et al (2000) Physical activity and postmenopausal endometrial cancer risk (Sweden). Cancer Causes Control 11:829–837

Mota F, De Oliveira C (2003) Symptoms, signs and clinico-pathological prognostic factors. In: Bösze Mayenne P (ed) Endometrial cancer. Elsevier, France, pp 55–65

National Center for Chronic Disease Prevention and Health Promotion; Centers for Disease Control and Prevention (1996). Physical activity and health: a report of the Surgeon General, Atlanta, GA

Nehlsen-Cannarella SL (1998) Cellular responses to moderate and heavy exercise. Can J Physiol Pharmacol 76:485–489

Nelson ME, Meredith CN, Dawson-Hughes B et al (1988) Hormone and bone mineral status in endurance-trained and sedentary postmenopausal women. J Clin Endocrinol Metab 66: 927–933

Ness RB, Cottreau C (1999) Possible role of ovarian epithelial inflammation in ovarian cancer. J Natl Cancer Inst 91:1459–1467

Nieman DC (1997) Exercise immunology: practical applications. Int J Sports Med 18(Suppl 1): S91–S100

Olsen CM, Bain CJ, Jordan SJ et al (2007a) Recreational physical activity and epithelial ovarian cancer: a case-control study, systematic review, and meta-analysis. Cancer Epidemiol Biomark Prev 16:2321–2330

Olsen CM, Green AC, Whiteman DC et al (2007b) Obesity and the risk of epithelial ovarian cancer: a systematic review and meta-analysis. Eur J Cancer 43:690–709

Olsen CM, Green AC, Nagle CM et al (2008) Epithelial ovarian cancer: testing the 'androgens hypothesis'. Endocr Relat Cancer 15: 1061–1068

Olson SH, Vena JE, Dorn JP et al (1997) Exercise, occupational activity, and risk of endometrial cancer. Ann Epidemiol 7:46–53

Pan SY, Ugnat AM, Mao Y (2005) Physical activity and the risk of ovarian cancer: a case-control study in Canada. Int J Cancer 117:300–307

Parkin DM, Bray F, Ferlay J et al (2005) Global cancer statistics, 2002. CA Cancer J Clin 55: 74–108

Pate RR, Pratt M, Blair SN et al (1995) Physical activity and public health. A recommendation from the Centers for Disease Control and Prevention and the American College of Sports Medicine. JAMA 273:402–407

Patel AV, Rodriguez C, Pavluck AL et al (2006) Recreational physical activity and sedentary behavior in relation to ovarian cancer risk in a large cohort of US women. Am J Epidemiol 163:709–716

Patel AV, Feigelson HS, Talbot JT et al (2008) The role of body weight in the relationship between physical activity and endometrial cancer: results from a large cohort of US women. Int J Cancer 123:1877–1882

Pecorelli S, Benedet JL, Creasman WT et al (1999) FIGO staging of gynecologic cancer. 1994–1997 FIGO Committee on Gynecologic Oncology. International Federation of Gynecology and Obstetrics. Int J Gynaecol Obstet 64:5–10

Pedersen BK, Ostrowski K, Rohde T et al (1998) The cytokine response to strenuous exercise. Can J Physiol Pharmacol 76:505–511

Peeters PH, Lukanova A, Allen N et al (2007) Serum IGF-I, its major binding protein (IGFBP-3) and epithelial ovarian cancer risk: the European Prospective Investigation into Cancer and Nutrition (EPIC). Endocr Relat Cancer 14: 81–90

Pischon T, Hankinson SE, Hotamisligil GS et al (2003) Leisure-time physical activity and reduced plasma levels of obesity-related inflammatory markers. Obes Res 11:1055–1064

Pukkala E, Poskiparta M, Apter D et al (1993) Life-long physical activity and cancer risk among Finnish female teachers. Eur J Cancer Prev 2: 369–376

Purdie DM, Bain CJ, Siskind V et al (2003) Ovulation and risk of epithelial ovarian cancer. Int J Cancer 104:228–232

Purohit A, Newman SP, Reed MJ (2002) The role of cytokines in regulating estrogen synthesis: implications for the etiology of breast cancer. Breast Cancer Res 4:65–69

Rajaram S, Baylink DJ, Mohan S (1997) Insulin-like growth factor-binding proteins in serum and other biological fluids: regulation and functions. Endocr Rev 18:801–831

Ravussin E (2005) Physiology. A NEAT way to control weight? Science 307:530–531

Riman T, Dickman PW, Nilsson S et al (2004) Some life-style factors and the risk of invasive epithelial ovarian cancer in Swedish women. Eur J Epidemiol 19:1011–1019

Rinaldi S, Key TJ, Peeters PH et al (2006) Anthropometric measures, endogenous sex steroids and breast cancer risk in postmenopausal women: a study within the EPIC cohort. Int J Cancer 118:2832–2839

Rinaldi S, Dossus L, Lukanova A et al (2007) Endogenous androgens and risk of epithelial ovarian cancer: results from the European Prospective Investigation into Cancer and Nutrition (EPIC). Cancer Epidemiol Biomark Prev 16:23–29

Risch HA (1998) Hormonal etiology of epithelial ovarian cancer, with a hypothesis concerning the role of androgens and progesterone. J Natl Cancer Inst 90:1774–1786

7

Robertson JD, Maughan RJ, Duthie GG et al (1991) Increased blood antioxidant systems of runners in response to training load. Clin Sci (Lond) 80:611–618

Rogol AD, Weltman A, Weltman JY et al (1992) Durability of the reproductive axis in eumenorrheic women during 1 yr of endurance training. J Appl Physiol 72:1571–1580

Rose PG (1996) Endometrial carcinoma. N Engl J Med 335:640–649

Ross R, Dagnone D, Jones PJ et al (2000) Reduction in obesity and related comorbid conditions after diet-induced weight loss or exercise-induced weight loss in men. A randomized, controlled trial. Ann Intern Med 133:92–103

Ross R, Janssen I, Dawson J et al (2004) Exercise-induced reduction in obesity and insulin resistance in women: a randomized controlled trial. Obes Res 12:789–798

Rossing MA, Cushing-Haugen KL, Wicklund KG et al (2010) Recreational physical activity and risk of epithelial ovarian cancer. Cancer Causes Control 21:485–491

Salazar-Martinez E, Lazcano-Ponce EC, Lira-Lira GG et al (2000) Case-control study of diabetes, obesity, physical activity and risk of endometrial cancer among Mexican women. Cancer Causes Control 11:707–711

Schnohr P, Gronbaek M, Petersen L et al (2005) Physical activity in leisure-time and risk of cancer: 14-year follow-up of 28,000 Danish men and women. Scand J Public Health 33: 244–249

Schouten LJ, Goldbohm RA, van den Brandt PA (2004) Anthropometry, physical activity, and endometrial cancer risk: results from the Netherlands cohort study. J Natl Cancer Inst 96: 1635–1638

Schouten LJ, Rivera C, Hunter DJ et al (2008) Height, body mass index, and ovarian cancer: a pooled analysis of 12 cohort studies. Cancer Epidemiol Biomark Prev 17:902–912

Shephard RJ, Shek PN (1998) Associations between physical activity and susceptibility to cancer: possible mechanisms. Sports Med 26: 293–315

Sherman B, Wallace R, Bean J et al (1981) Relationship of body weight to menarcheal and menopausal age: implications for breast cancer risk. J Clin Endocrinol Metab 52:488–493

Shu XO, Hatch MC, Zheng W et al (1993) Physical activity and risk of endometrial cancer. Epidemiology 4:342–349

Smith JS, Green J, Berrington de Gonzalez A et al (2003) Cervical cancer and use of hormonal contraceptives: a systematic review. Lancet 361: 1159–1167

Steben M, Duarte-Franco E (2007) Human papillomavirus infection: epidemiology and pathophysiology. Gynecol Oncol 107:S2–S5

Sturgeon SR, Brinton LA, Berman ML et al (1993) Past and present physical activity and endometrial cancer risk. Br J Cancer 68:584–589

Stuver S, Adami H (2002) Cervical cancer. In: Adami HO, Hunter D, Trichopoulos D (eds) Textbook of cancer epidemiology. Oxford University Press, Oxford, pp 340–354

Tavani A, Gallus S, La Vecchia C et al (2001) Physical activity and risk of ovarian cancer: an Italian case-control study. Int J Cancer 91: 407–411

Tavani A, Bravi F, Dal Maso L et al (2009) Physical activity and risk of endometrial cancer: an Italian case-control study. Eur J Cancer Prev 18:303–306

Terry P, Baron JA, Weiderpass E et al (1999) Lifestyle and endometrial cancer risk: a cohort study from the Swedish Twin Registry. Int J Cancer 82:38–42

Thune I, Furberg AS (2001) Physical activity and cancer risk: dose-response and cancer, all sites and site-specific. Med Sci Sports Exerc 33:S530–S550, discussion S609–510

Tworoger SS, Eliassen AH, Missmer SA et al (2006) Birthweight and body size throughout life in relation to sex hormones and prolactin concentrations in premenopausal women. Cancer Epidemiol Biomark Prev 15:2494–2501

van Gils CH, Peeters PH, Schoenmakers MC et al (2009) Physical activity and endogenous sex hormone levels in postmenopausal women: a cross-sectional study in the Prospect-EPIC Cohort. Cancer Epidemiol Biomark Prev 18: 377–383

Verkasalo PK, Thomas HV, Appleby PN et al (2001) Circulating levels of sex hormones and their relation to risk factors for breast cancer: a cross-sectional study in 1092 pre- and postmenopausal women (United Kingdom). Cancer Causes Control 12:47–59

Voskuil DW, Monninkhof EM, Elias SG et al (2007) Physical activity and endometrial cancer risk, a systematic review of current evidence. Cancer Epidemiol Biomark Prev 16:639–648

Waggoner SE (2003) Cervical cancer. Lancet 361: 2217–2225

Warren MP (1980) The effects of exercise on pubertal progression and reproductive function in girls. J Clin Endocrinol Metab 51:1150–1157

Weiderpass E, Margolis KL, Sandin S et al (2006) Prospective study of physical activity in different periods of life and the risk of ovarian cancer. Int J Cancer 118:3153–3160

Willett W (1989) An overview of issues related to the correction of non-differential exposure measurement error in epidemiologic studies. Stat Med 8:1031–1040, discussion 1071–1033

World Cancer Research Fund & American Institute for Cancer Research (2007) Food, nutrition, physical activity, and the prevention of cancer: a global perspective. American Institute for Cancer Research, Washington, DC

Zhang M, Lee AH, Binns CW (2003) Physical activity and epithelial ovarian cancer risk: a case-control study in China. Int J Cancer 105: 838–843

Zhang M, Xie X, Lee AH et al (2004) Sedentary behaviours and epithelial ovarian cancer risk. Cancer Causes Control 15:83–89

Zheng W, Shu XO, McLaughlin JK et al (1993) Occupational physical activity and the incidence of cancer of the breast, corpus uteri, and ovary in Shanghai. Cancer 71:3620–3624

Part II

Physical Activity and Cancer Survivorship

Physical Activity and Breast Cancer Survivorship

8

Kathryn Schmitz

Abstract A diagnosis of breast cancer is associated with treatments that have physiologic effects beyond the intended curative therapy. The first section of this chapter provides and integrative physiology review of the effects of breast cancer treatment on the body systems used by and affected by physical activity, including effects of chemotherapy, radiation, and surgery. In later sections, we review the literature on physical activity and breast cancer from the point of diagnosis and for the balance of life. The efficacy of physical activity for supportive cancer care outcomes is reviewed separately from the purported usefulness of physical activity for disease-free and overall survival from breast cancer. The current evidence supports the safety of physical activity during and after breast cancer therapy. The supportive cancer care outcomes for which there is sufficient evidence of efficacy during and after breast cancer treatment include fitness, fatigue, body size, and quality of life. Further, there is growing evidence that upper body exercise does not pose additional risk for negative lymphedema outcomes among survivors with and at risk for lymphedema. For overall survival, the evidence is largely observational, with sufficient evidence that physical activity does confer benefit. Finally, we outline future directions for research on physical activity among breast cancer survivors, including expanding to focus on subsets of the population not included in most prior studies (minority women and older women), tailoring of interventions to stages of cancer most likely to benefit, expanding to study women with metastatic cancer, and new modes of exercise, such as team sports, martial arts, and Pilates.

K. Schmitz
Department of Biostatistics and Epidemiology
University of Pennsylvania School of Medicine,
903 Blockley Hall, 423 Guardian Drive,
Philadelphia, PA, 19104-6021, USA
e-mail: Schmitz@mail.med.upenn.edu

8.1 Introduction

There are nearly 200,000 new cases of breast cancer diagnosed in the USA every year (Jemal et al. 2009). Each year, almost one million women are diagnosed worldwide (Boyle and Levin 2008). Nearly 90% of women diagnosed with breast cancer in the USA will live 5 or more years (Jemal et al. 2009). The increasing success of earlier diagnosis and better treatment has resulted in a welcome shift of focus to new challenges of addressing persistent adverse

K.S. Courneya and C.M. Friedenreich (eds.), *Physical Activity and Cancer*,
Recent Results in Cancer Research 186, DOI: 10.1007/978-3-642-04231-7_8,

effects of treatment in addition to ongoing risk for recurrence. There is evidence from both observational and intervention research that physical activity may reduce the burden of both of these challenges. The goal of this chapter is to review all physical activity research in breast cancer survivors during the post-diagnosis time period, including research focused on both supportive care and disease outcomes. Motivational and behavior change research is covered in a separate chapter.

8.2 Clinical Aspects: Effects of Treatment that Might Be Altered by Physical Activity

When prescribing physical activity for a breast cancer survivor, one must consider the adverse effects of cancer treatment. Adverse effects may be acute, resolving over a period of days, weeks, or months, or they may be persistent, lasting years after treatment is completed or even for the remainder of life. For the purpose of this chapter, we use the term "persistent effects" as per the definition from Aziz and Rowland (2003). "Persistent effects" is an umbrella term that includes long-term and late effects. Long-term effects are persistent side effects or complications of treatment for which the cancer survivor must compensate. Long-term effects are distinct from late effects in that the long-term effects begin during treatment and persist after treatment, while late effects appear months or years after the end of treatment (e.g., arrhythmias or cardiomyopathies experienced by breast cancer survivors many years after exposure to cardiotoxic drugs) (Hewitt et al. 2006). Here we provide a brief review of persistent effects of the five common types of breast cancer treatments, including chemotherapy, radiation, surgery, hormonal therapies, and targeted therapies. Within sections on each treatment type, we focus on the effects on five body systems relevant to exercise training effects: cardiovascular, musculoskeletal, nervous, endocrine, and immune. The reader is referred to a recent IOM report on adult cancer survivorship for a more in-depth review of this topic than is possible here (Hewitt et al. 2006). We use the term "persistent effects" to avoid needing to delineate between long-term versus late effects in this chapter. It is acknowledged that for all persistent adverse effects of cancer treatment, there are well-established predisposing host factors, including age, gender, and other comorbid health conditions, and that the predisposing host factors and combinations of treatments can be synergistic with regard to incidence and severity of persistent adverse treatment effects.

8.2.1 Chemotherapy

Over half of breast cancer patients receive chemotherapy, and the most common agents used include alkylating agents (e.g., platinum-based drugs), antimetabolites (e.g., methotrexate), antitumor antibiotics (e.g., anthracyclines), mitotic inhibitors (taxanes), and corticosteroids. The persistent effects of chemotherapy vary according to mechanism of action and the specific agent(s) and dosages used. Change in body composition is common (Demark-Wahnefried et al. 2001; Harvie et al. 2004); however, the specific gains and losses (total weight, lean body mass, fat mass, etc.) may differ by chemotherapeutic agent (Heasman et al. 1985; Heideman et al. 2009). Several other treatment-related factors are associated with weight gain after breast cancer treatment as well, including treatment-induced menopause and hormone therapy.

Immunologic suppression can be persistent beyond the end of chemotherapy (Stricker and Jacobs 2008). Treatment with anthracyclines is associated with cardiotoxicity (Carver et al. 2007). Several chemotherapeutic agents used to treat breast cancer are associated with pulmonary damage (e.g., cyclophosphamide, paclitaxel) (Carver et al. 2007). There is also the potential for chemotherapy-related amenorrhea and/or premature menopause, particularly after treatment with alkylating agents (e.g., cyclophosphamide) (Stricker and Jacobs 2008). Taxanes are associated with peripheral sensory neuropathies that often take the form of numbness on the palms of the hands and/or the soles of the feet and can negatively affect balance (Stricker and Jacobs 2008). It is increasingly accepted that there are negative short- and long-term cognitive effects of chemotherapy as well (so-called chemo brain) (Stricker and Jacobs 2008).

8.2.2 Radiation

The treatment-related factors associated with incidence of persistent radiation toxicities include dose, volume of tissue irradiated, severity of acute effects, previous surgery, and concomitant chemotherapy (Mohanti and Bansal 2005). Organ systems not targeted for treatment may experience negative effects of radiation because they are located in the same region of the body. Examples are the pulmonary scarring and cardiac changes that can appear as late effects after radiation treatment to the chest wall. Severe, long-term side effects include lymphedema onset (Hinrichs et al. 2004), pulmonary (Lingos et al. 1991) and cardiac toxicities (Paszat et al. 1998), as well as damage to gastrointestinal tissues (Stricker and Jacobs 2008) and sustained immune suppression (Mohanti and Bansal 2005). The risk of radiation pneumonitis is higher in survivors treated with combination or sequential chemotherapy. Some chemotherapy drugs are thought to increase the radiosensitivity of the tissues, increasing the likelihood that the tumor will be damaged by ionizing radiation, increasing both the therapeutic value of and potential negative effects (Taghian et al. 2001). Radiation also may contribute to the arm and shoulder morbidities seen after breast cancer treatment through fibrotic damage to soft and/or contractile tissue (Stricker and Jacobs 2008).

8.2.3 Surgery

With any surgical procedure, it is possible to have long-term lingering pain, changes in appearance, psychosocial effects, and impaired wound healing or tightness of skin at the site of the surgery. The rate of wound healing varies by host factors (e.g., presence of underlying medical conditions such as diabetes, personal lifestyle choices) and the extent of surgery. Body systems other than the organ or tissue where the surgery is performed may also be affected by the trauma of surgery. For example, breast cancer surgeries may result in significant shoulder and arm morbidity due to cutting of muscles and other soft tissue effects of surgery (and radiotherapy). Estimated prevalence of long-term arm and shoulder morbidity is 35–58% in breast cancer survivors (Lauridsen et al. 2008; Nesvold et al. 2008). One common and feared persistent effect of breast cancer surgeries on the arms and shoulders is lymphedema, which is defined as a protein-rich swelling of the affected body part (Rockson and Rivera 2008). It is estimated that 20–30% of breast cancer survivors develop lymphedema in the affected arm or torso, though estimates vary according to whether women have sentinel lymph node biopsy (17%) versus axillary node dissection (47%) (Francis et al. 2006). Nearly one third of breast cancer survivors (and half of all African American survivors) are diagnosed with distantly invasive disease associated with axillary dissection (Jemal et al. 2009). Lymphedema is a chronic, progressive condition with no known cure and which has negative effects on wound healing, local blood flow, and tissue oxygenation (Petrek et al. 2000; Szuba and Rockson

1997). Function of the affected limb, quality of life, and finances are also negatively impacted (Cheville et al. 2010; Shih et al. 2009).

Surgery to remove cancerous tissue can require severing muscles and nerves, and cutting through multiple layers soft tissue that can result in scarring, altered range of motion, and altered muscle strength and function of the affected site. At some institutions, a physical therapist comes to visit within a day or two after surgery to get survivors moving. However, rehabilitative exercises for recovery of full function are not always prescribed and the extent to which they are needed after specific types of breast cancer surgeries is not well established.

8.2.4 Hormone Therapies

Hormonal therapies include antiestrogens and aromatase inhibitors, as well as some surgical procedures (e.g., oophorectomy). The magnitude of the side effects and symptoms vary by host and treatment factors, including the mechanisms of action. Common side effects from antiestrogens (e.g., tamoxifen) or oophorectomy are similar to the symptoms of menopause and include fatigue, hot flashes, bone loss, joint pain, vaginal discharge, weight gain, mood swings, and unfavorable changes in serum lipids (i.e., LDL, HDL, TGs). Premenopausal women who take tamoxifen may experience changes in their menstrual cycles. The side effects associated with aromatase inhibitors (prescribed for postmenopausal women with estrogen-linked cancers) include bone loss, joint stiffness, and muscle pain (Zivian and Salgado 2008). Oophorectomy or medically induced ovarian ablation with LHRH analogues may be used in premenopausal women with hormone sensitive breast cancers. Currently, research studies are evaluating the use of these agents in association with either tamoxifen or an aromatase inhibitor to see if there is additional benefit in the adjuvant or preventive setting. They may be used in the advanced (metastatic setting) as a standard and established therapy. This treatment induces premature menopause in these women. Changes expected with a sudden decrease in ovarian steroid hormones include increases in body weight or body composition, cardiovascular risk, vasomotor symptoms, bone loss, skin changes, and vaginal dryness. These changes are reversible after ovarian ablation with medications, but not after bilateral oophorectomy.

8.2.5 Targeted Therapies

Recent additions to the arsenal of breast cancer treatment include agents that target cancer, its vasculature, or its products more specifically. These agents can be delivered either alone or in combination with chemotherapy, orally or through an intravenous infusion. As these treatments are fairly new, their acute effects are only now being understood. Because cancer treatment modalities change rapidly, it is important to consult a physician about any potential risks prior to prescribing exercise in patients who are receiving a new form of targeted therapy. Some of the more common targeted therapies include trastuzumab, lapatinib, and, bevacizumab. The main side effect of trastuzumab therapy is a reversible type of cardiac dysfunction. The degree and severity of the dysfunction is a result of survivor medical factors, and the setting of treatment (e.g., adjuvant versus metastatic) and drugs previously or concurrently being used. The main side effects of lapatinib are diarrhea, flu-like symptoms, fatigue, and rash (foot-hand syndrome). Important complications of bevacizumab include gastrointestinal perforation, wound healing complications, and hemorrhage. Each of these side effects may impact ability to perform exercise and/or the usefulness of exercise.

8.2.6 Second Cancer Risk

Finally, another important late effect from chemotherapy and/or radiotherapy includes the increased risk for second cancers caused by the treatment. Numerous types of chemotherapeutic agents, including alkylating agents and anthracyclines, are linked to the development of leukemia. Specific links have been noted between radiation to the breast and the later development of lung cancer and leukemia (Matesich and Shapiro 2003). The potential for exercise to prevent second cancers among survivors treated with chemotherapy or radiation has been addressed in numerous observational studies. In addition, exercise has been hypothesized to be useful for preventing, attenuating, or in the rehabilitation of many of the persistent effects of cancer treatment. The remainder of this chapter is focused on reviewing this observational and interventional research.

8.3 Effects of Physical Activity on Supportive Care Outcomes

There are short and persistent adverse, even toxic effects of breast cancer treatment that might be prevented, attenuated, treated, or rehabilitated through regular physical activity. Herein, we review the evidence for safety of physical activity during treatment, as well as effects on several common adverse effects of treatment, including aerobic fitness, fatigue, body weight, lymphedema, and quality of life. There are multiple reviews available that comment on a broader array of supportive care outcomes than will be reviewed herein. Readers interested in knowing more about the effects of physical activity on breast cancer survivorship supportive care outcomes not reviewed here are directed to these other sources (Schmitz et al. 2010; Schmitz and Speck 2010; Speck et al. 2010).

8.3.1 Safety of Exercise During and After Breast Cancer Therapies

Activity-related advice from oncologists has historically been to "take it easy" and "pace yourself: do what you can, but don't push yourself" during the period of active breast cancer treatment. Therefore, it is not particularly surprising that there is empirical evidence that women decrease their activity level during the period between diagnosis and 1 year later, though most return to pre-diagnosis activity levels by 3 years post-diagnosis (Irwin et al. 2003). However, these decreases in activity may not be needed. There have been 21 randomized controlled trials (RCTs) that have prescribed various modes and doses of physical activity *during active breast cancer treatment* that evaluated the outcomes reviewed in this chapter (see Table 8.1). Fourteen of these have specifically reported on the safety of physical activity during active treatment, all concluded that the physical activity programming was safe during active breast cancer treatments such as radiation or chemotherapy or even bone marrow transplant. The modes of activity prescribed have varied from mild hatha yoga asanas and stretching activities to vigorous intensity resistance and aerobic exercise training. Frequency of activity has varied from one to five times per week, with an average of three times weekly. Duration of sessions is most commonly between 20 and 50 min.

Since the conclusion is that physical activity of multiple modes and doses appears to be safe during active treatment, it is not surprising that the same conclusion can be drawn for survivors who have completed active treatment. Thirty-six randomized controlled trials have tested effects of physical activity interventions among breast cancer survivors who have completed surgery, chemotherapy, and radiation treatments (see Table 8.2). Of these, 16 reported on adverse effects of physical activity. As with the studies

Table 8.1 Summary of 21 randomized controlled exercise intervention trials in breast cancer survivors during active treatment

First author (Year published)	Sample size[a]	Intervention length	Exercise mode	Exercise dose (frequency, intensity, duration)[b]	Safety	Fitness	Fatigue	Body Size	Lymph-edema	QOL
Dimeo et al. (1997a)	33	6 weeks	Aerobic	5× weekly, moderate intensity, 15–30 min sessions	✓	✔				
Mock et al. (1997)	46	6 weeks	Aerobic	5–6× weekly, moderate intensity, 15–30 min sessions		✔	✔			
Dimeo et al. (1999)	59	While hospitalized for Bone Marrow Transplant	Aerobic	Daily, moderate intensity, 30 min sessions			✔			
Segal et al. (2001)	123	26 weeks	Aerobic	5× weekly, moderate intensity	✓	✔		✔		
Headley et al. (2004)	24	12 weeks	Seated Exercises	3× weekly, light intensity, 30 min. sessions	✓		✔			✔
Campbell et al. (2005)	22	12 weeks	Aerobic	2× weekly, moderate intensity	✓	✔				✔
Mock et al. (2005)	119	6 months	Aerobic	5–6× weekly, moderate intensity, 15–30 min sessions			✓			
Drouin et al. (2006)	21	7 weeks	Aerobic	3–5× weekly, moderate intensity, 20–45 min. sessions	✓	✔				
Kim et al. (2006)	41	8 weeks	Aerobic	3× weekly, moderate intensity, 30–90 min. sessions		✓				
Battaglini et al. (2007)	20	15 weeks	Aerobic, strength, flexibility	2× weekly, moderate intensity, 60 min sessions	✓			✔		
Courneya et al. (2007)	219	17 weeks	Aerobic or Strength	3× weekly, moderate intensity, 15–45 min	✓	✔	✓	✔	✓	✓

Mutrie et al. (2007)	174	12 weeks	Group exercise class	2× weekly, 45 min sessions						✔
Schwartz et al. (2007)	66	6 months	Aerobic or Strength	4× weekly, moderate intensity, 15–30 min sessions	✓	✔				
Battaglini et al. (2008)	20	15 weeks	Aerobic, strength, flexibility	2× weekly, moderate intensity, 60 min sessions			✓	✓		
Courneya et al. (2008)	55	12 weeks	Aerobic	3× weekly, moderate to vigorous intensity	✓	✔	✓			
Demark-Wahnefried et al. (2008)	53	6 months	Aerobic, Strength	3× weekly, moderate intensity, 30 min. sessions	✓			✓		✓
Adamsen et al. (2009)	119	6 weeks	Aerobic, strength, flexibility	3× weekly, moderate to vigorous intensity, 90 min sessions	✓	✔	✔			✔
Cadmus et al. (2009)	50	6 months	Aerobic	Goal of 150 min/week moderate intensity	✓					✓
Mustian et al. (2009)	27	4 weeks	Aerobic, Strength	7× weekly, moderate intensity, 10,000 steps/week, daily resistance band exercises		✓	✔			✔
Sagen et al. (2009)	204	6 months, 2 years follow-up	Strength	2–3× weekly, moderate intensity, 45 min sessions	✓				✓	
Schwartz and Winters-Stone (2009)	101	12 months	Aerobic or Strength	4× weekly, moderate intensity, 20–30 min sessions	✓	✔		✔		

A ✓ indicates that the trial assessed the outcome. A bolded, larger ✔ indicates that the trial showed a statistically significant positive effect on the outcome. In the case of SAFETY and LYMPHEDEMA, a smaller check mark is the desired outcome

[a]Sample sizes reflect the number of breast cancer survivors. Some studies included other diagnoses as well

[b]If frequency, intensity, or duration of session is not provided in this column that detail was not provided in the published work

Table 8.2 Summary of 36 randomized controlled exercise intervention trials in breast cancer survivors conducted after completion of active treatment

First author (year published)	Sample size[a]	Intervention length	Exercise mode	Exercise dose (frequency, intensity, duration)[b]	Safety	Fitness	Fatigue	Body Size	Lymph-edema	QOL
Berglund et al. (1994)	160	4 weeks	Strength, flexibility	1× week			✓			✓
Nieman et al. (1995)	16	8 weeks	Aerobic, strength	3× weekly, 60 min/session, moderate intensity		✔				
Dimeo et al. (1997b)	17	7 weeks	Aerobic	5× weekly, intensity progressed from moderate to vigorous, session duration progressed from 15 to 30 min						✔
Burnham and Wilcox (2002)	15	10 weeks	Aerobic	3× weekly, moderate intensity, increa sed to 32 min/session by week 10		✔		✔		✔
Djuric et al. (2002)	48	12 months	Aerobic	Most days of the week, moderate intensity 30–45 min/session				✔		
Courneya et al. (2003); Fairey et al. (2005)	53	15 weeks	Aerobic	3× weekly, moderate intensity, 35 min/session	✓	✔	✔	✓		✔
Courneya et al. (2003b)	44	10 weeks	Aerobic	3–5× weekly, 65–75% max. heart rate, 20–30 min/session			✔	✔		✔
McKenzie and Kalda (2003)	14	8 weeks	Aerobic, strength, flexibility upper body only	3× weekly, moderate intensity	✓				✓	✓

Pinto et al. (2003)	24	12 weeks	Aerobic, strength	3× weekly, moderate intensity, 50 min/session		✔	✓			
Pinto et al. (2005)	86	12 weeks	Aerobic	5× weekly, moderate intensity, 30 min/session		✔	✔	✓		
Sandel et al. (2005)	38	12 weeks	Dance	1–2× weekly, 60 min/session	✓				✓	✔
Schmitz et al. (2005); Ahmed et al. (2006); Ohira et al. (2006)	86	6 months	Strength	2× weekly, 60–90 min/session	✓			✔	✓	✔
Thorsen et al. (2005)	80	14 weeks	Aerobic, strength, or flexibility – at discretion of participant	2× weekly, moderate to vigorous intensity, 30 min/session		✔	✓			✓
Basen-Engquist et al. (2006)	60	6 months	Lifestyle intervention	Tailored to stage of readiness	✓	✔		✓	✓	✔
Cho et al. (2006)	55	10 weeks	Lifestyle intervention, Aerobic, Stretching	2× weekly, 90 min/session						✔
Culos-Reed et al. (2006)	38	7 weeks	Yoga	75 min/session						✔
Demark-Wahnefried et al. (2006)	104	6 months	Aerobic	5× weekly, moderate intensity, 30 min/session	✓			✓		✓
Herrero et al. (2006)	16	8 weeks	Aerobic, Strength	3× weekly, 90 min. per session, moderate to vigorous intensity	✓	✔		✔		✔

(*continued*)

Table 8.2 (continued)

First author (year published)	Sample size[a]	Intervention length	Exercise mode	Exercise dose (frequency, intensity, duration)[b]	Safety	Fitness	Fatigue	Body Size	Lymph-edema	QOL
Bennett et al. (2007)	56	6 months	Lifestyle intervention	Goal of 30 min moderate intensity most days		✓	✓			
Daley et al. (2007)	108	8 weeks	Aerobic	3× weekly, moderate intensity, 50 min/session		✔	✓	✓		✔
Demark-Wahnefried et al. (2007)	306	10 months	Aerobic	5× weekly, moderate intensity, 30 min/session	✓			✔		✓
Matthews et al. (2007)	36	12 weeks	Lifestyle intervention, Walking training	3–5× weekly, moderate intensity, 20–40 min/session				✓		
Mefferd et al. (2007)	85	16 weeks	Aerobic, Strength	1 h daily moderate intensity aerobic, 2–3× weekly strength training				✔		
Moadel et al. (2007)	128	12	Yoga	1× weekly, 1.5 h/session			✓			✔
Nikander et al. (2007)	28	12 weeks	Aerobic	3× weekly, moderate intensity, 30–40 min/session	✓	✔				
Vallance et al. (2007)	377	12 weeks	Aerobic	30 min 5× weekly						✔
Fillion et al. (2008)	87	4 weeks	Lifestyle intervention, Walking training, Stress management	Tailored by physical condition and personal goal. 2.5 h/week session		✓	✔			✔
Kilgour et al. (2008)	27	11 days	Shoulder stretches	Daily, light intensity, 15–30 min/session	✓				✓	

Ligibel et al. (2008)	101	16 weeks	Aerobic, Strength	90 min weekly aerobic activity, 2× weekly strength training				✓		
Milne et al. (2008)	58	12 weeks	Aerobic, Strength	3× weekly, 30–45 min/session		✓	✓			✓
Carson et al. (2009)	37	8 weeks	Yoga	1× weekly, light intensity, 120 min/sessions			✓			
Hayes et al. (2009)	32	12 weeks	Aerobic, Strength	3–4× weekly, intensity and duration progressed over 12 weeks	✓				✓	
Irwin et al. (2009b)	75	6 months	Aerobic	150 min/week, moderate intensity	✓			✓		✓
Morey et al. (2009)	289	12 months	Aerobic, Strength	15 min strength training 3–4× weekly, 30 min aerobic exercise daily	✓			✓		✓
Rogerset al. (2009)	41	12 weeks	Aerobic	3–5× weekly, moderate intensity	✓	✓		✓		✓
Schmitz (2009)	141	12 months	Strength	2× weekly, 90 min/session	✓			✓	✓	

[a]Sample sizes reflect the number of breast cancer survivors. Some studies included other diagnoses as well

[b]If frequency, intensity, or duration of session is not provided in this column that detail was not provided in the published work

conducted during active cancer treatment, physical activity interventions after completion of surgery, radiation, and chemotherapy were found to be safe, with very few reports of adverse effects. The adverse effects noted tended to be mild activity-related injuries from which participants recovered quickly, such as foot pain from walking programs or shoulder pain from upper body resistance training. As with the studies conducted during active cancer therapy, the vast majority of the interventions were aerobic exercise, with walking as the most common form of activity prescribed. Other modes of activity that have been tried with post-treatment breast cancer survivors include upper body and total body resistance training, yoga, dance programs, and stretching activities. The intensity prescribed is generally moderate to vigorous, frequency is most commonly three to five times a week, and the duration of sessions is usually between 20 and 60 min.

Treatment for breast cancer results in substantive physical and emotional challenges for patient. Clinicians interacting with breast cancer survivors (during and after active treatment) will want to give advice that will minimize these challenges in the short and long run. Until relatively recently, oncology clinicians could advise their patients to "take it easy," "rest," and to avoid pushing themselves, particularly during active treatment, with the common sense logic that until it was proven safe, additional physical challenges from physical activity (leisure or otherwise) should be avoided. However, there is now overwhelming evidence that being physically active during and after active cancer treatments IS safe and poses no adverse risk for treatment outcomes or patient side effects during or after active cancer treatment. The available evidence supports a change in advice from clinicians to breast cancer survivors. Clinicians should advise breast cancer patients undergoing treatment to avoid inactivity and to remain physically active during and after treatment, to the extent that they are physically able to do so. This advice is in keeping with the new ACSM/ACS guidelines for cancer survivors during and after active treatment to follow age-appropriate guidance for physical activity levels from the US Department of Health and Human Services to the extent that they are able to do so (Schmitz et al. 2010) (presented in Tables 8.3 and 8.4). In addition to being safe, there are benefits to this level of activity for breast cancer survivors. In the remainder of this chapter, we review these effects, focusing on outcomes for which there is the greatest amount of evidence, including: aerobic fitness, fatigue, body size, lymphedema, and quality of life.

8.3.2 Aerobic Fitness

At first glance, it seems obvious that an aerobic exercise intervention would improve aerobic fitness. However, cancer treatments involve exposures that may alter the body's response to training (e.g., increases in cell death for rapidly dividing cells during chemotherapy and radiation) and/or alter the body in ways that alters response to or need for training (e.g., cardiotoxicity and pulmonary toxicity of chemotherapy and radiation therapy). There may also be biochemical changes associated with cancer-related fatigue (CRF) that alter exercise tolerance and/or response to training. Finally, the physical challenges of cancer treatment may result in decreases in fitness level due to reduced activity levels, which may further exacerbate effects of treatment on fatigue and quality of life. Therefore, it is of interest to know whether physical activity can assist with maintaining or improving fitness among breast cancer survivors during and after active treatment. It can be hypothesized that an aerobically fit breast cancer survivor will be more physically capable of withstanding the physical challenges of active treatment.

Table 8.3 Review of US DHHS Physical Activity Guidelines (PAGs) for Americans and alterations needed for breast cancer survivors

General statements	Avoid inactivity 1. Return to normal daily activities as quickly as possible after surgery 2. Continue normal daily activities and exercise as much as possible during and after nonsurgical treatments. Individuals with known metastatic bone disease will require modifications to avoid fractures 3. Individuals with cardiac conditions (secondary to cancer or not) may require modifications and may require greater supervision for safety
Aerobic exercise training (volume, intensity, progression)	1. Recommendations are the same as age-appropriate guidelines from PAGs for Americans (see Table 8.4) 2. Be aware of fracture risk
Resistance training (volume, intensity, progression)	Recommendations in Table 8.4 should be altered as follows 1. Start with a supervised program of at least 16 sessions and very low resistance 2. Progress resistance at small increments 3. No upper limit on the amount of weight to which survivors can progress 4. Watch for arm/shoulder symptoms, including lymphedema, and reduce resistance or stop specific exercises according to symptom response 5. If a break is taken, back off the level of resistance by 2 weeks worth for every week of no exercise (e.g. a 2 week exercise vacation = back off to resistance used 4 weeks ago) 6. Be aware of risk for fracture in this population
Flexibility training (volume, intensity, progression)	Recommendations are the same as age appropriate PAGs for Americans (see Table 8.4)
Exercises with special considerations (e.g. yoga, organized sports, Pilates)	1. Yoga appears safe as long as arm and shoulder morbidities are taken into consideration 2. Dragon boat racing not empirically tested, but the volume of participants worldwide provides face validity of safety for this activity 3. No evidence on organized sport or Pilates

There have been 12 RCTs that have examined effects of physical activity interventions during chemotherapy and/or radiation. All but two RCTs (Kim et al. 2006; Mustian et al. 2009), have reported significant aerobic capacity improvements. The interventions ranged from home-based walking programs to structured, supervised fitness sessions that included aerobic, resistance, and flexibility activities. The interventions that did not show an effect on aerobic fitness were particularly short (4 weeks and 6 weeks), which may be too short to see a training effect on cardiorespiratory fitness.

Timed distance tests and maximal oxygen consumption have been used to evaluate improvements in aerobic fitness in 14 exercise interventions for breast cancer survivors post-treatment (Basen-Engquist et al. 2006; Bennett

8

Table 8.4 Key guidelines for adults and older adults from the US Department of Health and Human Services

Key guidelines for adults from the US Department of Health and Human Services
• All adults should avoid inactivity. Some physical activity is better than none, and adults who participate in any amount of physical activity gain some health benefits • For substantial health benefits, adults should do at least 150 min (2 h and 30 min) a week of moderate-intensity, or 75 min (1 h and 15 min) a week of vigorous-intensity aerobic physical activity, or an equivalent combination of moderate- and vigorous intensity aerobic activity. Aerobic activity should be performed in episodes of at least 10 min, and preferably, it should be spread throughout the week • For additional and more extensive health benefits, adults should increase their aerobic physical activity to 300 min (5 h) a week of moderate intensity, or 150 min a week of vigorous intensity aerobic physical activity, or an equivalent combination of moderate- and vigorous-intensity activity. Additional health benefits are gained by engaging in physical activity beyond this amount • Adults should also do muscle-strengthening activities that are moderate or high intensity and involve all major muscle groups on two or more days a week, as these activities provide additional health benefits.
The key guidelines for adults also apply to older adults. In addition, the following guidelines are just for older adults
• When older adults cannot do 150 min of moderate-intensity aerobic activity a week because of chronic conditions, they should be as physically active as their abilities and conditions allow • Older adults should do exercises that maintain or improve balance if they are at risk of falling • Older adults should determine their level of effort for physical activity relative to their level of fitness • Older adults with chronic conditions should understand whether and how their conditions affect their ability to do regular physical activity safely

et al. 2007; Burnham and Wilcox 2002; Courneya et al. 2003b; Daley et al. 2007; Fillion et al. 2008; Herrero et al. 2006; Nieman et al. 1995; Nikander et al. 2007; Pinto et al. 2003, 2005; Rogers et al. 2009; Thorsen et al. 2005). All but three of these studies (Bennett et al. 2007; Fillion et al. 2008; Rogers et al. 2009) observed statistically significant improvements in aerobic capacity in the treatment compared to control participants.

In summary, the majority of physical activity interventions that have examined effects on aerobic fitness have demonstrated that breast cancer survivors during and posttreatment do exhibit training effects, and the changes are of similar magnitude to what might be expected among those who do not have cancer. It might be hypothesized that a more fit breast cancer survivor would be less likely to suffer from cancer-related fatigue (Kangas et al. 2008). In the next section, we examine effects of physical activity interventions on fatigue among breast cancer survivors.

8.3.3 Fatigue

Cancer-related fatigue (CRF) has been defined as "an unusual, persistent, subjective sense of tiredness related to cancer or cancer treatment that interferes with usual functioning" (Mock 2001). CRF is a common complaint from breast cancer patients during and after systemic therapies (Lawrence et al. 2004). There have been nine RCTs that have examined the efficacy of exercise to mitigate fatigue during chemotherapy for breast cancer: five showed a significant positive effect (Dimeo et al. 1999; Headley et al. 2004; Mock et al. 1997; Mustian et al. 2009;

Schwartz et al. 2007) and four showed no effect or failed to achieve statistical significance (Battaglini et al. 2008; Courneya et al. 2007, 2008; Mock et al. 2005). The largest of these seven studies (N = 242) was the Supervised Trial of Aerobic versus Resistance Training (START) trial, which showed no effect of aerobic exercise or resistance training on fatigue during chemotherapy for breast cancer survivors (Courneya et al. 2007). These mixed results for studies conducted during active treatment are matched by equally mixed results among survivors who have completed treatment. There have been 12 RCTs that have assessed the effects of exercise training on fatigue after breast cancer treatment. Of these, six observed that exercise improved fatigue (Carson et al. 2009; Courneya et al. 2003b; Fillion et al. 2008; Pinto et al. 2005), five observed no significant effect of exercise compared to no exercise (Bennett et al. 2007; Berglund et al. 1994; Daley et al. 2007; Pinto et al. 2003; Rogers et al. 2009), and one observed worse fatigue after an exercise intervention than with exercise (Thorsen et al. 2005).

There are multiple possible reasons for the mixed results on the effects of physical activity interventions on CRF. First, it has been noted in a recent systematic review (Jacobsen et al. 2007) that few of the studies on this topic specifically recruited breast cancer survivors who reported significant levels of fatigue. It would be difficult to reduce fatigue in a woman who is not fatigued at study entry! Second, the studies varied with regard to whether fatigue was the primary outcome of interest, which may mean that there may have been limited statistical power to detect an effect. Third, few of these studies have specifically designed the physical activity intervention to address one or more of the hypothesized causes of CRF, such as decreased muscle mass (Demark-Wahnefried et al. 2001), increases in pro-inflammatory cytokines (Bower et al. 2002; Bower 2007; Greenberg et al. 1993), psychological distress, sleep problems, or decreased physical function (Payne 2002; Ramsey et al. 2002) (Schmitz et al. 2007) Therefore, prior to concluding that physical activity is ineffective for CRF, future research is needed to address these limitations. Further, it *can* be concluded that physical activity does not make CRF worse during or after breast cancer treatment. Given the history of clinicians advising breast cancer survivors to “take it easy” and “avoid overdoing it,” this is important information.

8.3.4 Body Size

Breast cancer survivors may gain weight as a result of treatment, and there is empirical evidence that body fat increases and lean muscle mass decreases as a result of treatment (Demark-Wahnefried et al. 2001). In addition to being upsetting to survivors, weight gain predicts multiple negative health consequences for cardiovascular and metabolic disease outcomes (Obunai et al. 2007). There is also some evidence that weight gain post-diagnosis is associated with worse prognosis and overall survival after breast cancer (Kroenke et al. 2005), though not all studies agree regarding the influence of post-diagnosis weight gain and altered breast cancer survival (Caan et al. 2006). It could be that women who enter breast cancer diagnosis with a higher weight already have a hormonal milieu consistent with higher risk for recurrence and worse overall survival (Daniell 2009). The wake-up call of a cancer diagnosis may increase motivation to change health behaviors and lose weight, resulting in what is commonly termed “the teachable moment” for breast cancer survivors. Weight control is also a key factor for reducing risk for onset or worse clinical course of breast cancer-related lymphedema (Bar Ad et al. 2010; Petrek et al. 2001). Physical activity is acknowledged to be an important adjunct to dietary changes for weight control efforts in adults who have not had cancer (Donnelly et al. 2009).

There have been 18 randomized controlled trials that have examined the potential for physical activity to alter weight or body composition (fat mass and or lean mass) during or posttreatment in breast cancer survivors. Six of these specifically examined the effect of exercise to improve body size (e.g., weight, BMI) or body composition (e.g., fat mass, lean mass) during treatment for breast cancer (Battaglini et al. 2007, 2008; Courneya et al. 2007; Demark-Wahnefried et al. 2008; Schwartz and Winters-Stone 2009; Segal et al. 2001). Two of these studies showed no effect of exercise on body size or composition endpoints (Battaglini et al. 2008; Demark-Wahnefried et al. 2008). Percent body fat was improved in three interventions (Battaglini et al. 2007; Courneya et al. 2007; Schwartz and Winters-Stone 2009), body weight was reduced by exercisers more than usual care participants in two interventions (Schwartz and Winters-Stone 2009; Segal et al. 2001), and lean mass was improved among women who did supervised resistance training during chemotherapy (Courneya et al. 2007). Changes in body weight, body mass index (BMI), fat mass, lean mass, body fat percentage, and waist circumference were assessed in 18 exercise interventions for breast cancer survivors posttreatment. The effects vary widely, with ten of the studies showing statistically significant positive effects on one or more variables related to body size or body composition (Ahmed et al. 2006; Burnham and Wilcox 2002; Courneya et al. 2003b; Demark-Wahnefried et al. 2007; Djuric et al. 2002; Herrero et al. 2006; Irwin et al. 2009a; Mefferd et al. 2007; Morey et al. 2009; Rogers et al. 2009). A complete review of the effects of each type of intervention on specific body composition variables is beyond the scope of this chapter but can be found elsewhere (Ingram et al. 2006; Kim et al. 2009; Speck et al. 2010).

In general, effects of exercise interventions among breast cancer survivors on body weight and body composition concur with results from studies of adults who have not had cancer. The 2009 ACSM position stand on appropriate physical activity intervention strategies for weight loss and prevention of weight regain for adults includes concluding evidence statements that activity of less than 150 min/week is insufficient to reduce weight, while 150–250 min/week of moderate intensity aerobic activity results in 2–3 kg of weight loss, and that exercise of 225–420 min/week results in a 5–7 kg weight loss (Donnelly et al. 2009). There is a clear dose–response relationship noted between amount of exercise and weight loss, but increasing levels of exercise also increase risk of injury. Therefore, breast cancer survivors who are overweight and wish to lose weight should be guided to approach weight loss through a combined program of dietary and physical activity changes, as sustainable levels of exercise are not likely to result in significant weight loss. That said, weight loss through dietary changes alone, with no exercise, may be less likely to be maintained in the long term. There is also more consistent evidence for a role of exercise than weight loss for overall survival benefit in breast cancer survivors as well, as reviewed in a later section of this chapter.

8.3.5 Lymphedema

As noted earlier, lymphedema is a common and feared adverse effect of breast cancer treatment. Upper body exercise has been historically discouraged for women who have had axillary lymph nodes removed and/or radiation to the axilla. In light of this, it is notable that there have been eight randomized controlled trials that have all shown that upper body exercise (aerobic and/or resistance training) does *not* contribute to the onset or worsening of lymphedema among survivors at risk (Ahmed et al. 2006; Basen-Engquist et al. 2006; Hayes et al. 2009; Kilgour et al. 2008; McKenzie and Kalda 2003; Sagen et al. 2009; Sandel et al. 2005;

Schmitz et al. 2009). Though most of these were relatively small, with sample sizes of 81 or fewer, two of these trials were particularly large (Sagen et al. 2009; Schmitz et al. 2009). In one of these trials, which was conducted in Norway, survivors who had axillary dissection were randomized to receive advice to restrict use of the affected limb ($N = 100$) or to do slowly progressive strength training activity with the affected limb and "not" to restrict use of the affected limb ($N = 104$). At the end of 2 years of follow-up, there were no differences in the onset of lymphedema, with a rate of 13% onset in both groups (Sagen et al. 2009). The only variable that was shown to predict onset of lymphedema was a baseline body mass index over 25 kg/m^2, with an Odds Ratio of 3.42 for lymphedema onset when compared to women who had a BMI less than 25 at baseline (Sagen et al. 2009). The other large trial on this topic was called the Physical Activity and Lymphedema (PAL) Trial. The PAL trial randomized 141 breast cancer survivors with preexisting lymphedema into a slowly progressive resistance training intervention or a wait-list control condition and demonstrated that slowly progressive resistance training undertaken with a compression garment is actually protective against lymphedema flare-ups (Schmitz et al. 2009). The Norwegian trial only included women who had axillary dissection, but the PAL trial included women who had both axillary node dissection and sentinel node biopsy. In all of the completed trials that have specifically focused on the safety of upper body exercise among women with or at-risk for lymphedema, the protocols all started with eight or more weeks of supervised training with a certified fitness professional.

8.3.6 Quality of Life

The physical and psychological challenges introduced with a diagnosis and treatment for breast cancer can alter a woman's sense of purpose and meaning in life, as well as her sense of well-being (Hewitt et al. 2006). A correlation has been noted between the extent of symptoms, side effects, pain, and other persistent adverse effects of treatment and the impact of cancer on quality of life (Speck et al. 2009). There is observational evidence that survivors who are more physically active report higher quality of life (Chen et al. 2009) and that these effects may be more pronounced among younger than older survivors (Harrison et al. 2010). There have been 31 randomized controlled trials that assessed the effects of physical activity interventions on quality of life within breast cancer survivors during and after active treatments. Five RCTs have shown that supervised and unsupervised exercise (aerobic, resistance, and stretching interventions) improves QOL in breast cancer survivors during chemotherapy or radiotherapy (Adamsen et al. 2009; Campbell et al. 2005; Headley et al. 2004; Mustian et al. 2009; Mutrie et al. 2007). Three RCTs conducted during active breast cancer therapy observed no such effect (Cadmus et al. 2009; Courneya et al. 2007; Demark-Wahnefried et al. 2008). The most recent of these studies during active treatment was a 4-week long, daily, home-based walking and resistance band intervention during radiation therapy that resulted in substantive improvements in the Functional Assessment of Chronic Illness Therapy scale. It is notable that this intervention was designed with broad disseminability in mind – participants were given instruction on the intervention in a single 45-min session, yet adherence to daily walking and achieving the goal of 10,000 steps/day was achieved (Mustian et al. 2009).

Among breast cancer survivors who have completed treatment, QOL outcomes have been assessed using a wide variety of instruments in 23 exercise interventions. Of these, 17 noted statistically significant improvements (Basen-Engquist et al. 2006; Burnham and Wilcox 2002; Cho et al. 2006; Courneya et al. 2003b; Culos-Reed et al. 2006; Daley et al. 2007; Dimeo et al. 1997a; Fillion et al. 2008; Herrero et al. 2006; Milne et al. 2008; Moadel et al. 2007; Morey et al. 2009; Ohira et al. 2006; Rogers et al. 2009; Sandel et al. 2005; Vallance et al. 2007), and six did not (Berglund et al. 1994; Demark-Wahnefried et al. 2006, 2007; Irwin et al. 2009a; McKenzie and Kalda 2003; Thorsen et al. 2005). More consistent improvements have been noted in posttreatment studies on scores for the Breast Cancer Subscale of the Functional Assessment of Cancer Therapy (FACT)-Breast (Brady et al. 1997), than for other, more generic quality of life assessment tools. The questions on the FACT-Breast scale are geared specifically to issues faced by breast cancer survivors, such as reporting feeling short of breath, self-consciousness about appearance, arm and shoulder symptoms, body image, and pain. Overall, there is evidence that physical activity interventions among breast cancer survivors can lead to improved quality of life.

8.3.7 Summary and Conclusions Regarding Effects of Physical Activity on Supportive Care Outcomes

There is overwhelming evidence that physical activity is safe for breast cancer survivors to perform during and after the completion of active treatment (e.g., chemotherapy and radiation therapy). Advice to "take it easy" might be taken as a recommendation to reduce activity level during or after active cancer treatment. This could result in worse supportive care outcomes, including body size, quality of life, fatigue, and aerobic fitness. Each of these outcomes, and many others (reviewed elsewhere) (Schmitz et al. 2010; Schmitz and Speck 2010; Speck et al. 2010) have been shown to be positively influenced by a program of physical activity, both during and after the end of active treatment. Finally, the long-held advice to limit use of an arm at risk for or with breast cancer–related lymphedema appears to be unwarranted. There is ample evidence from multiple well-controlled trials that upper body exercise is safe and may help with symptoms of lymphedema secondary to breast cancer.

8.4 Disease Outcomes

Once initial curative treatment is completed, many breast cancer survivors are eager to learn what predicts the likelihood of recurrence and promotes long-term survival. There is an emerging body of literature on the effects of pre- and post-diagnosis levels of physical activity on disease outcomes among breast cancer survivors. Six studies have examined whether pre-diagnosis lifetime physical activity levels affect breast cancer survival. Four of these have observed a protective effect of pre-diagnosis physical activity (Abrahamson et al. 2006; Friedenreich et al. 2009; Irwin et al. 2008; West-Wright et al. 2009). By contrast, two others showed no such association (Enger and Bernstein 2004; Rohan et al. 1995). Though information on pre-diagnosis lifetime activity levels may bring comfort to those who happened to be active before diagnosis, these women are in the minority: The majority of women do not meet the current recommendations for regular physical activity (CDC 2008). Therefore, it is of equal or greater importance to learn whether post-diagnostic activity levels are associated with recurrence and survival. There have been four cohorts of breast cancer survivors that have addressed this question. In contrast to the studies on pre-diagnostic activity levels, the results of these four studies of post-diagnosis physical activity levels and protection from recurrence or mortality after breast cancer have been more consistent in showing a protective effect. The first of these studies was based on the Nurses' Health Study (NHS), a large cohort study of nursing professionals (Holmes et al. 2005). Nursing professionals who had had a diagnosis of breast cancer

(N = 2,987) were followed for an average of 8 years, during which time 280 breast cancer deaths occurred. In the NHS cohort, survivors who exercised at a level approximating 3–5 h of weekly walking had a 50% reduced risk of dying from breast cancer (95% confidence interval of 0.38–0.84). The benefit was especially noted among women with hormone-sensitive tumors. The Collaborative Women's Longevity Study (CWLS), followed 4,482 breast cancer survivors over 6 years (Holick et al. 2008). There were 109 deaths. The reduction in risk from breast cancer and total deaths was similar to the 50% reduction observed in the Nurses' Health Study, with similar levels of activity (3–5 h of weekly walking). In the Life After Cancer Epidemiology (LACE) study, 1,970 women were followed an average of 7.25 years after breast cancer diagnosis (Sternfeld et al. 2009). During the follow-up, there were 225 recurrences, 102 breast cancer deaths, and 187 total deaths. The results in this slightly smaller study were not quite as clear, as in the NHS and CWLS studies. Though there was indication that moderate-to-vigorous intensity activity attenuated risk for recurrence and breast cancer mortality, the associations disappeared when adjusting for other prognostic factors such as number of positive nodes and treatment types. The association with overall mortality was robust after these same adjustments. The authors reported a 30–40% decrease in the risk of overall mortality among breast cancer survivors who performed moderate intensity activity of at least 1 h/week (hazard ratio of 0.71, 0.66, 0.66 for activity levels of 1–<3, 3–<6, and $^{3}6$ weekly hours of moderate intensity physical activity, p for trend = 0.04). Finally, the Health, Eating, Activity, and Lifestyle (HEAL) study examined post-diagnosis physical activity among 688 survivors followed a median of 6 years. Similar to the LACE study results, the significant effects were present for overall mortality but not breast cancer specific mortality (Irwin et al. 2008), with a 45% decreased risk of death among survivors who increased activity after diagnosis. Another recent observational study examined the effect of acquired comorbidities after a breast cancer diagnosis on overall mortality in 689 survivors followed for an average of 7 years (Ahern et al. 2009). Comorbidities were evaluated using the Charlson Index, which grades comorbidity presence on a scale from 0 to 4 and includes conditions such as cardiovascular disease and events, pulmonary disease, and Alzheimer's disease, as well as arthritis, liver, kidney, and endocrine conditions. The results indicated that for each comorbidity at the time of breast cancer diagnosis and newly acquired after diagnosis, there is a 30–40% increased risk for mortality. Taken as a whole, it appears safe to conclude that increasing physical activity after breast cancer diagnosis does confer benefit to survival.

8.5 Future Research Directions

8.5.1 Overall

The methodologic quality of studies on exercise in breast cancer survivors has improved over time. However, the published research can still be viewed critically. Some potential limitations to the ability to exercise during treatment have yet to be studied to reassure oncologists who have the opportunity to prescribe exercise to their patients. These include dyspnea, nausea, ataxia, dizziness, and peripheral neuropathy. In order for oncologists to recommend or refer their patients for exercise counseling, a better understanding of the impact of exercise on attenuating side effects during treatment is needed.

Studies are also needed to examine the relationship between exercise and quality of life in segments of the population of breast cancer survivors who have been largely absent from previous research. These survivors include racial and ethnic minorities, those with low educational attainment and or low socioeconomic position. These types of studies will contribute important information about the generalizability of the effects of exercise on the outcomes reviewed herein.

8.5.2 During Chemotherapy and Radiotherapy

The effect of exercise on body composition changes, immune and hormonal changes for breast cancer survivors undergoing treatment is as yet unclear. There are too few studies on these outcomes to draw firm conclusions. For outcomes with inconsistent findings, such as QOL, there is also the possibility exercise interventions may need to be further targeted to become more effective. For example, increases in QOL are most often seen in exercise studies with younger women. Future research should consist of larger RCTs with long intervention periods that would allow an opportunity to examine several as yet unaddressed questions, including a comprehensive array of psychosocial measures to provide more conclusive answers regarding the aspects of quality of life that are most amenable to change via exercise. Similarly, such a study would provide valuable information about how long it takes to observe maximum quality of life benefits from exercise, and whether benefits persist over time.

Authors have repeatedly speculated that the effects of exercise on certain endpoints is likely to differ based on moderating factors such as stage at diagnosis, treatment type, age, weight, and body composition. No studies have reported analyses of these potential interactions, possibly due to small sample sizes. Better understanding of these relationships will aid in the tailoring of exercise programs for specific subgroups of breast cancer survivors.

Little is known about which features of physical activity are most important for psychosocial outcomes and what type, duration, and frequency of activity is necessary to achieve specific types of benefits. Most interventions to date have focused on walking or other moderate-intensity aerobic interventions, but often do not include enough activity to meet generally recommended levels. More research is needed to understand the impact of greater amounts of exercise as well as the potential benefits of strength training for therapeutic outcomes.

8.5.3 After Chemotherapy and Radiotherapy

Despite the 36 RCTs reviewed in Table 8.2 that have assessed the efficacy of exercise training among breast cancer survivors who have completed surgery, chemotherapy, and radiotherapy, there are still gaps in the literature. For example, there is a need for assessing the safety and efficacy of alternate types of physical activity, such as Pilates, various forms of yoga, martial arts, Curves™, and organized sport activities. There is also a need for deeper clarification of specifics regarding the level of supervision needed for effective interventions for a variety of outcomes, including lymphedema and quality of life. Perhaps the most pressing need, however, is for a large randomized controlled trial to discern whether exercise alone, or in concert with dietary changes, would lead to a reduction in breast cancer recurrence.

8.6 Clinical Recommendations

Clinicians who treat breast cancer can feel comfortable with advising their patients to stay physically active during and after active treatment, given ample empirical evidence from dozens of randomized trials of the safety of a variety of modes and intensities of exercise programming. Women with and at risk for lymphedema can and should participate in upper body exercise in order to gain the well-established health benefits. The specific benefits of physical activity programming among breast cancer survivors include improved fitness, quality of life, and body weight or body composition. Weight loss effects will be most evident in physical activity programs combined with caloric restriction. Effects of physical activity interventions on cancer-related fatigue are mixed, in part due to methodologic limitations of the research completed to date. It can be concluded, however, that being physically active will not make fatigue worse. Clinicians are urged to prescribe that their patients "avoid inactivity" both during and after active breast cancer treatment, in keeping with the soon-to-be released guidance for exercise prescription among cancer survivors from the American College of Sports Medicine (Schmitz et al. 2010). These guidelines are presented in Tables 8.3 and 8.4.

8.7 Summary and Conclusion

Curative treatments for breast cancer pose significant physiologic and psychological challenges. There is some evidence that there are long-lasting changes in physical function as a result of breast cancer treatment and it has been hypothesized that there may be a permanent alteration in the aging trajectory toward frank disability as a result (Schmitz et al. 2007). Exercise training has been shown to be safe during and after breast cancer treatments and the soon-to-be released guidance from the American Cancer Society and the American College of Sports Medicine recommend that women should remain as active as possible during their treatments. Exercise has been shown to be efficacious for multiple physiologic and psychosocial outcomes in this population. Clinicians are urged to recommend that their patients "avoid inactivity" during and after treatment, in order to minimize the functional decline that can accompany curative breast cancer treatments. Resistance training can be performed safely by breast cancer survivors with and at risk for lymphedema.

Multiple research gaps remain in this field, including the need for greater specificity with regard to the dose–response effects of specific modes of exercise training on specific endpoints and within more diverse populations of breast cancer survivors. Perhaps most importantly, there is outstanding observational evidence for a role of physical activity in preventing, attenuating, or delaying breast cancer recurrence. A large clinical trial on this topic is needed to establish that the observational findings are causal.

References

Abrahamson PE, Gammon MD, Lund MJ, Britton JA, Marshall SW, Flagg EW et al (2006) Recreational physical activity and survival among young women with breast cancer. Cancer 107(8):1777–1785

Adamsen L, Quist M, Andersen C, Moller T, Herrstedt J, Kronborg D et al (2009) Effect of a multimodal high intensity exercise intervention in cancer patients undergoing chemotherapy: randomised controlled trial. BMJ 339:b3410

Ahern TP, Lash TL, Thwin SS, Silliman RA (2009) Impact of acquired comorbidities on all-cause mortality rates among older breast cancer survivors. Med Care 47(1):73–79

Ahmed RL, Thomas W, Yee D, Schmitz K (2006) Weight training does not increase incidence of lymphedema in breast cancer survivors. J Clin Oncol 24:2765–2772

Aziz NM, Rowland JH (2003) Trends and advances in cancer survivorship research: challenge and

8

opportunity. Semin Radiat Oncol 13(3): 248–266

Bar Ad V, Cheville A, Solin LJ, Dutta P, Both S, Harris EE (2010) Time course of mild arm lymphedema after breast conservation treatment for early-stage breast cancer. Int J Radiat Oncol Biol Phys 76(1):85–90

Basen-Engquist K, Taylor CL, Rosenblum C, Smith MA, Shinn EH, Greisinger A et al (2006) Randomized pilot test of a lifestyle physical activity intervention for breast cancer survivors. Patient Educ Couns 64(1–3):225–234

Battaglini C, Bottaro M, Dennehy C, Rae L, Shields E, Kirk D et al (2007) The effects of an individualized exercise intervention on body composition in breast cancer patients undergoing treatment. São Paulo Med J 125(1):22–28

Battaglini CL, Mihalik JP, Bottaro M, Dennehy C, Petschauer MA, Hairston LS et al (2008) Effect of exercise on the caloric intake of breast cancer patients undergoing treatment. Braz J Med Biol Res 41(8):709–715

Bennett JA, Lyons KS, Winters-Stone K, Nail LM, Scherer J (2007) Motivational interviewing to increase physical activity in long-term cancer survivors: a randomized controlled trial. Nurs Res 56(1):18–27

Berglund G, Bolund C, Gustafsson UL, Sjoden PO (1994) One-year follow-up of the 'Starting Again' group rehabilitation programme for cancer patients. Eur J Cancer 30A(12):1744–1751

Bower JE (2007) Cancer-related fatigue: links with inflammation in cancer patients and survivors. Brain Behav Immun 21(7):863–871

Bower J, Ganz P, Aziz N, Fahey J (2002) Fatigue and proinflammatory cytokine activity in breast cancer survivors. Psychosom Med 64:604–611

Boyle P, Levin B (2008) World cancer report 2008. World Health Orgnization, International Agency for Research on Cancer, Lyon

Brady MJ, Cella DF, Mo F, Bonomi AE, Tulsky DS, Lloyd SR et al (1997) Reliability and validity of the functional assessment of cancer therapy-breast quality-of-life instrument. J Clin Oncol 15(3):974–986

Burnham TR, Wilcox A (2002) Effects of exercise on physiological and psychological variables in cancer survivors. Med Sci Sports Exerc 34(12):1863–1867

Caan BJ, Emond JA, Natarajan L, Castillo A, Gunderson EP, Habel L et al (2006) Post-diagnosis weight gain and breast cancer recurrence in women with early stage breast cancer. Breast Cancer Res Treat 99(1):47–57

Cadmus LA, Salovey P, Yu H, Chung G, Kasl S, Irwin ML (2009) Exercise and quality of life during and after treatment for breast cancer: results of two randomized controlled trials. Psychooncology 18(4):343–352

Campbell A, Mutrie N, White F, McGuire F, Kearney N (2005) A pilot study of a supervised group exercise programme as a rehabilitation treatment for women with breast cancer receiving adjuvant treatment. Eur J Oncol Nurs 9(1):56–63

Carson JW, Carson KM, Porter LS, Keefe FJ, Seewaldt VL (2009) Yoga of Awareness program for menopausal symptoms in breast cancer survivors: results from a randomized trial. Support Care Cancer 17(10):1301–1309

Carver JR, Shapiro CL, Ng A, Jacobs L, Schwartz C, Virgo KS et al (2007) American Society of Clinical Oncology clinical evidence review on the ongoing care of adult cancer survivors: cardiac and pulmonary late effects. J Clin Oncol 25(25):3991–4008

Centers for Disease Control and Prevention (CDC) (2008) Prevalence of self-reported physically active adults – United States. Morb Mortal Wkly Rep 57(48):1297–1300

Chen X, Zheng Y, Zheng W, Gu K, Chen Z, Lu W et al (2009) The effect of regular exercise on quality of life among breast cancer survivors. Am J Epidemiol 170(7):854–862

Cheville AL, Almoza M, Courmier JN, Basford JR (2010) A prospective cohort study defining utilities using time trade-offs and the Euroqol-5D to assess the impact of cancer-related lymphedema. Cancer 116(15):3722–3731

Cho OH, Yoo YS, Kim NC (2006) Efficacy of comprehensive group rehabilitation for women with early breast cancer in South Korea. Nurs Health Sci 8(3):140–146

Courneya KS, Friedenreich CM, Sela RA, Quinney HA, Rhodes RE, Handman M (2003a) The group psychotherapy and home-based physical exercise (group-hope) trial in cancer survivors: physical fitness and quality of life outcomes. Psychooncology 12:357–374

Courneya KS, Mackey JR, Bell GJ, Jones LW, Field CJ, Fairey AS (2003b) Randomized controlled trial of exercise training in postmenopausal breast cancer survivors: cardiopulmonary and quality of life outcomes [comment]. J Clin Oncol 21(9):1660–1668

Courneya KS, Segal RJ, Mackey JR, Gelmon K, Reid RD, Friedenreich CM et al (2007) Effects of aerobic and resistance exercise in breast cancer patients receiving adjuvant chemotherapy: a multicenter randomized controlled trial. J Clin Oncol 25(28):4396–4404

Courneya KS, Jones LW, Peddle CJ, Sellar CM, Reiman T, Joy AA et al (2008) Effects of aerobic exercise training in anemic cancer patients receiving darbepoetin alfa: a randomized controlled trial. Oncologist 13(9):1012–1020

Culos-Reed SN, Carlson LE, Daroux LM, Hately-Aldous S (2006) A pilot study of yoga for breast cancer survivors: physical and psychological benefits. Psychooncology 15(10):891–897

Daley AJ, Crank H, Saxton JM, Mutrie N, Coleman R, Roalfe A (2007) Randomized trial of exercise therapy in women treated for breast cancer. J Clin Oncol 25(13):1713–1721

Daniell HW (2009) Weight loss after breast cancer diagnosis may not improve prognosis. J Clin Oncol 27(5):829–830, author reply 830-821

Demark-Wahnefried W, Peterson B, Winer E, Marks L, Aziz N, Marcom P et al (2001) Changes in weight, body composition, and factors influencing energy balance among premenopausal breast cancer patients receiving adjuvant chemotherapy. J Clin Oncol 19(9):2381–2389

Demark-Wahnefried W, Clipp EC, Morey MC, Pieper CF, Sloane R, Snyder DC et al (2006) Lifestyle intervention development study to improve physical function in older adults with cancer: outcomes from Project LEAD. J Clin Oncol 24(21):3465–3473

Demark-Wahnefried W, Clipp EC, Lipkus IM, Lobach D, Snyder DC, Sloane R et al (2007) Main outcomes of the FRESH START trial: a sequentially tailored, diet and exercise mailed print intervention among breast and prostate cancer survivors. J Clin Oncol 25(19):2709–2718

Demark-Wahnefried W, Case LD, Blackwell K, Marcom PK, Kraus W, Aziz N et al (2008) Results of a diet/exercise feasibility trial to prevent adverse body composition change in breast cancer patients on adjuvant chemotherapy. Clin Breast Cancer 8(1):70–79

Dimeo F, Fetscher S, Lange W, Mertelsmann R, Keul J (1997a) Effects of aerobic exercise on the physical performance and incidence of treatment-related complications after high-dose chemotherapy. Blood 90(9):3390–3394

Dimeo FC, Tilmann MH, Bertz H, Kanz L, Mertelsmann R, Keul J (1997b) Aerobic exercise in the rehabilitation of cancer patients after high dose chemotherapy and autologous peripheral stem cell transplantation. Cancer 79(9): 1717–1722

Dimeo FC, Stieglitz RD, Novelli-Fischer U, Fetscher S, Keul J (1999) Effects of physical activity on the fatigue and psychologic status of cancer patients during chemotherapy. Cancer 85(10):2273–2277

Djuric Z, DiLaura NM, Jenkins I, Darga L, Jen CK, Mood D et al (2002) Combining weight-loss counseling with the weight watchers plan for obese breast cancer survivors. Obes Res 10(7): 657–665

Donnelly JE, Blair SN, Jakicic JM, Manore MM, Rankin JW, Smith BK (2009) American College of Sports Medicine Position Stand. Appropriate physical activity intervention strategies for weight loss and prevention of weight regain for adults. Med Sci Sports Exerc 41(2):459–471

Drouin JS, Young TJ, Beeler J, Byrne K, Birk TJ, Hryniuk WM et al (2006) Random control clinical trial on the effects of aerobic exercise training on erythrocyte levels during radiation treatment for breast cancer. Cancer 107(10): 2490–2495

Enger SM, Bernstein L (2004) Exercise activity, body size and premenopausal breast cancer survival. Br J Cancer 90(11):2138–2141

Fairey AS, Courneya KS, Field CJ, Bell GJ, Jones LW, Martin BS et al (2005) Effect of exercise training on C-reactive protein in postmenopausal breast cancer survivors: a randomized controlled trial. Brain Behav Immun 19(5):381–388

Fillion L, Gagnon P, Leblond F, Gelinas C, Savard J, Dupuis R et al (2008) A brief intervention for fatigue management in breast cancer survivors. Cancer Nurs 31(2):145–159

Francis WP, Abghari P, Du W, Rymal C, Suna M, Kosir MA (2006) Improving surgical outcomes: standardizing the reporting of incidence and severity of acute lymphedema after sentinel lymph node biopsy and axillary lymph node dissection. Am J Surg 192(5):636–639

Friedenreich CM, Gregory J, Kopciuk KA, Mackey JR, Courneya KS (2009) Prospective cohort

8

study of lifetime physical activity and breast cancer survival. Int J Cancer 124(8):1954–1962

Greenberg DB, Gray JL, Mannix CM, Eisenthal S, Carey M (1993) Treatment-related fatigue and serum interleukin-1 levels in patients during external beam irradiation for prostate cancer. J Pain Symptom Manage 8(4):196–200

Harrison SA, Hayes SC, Newman B (2010) Age-related differences in exercise and quality of life among breast cancer survivors. Med Sci Sports Exerc 42(1):67–74

Harvie MN, Campbell IT, Baildam A, Howell A (2004) Energy balance in early breast cancer patients receiving adjuvant chemotherapy. Breast Cancer Res Treat 83(3):201–210

Hayes SC, Reul-Hirche H, Turner J (2009) Exercise and secondary lymphedema: safety, potential benefits, and research issues. Med Sci Sports Exerc 41(3):483–489

Headley JA, Ownby KK, John LD (2004) The effect of seated exercise on fatigue and quality of life in women with advanced breast cancer. Oncol Nurs Forum 31(5):977–983

Heasman KZ, Sutherland HJ, Campbell JA, Elhakim T, Boyd NF (1985) Weight gain during adjuvant chemotherapy for breast cancer. Breast Cancer Res Treat 5(2):195–200

Heideman WH, Russell NS, Gundy C, Rookus MA, Voskuil DW (2009) The frequency, magnitude and timing of post-diagnosis body weight gain in Dutch breast cancer survivors. Eur J Cancer 45(1):119–126

Herrero F, San Juan AF, Fleck SJ, Balmer J, Perez M, Canete S et al (2006) Combined aerobic and resistance training in breast cancer survivors: a randomized, controlled pilot trial. Int J Sports Med 27(7):573–580

Hewitt M, Greenfield S, Stovall E (eds) (2006) From cancer patient to cancer survivor: lost in transition. National Academies Press, Washington, DC

Hinrichs CS, Watroba NL, Rezaishiraz H, Giese W, Hurd T, Fassl KA et al (2004) Lymphedema secondary to postmastectomy radiation: incidence and risk factors. Ann Surg Oncol 11(6): 573–580

Holick CN, Newcomb PA, Trentham-Dietz A, Titus-Ernstoff L, Bersch AJ, Stampfer MJ et al (2008) Physical activity and survival after diagnosis of invasive breast cancer. Cancer Epidemiol Biomark Prev 17(2):379–386

Holmes M, Chen WDF, Kroenke C, Colditz G (2005) Physical activity and survival after breast cancer diagnosis. JAMA 293:2479–2486

Ingram C, Courneya KS, Kingston D (2006) The effects of exercise on body weight and composition in breast cancer survivors: an integrative systematic review. Oncol Nurs Forum 33(5):937–947, quiz 948-950

Irwin ML, Crumley D, McTiernan A, Bernstein L, Baumgartner R, Gilliland FD et al (2003) Physical activity levels before and after a diagnosis of breast carcinoma: the Health, Eating, Activity, and Lifestyle (HEAL) study. Cancer 97(7):1746–1757

Irwin ML, Smith AW, McTiernan A, Ballard-Barbash R, Cronin K, Gilliland FD et al (2008) Influence of pre- and postdiagnosis physical activity on mortality in breast cancer survivors: the health, eating, activity, and lifestyle study. J Clin Oncol 26(24):3958–3964

Irwin ML, Alvarez-Reeves M, Cadmus L, Mierzejewski E, Mayne ST, Yu H et al (2009a) Exercise improves body fat, lean mass, and bone mass in breast cancer survivors. Obesity (Silver Spring) 17(8):1534–1541

Irwin ML, Varma K, Alvarez-Reeves M, Cadmus L, Wiley A, Chung GG et al (2009b) Randomized controlled trial of aerobic exercise on insulin and insulin-like growth factors in breast cancer survivors: the Yale Exercise and Survivorship study. Cancer Epidemiol Biomark Prev 18(1):306–313

Jacobsen PB, Donovan KA, Vadaparampil ST, Small BJ (2007) Systematic review and meta-analysis of psychological and activity-based interventions for cancer-related fatigue. Health Psychol 26(6):660–667

Jemal A, Siegel R, Ward E, Hao Y, Xu J, Thun MJ (2009) Cancer statistics, 2009. CA Cancer J Clin 59(4):225–249

Kangas M, Bovbjerg DH, Montgomery GH (2008) Cancer-related fatigue: a systematic and meta-analytic review of non-pharmacological therapies for cancer patients. Psychol Bull 134(5):700–741

Kilgour RD, Jones DH, Keyserlingk JR (2008) Effectiveness of a self-administered, home-based exercise rehabilitation program for women following a modified radical mastectomy and axillary node dissection: a preliminary study. Breast Cancer Res Treat 109(2):285–295

Kim CJ, Kang DH, Smith BA, Landers KA (2006) Cardiopulmonary responses and adherence to exercise in women newly diagnosed with breast cancer undergoing adjuvant therapy. Cancer Nurs 29(2):156–165

Kim CJ, Kang DH, Park JW (2009) A meta-analysis of aerobic exercise interventions for women with breast cancer. West J Nurs Res 31(4):437–461

Kroenke CH, Chen WY, Rosner B, Holmes MD (2005) Weight, weight gain, and survival after breast cancer diagnosis. J Clin Oncol 23(7): 1370–1378

Lauridsen MC, Overgaard M, Overgaard J, Hessov IB, Cristiansen P (2008) Shoulder disability and late symptoms following surgery for early breast cancer. Acta Oncol 47(4):569–575

Lawrence DP, Kupelnick B, Miller K, Devine D, Lau J (2004) Evidence report on the occurrence, assessment, and treatment of fatigue in cancer patients. J Natl Cancer Inst Monogr 32:40–50

Ligibel JA, Campbell N, Partridge A, Chen WY, Salinardi T, Chen H et al (2008) Impact of a mixed strength and endurance exercise intervention on insulin levels in breast cancer survivors. J Clin Oncol 26(6):907–912

Lingos TI, Recht A, Vicini F, Abner A, Silver B, Harris JR (1991) Radiation pneumonitis in breast cancer patients treated with conservative surgery and radiation therapy. Int J Radiat Oncol Biol Phys 21(2):355–360

Matesich SM, Shapiro CL (2003) Second cancers after breast cancer treatment. Semin Oncol 30(6):740–748

Matthews CE, Wilcox S, Hanby CL, Der Ananian C, Heiney SP, Gebretsadik T et al (2007) Evaluation of a 12-week home-based walking intervention for breast cancer survivors. Support Care Cancer 15(2):203–211

McKenzie DC, Kalda AL (2003) Effect of upper extremity exercise on secondary lymphedema in breast cancer patients: a pilot study. J Clin Oncol 21(3):463–466

Mefferd K, Nichols JF, Pakiz B, Rock CL (2007) A cognitive behavioral therapy intervention to promote weight loss improves body composition and blood lipid profiles among overweight breast cancer survivors. Breast Cancer Res Treat 104(2):145–152

Milne HM, Wallman KE, Gordon S, Courneya KS (2008) Effects of a combined aerobic and resistance exercise program in breast cancer survivors: a randomized controlled trial. Breast Cancer Res Treat 108(2):279–288

Moadel AB, Shah C, Wylie-Rosett J, Harris MS, Patel SR, Hall CB et al (2007) Randomized controlled trial of yoga among a multiethnic sample of breast cancer patients: effects on quality of life. J Clin Oncol 25(28):4387–4395

Mock V (2001) Fatigue management: evidence and guidelines for practice. Cancer 92(6 Suppl): 1699–1707

Mock V, Dow KH, Meares CJ, Grimm PM, Dienemann JA, Haisfield-Wolfe ME et al (1997) Effects of exercise on fatigue, physical functioning, and emotional distress during radiation therapy for breast cancer. Oncol Nurs Forum 24(6): 991–1000

Mock V, Frangakis C, Davidson NE, Ropka ME, Pickett M, Poniatowski B et al (2005) Exercise manages fatigue during breast cancer treatment: a randomized controlled trial. Psychooncology 14(6):464–477

Mohanti BK, Bansal M (2005) Late sequelae of radiotherapy in adults. Support Care Cancer 13(10):775–780

Morey MC, Snyder DC, Sloane R, Cohen HJ, Peterson B, Hartman TJ et al (2009) Effects of home-based diet and exercise on functional outcomes among older, overweight long term cancer survivors: RENEW: a randomized controlled trial. JAMA 301(18):1883–1891

Mustian KM, Peppone L, Darling TV, Palesh O, Heckler CE, Morrow GR (2009) A 4-week home-based aerobic and resistance exercise program during radiation therapy: a pilot randomized clinical trial. J Support Oncol 7(5): 158–167

Mutrie N, Campbell AM, Whyte F, McConnachie A, Emslie C, Lee L et al (2007) Benefits of supervised group exercise programme for women being treated for early stage breast cancer: pragmatic randomised controlled trial. BMJ 334(7592):517

Nesvold IL, Dahl AA, Lokkevik E, Marit AM, Fossa SD (2008) Arm and shoulder morbidity in breast cancer patients after breast-conserving therapy versus mastectomy. Acta Oncol 47(5):835–842

Nieman DC, Cook VD, Henson DA, Suttles J, Rejeski WJ, Ribisl PM et al (1995) Moderate exercise training and natural killer cell cytotoxic activity in breast cancer patients. Int J Sports Med 16(5):334–337

Nikander R, Sievanen H, Ojala K, Oivanen T, Kellokumpu-Lehtinen PL, Saarto T (2007)

8

Effect of a vigorous aerobic regimen on physical performance in breast cancer patients – a randomized controlled pilot trial. Acta Oncol 46(2):181–186

Obunai K, Jani S, Dangas GD (2007) Cardiovascular morbidity and mortality of the metabolic syndrome. Med Clin North Am 91(6):1169–1184, x

Ohira T, Schmitz KH, Ahmed RL, Yee D (2006) Effects of weight training on quality of life in recent breast cancer survivors: the weight training for breast cancer survivors (WTBS) study. Cancer 106(9):2076–2083

Paszat LF, Mackillop WJ, Groome PA, Boyd C, Schulze K, Holowaty E (1998) Mortality from myocardial infarction after adjuvant radiotherapy for breast cancer in the surveillance, epidemiology, and end-results cancer registries. J Clin Oncol 16(8):2625–2631

Payne JK (2002) The trajectory of fatigue in adult patients with breast and ovarian cancer receiving chemotherapy. Oncol Nurs Forum 29(9): 1334–1340

Petrek JA, Pressman PI, Smith RA (2000) Lymphedema: current issues in research and management. CA Cancer J Clin 50(5):292–307, quiz 308-211

Petrek JA, Senie RT, Peters M, Rosen PP (2001) Lymphedema in a cohort of breast carcinoma survivors 20 years after diagnosis. Cancer 92:1368–1377

Pinto BM, Clark MM, Maruyama NC, Feder SI (2003) Psychological and fitness changes associated with exercise participation among women with breast cancer. Psychooncology 12(2): 118–126

Pinto BM, Frierson GM, Rabin C, Trunzo JJ, Marcus BH (2005) Home-based physical activity intervention for breast cancer patients. J Clin Oncol 23(15):3577–3587

Ramsey SD, Berry K, Moinpour C, Giedzinska A, Andersen MR (2002) Quality of life in long term survivors of colorectal cancer. Am J Gastroenterol 97(5):1228–1234

Rockson SG, Rivera KK (2008) Estimating the population burden of lymphedema. Ann NY Acad Sci 1131:147–154

Rogers LQ, Hopkins-Price P, Vicari S, Pamenter R, Courneya KS, Markwell S et al (2009) A randomized trial to increase physical activity in breast cancer survivors. Med Sci Sports Exerc 41(4):935–946

Rohan TE, Fu W, Hiller JE (1995) Physical activity and survival from breast cancer. Eur J Cancer Prev 4(5):419–424

Sagen A, Karesen R, Risberg MA (2009) Physical activity for the affected limb and arm lymphedema after breast cancer surgery. A prospective, randomized controlled trial with two years follow-up. Acta Oncol 48(8):1102–1110

Sandel SL, Judge JO, Landry N, Faria L, Ouellette R, Majczak M (2005) Dance and movement program improves quality-of-life measures in breast cancer survivors. Cancer Nurs 28(4):301–309

Schmitz KH, Speck RM (2010) Risks and benefits of physical activity among breast cancer survivors who have completed treatment. Womens Health (Lond Engl) 6(2):221–238

Schmitz KH, Ahmed RL, Hannan PJ, Yee D (2005) Safety and efficacy of weight training in recent breast cancer survivors to alter body composition, insulin, and insulin-like growth factor axis proteins. Cancer Epidemiol Biomark Prev 14(7):1672–1680

Schmitz KH, Cappola AR, Stricker CT, Sweeney C, Norman SA (2007) The intersection of cancer and aging: establishing the need for breast cancer rehabilitation. Cancer Epidemiol Biomark Prev 16(5):866–872

Schmitz K, Ahmed RL, Troxel A, Cheville A, Smith R, Grant LL, Bryan CJ, Williams-Smith CT, Greene QP (2009) Weight lifting in women with breast cancer-related lymphedema. N Engl J Med 361:664–673

Schmitz KH, Courneya KS, Matthews C, Demark-Wahnefried W, Galvao DA, Pinto BM et al (2010) American College of Sports Medicine roundtable on exercise guidelines for cancer survivors. Med Sci Sports Exerc 42(7):1409–1426

Schwartz AL, Winters-Stone K (2009) Effects of a 12-month randomized controlled trial of aerobic or resistance exercise during and following cancer treatment in women. Phys Sports Med 37(3):1–6

Schwartz AL, Winters-Stone K, Gallucci B (2007) Exercise effects on bone mineral density in women with breast cancer receiving adjuvant chemotherapy. Oncol Nurs Forum 34(3):627–633

Segal R, Evans W, Johnson D, Smith J, Colletta S, Gayton J et al (2001) Structured exercise improves physical functioning in women with stages I and II breast cancer: results of a randomized controlled trial. J Clin Oncol 19(3):657–665

Shih YC, Xu Y, Cormier JN, Giordano S, Ridner SH, Buchholz TA et al (2009) Incidence, treatment costs, and complications of lymphedema after breast cancer among women of working age: a 2-year follow-up study. J Clin Oncol 27(12):2007–2014

Speck RM, Gross CR, Hormes JM, Ahmed RL, Lytle LA, Hwang WT et al (2009) Changes in the Body Image and Relationship Scale following a one-year strength training trial for breast cancer survivors with or at risk for lymphedema. Breast Cancer Res Treat 121(2):421–430

Speck RM, Courneya KS, Masse LC, Duval S, Schmitz KH (2010) An update of controlled physical activity trials in cancer survivors: a systematic review and meta-analysis. J Cancer Surviv 4(2):87–100

Sternfeld B, Weltzien E, Quesenberry CP Jr, Castillo AL, Kwan M, Slattery ML et al (2009) Physical activity and risk of recurrence and mortality in breast cancer survivors: findings from the LACE study. Cancer Epidemiol Biomark Prev 18(1): 87–95

Stricker CT, Jacobs LA (2008) Physical late effects in adult cancer survivors. Oncol Nurse Ed 22(8): 33–42

Szuba A, Rockson SG (1997) Lymphedema: anatomy, physiology and pathogenesis. Vasc Med 2(4):321–326

Taghian A, Assaad S, Niemierko A, Kuter I, Younger J, Schoenthaler R et al (2001) Risk of pneumonitis in breast cancer patients treated with radiation therapy and combination chemotherapy with paclitaxel. J Natl Cancer Inst 93: 1806–1811

Thorsen L, Skovlund E, Stromme SB, Hornslien K, Dahl AA, Fossa SD (2005) Effectiveness of physical activity on cardiorespiratory fitness and health-related quality of life in young and middle-aged cancer patients shortly after chemotherapy. J Clin Oncol 23(10):2378–2388

Vallance JK, Courneya KS, Plotnikoff RC, Yasui Y, Mackey JR (2007) Randomized controlled trial of the effects of print materials and step pedometers on physical activity and quality of life in breast cancer survivors. J Clin Oncol 25(17): 2352–2359

West-Wright CN, Henderson KD, Sullivan-Halley J, Ursin G, Deapen D, Neuhausen S et al (2009) Long-term and recent recreational physical activity and survival after breast cancer: the California Teachers Study. Cancer Epidemiol Biomarkers Prev 18(11):2851–2859

Zivian MT, Salgado B (2008) *Side effects revisited: Women's Experiences with aromatase inhibitors*. Breast Cancer Action, San Francisco

Physical Activity and Genitourinary Cancer Survivorship 9

Daniel A. Galvão, Dennis R. Taaffe, Nigel Spry, and Robert U. Newton

Abstract In this chapter we discuss common toxicities arising from genitourinary cancer treatments, in particular the adverse effects from androgen deprivation therapy (ADT) for prostate cancer given its well established detrimental effects on physical, physiological, and psychological function, and existing physical activity research in the postdiagnosis period including studies focusing on supportive care and some limited data on disease outcomes. Overall, consistent positive outcomes have been reported across studies showing that exercise is beneficial to reduce a number of treatment-related toxicities and improve symptoms. Additional studies are needed in genitourinary cancers other than prostate to establish specific physical activity requirements and implementation strategies.

D.A. Galvão (✉) and R.U. Newton
Edith Cowan University Health and Wellness Institute, School of Exercise, Biomedical and Health Sciences, Edith Cowan University, Joondalup, WA, Australia
e-mail: d.galvao@ecu.edu.au

D.R. Taaffe
School of Human Movement Studies, University of Queensland, Brisbane, QLD, Australia

N. Spry
Department of Radiation Oncology, Sir Charles Gairdner Hospital, Nedlands, WA, Australia

9.1 Introduction

Cancers of the genitourinary system include those of the prostate, bladder, and kidneys, and less common cancers such as those of the urethra and ureters (Winer et al. 2009). Prostate cancer represents the major cause of genitourinary malignancy (25%) in men with approximately 91% of new cases diagnosed at local or regional stages and a 5-year relative survival rate approaching 100% (Jemal et al. 2008). This cancer increases in prevalence with age, and about 85% of patients are diagnosed after 65 years (Gronberg 2003). Advancing age also increases the risk for other comorbid conditions (e.g., cardiovascular disease, diabetes, osteoporosis, arthritis, and sarcopenia) (Yancik et al. 2001), which can compromise physical function and independent living. Bladder cancer is the fourth leading cancer in men, accounting for 7% of new estimated cases with approximately 75% of new cases expected to be diagnosed at local stages with a 5-year relative survival rate of 80%. In women, the

K.S. Courneya and C.M. Friedenreich (eds.), *Physical Activity and Cancer*, Recent Results in Cancer Research 186, DOI: 10.1007/978-3-642-04231-7_9,

incidence of new cases are estimated to be lower (~2.5%), placing bladder cancer just outside the ten most common cancer types for women (Jemal et al. 2008). Kidney cancer accounts for 4% and 3% of new estimated cancer cases for men and women, respectively, with a 5-year relative survival rate of 66% (Jemal et al. 2008).

The role of physical exercise as a possible adjuvant therapy for cancer survivors has been gaining recognition with the majority of studies conducted with breast cancer survivors (Courneya 2003; Galvão and Newton 2005; Schmitz et al. 2005; Doyle et al. 2006). Since the initial exercise trial conducted by Segal et al. (2003) several exercise studies have been conducted with prostate cancer survivors (Blanchard et al. 2004; Demark-Wahnefried et al. 2004; Windsor et al. 2004; Dahn et al. 2005; Galvão et al. 2006, 2008b, 2009b, 2010; Culos-Reed et al. 2007; Monga et al. 2007; Culos-Reed et al. 2009; Morey et al. 2009; Segal et al. 2009). Overall, consistent positive outcomes have been reported across studies, strongly indicating that resistance and aerobic exercise is beneficial to reduce a number of treatment-related toxicities and improve symptoms in prostate cancer survivors. However, there is an absence or paucity of work in the other genitourinary cancers, and is an area of research that needs to be addressed.

In this chapter we discuss: (1) common toxicities arising from genitourinary cancer treatments, in particular the adverse effects from hormone suppression for prostate cancer given its well established detrimental effects on physical, physiological, and psychological function; (2) physical activity research primarily for prostate cancer, and some limited information on bladder cancer in the postdiagnosis period (during and following treatment) including studies focusing on supportive care (e.g., quality of life, fatigue, physical function) and disease outcomes; and (3) future directions for research work in this area.

9.2 Treatment of Prostate Cancer and Common Adverse Effects

The introduction of the prostate specific antigen (PSA) blood test into routine clinical practice in the 1990s has led to earlier diagnosis of prostate cancer (McCredie and Cox 1998; Moul 2000). Men are often minimally symptomatic or completely asymptomatic and can be expected to survive substantially longer than their historical counterparts (Moul 2000; Rashid and Chaudhary 2004). Full characterization of toxicity arising from treatment is now seen to be an important priority for research (Chodak 1998; Ransohoff et al. 2002; Rashid and Chaudhary 2004).

Common treatments for prostate cancer involve active surveillance, surgical removal of the prostate, radiation therapy, androgen deprivation therapy (ADT), and chemotherapy. Active surveillance is a nontreatment approach that leads to no specific treatment induced adverse effects but may permit the progression of disease and is accompanied by psychological effects of living with untreated prostate cancer (Herr 1997). Radical prostatectomy (e.g., retropubic, perineal, or laparoscopic) is a surgical procedure known as definitive therapy for localized prostate cancer and more commonly performed in younger patients (Catalona et al. 1999; Yan et al. 2000). Common postoperative adverse effects include urinary (incontinence) and sexual dysfunction (impotence) (Catalona et al. 1999; Stanford et al. 2000; Michaelson et al. 2008) and these complications are increased with age (Stanford et al. 2000). Radiation therapy in the form of external beam radiation therapy or interstitial brachytherapy (implantation of radioactive seeds into the prostate) is commonly used in the treatment of early disease and locally advanced prostate cancer (Lu-Yao and Yao 1997; Michaelson et al. 2008). Common adverse effects of radiation therapy include urinary, bowel, and sexual dysfunction (Miller et al. 2005; Michaelson et al. 2008) and increased fatigue (Hickok et al. 2005). Chemotherapy is used in men with metastatic castration-resistant prostate cancer (Petrylak et al. 2004; Oudard et al. 2005). Adverse effects include neutropenic fevers, cardiovascular and neurological complications, metabolic disturbances, infection, nausea and vomiting, diarrhea, and fatigue (Petrylak et al. 2004). Androgen deprivation therapy (ADT), also known as hormone suppression or hormone treatment, is a widely employed means of treating prostate cancer and is achieved by either surgical castration or more commonly by administering LHRHa (luteinizing hormone-releasing hormone agonist) and/or anti-androgen medications that block the androgen receptors (Kaisary 2005). There has been a substantial increase in the use of temporary ADT in the adjuvant management of prostate cancer (Shahinian et al. 2005b). Well recognized side effects of hormone treatment include vasomotor flushing, anemia, fatigue, gynecomastia, osteoporosis and skeletal fractures, reduced muscle mass and strength, increased fat mass and abdominal obesity, hyperglycemia, reduced insulin sensitivity and altered lipoprotein profile, and reduced quality of life (Smith et al. 2002, 2006; Shahinian et al. 2005 A; Sharifi et al. 2005; Basaria et al. 2006; Braga-Basaria et al. 2006b; Spry et al. 2006; Galvao et al. 2008b, 2009a). This array of side effects related to ADT affecting the musculoskeletal system and physiological function or "Androgen Deprivation and Sarcopenia-Related Disorders" are presented in Table 9.1. ADT has also been shown to contribute to emotional disturbances, fatigue, and memory difficulties, with these cognitive ADT-related disorders referred to as "Androgen Deprivation Syndrome" (Shahinian et al. 2006) (Table 9.1). Apart from these well-established adverse effects of ADT, evidence is accumulating that substantial cardiovascular and metabolic complications also result (Braga-Basaria et al. 2006a; Keating et al. 2006, 2009; D'Amico et al. 2007; Saigal et al. 2007; Tsai et al. 2007), which may impact quality of life and overall survival. Moreover, this may be compounded by the failure of testosterone to recover in some men following cessation of ADT (Kaku et al. 2006; Bong et al. 2008; Spry et al. 2009); hence, the ADT-related complications that arise may not be temporary.

9.3 Androgen Deprivation and Sarcopenia-Related Disorders

9.3.1 Body Composition

Several studies have documented marked alterations in body composition in men receiving ADT for prostate cancer (Smith et al. 2001, 2002, 2006, 2008; Smith 2004; Greenspan et al. 2005; Lee et al. 2005; Galvao et al. 2008) (Table 9.2). Smith et al. (2002) reported a 9.4% increase in whole body fat and a 2.7% reduction in whole body lean mass assessed by dual-energy X-ray absorptiometry (DXA) following 48 weeks of ADT. Similarly, Galvão et al. (2008) recently reported a reduction of 1.4 kg in total body lean mass and an increase of 2.3 kg in fat mass following 36 weeks of ADT while continued loss of lean mass following 2 years of interrupted ADT has also been reported (van Londen et al. 2008). Cross-sectional studies comparing ADT treated versus non-ADT treated prostate cancer patients and healthy matched individuals have also indicated lower whole body lean mass and higher fat mass in ADT-treated men (Basaria et al. 2002; Chen et al. 2002; Galvao et al. 2009). Importantly, reduction of lean mass following ADT can reduce musculoskeletal fitness, compromising muscle

9

Table 9.1 Side effects from androgen deprivation therapy (ADT) (Redraw from Galvão et al. 2007)

Reference	Androgen Deprivation and Sarcopenia-Related Disorders
Smith et al. 2002, Galvão et al. 2008 C	Decrease whole body lean mass
Smith et al. 2002, Galvão et al. 2008 C	Increase whole body fat mass
Greenspan et al 2005, Galvão et al. 2008 C	Decrease bone mass
Shahinian et al. 2005 A, Smith et al. 2005	Increase fracture risk
Basaria et al. 2002, Galvão et al. 2009	Decrease muscle strength
Basaria et al. 2006	Increase insulin resistance
Smith et al. 2002, Braga-Basaria et al. 2006	Negative lipoprotein profile
	Androgen Deprivation Syndrome
Shahinian et al. 2006	Increase depression
Shahinian et al. 2006	Decrease cognitive function
Shahinian et al. 2006, Spry et al. 2006	Increase fatigue
	Other Side-Effects from Androgen Deprivation
Spry et al. 2006	Decrease health-related quality of life
Spry et al. 2006	Hot flashes
Spry et al. 2006	Decrease libido

strength, physical function, and physical reserve capacity (Galvão et al. 2007) (Fig. 9.1). Such changes have implications in terms of reducing the age at which the individual falls below the functional capacity threshold, requiring a shift away from independent living and a reduced quality of life. Moreover, the increase in fat mass during ADT can lead to increased levels of total cholesterol and triglycerides (Smith et al. 2002; Braga-Basaria et al. 2006b) and consequently the possible development of cardiovascular complications (Keating et al. 2006; D'Amico et al. 2007; Saigal et al. 2007; Tsai et al. 2007). Lastly, it should not be forgotten the detrimental effect that these body composition changes may have on the psychological status of these men.

9.3.2 Bone Mass and Skeletal Fracture

Apart from a decline in muscle mass and strength, ADT-treated men suffer a reduction in bone mass and consequently bone strength, which contributes to an increased incidence of fracture and associated disability (Shahinian et al. 2005a; Smith et al. 2005). The ADT-related bone loss is significant and exceeds that of women experiencing early menopause (Higano 2003). Recently, Greenspan et al. (2005) indicated that men with prostate cancer initiating ADT have a five- to tenfold loss of bone mineral density compared to healthy controls or men with prostate cancer not on ADT. Importantly, following ADT, there is a significant dose–response relationship between fracture risk and the number of LHRHa doses administrated (Shahinian et al. 2005a). The reduced structural bone strength is compounded by the reduction in muscle strength and power which has been related to increased incidence of falls (Petrella et al. 2005), resulting in two separate side effects of ADT combining to greatly increase fractures due to falls.

Table 9.2 Prospective studies examining body composition alterations during androgen deprivation therapy (ADT)

Study	Study Design/ Duration	*n*/Age	Therapy mode	Body composition
Smith et al. 2001	Prospective 24 weeks	*n* = 22 (67 years)	LHRHa Bilateral orchiectomy	% Body fat 8.4% Lean mass 2.6%
Smith et al. 2002	Prospective 48 weeks	*n* = 40 (66 years)	LHRHa	% Body fat ↑ 9.4%, Abdominal fat ↑ 3.9% Abdominal sc fat ↑ 11.1%, Lean body mass ↓ 2.7%
Smith et al. 2004	Prospective 48 weeks	*n* = 79 (71 years)	Bilateral orchiectomy/ LHRHa LHRHa + antiandrogen	Fat mass ↑ 11% Lean body mass ↓ 3.8%
Greenspan et al. 2005	Prospective Controlled trial 52 weeks	*n* = 30, PCA (69 years)	LHRHa/antiandrogen LHRHa + antiandrogen	Fat mass ↑ 10.4% PCA Lean body mass ↓ 3.5% PCA
		n = 40, PCC (71 years)	Bilateral orchiectomy/ LHRHa LHRHa + antiandrogen	Fat mass ↔ PCC, PCN, CO Lean body mass ↔ PCC, PCN, CO
		n = 72, PCN (66 years)	No ADT	
		n = 43, CO (67 years)	No treatment	
Lee et al. 2005	Prospective 52 weeks	*n* = 65 (66 years)	LHRHa	Fat mass ↑ 6.6% Lean body mass ↓ 2%
Smith et al. 2006	Prospective 12 weeks	*n* = 25 (68 years)	LHRHa + antiandrogen	% Body fat ↑ 4.3% Lean mass ↓ 1.4%
Galvão et al. 2008 C	Prospective 36 weeks	*n* = 72 (73 years)	LHRHa + antiandrogen	Fat mass ↑ 13.8%, trunk fat ↑ 12% Lean mass ↓ 2.4%, ASM ↓ 4.2%
Smith et al. 2008	Prospective 52 weeks	*n* = 26 (65 years)	LHRHa + antiandrogen	Fat mass ↑ 11.2% Lean mass ↓ 3.6% Abdominal fat ↑ 16.5%

↑ = Increase, ↓ = decrease, ↔ = no change, *PC* prostate cancer patients on ADT; *PCN* prostate cancer patients not on ADT, *CO* nonprostate cancer patients controls, *PCA* prostate cancer patients on acute ADT (<6 months), *PCC* prostate cancer patients on chronic ADT (≥6 months); *SAC* systemic arterial compliance; *LHRHa* luteinizing hormone releasing hormone agonist; *ASM* appendicular skeletal muscle

9.3.3 Insulin Resistance and Lipoprotein Profile

Basaria et al. (2006) suggested that men with prostate cancer undergoing long-term ADT can develop insulin resistance and hyperglycemia and these metabolic alterations are independent of age and body mass index. In this cross-sectional study (Basaria et al. 2006), ADT-treated men had significantly higher fasting levels of glucose, insulin, and leptin when compared to healthy age-matched controls and prostate cancer patients not on ADT. Moreover, significant negative correlations were reported between

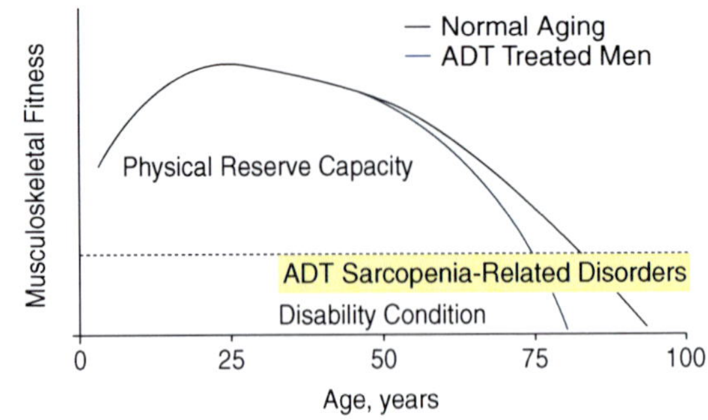

Fig. 9.1 Theoretical model of musculoskeletal fitness reduction during aging and androgen deprivation therapy (ADT) (Redrawn from Galvão et al. 2007)

total and free testosterone levels with fasting glucose, insulin, and leptin. Further, data from the same research group also indicated that long-term ADT-induced hypogonadal men have higher fasting levels of total cholesterol, LDL cholesterol, and non-HDL cholesterol than non-ADT prostate cancer men and age-matched controls (Braga-Basaria et al. 2006b). Other studies (Smith et al. 2002) have also indicated that long-term negative alterations in the lipoprotein profile occur in men treated with ADT with increases in serum total cholesterol (9%) and triglycerides (26.5%) following 48 weeks of therapy.

9.4 Other Side Effects from Androgen Deprivation

9.4.1 Quality of Life

Testosterone suppression for prostate cancer has been shown to negatively affect health-related quality of life. As such, reduced physical function and general health has also been reported in men on ADT compared to non-ADT treated men and healthy matched controls (Fowler et al. 2002). For example, Spry et al. (2006) reported results from a large longitudinal, multicentre study examining the dynamic change in quality of life and testosterone in men initiating an intermittent maximal androgen blockade program. ADT leads to a significant reduction in health-related quality of life during the initial 9 months of therapy with substantial changes occurring by 3 months. Further, during the recovery phase (off-ADT), improvements in quality of life occurred in a more gradual fashion and were of smaller magnitude than the changes observed during the ADT phase.

9.5 Treatment of Bladder and Kidney Cancers and Common Adverse Effects

Bladder cancer includes nonmuscle-invasive (superficial), muscle-invasive, and metastatic disease. Common treatments of superficial bladder cancer are surgery (transurethral resection of bladder tumor) and adjuvant therapy with intravesical chemotherapy or immunotherapy (Hussain et al. 2009). For muscle-invasive bladder cancer, primary treatment includes surgery to remove the bladder and nearby organs (radical cystectomy) and neoadjuvant chemotherapy (Hussain et al. 2009). Urinary and sexual dysfunction are common side effects from radical cystectomy (Hara et al. 2002). Systemic chemotherapy is the standard approach for patients with inoperable metastatic disease (von der Maase et al. 2000). The most common form of kidney cancer in adults is renal cell carcinoma with the preferred treatment being surgical resection (to remove part or all of the kidney) for patients with stage I, II, or III cancer (Vogelzang and Stadler 1998).

9.6 Exercise Interventions During Prostate Cancer Treatment

A summary of the exercise interventions examining the effect of resistance, cardiovascular, or both training modalities in prostate cancer survivors undergoing treatment is shown in Table 9.3. In most cases survivors were receiving ADT, radiation, or sometimes the combination of the two treatment modalities (Segal et al. 2003, 2009; Windsor et al. 2004; Carmack Taylor et al. 2006; Galvão et al. 2006, 2008b, 2010; Culos-Reed et al. 2007, 2009; Monga et al. 2007).

Segal et al. (2003) conducted the largest randomized controlled trial with 155 men with localized and nonlocalized prostate cancer undertaking or scheduled to receive ADT for at least the 12-week exercise training period. Participants were assigned to either whole body resistance training that incorporated three upper and four lower body exercises ($n = 82$) or a nonexercise control group ($n = 73$). Training intensity was set at 60–70% of one repetition maximum (1-RM; the maximal weight that can be lifted once only) for two sets of 12 repetitions (sets refers to a series of repetitions performed without stopping; e.g., eight repetitions per set) three times per week. Progression was incorporated by increasing load (~ 2.5 kg) when subjects were able to pass the 12-repetition mark. The exercise group experienced improved symptoms of fatigue and health-related quality of life compared to the nonexercise group. Moreover, submaximal muscle strength increased by 42% and 32% for the chest press and leg press, respectively. The observed changes for fatigue and quality of life are extremely relevant given that they are negatively affected during ADT (Herr 1997; Spry et al. 2006). Importantly, information from this study provides support that even a low volume training program at a moderate intensity undertaken for a relatively short time period can confer substantial benefits to this group of cancer patients on therapy.

Windsor et al. (2004) examined the effects of a cardiovascular training mode incorporating a home-based walking program, at least 3 days per week at 60–70% maximum heart rate, in prostate cancer patients initiating a 4-week external beam radiotherapy program. In this randomized controlled trial, 66 patients were assigned to standard care (control) or exercise. While fatigue levels for the control group increased following the radiotherapy regimen, there was no change in the exercise group who also experienced a significant improvement in walking endurance of 13%. This study indicates that beneficial effects can be derived from even a modest short-term unsupervised, home-based exercise program.

Galvão et al. (2006) examined the effects of a longer (20 weeks) progressive resistance exercise intervention in a group of men receiving ADT for prostate cancer. Training intensity, volume, and frequency were set at 12–6-RM (RM refers to the maximal number of repetitions that can be performed at a given resistance load) using two to four sets for 10–12 exercises undertaken twice weekly. This extended the work of Segal et al. (2003) by examining the physical, functional, morphological, and physiological outcomes of the intervention. Dramatic improvements in muscle strength (chest press 41%, seated row 42%, leg press 96%) and muscle endurance (chest press 115%, leg press 167%) resulted, as well as improvements in a number of physical performance tasks including the 6-m usual walk, 6-m backward walk, chair rise, stair climbing, 400-m walk and balance ranging from 7% to 27%. Further, changes

Table 9.3 Exercise interventions during prostate cancer treatment

Study	Study Design/ Duration	*n*/Age	Therapy Mode/Time	Exercise program	Intensity/Volume/ Frequency	Key outcome measures
Segal et al. 2003	Randomized controlled trial 12 weeks	$n = 155$ (68 years)	Receiving or scheduled to receive ADT for at least 12 weeks	Resistance training (Clinic-based)	12-RM, two sets Eight exercises ×3 week	↓ Fatigue[a] ↑ Quality of life[a] ↑ Muscle fitness[a] ↔ Body composition[a] ↔ Testosterone[a] ↔ PSA[a]
Windsor. et al. 2004	Randomized controlled trial 4 weeks	$n = 66$ (69 years)	Radiotherapy	Cardiovascular walking (Home-based)	60–70% MHR 30 min ×3 week	↔ Fatigue[a], ↑ Fatigue[b] ↑ Walking distance[a]
Galvão et al. 2006	Uncontrolled trial 20 weeks	$n = 10$ (70 years)	Minimum 8 weeks on ADT prior to entering the study and scheduled to receive ADT for at least 20 weeks	Resistance training (Clinic-based)	12–6-RM, two to four setsw 10–12 Exercises ×2 week	↑ Muscle strength ↑ Muscle endurance ↑ Functional performance ↔ Body composition ↑ ↔ Muscle thickness ↑ Balance ↔ Testosterone ↔ PSA
Carmack Taylor et al. (2006)	Randomized controlled trial 48 weeks	$n = 134$ (69 years)	Continuous ADT and scheduled to receive ADT for at least 1 year	6-month group-based lifestyle program aiming to increase physical activity	Not defined	↔ Quality of life[a] ↔ Walking distance[a]
Culos-Reed et al. 2007	Uncontrolled trial 12 weeks	$n = 31$ (67 years)	Receiving ADT	Resistance training Cardiovascular walking (Home-based)	Intensity/volume not determined ×3–5 week	↑ Levels of PA ↓ Fatigue ↑ Walking distance ↔ Quality of life ↑ BMI

Monga et al. 2007	Randomized controlled trial 8 weeks	$n = 21$ (68 years)	Radiotherapy	Cardiovascular walking (Clinic-based)	65% MHR 30–45 min ×3 week	↓ Fatigue[a] ↑ Quality of life[a] ↑ Aerobic fitness[a] ↑ Flexibility[a]
Galvão et al. 2008 B	Uncontrolled trial Single session	$n = 10$ (70 years)	Minimum 28 weeks on ADT prior undertaking session	Resistance training (Clinic-based)	6-RM, four sets Eight exercises Single session	↔ Testosterone ↔ PSA ↑ GH, ↑ DHEA ↑ Leukocyte counts
Segal et al. 2009	Randomized controlled trial 24 weeks	$n = 121$ (66 years)	Initiating Radiotherapy (all sample) Initiating ADT (60% of sample)	Resistance training (Clinic-based) or Cardiovascular Walking/cycling/ elliptical (Clinic-based)	8–12 Repetitions 60–70%-1-RM Ten exercises ×3 week or 50–75% VO2peak 15–45min ×3 week	↓ Fatigue week-12 (r/a) ↓ Fatigue week-24 (r) ↑ Quality of life (r) ↑ Aerobic fitness (r/a) ↑ Muscle strength (r) ↓ Triglycerides (r) ↔ Body fat (r) ↓ PSA (all groups)
Culos-Reed et al. 2009	Randomized controlled trial 16 weeks	$n = 100$ (67 years)	Minimum 36 weeks on ADT	Resistance training Cardiovascular walking (Home-based)	Intensity/Volume Not determined ×3–5 week	↑ Levels of PA[a] ↓ Waist[a] ↓ Blood pressure[a] ↔ Fatigue[a] ↔ Depression[a] ↔ Quality of life[a] ↔ PSA[a]

(*continued*)

Table 9.3 (continued)

Study	Study Design/ Duration	*n*/Age	Therapy Mode/Time	Exercise program	Intensity/Volume/ Frequency	Key outcome measures
Galvão et al. 2010	Randomized controlled trial 12 weeks	*n* = 57 (70 years)	Minimum 8 weeks on ADT prior to entering the study and scheduled to receive ADT for at least 12 weeks	Resistance training Cardiovascular Walking/cycling (Clinic-based)	12–6-RM, two to four sets 10–12 Exercises 15–20 min 65–80% MHR 11–13RPE ×2 week	↑ Muscle strength[a] ↑ Lean mass[a] ↓ Fatigue[a] ↑ Physical function[a] ↑ Quality of life[a] ↔ Testosterone[a] ↔ PSA[a] ↓ CRP[a]

↓ = No change, ↑ = increase, ↔ = decrease, *ADT* androgen deprivation therapy; *PSA* prostate-specific antigen; *GH* growth hormone; *DHEA* dehydroepiandrosterone; *CRP* C-reactive protein; *MHR* maximum heart rate; *RPE* rate of perceived exertion; *PA* physical activity, (r) resistance versus controls, (a) aerobic versus control

[a] Exercise intervention group

[b] Control group

in muscle endurance and functional capacity indicated that ADT-treated men may carry out functional daily activities with less fatigue following resistance exercise regimes and could partially explain the reduced levels of fatigue in resistance-trained men reported by Segal et al. (2003). The results also indicated that muscle thickness increased at the quadriceps site, and whole body lean mass by DXA was preserved with no change in fat mass. Considering that detrimental alterations in body composition are well-established side effects from ADT, these results provide support for the role of resistance exercise to preserve soft-tissue mass and enhance physical function in prostate cancer patients undergoing therapy.

Carmack Taylor et al. (2006) examined the effects of a lifestyle physical activity program over 12 months in prostate survivors receiving continuous ADT. Participants were randomly assigned to lifestyle ($n = 46$), educational support ($n = 51$), or usual care ($n = 37$) groups. The lifestyle group attended weekly sessions and received cognitive–behavioural intervention focused on increasing physical activity (no physical activity skills or supervision were provided). The educational support group also attended weekly sessions and undertook facilitated discussion. The usual care did not attend support meetings but received mailed educational material. The authors reported no improvements in quality of life for any of the groups following the program.

The effects of a home-based aerobic and low intensity resistance exercise in 31 prostate cancer survivors with localized and metastatic disease undergoing ADT have been reported by Culos-Reed et al. (2007). This was a 12-week intervention program incorporating home exercises and biweekly group exercise sessions. The authors reported improvements in physical activity levels, improvements in the 6-min walk test and reduced fatigue following the intervention.

Monga et al. (2007) examined the effects of aerobic exercise in men undergoing radiation therapy for prostate cancer. Participants were randomly assigned to exercise and radiation ($n = 11$) or radiation therapy alone ($n = 10$). The intervention program consisted of 45 min of supervised aerobic exercise at 65% of their maximal heart rate reserve undertaken three times per week for 8 weeks. Following the intervention the exercise group improved aerobic capacity, lower body physical function, overall quality of life, and were not subject to increased levels of fatigue.

Another recent, large randomized controlled trial conducted by Segal et al. (2009) compared for the first time the effects of resistance ($n = 40$) or aerobic ($n = 40$) exercise versus usual care ($n = 41$) in men receiving radiation therapy for prostate cancer (60% of participants were also on ADT). The resistance exercise program comprised 8–12 repetitions at 60–70% of 1-RM and the aerobic exercise incorporated 15–45 min at 50–75% of maximal oxygen uptake (VO_{2max}) using cycling, walking, or elliptical training. Both exercise programs were undertaken three times per week over 24 weeks. The aerobic exercise group reduced fatigue following 12 weeks and improved aerobic capacity following 24 weeks of training compared to usual care. The resistance exercise group also reduced fatigue following 12 weeks with further long-term improvement following 24 weeks of exercise. Further, resistance training improved aerobic capacity, muscle strength, triglyceride levels, quality of life, and preserved body composition. There was one serious adverse effect in the aerobic group where a participant without previous cardiac disease history suffered an acute myocardial infarction following 15 min of aerobic exercise.

Culos-Reed and co-workers (2009) recently examined the effect of a 16-week home-based exercise program with weekly group sessions in men receiving ADT for prostate cancer. Participants were randomized to the intervention ($n = 53$) or nonexercise control ($n = 47$) groups. The intervention program was designed to increase daily levels of physical activity and comprised of low intensity aerobic, resistance, and stretching exercises. Following 16 weeks there was an overall dropout rate of 34%, where 33% of these participants were from the exercise group and 67% were controls. The authors reported increased levels of physical activity, reduction in waist circumference, and blood pressure in the intervention group compared to controls.

Galvão et al. (2010) also recently reported the effects of a 12-week combined resistance and low volume aerobic exercise program versus usual care in hypogonadal prostate cancer survivors. Using a randomized controlled design, prostate cancer survivors were assigned to exercise (n =29) or a nonexercise control group (n = 28). The resistance exercise program was designed to progress from 12- to 6-RM for two to four sets per exercise. The aerobic component of the training program included 15–20 min of cardiovascular exercises (cycling and walking/jogging) at 65–80% maximum heart rate and perceived exertion at 11–13 (6–20 point, Borg scale). Total body and regional lean mass significantly increased in the exercise group compared with controls (~ 1 kg, Fig. 9.2a). As mentioned earlier in the chapter, loss of lean mass following the first year of ADT has been extensively documented (Smith et al. 2002; Galvao et al. 2008c). In addition, accretion of lean mass was accompanied by a significant improvement in upper and lower body muscle strength (Fig. 9.2b). These findings are consistent with previous studies described earlier examining resistance training as an individual exercise mode (Segal et al. 2003, 2009; Galvão et al. 2006). The exercise program also improved functional performance (e.g., gait speed) and balance measures compared to usual care. These changes in functional performance and balance are similar to those achieved in an earlier study of survivors on ADT undertaking resistance training (Galvão et al. 2006) and comparable to previous studies in healthy older men undertaking resistance training alone. Lastly, several aspects of quality of life including

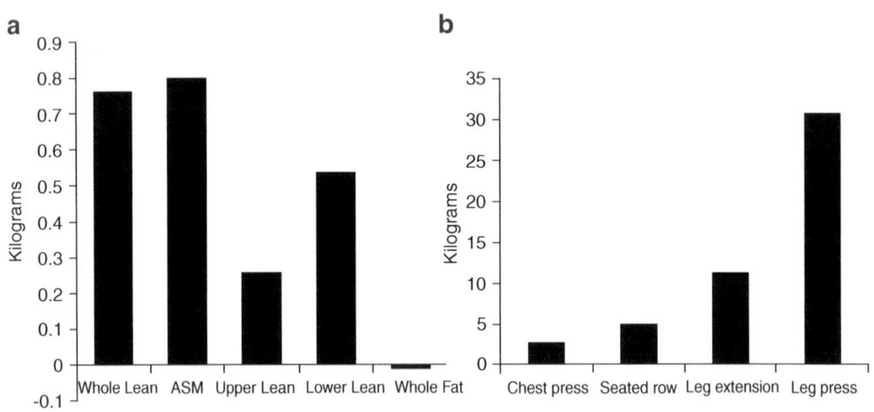

Fig. 9.2 (a) Total and regional body composition between group change over 12 weeks. ASM appendicular skeletal muscle. (b) Muscle strength between group change over 12 weeks (adjusted for baseline, ADT time, use of antiandrogen, number of medications, and education) (Redrawn from Galvão et al. 2010), Epub 2009 30 Nov

general health and reduced fatigue were significantly enhanced following exercise in comparison with the control group.

In addition to the prospective intervention studies listed above, a recent observational study examined the impact of physical activity levels prior to radical prostatectomy and found higher incontinence in survivors who were obese and sedentary compared to those normal weight and physically active (Wolin et al. 2010).

9.7 Exercise Studies and Effects on Testosterone and PSA (Disease Outcomes)

PSA is the most commonly used serum marker for prostate cancer disease from both diagnostic and disease progression perspectives (Thompson et al. 2004). A number of studies have indicated that PSA remains unchanged following resistance or aerobic training (Segal et al. 2003, 2009; Galvão et al. 2006, 2010; Culos-Reed et al. 2009). Additionally, Galvão et al. (2008b) have also reported that testosterone remains suppressed even immediately following an acute bout of high intensity resistance exercise. This is important given that several studies have demonstrated considerable elevation of testosterone in older men as a result of an acute bout of resistance training (Kraemer et al. 1999; Hakkinen et al. 2000). These findings collectively suggest that nonandrogen mediated mechanisms, such as neurological adaptations to training, and possible acute exercise-induced elevations in other muscle growth mediators such as growth hormone and insulin-like growth factor-1 are likely responsible for the observed changes in muscle function and hence physical performance following resistance training (Galvão et al. 2008b).

9.8 Exercise Interventions Post-treatment of Prostate Cancer

A limited body of information exists regarding the effects of physical activity posttreatment. Cross-sectional work undertaken by Dahn and colleagues (2005) indicated that for men who received external beam radiation therapy within the past 18 months, levels of physical activity were positively associated with sexual functioning. Similarly, Blanchard et al. (2004) reported an association between higher health-related quality of life in survivors who were undergoing 30 min of physical activity five times per week while Demark-Wahnefried et al. (2004) found better physical function in those undergoing vigorous continuous physical activity for at least 20 min three times per week.

In a randomized controlled study with men who had undergone radical prostatectomy, a program of pelvic-floor exercises for a maximum of 1 year was found to significantly reduce rates of incontinence (Van Kampen et al. 2000). Patients received individual treatment in an outpatient clinic once per week and also performed daily pelvic-floor exercises at home. By 3 months following surgery, 88% of the treatment group had achieved continence compared to only 56% of the control group.

Demark-Wahnefried et al. (2006) examined the effects of a 6-month telephone counseling and tailored printed materials intervention aimed at increasing physical activity and enhancing overall diet in 182 older (≥65 years) prostate and breast cancer survivors. Measures of physical activity, physical functional status (SF-36 Physical Function Scale), and quality of life were undertaken at baseline and at 6 and 12 months (6 months following the intervention). Although the study did not achieve the original target participant number ($n = 420$), the intervention group did show a trend toward improvements in physical function and physical activity energy expenditure.

9

In a similar study, Demark-Wahnefried et al. (2007) examined the effect of a longer (10 months) intervention using tailored mailed material aimed to increase physical activity and improve diet in a larger cohort of early stage prostate ($n = 237$) and breast cancer ($n = 306$) survivors. Participants were randomly allocated to the intervention group or an attention control arm that received nontailored mailed material. The authors reported that both groups improved their lifestyle behaviour but greater gains occurred for the intervention arm for the amount of exercise in minutes per week and fruit and vegetables consumed, and reduction in total and saturated fat consumption.

Lastly, in a recent large multicentre randomized controlled trial examining the effects of a 12-month diet and exercise intervention delivered via telephone counseling and tailored mailed material with 641 long-term (≥5 years) cancer survivors (261 with prostate cancer), a reduction in the rate of physical function decline was observed compared to a nonintervention control condition (Morey et al. 2009).

9.9 Physical Activity and Bladder Cancer

Physical activity research in postdiagnosis bladder cancer has been limited to a few reports including a population-based study examining associations between exercise and quality of life (Karvinen et al. 2007a), a prospective study of determinants of exercise using the theory of planned behavior (Karvinen et al. 2009), and a population-based study on exercise programming and counseling preferences (Karvinen et al. 2007b). Collectively, the results from these studies indicate that ~22% (similar to other cancer survivor groups) of bladder cancer survivors are meeting public health exercise guidelines and that exercise is positively associated with quality of life in this group of cancer survivors. Future prospective studies particularly randomized controlled trials examining causal effects are clearly needed to help establish specific physical activity requirements and implementation strategies for this group of cancer survivors.

9.10 Clinical Recommendations

Prostate cancer survivors, particularly those undergoing ADT, should initiate a program of resistance training incorporating seven to ten exercises, undertaken one to three times per week, using one to four sets per muscle group, at an intensity of 60–80% of 1-RM or 6–12-RM (Galvão et al. 2007). It is also recommended that survivors undertake aerobic exercise (e.g., walking, cycling) programs with intensity, volume, and frequency similar to those we have previously reported (50–90% maximal heart rate, 20–60 min of continuous or intermittent exercise, and three to five times per week) (Galvão and Newton 2005). Aerobic and resistance training activities when undertaken during therapy are safe and feasible for cancer patients and can lead to a range of positive physiological and psychological benefits (Courneya 2003; Galvão and Newton 2005). While not definitively confirmed at this stage, these benefits should extend to a reduction in cardiovascular and metabolic morbidity in this population (Keating et al. 2006; D'Amico et al. 2007; Saigal et al. 2007; Tsai et al. 2007). Further details on exercise training variables, practical examples of structured resistance programs based on previous studies with ADT-treated men (Segal et al. 2003; Galvão et al. 2006), as well as availability of resources (e.g., free weights, elastic bands, gravitational weight force machines) have been published elsewhere (Galvão et al. 2007). Pictorial examples of resistance exercises tailored to cancer patients are available on request from The Cancer Council of Western Australia – http://www.cancerwa.asn.au/. Undertaking resistance exercise in small groups will facilitate adherence and compliance, and also reduce the financial cost to the patient, and this should be mentioned to patients. In addition, varying components of the program from time to time will assist with motivation. However, it is important for both the specialists involved and the general/family practitioner to provide a consistent message regarding exercise and physical activity, and to monitor the patient's progress.

In the United States, the American College of Sports Medicine (ACSM – www.acsm.org) provides registered professionals with University qualifications in exercise science or related areas. Similarly, other countries such as Australia and United Kingdom possess organizations (Exercise and Sports Science Australia, ESSA – www.essa.org.au – British Association of Sport and Exercise Sciences, BASES – www.bases.org.uk/) that provide registered exercise professionals with University qualifications who are able to conduct exercise training with this patient population.

9.11 Future Directions

Ideally, research initiatives should be coordinated, and sequential, to ensure optimal coverage of the highest priority issues, avoiding unnecessary duplication. At the point that benefit is established, research should be directed toward profiling the relative importance of intensity, duration, timing and nature of exercise interventions, taking into account the interplay of common comorbidities.

There is a clear need to determine the long-term effects of exercise on reducing risk factors and incidence of comorbidities associated with treatments such as reduced bone mineral density and risk of fracture, metabolic complications, and cardiovascular disease, and large trials are underway (Galvão et al. 2009a; Newton et al. 2009). The effect of exercise at the onset of ADT may significantly attenuate the initial adverse effects and lead to better patient outcomes and treatment acceptance, but is yet to be studied. In addition, the effects of exercise during intermittent regimens of ADT to improve and maintain physical function, in particular during off-ADT phases to enhance physical reserve capacity when undergoing periods of testosterone suppression is a potentially important strategy that should be considered in the future. Although a recent randomized controlled study in men with prostate cancer compared the effects of aerobic versus resistance training, no information is available regarding the combined effects of resistance and aerobic exercises against resistance or aerobic exercise alone during practically all different treatment settings. Further, there is no information on the independent effect of exercise on treatment efficacy.

Available data on the effects of exercise during the posttreatment phase are limited. There is a need to determine the effects of exercise on reducing risk factors and incidence of long-term musculoskeletal, metabolic and cardiovascular toxicities, and psychological distress (Galvão et al. 2008a). This would be very important given that testosterone may fail to recover in some men following cessation of ADT, particularly in older men. Further, the effects of exercise for those who have undertaken radical prostatectomy, radiation, brachytherapy, and chemotherapy on physical, functional, and quality of life endpoints are understudied. Lastly, alternative strategies to deliver effective and safe exercise programs are needed as a priority in this group of cancer survivors given the high rates of survivorship following prostate cancer treatment.

Given the limited data in other genitourinary cancers (e.g., bladder, kidney) and the potential role of physical activity to promote physiological and psychological well being, there is a clear need to establish the feasibility and specific physical activity requirements, as well as the implementation strategies for these cancer survivors.

9.12 Summary

Physical activity research in genitourinary cancer as an adjunct to cancer treatment has only recently commenced and has focused on prostate cancer with limited data available on bladder cancer. However, the beneficial effect of physical activity in this population on attenuating the effects of treatment-related toxicities and disease symptoms is likely to be applicable to those with other genitourinary conditions. Specifically in relation to prostate cancer survivors, resistance and aerobic exercises have been successfully incorporated as an important adjuvant therapy to counteract the catabolic side effects of treatment. Larger ongoing randomized controlled trials are needed to confirm and expand these findings, and to establish the optimal timing and dosage of exercise. Moreover, nonsupervised physical activity alternative strategies, such as telephone counseling and tailored mailed material, have also been shown to reduce the rate of physical function decline in this cancer group.

Consequently, prostate cancer survivors, especially those undertaking hormone treatment, should be actively encouraged to engage in physical activity, preferably one that incorporates some form of resistance training to counter an array of adverse effects associated with treatment and the disease. Treating physicians should refer the patient to appropriately qualified exercise professionals who will not only be able to deliver a safe and effective program but also be able to utilize strategies to ensure on-going adherence so that benefits can be maintained. Moreover, the physician and associated health care professionals need to monitor the patients exercise progress and reinforce the importance of exercise in their treatment whenever possible to aid in exercise adherence.

References

Basaria S, Lieb J 2nd, Tang AM et al (2002) Long-term effects of androgen deprivation therapy in prostate cancer patients. Clin Endocrinol (Oxf) 56(6):779–786

Basaria S, Muller DC, Carducci MA, Egan J, Dobs AS (2006) Hyperglycemia and insulin resistance in men with prostate carcinoma who receive androgen-deprivation therapy. Cancer 106(3): 581–588

Blanchard MC, Stein KD, Baker F et al (2004) Association between current lifestyle behaviors and health-related quality of life in breast, colorectal, and prostate cancer survivors. Psychol Health 19(1):1–13

Bong GW, Clarke HS Jr, Hancock WC, Keane TE (2008) Serum testosterone recovery after cessation of long-term luteinizing hormone-releasing hormone agonist in patients with prostate cancer. Urology 71(6):1177–1180

Braga-Basaria M, Dobs AS, Muller DC et al (2006a) Metabolic syndrome in men with prostate cancer undergoing long-term androgen-deprivation therapy. J Clin Oncol 24(24):3979–3983

Braga-Basaria M, Muller DC, Carducci MA, Dobs AS, Basaria S (2006b) Lipoprotein profile in men with prostate cancer undergoing androgen deprivation therapy. Int J Impot Res 18: 494–498

Carmack Taylor CL, Demoor C, Smith MA et al (2006) Active for life after cancer: a randomized trial examining a lifestyle physical activity program for prostate cancer patients. Psychooncology 15(10):847–862

Catalona WJ, Ramos CG, Carvalhal GF (1999) Contemporary results of anatomic radical prostatectomy. CA Cancer J Clin 49(5):282–296

Chen Z, Maricic M, Nguyen P et al (2002) Low bone density and high percentage of body fat among men who were treated with androgen deprivation therapy for prostate carcinoma. Cancer 95(10):2136–2144

Chodak GW (1998) Comparing treatments for localized prostate cancer–persisting uncertainty. JAMA 280(11):1008–1010

Courneya KS (2003) Exercise in cancer survivors: an overview of research. Med Sci Sports Exerc 35(11):1846–1852

Culos-Reed SN, Robinson JL, Lau H, O'Connor K, Keats MR (2007) Benefits of a physical activity intervention for men with prostate cancer. J Sport Exerc Psychol 29(1):118–127

Culos-Reed SN, Robinson JW, Lau H et al (2009) Physical activity for men receiving androgen deprivation therapy for prostate cancer: benefits from a 16-week intervention. Support Care Cancer 18(5):591–599

D'Amico AV, Denham JW, Crook J et al (2007) Influence of androgen suppression therapy for prostate cancer on the frequency and timing of fatal myocardial infarctions. J Clin Oncol 25(17):2420–2425

Dahn JR, Penedo FJ, Molton I et al (2005) Physical activity and sexual functioning after radiotherapy for prostate cancer: beneficial effects for patients undergoing external beam radiotherapy. Urology 65(5):953–958

Demark-Wahnefried W, Clipp EC, Lipkus IM et al (2007) Main outcomes of the FRESH START trial: a sequentially tailored, diet and exercise mailed print intervention among breast and prostate cancer survivors. J Clin Oncol 25(19): 2709–2718

Demark-Wahnefried W, Clipp EC, Morey MC et al (2004) Physical function and associations with diet and exercise: Results of a cross-sectional survey among elders with breast or prostate cancer. Int J Behav Nutr Phys Act 1(1):16

Demark-Wahnefried W, Clipp EC, Morey MC et al (2006) Lifestyle intervention development study to improve physical function in older adults with cancer: outcomes from Project LEAD. J Clin Oncol 24(21):3465–3473

Doyle C, Kushi LH, Byers T et al (2006) Nutrition and physical activity during and after cancer treatment: an American Cancer Society guide for informed choices. CA Cancer J Clin 56(6): 323–353

Fowler FJ Jr, McNaughton Collins M, Walker Corkery E, Elliott DB, Barry MJ (2002) The impact of androgen deprivation on quality of life after radical prostatectomy for prostate carcinoma. Cancer 95(2):287–295

Galvão DA, Newton RU (2005) Review of exercise intervention studies in cancer patients. J Clin Oncol 23(4):899–909

Galvão DA, Newton RU, Taaffe DR, Spry N (2008a) Can exercise ameliorate the increased risk of cardiovascular disease and diabetes associated with ADT? Nat Clin Pract Urol 5(6):306–307

Galvão DA, Nosaka K, Taaffe DR et al (2008b) Endocrine and immune responses to resistance training in prostate cancer patients. Prostate Cancer Prostatic Dis 11(2):160–165

Galvão DA, Nosaka K, Taaffe DR et al (2006) Resistance training and reduction of treatment side effects in prostate cancer patients. Med Sci Sports Exerc 38(12):2045–2052

Galvão DA, Spry N, Taaffe DR et al (2009a) A randomized controlled trial of an exercise intervention targeting cardiovascular and metabolic risk factors for prostate cancer patients from the RADAR trial. BMC Cancer 9(1):419

Galvão DA, Spry NA, Taaffe DR et al (2008c) Changes in muscle, fat and bone mass after 36 weeks of maximal androgen blockade for prostate cancer. BJU Int 102(1):44–47

Galvão DA, Taaffe DR, Spry N, Joseph D, Newton RU (2010) Combined resistance and aerobic exercise program reverses muscle loss in men undergoing androgen suppression therapy for prostate cancer without bone metastases: a randomized controlled trial. J Clin Oncol 28(2): 340–347

Galvão DA, Taaffe DR, Spry N et al (2009b) Reduced muscle strength and functional performance in men with prostate cancer undergoing androgen suppression: a comprehensive cross-sectional investigation. Prostate Cancer Prostatic Dis 12(2):198–203

Galvão DA, Taaffe DR, Spry N, Newton RU (2007) Exercise can prevent and even reverse adverse effects of androgen suppression treatment in men with prostate cancer. Prostate Cancer Prostatic Dis 10(4):340–346

Greenspan SL, Coates P, Sereika SM et al (2005) Bone loss after initiation of androgen deprivation therapy in patients with prostate cancer. J Clin Endocrinol Metab 90(12):6410–6417

Gronberg H (2003) Prostate cancer epidemiology. Lancet 361(9360):859–864

Hakkinen K, Pakarinen A, Kraemer WJ, Newton RU, Alen M (2000) Basal concentrations and acute responses of serum hormones and strength

9

development during heavy resistance training in middle-aged and elderly men and women. J Gerontol A Biol Sci Med Sci 55(2):B95–B105

Hara I, Miyake H, Hara S et al (2002) Health-related quality of life after radical cystectomy for bladder cancer: a comparison of ileal conduit and orthotopic bladder replacement. BJU Int 89(1): 10–13

Herr HW (1997) Quality of life in prostate cancer patients. CA Cancer J Clin 47(4):207–217

Hickok JT, Roscoe JA, Morrow GR et al (2005) Frequency, severity, clinical course, and correlates of fatigue in 372 patients during 5 weeks of radiotherapy for cancer. Cancer 104(8): 1772–1778

Higano CS (2003) Bone loss and the evolving role of bisphosphonate therapy in prostate cancer. Urol Oncol 21(5):392–398

Hussain MH, Wood DP, Bajorin DF et al (2009) Bladder cancer: narrowing the gap between evidence and practice. J Clin Oncol 27(34): 5680–5684

Jemal A, Siegel R, Ward E et al (2008) Cancer statistics, 2008. CA Cancer J Clin 58(2):71–96

Kaisary AV (2005) Evaluating the use of early hormonal therapy in patients with localised or locally advanced prostate cancer. Prostate Cancer Prostatic Dis 8(2):140–151

Kaku H, Saika T, Tsushima T et al (2006) Time course of serum testosterone and luteinizing hormone levels after cessation of long-term luteinizing hormone-releasing hormone agonist treatment in patients with prostate cancer. Prostate 66(4):439–444

Karvinen KH, Courneya KS, North S, Venner P (2007a) Associations between exercise and quality of life in bladder cancer survivors: a population-based study. Cancer Epidemiol Biomark Prev 16(5):984–990

Karvinen KH, Courneya KS, Plotnikoff RC et al (2009) A prospective study of the determinants of exercise in bladder cancer survivors using the Theory of Planned Behavior. Support Care Cancer 17(2):171–179

Karvinen KH, Courneya KS, Venner P, North S (2007b) Exercise programming and counseling preferences in bladder cancer survivors: a population-based study. J Cancer Surviv 1(1): 27–34

Keating NL, O'Malley AJ, Freedland SJ, Smith MR (2009) Diabetes and cardiovascular disease during androgen deprivation therapy: observational study of veterans with prostate cancer. J Natl Cancer Inst 102(1):39–46

Keating NL, O'Malley AJ, Smith MR (2006) Diabetes and cardiovascular disease during androgen deprivation therapy for prostate cancer. J Clin Oncol 24(27):4448–4456

Kraemer WJ, Hakkinen K, Newton RU et al (1999) Effects of heavy-resistance training on hormonal response patterns in younger vs. older men. J Appl Physiol 87(3):982–992

Lee H, McGovern K, Finkelstein JS, Smith MR (2005) Changes in bone mineral density and body composition during initial and long-term gonadotropin-releasing hormone agonist treatment for prostate carcinoma. Cancer 104(8): 1633–1637

Lu-Yao GL, Yao SL (1997) Population-based study of long-term survival in patients with clinically localised prostate cancer. Lancet 349(9056): 906–910

McCredie M, Cox B (1998) Prostate-specific antigen testing for prostate cancer: the case for informed consent. Med J Aust 169(1):9–10

Michaelson MD, Cotter SE, Gargollo PC et al (2008) Management of complications of prostate cancer treatment. CA Cancer J Clin 58(4): 196–213

Miller DC, Sanda MG, Dunn RL et al (2005) Long-term outcomes among localized prostate cancer survivors: health-related quality-of-life changes after radical prostatectomy, external radiation, and brachytherapy. J Clin Oncol 23(12): 2772–2780

Monga U, Garber SL, Thornby J et al (2007) Exercise prevents fatigue and improves quality of life in prostate cancer patients undergoing radiotherapy. Arch Phys Med Rehabil 88(11): 1416–1422

Morey MC, Snyder DC, Sloane R et al (2009) Effects of home-based diet and exercise on functional outcomes among older, overweight long-term cancer survivors: RENEW: a randomized controlled trial. Jama 301(18):1883–1891

Moul JW (2000) Prostate specific antigen only progression of prostate cancer. J Urol 163(6): 1632–1642

Newton RU, Taaffe DR, Spry N et al (2009) A phase III clinical trial of exercise modalities on treatment side-effects in men receiving therapy for prostate cancer. BMC Cancer 9:210

Oudard S, Banu E, Beuzeboc P et al (2005) Multicenter randomized phase II study of two schedules of docetaxel, estramustine, and prednisone versus mitoxantrone plus prednisone in patients with metastatic hormone-refractory prostate cancer. J Clin Oncol 23(15): 3343–3351

Petrella JK, Kim JS, Tuggle SC, Hall SR, Bamman MM (2005) Age differences in knee extension power, contractile velocity, and fatigability. J Appl Physiol 98(1):211–220

Petrylak DP, Tangen CM, Hussain MH et al (2004) Docetaxel and estramustine compared with mitoxantrone and prednisone for advanced refractory prostate cancer. N Engl J Med 351(15): 1513–1520

Ransohoff DF, McNaughton Collins M, Fowler FJ (2002) Why is prostate cancer screening so common when the evidence is so uncertain? A system without negative feedback. Am J Med 113(8):663–667

Rashid MH, Chaudhary UB (2004) Intermittent androgen deprivation therapy for prostate cancer. Oncologist 9(3):295–301

Saigal CS, Gore JL, Krupski TL et al (2007) Androgen deprivation therapy increases cardiovascular morbidity in men with prostate cancer. Cancer 110(7):1493–500

Schmitz KH, Holtzman J, Courneya KS et al (2005) Controlled physical activity trials in cancer survivors: a systematic review and meta-analysis. Cancer Epidemiol Biomark Prev 14(7): 1588–1595

Segal RJ, Reid RD, Courneya KS et al (2003) Resistance exercise in men receiving androgen deprivation therapy for prostate cancer. J Clin Oncol 21(9):1653–1659

Segal RJ, Reid RD, Courneya KS et al (2009) Randomized controlled trial of resistance or aerobic exercise in men receiving radiation therapy for prostate cancer. J Clin Oncol 27(3): 344–351

Shahinian VB, Kuo YF, Freeman JL, Goodwin JS (2005a) Risk of fracture after androgen deprivation for prostate cancer. N Engl J Med 352(2): 154–164

Shahinian VB, Kuo YF, Freeman JL, Goodwin JS (2006) Risk of the "androgen deprivation syndrome" in men receiving androgen deprivation for prostate cancer. Arch Intern Med 166(4): 465–471

Shahinian VB, Kuo YF, Freeman JL, Orihuela E, Goodwin JS (2005b) Increasing use of gonadotropin-releasing hormone agonists for the treatment of localized prostate carcinoma. Cancer 103(8):1615–1624

Sharifi N, Gulley JL, Dahut WL (2005) Androgen deprivation therapy for prostate cancer. Jama 294(2):238–244

Smith JC, Bennett S, Evans LM et al (2001) The effects of induced hypogonadism on arterial stiffness, body composition, and metabolic parameters in males with prostate cancer. J Clin Endocrinol Metab 86(9):4261–4267

Smith MR (2004) Changes in fat and lean body mass during androgen-deprivation therapy for prostate cancer. Urology 63(4):742–745

Smith MR, Finkelstein JS, McGovern FJ et al (2002) Changes in body composition during androgen deprivation therapy for prostate cancer. J Clin Endocrinol Metab 87(2):599–603

Smith MR, Lee H, McGovern F et al (2008) Metabolic changes during gonadotropin-releasing hormone agonist therapy for prostate cancer: differences from the classic metabolic syndrome. Cancer 112(10):2188–2194

Smith MR, Lee H, Nathan DM (2006) Insulin sensitivity during combined androgen blockade for prostate cancer. J Clin Endocrinol Metab 91(4): 1305–1308

Smith MR, Lee WC, Brandman J et al (2005) Gonadotropin-releasing hormone agonists and fracture risk: a claims-based cohort study of men with nonmetastatic prostate cancer. J Clin Oncol 23(31):7897–7903

Spry NA, Galvão DA, Davies R et al (2009) Long-term effects of intermittent androgen suppression on testosterone recovery and bone mineral density: results of a 33-month observational study. BJU Int 104(6):806–812

Spry NA, Kristjanson L, Hooton B et al (2006) Adverse effects to quality of life arising from treatment can recover with intermittent androgen suppression in men with prostate cancer. Eur J Cancer 42(8):1083–1092

Stanford JL, Feng Z, Hamilton AS et al (2000) Urinary and sexual function after radical prostatectomy for clinically localized prostate cancer: the Prostate Cancer Outcomes Study. Jama 283(3):354–360

Thompson IM, Pauler DK, Goodman PJ et al (2004) Prevalence of prostate cancer among men with a

9

prostate-specific antigen level < or =4.0 ng per milliliter. N Engl J Med 350(22):2239–2246

Tsai HK, D'Amico AV, Sadetsky N, Chen MH, Carroll PR (2007) Androgen deprivation therapy for localized prostate cancer and the risk of cardiovascular mortality. J Natl Cancer Inst 99(20): 1516–1524

Van Kampen M, De Weerdt W, Van Poppel H et al (2000) Effect of pelvic-floor re-education on duration and degree of incontinence after radical prostatectomy: a randomised controlled trial. Lancet 355(9198):98–102

van Londen GJ, Levy ME, Perera S, Nelson JB, Greenspan SL (2008) Body composition changes during androgen deprivation therapy for prostate cancer: a 2-year prospective study. Crit Rev Oncol Hematol 68(2):172–177

Vogelzang NJ, Stadler WM (1998) Kidney cancer. Lancet 352(9141):1691–1696

von der Maase H, Hansen SW, Roberts JT et al (2000) Gemcitabine and cisplatin versus methotrexate, vinblastine, doxorubicin, and cisplatin in advanced or metastatic bladder cancer: results of a large, randomized, multinational, multicenter, phase III study. J Clin Oncol 18(17):3068–3077

Windsor PM, Nicol KF, Potter J (2004) A randomized, controlled trial of aerobic exercise for treatment-related fatigue in men receiving radical external beam radiotherapy for localized prostate carcinoma. Cancer 101(3):550–557

Winer E, Gralow J, Diller L et al (2009) Clinical cancer advances 2008: major research advances in cancer treatment, prevention, and screening–a report from the American Society of Clinical Oncology. J Clin Oncol 27(5):812–826

Wolin KY, Luly J, Sutcliffe S, Andriole GL, Kibel AS (2010) Risk of urinary incontinence following prostatectomy: the role of physical activity and obesity. J Urol 183(2):629–633

Yan Y, Carvalhal GF, Catalona WJ, Young JD (2000) Primary treatment choices for men with clinically localized prostate carcinoma detected by screening. Cancer 88(5):1122–1130

Yancik R, Ganz PA, Varricchio CG, Conley B (2001) Perspectives on comorbidity and cancer in older patients: approaches to expand the knowledge base. J Clin Oncol 19(4): 1147–1151

Physical Activity and Gastrointestinal Cancer Survivorship

10

Christopher M. Sellar and Kerry S. Courneya

Abstract Research examining physical activity in gastrointestinal cancer survivors is in its early stages and has focused primarily on colorectal cancer. Moreover, the majority of the research to date has been observational in nature, with very little interventional research. Though limited, the results of this research have been promising in nature, showing positive associations between physical activity and quality of life as well as disease outcomes, including improved disease-free and overall survival. The potential benefits of physical activity for gastrointestinal cancer survivors warrant further research on the underlying mechanisms of the relationship between physical activity and colorectal cancer disease outcomes, to determine if these associations extend to other gastrointestinal cancers, and to determine appropriate physical activity interventions to realize any potential supportive care benefits in various gastrointestinal cancer survivor groups.

C.M. Sellar and K.S. Courneya (✉)
E4-88 Van Vliet Centre, Behavioural Medicine Lab, University of Alberta, Edmonton, AB, Canada T6G 2H9
e-mail: kerry.courneya@ualberta.ca

10.1 Introduction

Cancers of the gastrointestinal (GI) tract, and more broadly the digestive system, present a large public health issue. As a group, these cancers represent the second highest number of new cases and deaths of any organ system (American Cancer Society 2009). The large number of new cases coupled with increasing survival rates through improved screening and treatment has resulted in a growing number of GI cancer survivors, with over 1 million in the United States alone (End Results 2008). Unfortunately, the survival rates for nearly all GI cancers fall below the average of about 66% for all cancer sites (American Cancer Society 2009). Currently, GI cancers are the second leading cause of cancer death trailing only respiratory system cancers (Jemal et al. 2009). This evidence suggests the need for interventions aimed at improving disease outcomes in GI cancer survivors. Further, the risk factors for many GI cancers include physical inactivity and/or being overweight/obese (Harriss et al. 2009; Samad et al. 2005; World Cancer Research Fund/American Institute for Cancer Research 2007), which are shared risk factors for many other chronic health issues including other cancers and cardiovascular and metabolic diseases,

K.S. Courneya and C.M. Friedenreich (eds.), *Physical Activity and Cancer*, Recent Results in Cancer Research 186, DOI: 10.1007/978-3-642-04231-7_10,

potentially elevating the risk of developing and/or dying from comorbidities (Baade et al. 2006). Exercise training has been shown to improve the health-related fitness of cancer survivors with other diagnoses (Speck et al. 2010), and therefore is a potential intervention to improve disease outcomes and supportive care outcomes in GI cancer survivors.

The purpose of the present chapter is to review the literature on physical activity (PA) and GI cancer survivorship. We begin by providing an overview of the clinical significance of GI cancers, the most common treatments for the various GI cancers, and the potential side effects of these treatments. Next, we review the research literature on PA in GI cancer survivors, discuss the potential biological mechanisms of any associations, provide some PA guidelines for GI cancer survivors, and end by offering some potential future research directions.

10.2 Clinical Significance of Gastrointestinal Cancers

For the purposes of this chapter, we have taken a broad definition of 'gastrointestinal' to include the organs of the entire digestive system. This includes the organs of the gastrointestinal tract: esophagus, stomach, small intestine, colon, rectum, and anus; and the digestive organs: pancreas, liver, and gall bladder. Taken together, GI cancers account for the second highest number of new cases diagnosed in the United States for any organ system, behind only cancers of the genital system (Jemal et al. 2009). Of the estimated 275,720 new cases of GI cancer in the USA in 2009, the most prevalent GI cancer site was the colon, with an estimated 106,100 cases or nearly 40% of all new GI cancers (Jemal et al. 2009). The next five most common GI cancers account for over 50% of all new GI cancer cases and are in order: pancreas, rectum, liver, stomach, and esophagus (Jemal et al. 2009).

GI cancers are the second leading cause of cancer-related death of any organ system, behind only cancers of the respiratory system (American Cancer Society 2009). Estimated deaths are combined for colon and rectal cancers and are the leading cause of GI cancer deaths, with 49,920 deaths or just over a third of all GI cancer deaths (American Cancer Society 2009). While only accounting for approximately 15% of new GI cancer cases, pancreatic cancer accounts for over a quarter of GI cancer deaths owing to its relatively low survival rate (American Cancer Society 2009).

The 5-year relative survival rates for GI cancers vary greatly by site and range from 5% for cancers of the pancreas to 67% for cancers of the rectum (American Cancer Society 2009). Rectal cancer is the only GI cancer with a survival rate above the 5-year survival rate for all cancers (66%), with colon (65%), stomach (25%), esophagus (17%), and liver (11%) all below average (American Cancer Society 2009). It is important to note that the survival rates for all GI cancers are improving, most likely due to improved methods of screening, detection, and treatment (American Cancer Society 2009). Furthermore, the survival rates are higher for all sites when the GI cancer is localized at diagnosis compared to regional or distant, stressing the importance of early detection (American Cancer Society 2009).

The high incidence of GI cancers combined with improving 5-year survival rates has resulted in a large number of GI cancer survivors in the population (End Results 2008). The only cancer sites that have larger numbers of cancer survivors are breast and prostate (End Results 2008). The latest estimates suggest that there are approximately 1.3 million GI cancer survivors in the USA, which is about 11% of all cancer survivors (End Results 2008). Individuals who were diagnosed with colorectal cancer make up about 86% of all GI cancer survivors (End Results 2008).

10.3 Treatment of Gastrointestinal Cancers

Owing to the large number of organs included within the GI system, the treatments for cancer diagnosed at each site differ greatly. Surgery, chemotherapy, radiation therapy, and biological and targeted treatments are used to varying degrees at each GI cancer site depending on the stage of the cancer at diagnosis (Oehler and Ciernik 2006; Willett and Czito 2009).

For individuals diagnosed with colon cancer, surgery is the primary form of treatment and may be curative by itself in early stage disease (Willett and Czito 2009 B). Surgery for colon cancer ranges from local excision to resection followed by anastomosis (or rarely colostomy) to the removal of tumors and/or organs at metastatic sites, depending on the stage of disease at the time of diagnosis (Wilkes and Hartshorn 2009). Chemotherapy regimens for colon cancer include both intravenous and oral drugs based on the drug fluorouracil (5-FU) (Andre and Schmiegel 2005). Adjuvant chemotherapy has been well established for Stage III colon cancer following surgery, but its use in Stage II colon cancer remains inconclusive (Willett and Czito 2009 B). Work is ongoing to establish definitive features that stratify Stage II patients into high- and low-risk categories, where high-risk patients would be recommended chemotherapy following surgery and low-risk patients would be monitored by surveillance only (Willett and Czito 2009 B). Radiation treatment is rarely used in individuals diagnosed with colon cancer, as it has shown no clear survival benefit for patients undergoing curative resection; however, it may assist in tumor control or play a palliative role in patients with recurrent or metastatic disease (Hung et al. 2006). Treatment for rectal cancer is similar to that of colon cancer, in that surgery is the most common treatment modality and curative on its own for early stage disease only (Wilkes and Hartshorn 2009). Total mesorectal excision is considered to be the standard surgical technique for rectal cancer (Wilkes and Hartshorn 2009). Currently, neoadjuvant radiation combined with chemotherapy (5-FU) is recommended for individuals diagnosed with Stages II–III rectal cancer (Willett and Czito 2009 B). Treatment for Stage IV colorectal cancer patients may include any combination of surgery, chemotherapy, radiation therapy and, more recently, targeted therapies (Wilkes and Hartshorn 2009).

As with cancers of the colon and rectum, surgical resection is the treatment of choice for all other GI cancers and often offers the best prognosis (Oehler and Ciernik 2006). Unfortunately, for many GI cancers surgery may provide the only option for curative treatment (Sauerland et al. 2009; Sweed et al. 2009) and survival rates remain low (American Cancer Society 2009). This includes cancers of the esophagus, stomach (gastric), pancreas, and liver (Oehler and Ciernik 2006; Quiros and Bui 2009; Samuel et al. 2009; Sauerland et al. 2009; Sweed et al. 2009; Willett and Czito 2009). The use of additional treatments has been shown to improve survival outcomes beyond surgery alone in these GI tumors, but the optimal sequence (pre-, post-, or perisurgical) and modality combinations (chemotherapy, radiation therapy, targeted, and/or biological therapies) are not currently known (Oehler and Ciernik 2006). To compound the lack of consensus for the definitive adjuvant treatments for these GI cancers, a majority of individuals with these cancer diagnoses are no longer candidates for resection due to the advanced stage of their disease at the time of diagnosis (American Cancer Society 2009). For individuals with nonresectable disease, the other treatment modalities may extend survival and/or provide palliation but are generally not curative.

Outcomes following GI cancer surgery vary greatly depending on the stage and site of the cancer at diagnosis. Surgery may temporarily or permanently effect postoperative digestive function, fecal continence, genitourinary function, and sexual function, all which may impact an individual's quality of life (Wilkes and Hartshorn 2009).

The chemotherapy treatments for colorectal cancer contain fluorouracil (5-FU) or a prodrug (capecitabine) that is activated to 5-FU in the body, which interferes with the normal division and functions of cells (Willett and Czito 2009 B). Common side effects of 5-FU-based chemotherapy can include myelosuppression, mucositis, diarrhea, nasal discharge, and eye irritation (Willett and Czito 2009 B). Less common side effects of 5-FU may include nausea, vomiting, hand-foot syndrome, and myocardial ischemia (Willett and Czito 2009). To enhance its antitumor effects in colon cancer, 5-FU can be combined with oxaliplatin (Andre and Schmiegel 2005). The possible side effects of oxaliplatin include neurotoxicity, nausea, diarrhea, mucositis, and mild myelosuppression (Willett and Czito 2009 B). The side effects of capecitabine are quite similar to intravenous 5-FU as they share the same active component, fluorouracil (Willett and Czito 2009 B). 5-FU is used alone or in combination for the treatment of many other GI cancers, including esophageal, pancreatic, and gastric (Sauerland et al. 2009; Sweed et al. 2009); therefore, patients receiving chemotherapy regimes containing 5-FU may experience the above side effects, in addition to side effects specific to the other drugs or therapies they are receiving.

The most common side effects of radiation treatment for rectal cancer are disturbed bowel function including diarrhea, cramping, and/or tenesmus (Hung et al. 2006). Less common side effects include local skin inflammation, cystitis, and myelosuppression (Hung et al. 2006). The side effects of radiation therapy used for other GI cancers are specific to the site being treated (Hung et al. 2006).

10.4 Physical Activity and Disease Outcomes in Gastrointestinal Cancer Survivorship

Research examining the associations of PA with disease outcomes in GI cancer survivors is relatively new, with all data being published since 2006. The most compelling results have come from observational data derived from individuals participating in four large cohort studies and who were diagnosed with colorectal cancer. These studies have shown a consistent association between higher levels of self-reported PA with improved disease outcomes in samples of colon and/or rectal cancer survivors. One study has examined the relationship of objectively measured fitness with GI cancers mortality, but the cohort was not limited to GI cancer survivors. Only one study has examined objectively measured fitness in relation to disease outcomes in a GI cancer survivors' group – esophageal – other than colorectal. Table 10.1 provides an overview of this research.

The results of four recent observational studies published by Meyerhardt et al. (Meyerhardt et al. 2006a; Meyerhardt et al. 2006b; Meyerhardt et al. 2009a; Meyerhardt et al. 2009b) have all suggested that postdiagnosis PA levels are positively associated with disease-specific and overall survival in colorectal survivors. This association between PA and improved disease outcomes in colorectal cancer survivors is further supported by the work of Haydon et al. (Haydon et al. 2006a), who found a protective effect of prediagnosis PA on disease specific survival. It is important to note that these authors also found that poor body composition (higher body fat%, body

Table 10.1 Observational studies examining association between PA and disease outcomes in GI cancer survivors

Authors	Sample	Design	Physical Activity Measure	Results
Haydon et al. (2006a)	526 cases of CRC from the Melbourne Collaborative Cohort Study	Prospective cohort study	Subjects classified as "Exercisers" (those who reported any regular exercise) vs. "Non-exercisers" (those who reported no exercise at all); PA assessed prediagnosis	• Decreased HR for disease-specific survival (HR = 0.73 [95%CI, 0.54–1.00], $p = 0.05$) for Exercisers vs. Nonexercisers. • Trend toward decreased HR for overall survival (HR = 0.77 [95%CI, 0.58–1.03], $p = 0.08$), for Exercisers vs. Nonexercisers. • Stronger association for right sided colon cancers and stage II–III disease. • Walking alone not associated with survival. • Higher body fat%, weight, and waist circumference associated with poorer disease-specific and overall survival. • Associations for PA with disease outcomes remained unchanged after adjusting for body composition, and vice versa.
Meyerhardt et al. (2006a)	573 female CRC cases (Stage I to III) from the Nurses' Health Study (NHS) cohort	Prospective cohort study	Leisure-time PA in MET-hours per week assessed both pre- and post diagnosis.	• Increasing levels of postdiagnosis PA reduced cancer-specific (p for trend =0.008) and overall (p for trend =0.003) mortality. • PA of ≥ 18 MET-hrs/wk was associated with reduced cancer-specific (HR = 0.39 [95%CI, 0.18–0.82]) and overall (HR = 0.43 [95% CI, 0.25 to 0.74]) mortality compared to <3 MET-hrs/wk. • Increasing activity level from pre- to postdiagnosis was associated with reduced cancer-specific (HR = 0.48 [95%CI, 0.24–0.97]) and overall (HR = 0.51 [95%CI, 0.30–0.85]) mortality compared to no change in PA. • Prediagnosis PA was not predictive of mortality.
Meyerhardt et al. (2006b)	832 patients with stage III colon cancer enroled in a chemotherapy trial (Cancer and Leukemia Group B 89803)	Prospective cohort study	Leisure-time PA in MET-hours per week assessed post diagnosis.	• Compared to PA of <3 MET-hrs/wk, the hazard ratio for disease-free survival was reduced for 18–26.9 MET-hrs/wk (0.51 (95% CI, 0.26 to 0.97]) and ≥ 27 MET-hrs/wk (0.55 (95% CI, 0.33 to 0.91]). The p for trend = 0.01 for increasing levels of PA. • Increasing levels of postdiagnosis PA were associated with improved disease-free survival (p for trend =0.01), recurrence-free survival (p for trend = 0.03), and overall survival (p for trend = 0.01).

(continued)

Table 10.1 (continued)

Authors	Sample	Design	Physical Activity Measure	Results
Murray et al. (2007)	51 preoperative esophageal cancer patients	Prospective cohort study	Preoperative shuttle walking distance in metres	• Overall mortality in the sample was 10% by 30 days post surgery. • Of patients who walked ≥ 350 m, none had died within 30 days post surgery. • Of the 8 patients who walked <350 m, 5 were dead and 2 were in critical care at 30 days post surgery. • Preoperative shuttle walk testing results may be indicative of operative risk in this group of patients.
Meyerhardt et al. (2009a)	668 men with stage I–III CRC from the Health Professionals Follow-up Study (HPFS)	Prospective cohort study	Leisure-time PA in MET-hours per week assessed post diagnosis.	• Compared to PA of <3 MET-hrs/wk, the hazard ratio for colorectal cancer-specific mortality was reduced for >27 MET-hrs/wk (HR = 0.47 [95%CI, 0.24–0.92]). • Increasing levels of PA were associated with improved colorectal cancer-specific mortality (p for trend = 0.002) and overall mortality (p for trend = 0.001). • 50.4% of sample exercised ≥ 18 MET-hrs/wk.
Meyerhardt et al. (2009b)	484 cases of stage I-III colon cancer from the NHS and HPFS cohorts, with both tumor sample and PA assessment	Prospective cohort study	Leisure-time PA in MET-hours per week assessed post diagnosis.	• Postdiagnosis PA of ≥ 18 MET-hrs/wk had a reduced hazard ratio for colon cancer-specific (0.64 [95%CI, 0.33–1.23]) and overall (HR = 0.60 [95%CI, 0.41–0.86]) mortality.
Peel et al. (2009)	38,801 men from Aerobics Center Longitudinal Study	Prospective cohort study	CRF as measured from a maximal treadmill exercise test	• The hazard ratios for overall digestive cancer deaths was reduced for those in the middle (HR = 0.66 [95%CI, 0.49–0.88) and upper (HR = 0.56 [95%CI, 0.40–0.80]) 40% of the distribution of CRF relative to those in the lowest 20%. • Being fit (upper 80% of CRF) was associated with a lower risk of mortality from colon [0.61 (0.37–1.00)], colorectal [HR = 0.58 [95%CI, 0.37–0.92]), and liver cancer (HR = 0.28 [95%CI, 0.11–0.72]) compared with being unfit (the lowest 20% of CRF).

CRC Colorectal Cancer; *PA* Physical Activity; *HR* Hazard Ratio; *CI* Confidence Interval; *MET-hrs/wk* Metabolic Equivalent Task-hours per Week; *CRF* Cardiorespiratory Fitness mass, and waist circumference) was associated with poorer disease-free and overall survival, with the associations of PA and body composition on disease outcomes independent of each other (Haydon et al. 2006a). Peel et al. (Peel et al. 2009) examined the association of cardiorespiratory fitness (CRF), an objective marker of habitual PA, on overall digestive cancer mortality, and suggested a protective role for CRF from total GI tract, colorectal, and liver cancer mortality in men (Peel et al. 2009). It should be noted that this sample did not comprise GI cancer survivors, and the benefit of higher CRF may lie entirely on the prediagnosis side of the cancer continuum. Again, only one study has examined the association between PA and disease outcomes in a GI cancer other than colorectal. Murray et al. (Murray et al. 2007) found a preoperative shuttle walking test to be a predictor of post-surgical outcomes in individuals diagnosed with esophageal cancer. This research also highlights another phase of the cancer continuum (pretreatment) where PA may play an important role for individuals diagnosed with GI cancer.

The research to date is very promising and points toward an important role for PA in individuals following a colorectal cancer diagnosis. However, much work is still needed to both confirm this association and its validity to determine if it extends to individuals with other GI cancer diagnoses. Future research examining PA in GI cancer survivors should incorporate objective measures of the components of health-related fitness to determine what associations, if any, exist on the postdiagnosis side of the cancer continuum. The Colon Health and Life-Long Exercise Change (CHALLENGE) trial will be the first study to attempt to do this (Courneya et al. 2008). The CHALLENGE trial is being conducted by the National Cancer Institute of Canada Clinical Trials Group and the Survivorship Research Group in Australia and will examine the effects of a structured PA intervention on disease outcomes in colon cancer survivors with high-risk stage II or III colon cancer who have completed adjuvant therapy (Courneya et al. 2008). This trial will enroll 962 participants who will be randomized to either a structured PA intervention consisting of a behavioral support program and supervised PA sessions or to receive general health education materials (Courneya et al. 2008). The primary outcome is disease-free survival, while secondary endpoints will include patient-reported outcomes, objectively measured physical functioning, and biological markers (Courneya et al. 2008). This will be the first behavioral intervention in a sample of GI cancer survivors to have a disease endpoint as its primary outcome.

10.4.1 Potential Mechanisms of Physical Activity for Improved Disease Outcomes in Gastrointestinal Cancer Survivors

A number of biological mechanisms have been proposed to account for the protective effect of PA in the primary prevention of colorectal cancer (Harriss et al. 2009; Samad et al. 2005; World Cancer Research Fund/American Institute for Cancer Research 2007), and it is plausible that these same mechanisms may account for the observed associations between PA and improved disease outcomes in colorectal cancer survivors. These potential mechanisms include decreased gut transit time, bile acid exposure, insulin resistance/hyperinsulinemia, insulin-like growth factor (and/or combined with increased insulin-like growth factor binding protein), prostaglandin (PG) E_2 concentration and/or PGE to PGF ratio, free radicals, and inflammation; and improved antioxidant status, immune function, and $PGF_2\alpha$ concentrations (Harriss et al. 2009; Samad et al. 2005). Further, PA may indirectly affect disease outcomes through the maintenance of a healthy weight and/or decreased obesity (i.e., negative energy balance) (World Cancer Research Fund/

10

American Institute for Cancer Research 2007). Unfortunately, very little data exist to support the mechanisms of PA in GI disease outcomes. Some initial work has been done in an attempt to elicit these mechanisms, but again has focused on individuals diagnosed with colorectal cancer. Table 10.2 outlines studies that have investigated potential mechanisms underlying the association of PA with GI cancer survivorship.

Additional biological data were collected from two large cohort studies to investigate potential mechanisms that may modify the observed association between PA and disease outcomes in colorectal cancer survivors. Meyerhardt et al. found that the association of PA with disease outcomes differed according to p27 status (Meyerhardt et al. 2009b). Based on their findings, Haydon et al. (2006b) suggest that a possible mechanism for the beneficial effect of PA on survival following colorectal diagnosis may be through the insulin-like growth factor (IGF) axis, particularly IGFBP-3.

Four studies have measured biological outcomes following exercise interventions, with two each in colorectal and gastric cancer survivors. Allgayer et al. (2004, 2008) have examined the effects of aerobic exercise training programs on the immune response and oxidative DNA damage. The authors suggest that a shift to a more proinflammatory state (Allgayer et al. 2004) and reduced oxidative DNA damage (Allgayer et al. 2008) via moderate exercise may have a potential clinical benefit, such as decreased rates of infection, relapses, and/or second tumors. The two studies examining exercise interventions in gastric cancer survivors have found conflicting effects on immune function (Lee et al. 2010; Na et al. 2000). One trial found that natural killer cell activity had increased significantly more in those who had completed an aerobic exercise training program (Na et al. 2000), whereas a recent single group study found a tai chi program to have no effect on immune function (Lee et al. 2010).

Additional research is still needed not only to further elicit the underlying mechanisms of PA on GI disease outcomes, but also to determine if the benefits of PA are the same and act through the same mechanisms in GI cancer survivors with diagnoses other than colorectal cancer, and to determine appropriate PA interventions to positively modify the underlying mechanisms with the hope of ultimately improving disease outcomes.

10.5 Physical Activity and Supportive Care Outcomes in Gastrointestinal Survivorship

Only 14 studies have examined PA and supportive care outcomes in samples consisting solely of GI cancer survivors. Nine of these have been observational in nature, including six cohort, and three cross-sectional studies. Table 10.3 summarizes studies examining the associations of PA with supportive care outcomes in GI cancer survivors. Five studies have examined the effects of exercise interventions on supportive care outcomes in GI cancer survivors. Table 10.4 summarizes studies examining the effects of exercise training on supportive care outcomes in GI cancer survivors.

10.5.1 Observational Studies

All of the observational studies examining the associations of PA with supportive care outcomes in GI cancer survivors have focused on colorectal cancer survivors. A majority of these have used the self-report of PA to examine patterns of exercise behavior in colorectal cancer survivors across the cancer continuum. The focus of much of this research has been on the association between PA levels and quality of life. Taken together, some consistent findings

Table 10.2 Studies examining potential mechanisms of PA on disease outcomes in GI cancer survivors

Authors	Sample	Design	Potential Mechanism	Results
Na et al. (2000)	35 stomach cancer patients who had curative surgery	Randomized, controled	Immune Function	• NCKA significantly decreased in both groups until day 7, at which time they began to increase. • At day 14, the mean NKCA of the exercise group demonstrated a significant increase compared with that of the control group.
Allgayer et al. (2004)	23 CRC patients after completion of treatment	Two-group, Quasi-experimental	Immune Function	• Both circulating and stimulated cytokines and antagonists did not significantly change during exercise training. • MI led to a decreased antagonist response suggesting a shift to a more proinflammatory state. • Suggest it is possible that these changes with MI may be of clinical benefit, such as decreased rates of infection, relapses, and/or second tumors.
Haydon et al. (2006b)	443 cases of CRC from the Melbourne Collaborative Cohort Study, with IGF-1/IGFBP-3 levels assessed	Prospective cohort study	Insulin and Insulin-like Growth Factor Axis	• For Exercisers, higher levels of IGFBP-3 associated with improved survival (HR = 0.52 [95%CI, 0.33–0.83], $p = 0.006$). • Suggest that the beneficial effects of PA in reducing CRC mortality may occur through interactions with the IGF axis, and more specifically with IGFBP-3.
Allgayer et al. (2008)	48 CRC patients after completion of treatment	Two-group, Quasi-experimental	Oxidative Stress and associated DNA damage	• MI was associated with decreased oxidative stress. • HI tended to increase DNA damage nonsignificantly. • The authors suggest further research to examine the potential role of MI in lowering the risk of relapse of colorectal cancer through reduced oxidative DNA damage.
Meyerhardt et al. (2009b)	484 cases of stage I–III colon cancer from the NHS and HPFS cohorts, with both tumor sample and PA assessment	Prospective cohort study	Genetic Marker associated with Cell Cycle Regulation	• The effect of PA on disease outcomes differed according to p27 status (p for interaction = 0.03). • For tumors with expression of p27, the hazard ratio for colon cancer mortality was 0.33 (95%CI, 0.12–0.85) for ≥ 8 MET-hrs/wk compared to <18 MET-hrs/wk. • PA had no benefit for tumors with loss of p27.
Lee et al. (2010)	33 gastric cancer patients after gastrectomy	One-group, pre-/post-test design	Immune Function	• Tai chi program had no significant effect on immune markers.

CRC Colorectal Cancer; *NKCA* Natural Killer Cell Activity; *PA* Physical Activity; *HR* Hazard Ratio; *CI* Confidence Interval; *IGF [BP]* Insulin-Like Growth Factor [Binding Protein]; *MET-hrs/wk* Metabolic Equivalent Task-hours per Week; *MI* Moderate Intensity Exercise; *HI* High Intensity Exercise

Table 10.3 Observational studies examining the association between PA and supportive care outcomes in GI cancer survivors

Authors	Sample	Design	Physical Activity Measure	Results
Courneya and Friedenreich (1997a)	130 CRC survivors	Retrospective Cohort	The Leisure Score Index of the Godin Leisure Time Exercise Questionnaire	• PA levels decreased during and increased following treatment, but did not return to prediagnosis levels. • Four main patterns of exercise behavior in CRC survivors were identified over the course of treatment: those who were active at all time points (maintainers), active before and after treatment, but not during (temporary relapsers), active before treatments but not during or after (permanent relapsers), or not active at any time point (nonexercisers) • Permanent relapsers had the lowest current QoL. • Functional QoL was the least possessed but most important dimension of QoL underlying overall satisfaction with life.
Courneya et al. (1999)	53 postsurgical CRC patients	Prospective Cohort	The Leisure Score Index of the Godin Leisure Time Exercise Questionnaire	• Changes in mild exercise from prediagnosis to post surgery correlated positively with QoL, suggesting only small changes in PA may be required to improve QoL. • Functional QoL was the least possessed but most important dimension of QoL underlying overall satisfaction with life.
Lynch et al. (2007a)	1966 CRC survivors from the CRC & QoL Study	Prospective Cohort	Active Australia Survey - Total weekly PA	• Study participants who were physically active after their diagnosis had a 17.0% higher total QoL score than those who were not. • PA levels were also associated with physical and functional well being and additional concerns subscales of the FACT-C questionnaire.
Lynch et al. (2007b)	1966 CRC survivors from the CRC & QoL Study	Prospective Cohort	Active Australia Survey – Total weekly PA	• 21% fewer participants were meeting PA public health guidelines postdiagnosis, compared to prediagnosis PA levels. • The% of participants meeting PA guidelines was less than the general population.

Hawkes et al. (2008)	1250 CRC survivors from the CRC & QoL Study	Prospective Cohort	Active Australia Survey – Total weekly PA	• 53% of CRC survivors were meeting public health guidelines for PA prediagnosis, 32% at 6 months, and 38% at 12 months postdiagnosis. • Compared with noncancer population controls, CRC survivors were more likely to be insufficiently active or inactive at 12 months post diagnosis.
Lynch et al. (2008)	1966 CRC survivors from the CRC & QoL Study	Prospective Cohort	Active Australia Survey – Total weekly PA	• A positive association between PA and QoL was found to be consistent over time. • Participants meeting the public health guidelines for PA had 18% higher QoL than those who reported no PA. • CRC survivors becoming more physically active may also experience greater QoL.
Peddle et al. (2008)	413 CRC survivors	Cross-sectional	The Leisure Score Index of the Godin Leisure Time Exercise Questionnaire	• 25.9% of participants reported meeting public health PA guidelines. • CRC survivors meeting the PA guidelines reported clinically & significantly better QoL & less fatigue.
Johnson et al. (2009)	843 CRC survivors ≥ 65 years old	Cross-sectional	The Community Healthy Activities Model Program (CHAMP) for Seniors PA questionnaire	• Higher SF-36 PF scores were associated with PA levels in a dose-dependent manner. • Moderate to vigorous intensity PA was associated with physical function; however, light intensity PA was not.
Stephenson et al. (2009)	67 CRC survivors currently receiving chemotherapy (63% metastatic)	Cross-sectional	The Leisure Score Index of the Godin Leisure Time Exercise Questionnaire	• 26% of participants reported meeting public health guidelines for PA and 12.3% reported no activity at all. • PA was not associated with QoL, suggesting that the relationship between these may be modified during treatment.

CRC Colorectal Cancer; *QoL* Quality of Life; *PA* Physical Activity; *SF-36* Medical Outcomes Study 36-Item Short-Form Health Status Survey; *PF* Physical Function; *FACT-C* Functional Assessment of Cancer Treatment-Colorectal

Table 10.4 Studies examining the effects of an exercise intervention on supportive care outcomes in gastrointestinal cancer survivors

Authors	Sample	Design	Exercise intervention	Duration	Frequency, Time and Intensity	Results
Courneya et al. (2005)	102 CRC patients following surgery	Randomized, controlled	HB aerobic exercise intervention	16 weeks	3–5 times/wk; for 20–30 min; Moderate Intensity	• Adherence in the exercise group was 75.8%, but a high level (51.6%).of exercise was completed by controls too. • No significant group differences were observed for change in FACT-C. • Participants who improved their CRF did improve on FACT-C, suggesting CRF is associated with QoL.
Allgayer et al. (2005)	95 CRC patients following completion of treatment	Two-group, nonrandomized	Pelvic exercises & biofeedback therapy supervised for 3 wks & then HB	1 year	Daily; 30–40 min for pelvic exercises & 1 h for biofeedback therapy	• A significant training effect was observed in both groups following as evidenced by decreased fecal incontinence. • This improvement was still evident at one year follow-up.
Jamal et al. (2009) and	119 CRC patients ≥ 60 years old following surgery	Randomized, controlled	Strength & aerobic training; supervised for 1st 10 days & then HB	3 months	5x/wk; 15–20 min of each: aerobic, and upper & lower extremity strength training]; strength training intensity: 50–80% of 1RM	• There was a significant group difference in lean body mass 7 days post surgery, which had increased in the exercise group and decreased in controls. • No other group differences were noted for weight, lean body mass, or fat mass at any other study time point.

Johnson et al. (2009) Houborg et al. (2009)							• Fatigue increased in both groups at 7 days post surgery, but increased less in the muscular strength group • Fatigue levels had returned to near preoperative levels by 90 days post surgery in both groups. • Physical function decreased in both groups at day 7 and had returned to preoperation levels by 90 days post surgery.
Lynch et al. (2008)	33 gastric cancer patients after gastrectomy	One-group, pre-/posttest design	Tai chi self-help education program	24 weeks	1 time/wk		• Tai chi exercise is safe & feasible for gastric cancer survivors, but had no significant effect on depression or QoL.

CRC Colorectal; *1RM* One Repetition Maximum; *QoL* Quality of Life; *FACT-C* Functional Assessment of Cancer Treatment-Colorectal; *CRF* cardiorespiratory fitness; *HB* Home based emerge from the above body of research. There is a positive association between PA and quality of life (specifically, the functional dimensions of the quality of life) in colorectal cancer survivors, and this relationship is consistent over the cancer continuum. Unfortunately, only a minority of colorectal cancer survivors report meeting public health guidelines for PA, and these numbers may be further diminished over the course of treatment.

10.5.2 Intervention Studies

Four of the intervention studies examining the effects of exercise training on supportive care outcomes in GI cancer survivors have consisted of samples of colorectal cancer survivors, and 1 included stomach cancer survivors. Three of these exercise trials employed a randomized controlled trial design. The interventions varied greatly in length from 3 months to 1 year, with a majority including aerobic exercise. While the outcomes assessed have varied greatly – including supportive care (quality of life and fatigue) and health-related fitness outcomes (cardiorespiratory fitness, body composition, and muscular strength) – in general the effect of exercise training on these outcomes has been positive.

10.6 Summary and Future Directions

Current evidence suggests that survival outcomes in individuals diagnosed with colorectal cancer may be associated with their PA levels and body composition. Exercise training has been shown to improve these and other aspects of health-related fitness, along with numerous other psychological and supportive care outcomes in other cancer patient groups, but there is little evidence that these benefits apply to GI cancer survivors. PA and exercise research in GI cancer survivorship have largely been restricted to observational studies of its association with quality of life, recurrence, and survival in colorectal cancer survivors. Furthermore, this research has focused on individuals diagnosed with colorectal cancer with very few studies examining the potential role of PA or exercise in helping GI cancer survivors cope with or recover following their treatments. Given the large public health issue presented by GI cancers and the positive results of the research conducted to date, the need for research in this area is still great.

While there are currently no guidelines for PA specific to individuals diagnosed with GI cancers or for cancer survivors in general, the mounting evidence of the benefits of regular exercise for cancer survivors, and specifically the promising early evidence for colorectal and other GI cancer survivors, suggests that these individuals should be encouraged to become (or continue to be) physically active. In the absence of any evidence-based guidelines, the PA guidelines provided by the US Department of Health and Human Services through the Centers for Disease Control and Prevention (CDC) provide an appropriate starting point for GI cancer survivors looking to become physically active (US Department of Health and Human Services 2008). The CDC has recommended that adults complete a minimum of 150 min per week of moderate-intensity or 75 min per week of vigorous-intensity aerobic PA (or an equivalent combination of the two), in addition to whole-body muscle-strengthening activities on two or more nonconsecutive days per week (US Department of Health and Human Services 2008). While the American Cancer Society (ACS) has provided PA guidelines for cancer survivors during and after treatment (Doyle et al. 2006), they have suggested that these individuals follow their physical activity guidelines for prevention (Kushi et al. 2006). The authors suggest that GI cancer survivors are likely to experience health benefits similar to that experienced by the general population by meeting these guidelines and, therefore, they provide an appropriate PA goal (Doyle et al. 2006). However, it is also noted that special concerns resulting from the specific disease and treatments may affect the ability of cancer survivors to complete PA (Doyle et al. 2006). While the ACS recommends a minimum of 150 min of moderate-intensity exercise per week, similarly to the CDC, they also suggest that 225–300 min per week may be preferred given that larger volumes of PA have been shown to have a greater protective effect against developing colon and breast cancer specifically, as well as having a greater impact on weight control (Kushi et al. 2006). The larger volume of exercise for improved disease outcomes following a GI cancer diagnosis is further supported by the work of Meyerhardt et al. (2006a, b, 2009a, b), where the greatest benefit was seen in those colorectal cancer survivors completing 18 or more MET hours per week, which is approximately equivalent to 300 min of moderate-intensity exercise per week.

GI cancer survivors attempting to improve their health-related fitness through structured exercise training again must look to resources developed for the general population. While not specific to cancer survivors, the American College of Sports Medicine recommends the frequency, intensity, duration, and type of exercise minimally required to improve all aspects of health-related fitness (American College of Sports Medicine 2009). In general, the exercise prescription should be individualized to the GI cancer survivor's current fitness level and health status, and follow the basic training principles that would be applied for an individual from the general population. However, as mentioned above, it is important to note that disease and/or treatment effects may impact a GI cancer survivor's ability to complete an exercise program (Doyle et al. 2006), and modifications may be required to achieve the desired fitness benefits.

Future research should attempt to determine the optimal role and timing that PA may play in the supportive care of individuals diagnosed with GI cancers at all sites and stages. In addition, research to elicit the mechanisms underlying the association of PA with colorectal cancer disease outcomes, and potentially other GI cancers, is needed. This will aid in designing appropriate interventions for GI cancer survivors, with the aim of maximizing both disease and supportive care outcomes for these individuals.

References

Allgayer H, Nicolaus S, Schreiber S (2004) Decreased interleukin-1 receptor antagonist response following moderate exercise in patients with colorectal carcinoma after primary treatment. Cancer Detect Prev 28:208–213

Allgayer H, Dietrich C, Rohde W, Koch G, Tuschhoff T (2005) Prospective comparison of short- and long-term effects of pelvic floor exercise/biofeedback training in patients with fecal incontinence after surgery plus irradiation versus surgery alone for colorectal cancer: clinical, functional and endoscopic/endosonographic findings. Scand J Gastroentero 40:1168–1175

Allgayer H, Owen R, Nair J, Spiegelhalder B, Streit J, Reichel C, Bartsch H (2008) Short-term moderate exercise programs reduce oxidative DNA damage as determined by high-performance liquid chromatography-electrospray ionization-mass spectrometry in patients with colorectal carcinoma following primary treatment. Scand J Gastroentero 43:971–978

American Cancer Society (2009) Cancer facts & figures 2009. American Cancer Society, Atlanta

American College of Sports Medicine (2009) ACSM's guidelines for exercise testing and prescription, 8th edn. Williams & Wilkins, Lippincott

Andre N, Schmiegel W (2005) Chemoradiotherapy for colorectal cancer. Gut 54:1194–1202

Baade P, Fritschi L, Eakin E (2006) Non-cancer mortality among people diagnosed with cancer (Australia). Cancer Cause Control 17:287–297

10

Courneya K, Friedenreich C (1997a) Relationship between exercise pattern across the cancer experience and current quality of life in colorectal cancer survivors. J Altern Complem Med 3 :215–226

Courneya K, Friedenreich C, Arthur K, Bobick T (1999) Physical exercise and quality of life in postsurgical colorectal cancer patients. Psychol Health Med 4:181–187

Courneya et al, 2005 in Table 10.4. The Courneya et al, 2005 reference should also be removed from the references.

Courneya K, Friedenreich C, Quinney H, Fields A, Jones L, Vallance J, Fairey A (2005) A longitudinal study of exercise barriers in colorectal cancer survivors participating in a randomized controlled trial. Ann Behav Med 29:147–153

Courneya K, Booth C, Gill S, O'Brien P, Vardy J, Friedenreich C, Au HJ, Brundage M, Tu D, Dhillon H, Meyer R (2008) The Colon Health and Life-Long Exercise Change trial: a randomized trial of the National Cancer Institute of Canada Clinical Trials Group. Curr Oncol 15:279–285

Doyle C, Kushi L, Byers T, Courneya K, Demark-Wahnefried W, Grant B, McTiernan A, Rock C, Thompson C, Gansler T, Andrews K, Nutrition, Physical Activity and Cancer Survivorship Advisory Committee; American Cancer Society (2006) (2006) Nutrition and physical activity during and after cancer treatment: an American Cancer Society guide for informed choices. CA Cancer J Clin 56:323–353

Harriss D, Atkinson G, Batterham A, George K, Cable N, Reilly T, Haboubi N, Renehan A, Colorectal Cancer, Lifestyle, Exercise And Research Group (2009) Lifestyle factors and colorectal cancer risk (2): a systematic review and meta-analysis of associations with leisure-time physical activity. Colorectal Dis 11: 689–701

Hawkes A, Lynch B, Youlden D, Owen N, Aitken J (2008) Health behaviors of Australian colorectal cancer survivors, compared with noncancer population controls. Support Care Cancer 16: 1097–1104

Haydon A, MacInnis R, English D, Giles G (2006a) Effect of physical activity and body size on survival after diagnosis with colorectal cancer. Gut 55:62–67

Haydon A, MacInnis R, English D, Giles G (2006b) Physical activity, insulin-like growth factor 1, insulin-like growth factor binding protein 3, and survival from colorectal cancer. Gut 55: 689–694

Houborg K, Jensen M, Hessov I, Laurberg S (2005) Little effect of physical training on body composition and nutritional intake following colorectal surgery-a randomised placebo-controlled trial. Eur J Clin Nutr 59:969–977

Houborg K, Jensen M, Rasmussen P, Gandrup P, Schroll M, Laurberg S (2006) Postoperative physical training following colorectal surgery: a randomised, placebo-controlled study. Scand J Surg 95:17–22

Hung A, Canning C, Patel K, Holland J, Kachnic L (2006) Radiation therapy for gastrointestinal cancer. Hematol Oncol Clin N 20:287–320

Jemal A, Siegel R, Ward E, Hao Y, Xu J, Thun MJ (2009) Cancer statistics, 2009. CA Cancer J Clin 59:225–249

Johnson B, Trentham-Dietz A, Koltyn K, Colbert L (2009) Physical activity and function in older, long-term colorectal cancer survivors. Cancer Cause Control 20:775–784

Kushi L, Byers T, Doyle C, Bandera E, McCullough M, McTiernan A, Gansler T, Andrews K, Thun M, Society AC (2006) Nutrition and Physical Activity Guidelines Advisory Committee (2006) American Cancer Society Guidelines on Nutrition and Physical Activity for cancer prevention: reducing the risk of cancer with healthy food choices and physical activity. CA Cancer J Clin 56:254–281

Lee E, Chae Y, Song R, Eom A, Lam P, Heitkemper M (2010) Feasibility and effects of a tai chi self-help education program for Korean gastric cancer survivors. Oncol Nurs Forum 37:E1–E6

Lynch B, Cerin E, Owen N, Aitken J (2007a) Associations of leisure-time physical activity with quality of life in a large, population-based sample of colorectal cancer survivors. Cancer Cause Control 18:735–742

Lynch B, Cerin E, Newman B, Owen N (2007b) Physical activity, activity change, and their correlates in a population-based sample of colorectal cancer survivors. Ann Behav Med 34: 135–143

Lynch B, Cerin E, Owen N, Hawkes A, Aitken J (2008) Prospective relationships of physical activity with quality of life among colorectal cancer survivors. J Clin Oncol 26:4480–4487

Meyerhardt J, Giovannucci E, Holmes M, Chan AT, Chan J, Colditz Fuchs C (2006a) Physical activity and survival after colorectal cancer diagnosis. J Clin Oncol 24:3527–3534

Meyerhardt J, Heseltine D, Niedzwiecki D, Hollis D, Saltz L, Mayer R, Thomas J, Nelson H, Whitton R, Hantel A, Schilsky RL, Fuchs C (2006b) Impact of physical activity on cancer recurrence and survival in patients with stage III colon cancer: findings from CALGB 89803. J Clin Oncol 24:3535–3541

Meyerhardt J, Giovannucci E, Ogino S, Kirkner G, Chan A, Willett W, Fuchs C (2009a) Physical activity and male colorectal cancer survival. Arch Intern Med 169:2102–2108

Meyerhardt J, Ogino S, Kirkner G, Chan A, Wolpin B, Ng K, Nosho K, Shima K, Giovannucci E, Loda M, Fuchs C (2009b) Interaction of molecular markers and physical activity on mortality in patients with colon cancer. Clin Cancer Res 15:5931–5936

Murray P, Whiting P, Hutchinson S, Ackroyd R, Stoddard C, Billings C (2007) Preoperative shuttle walking testing and outcome after oesophagogastrectomy. Brit J Anaesth 99:809–811

Na Y, Kim M, Kim Y, Ha Y, Yoon D (2000) Exercise therapy effect on natural killer cell cytotoxic activity in stomach cancer patients after curative surgery. Arch Phys Med Rehab 81:777–779

Oehler C, Ciernik I (2006) Radiation therapy and combined modality treatment of gastrointestinal carcinomas. Cancer Treat Rev 32:119–138

Peel J, Sui X, Matthews C, Adams S, Hébert J, Hardin J, Church T, Blair S (2009) Cardiorespiratory fitness and digestive cancer mortality: findings from the aerobics center longitudinal study. Cancer Epidem Biomar 18:1111–1117

Peddle C, Au HJ, Courneya K (2008) Associations between exercise, quality of life, and fatigue in colorectal cancer survivors. Dis Colon Rectum 51:1242–1248

Quiros R, Bui C (2009) Multidisciplinary approach to esophageal and gastric cancer. Surg Clin N Am 89:79–96

Samad A, Taylor R, Marshall T, Chapman M (2005) A meta-analysis of the association of physical activity with reduced risk of colorectal cancer. Colorectal Dis 7:204–213

Samuel M, Chow P, Chan Shih-Yen E, Machin D, Soo K (2009) Neoadjuvant and adjuvant therapy for surgical resection of hepatocellular carcinoma. Cochrane Db Sys Rev 2009(1):CD001199

Sauerland C, Engelking C, Wickham R, Pearlstone D (2009) Cancers of the pancreas and hepatobiliary system. Semin Oncol Nurs 25:76–92

Speck R, Courneya K, Mâsse L, Duval S, Schmitz K (2010) An update of controlled physical activity trials in cancer survivors: a systematic review and meta-analysis. J Cancer Surviv 4:87-100.

Stephenson L, Bebb D, Reimer R, Culos-Reed S (2009) Physical activity and diet behaviour in colorectal cancer patients receiving chemotherapy: associations with quality of life. BMC Gastroenterol 9:60

Surveillance Epidemiology and End Results (2008) Fast stats – statistics stratified by cancer site – prevalence. Retrieved February 1, 2010 from: http://seer.cancer.gov/faststats/selections.php?series=cancer

Sweed M, Edmonson D, Cohen S (2009) Tumors of the esophagus, gastroesophageal junction, and stomach. Semin Oncol Nurs 25:61–75

US Department of Health and Human Services (2008) 2008 physical activity guidelines for Americans. http://www.health.gov/PAGuidelines. Accessed 30 Apr 2010

Wilkes G, Hartshorn K (2009) Colon, rectal, and anal cancers. Semin Oncol Nurs 25:32–47

Willett C, Czito B (2009) Chemoradiotherapy in gastrointestinal malignancies. Clin Oncol 21:543–556

Wolpin B, Meyerhardt J, Mamon H, Mayer R (2007) Adjuvant treatment of colorectal cancer. CA Cancer J Clin 57:168–185

World Cancer Research Fund/American Institute for Cancer Research (2007) Food, Nutrition, Physical Activity, and the Prevention of Cancer: a Global Perspective. AICR, Washington

Physical Activity and Lung Cancer Survivorship

11

Lee W. Jones

Abstract A lung cancer diagnosis and associated therapeutic management is associated with unique and varying degrees of adverse physical/functional impairments that dramatically reduce a patient's ability to tolerate exercise. Poor exercise tolerance predisposes to increased susceptibility to other common age-related diseases, poor quality of life (QOL), and likely premature death. Here we review the putative literature investigating the role of exercise as an adjunct therapy across the lung cancer continuum (i.e., diagnosis to palliation). The current evidence suggests that exercise training is a safe and feasible adjunct therapy for operable lung cancer patients both before and after pulmonary resection. Among patients with inoperable disease, feasibility and safety studies of carefully prescribed exercise training are warranted. Preliminary evidence in this area supports that exercise therapy may be an important consideration in multidisciplinary management of patients diagnosed with lung cancer.

L.W. Jones (✉)
Department of Surgery, Duke University Medical Center, PO Box 3085, Durham, NC 27710, USA
email: lee.w.jones@duke.edu

11.1 Clinical Significance of Lung Cancer

Lung cancer is the second most commonly diagnosed malignancy among American adults and the leading cause of cancer-related death (Jemal et al. 2009). In 2009, a total of ~219,000 new cases were expected, accounting for 15% of all cancer diagnoses, and ~159,000 deaths, accounting for 20% of all cancer deaths (Jemal et al. 2009). Lung cancer accounts for more annual deaths than breast, prostate, and colorectal cancer combined. Approximately, 80% of lung cancer patients will be diagnosed with non–small cell lung cancer and ~25% will present with early-stage (operable) disease (Jemal et al. 2009). Improvements in surgical techniques together with more effective chemotherapeutic regimens have led to significant survival gains for individuals with early-stage disease (Butts et al. 2010; Arriagada et al. 2009; Douillard 2010) For example, the 3- and 5-year relative survival rates for localized disease are 58% and 49%, respectively. Approximately 26,000 individuals per year, in the U.S., will survive more than 5 years after initial diagnosis of lung cancer (Jemal et al. 2009). Given improving prognosis, long-term treatment-related morbidity, and overall QOL are becoming increasingly recognized as outcomes of

K.S. Courneya and C.M. Friedenreich (eds.), *Physical Activity and Cancer*,
Recent Results in Cancer Research 186, DOI: 10.1007/978-3-642-04231-7_11,

major clinical importance in the management of lung cancer (Woodward et al. 2007; Kenny et al. 2008; Fan et al. 2007; Paull et al. 2006; Rumble et al. 2005; Li et al. 2004).

Among patients diagnosed with inoperable disease, the median survival rate is only 8–10 months. The 2-, 3-, and 5-year overall survival rates are ~20%, 12%, and 7%, respectively (Blanchon et al. 2006; Brundage et al. 2002). Despite advancements in locoregional and palliative systemic therapy, concomitant improvements in survival have been modest and a unified, 'optimal' treatment protocol remains controversial. The purpose of this chapter is to review the evidence supporting the importance of cardiorespiratory fitness and application of exercise therapy as an adjunct therapy across the lung cancer continuum (i.e., prevention to palliation).

11.2 Lung Cancer Survivors Have Poor Cardiorespiratory Fitness

Irrespective of the clinical setting (i.e., operable or inoperable disease), all forms of regional (i.e., pulmonary resection or radiotherapy) and systemic therapies (i.e., chemotherapy and small molecule inhibitors) used in lung cancer are associated with unique and varying degrees of adverse physical/functional impairments that dramatically reduce a patient's ability to tolerate exercise (Jones et al. 2009a). Exercise tolerance, also known as cardiorespiratory fitness (these terms will be used interchangeably throughout this chapter), as measured by an objective exercise tolerance test, reflects the integrative capacity of components in the oxygen (O_2) cascade to supply adequate O_2 for adenosine triphosphate (ATP) resynthesis. Peak oxygen consumption (VO_{2peak}) provides the gold standard (direct) assessment of cardiorespiratory fitness (Jones et al. 2008a). Direct or estimated measurements of cardiorespiratory fitness are well established independent predictors of mortality in a broad range of noncancer, adult populations (Kavanagh et al. 2002; Myers et al. 2002).

Not surprisingly, lung cancer patients have significant and marked reductions in VO_{2peak}. These patients are subject to the effects of normal aging, age-related and/or disease-related comorbid conditions, and deconditioning that adversely impact components of the O_2 cascade. However, these 'normal' consequences are profoundly accelerated by disease pathophysiology and the use of conventional adjuvant therapy to create a 'perfect deconditioning storm', reducing either the body's ability to deliver and/or utilize O_2 and substrate leading to poor exercise tolerance (see Fig. 11.1) (Jones et al. 2008a).

The significant reduction in VO_{2peak} among patients with operable (early-stage) lung cancer has been known for over 3 decades. In the earliest published study, De Graff and colleagues (1965) reported that VO_{2peak} was 30–70% below age-matched normative data among eight lung cancer patients following pneumonectomy. More recently, in a prospective cohort study of 346 operable lung cancer patients, Loewen et al. (2007) reported that the VO_{2peak}, before pulmonary resection, was 17.0, 14.9, and 12.0 mL kg^{-1} min^{-1} in lung cancer patients at low risk, high risk, and very high risk of surgical complications, respectively. These values are equivalent to 25%, 29%, and 44% below age-matched normative data (Loewen et al. 2007). Following pulmonary resection, Jones et al. recently reported that mean VO_{2peak} was 38% below age–sex matched sedentary individuals without cancer (Jones et al. in press). Finally, further work by our group found VO_{2peak} to be 38% below age–sex matched values among patients with inoperable advanced disease undergoing cytotoxic therapy (e.g., systemic chemotherapy and/or regional radiotherapy) (Jones et al. 2007a). These findings demonstrate the following: (1) VO_{2peak} is

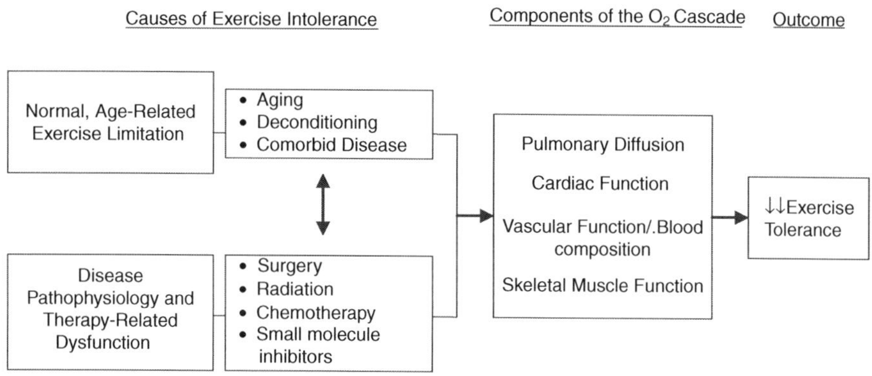

Fig. 11.1 Proposed causes of reduced exercise tolerance in cancer patients mediated by adverse changes in the components of the oxygen cascade

markedly reduced among lung cancer patients across the entire lung cancer survivorship continuum (i.e., presurgery to postsurgery to advanced disease), and (2) lung cancer surgery is associated with dramatic reductions in VO_{2peak}. However, the supplemental use of cytotoxic therapy may lead to additional detrimental effects on exercise tolerance.

11.3 Central Importance of Cardiorespiratory Fitness Across the Lung Cancer Continuum

In the preoperative setting, VO_{2peak} has been shown to be the strongest independent predictor of surgical complication rate (Loewen et al. 2007; Benzo et al. 2007; Bobbio et al. 2008; Bolliger et al. 1994; Brutsche et al. 2000; Villani et al. 2003; Win et al. 2006). Specifically, patients with a preoperative $VO_{2peak} < 20$ mL kg^{-1} min^{-1} are not at increased risk of complications; patients with a $VO_{2peak} < 15$ mL kg^{-1} min^{-1} are at an increased risk of perioperative complications; and patients with a $VO_{2peak} < 10$ mL kg^{-1} min^{-1} are at a very high risk of perioperative complications (Bobbio et al. 2005, 2008; Wang et al. 2006; Loewen et al. 2007; Benzo et al. 2007; Bolliger et al. 1994; Brutsche et al. 2000; Villani et al. 2003; Win et al. 2006). In the postoperative setting, Jones et al. reported that VO_{2peak} is a strong predictor of overall quality of life (QOL), fatigue, and other QOL domains (Jones et al. in press). In a prospective study among 173 postsurgical lung cancer patients, Kenny et al. (2008) reported significant decrements in QOL and higher lung cancer-related symptoms (i.e., fatigue, pain, sleep quality, etc.) following pulmonary resection. Importantly, physical functioning (a surrogate of exercise tolerance) was the strongest predictor of overall QOL. Although QOL generally improved 4 months after surgery, approximately half of patients continued to experience symptoms and functional limitations that persisted up to 2 years following initial resection (Kenny et al. 2008). Similarly, Clark et al. (2008) reported that higher levels of physical activity, a major correlate of exercise tolerance, were associated with higher overall QOL and fewer symptoms among 272 long-term (5 years post diagnosis) lung cancer survivors (Clark et al. 2008). Finally, Coups et al. (2009) reported that postsurgical lung cancer patients meeting national physical activity recommendations (i.e., at least moderate-intensity exercise, ≥30 min/session, on ≥5 days/week) reported significantly higher QOL relative to patients not meeting the recommendations.

In addition to the strong relationship between VO_{2peak} and perioperative and postoperative surgical complication rate, VO_{2peak} may also be an independent predictor of overall survival following a lung cancer diagnosis. Subjective measures of physical functioning (a surrogate of exercise tolerance) routinely used in the oncology setting [i.e., Karnofsky Performance Status (KPS), Eastern Cooperative Oncology Group (ECOG) performance status scoring systems] have been consistently demonstrated to be robust predictors of mortality in lung cancer with higher scores favoring better prognosis (Blanchon et al. 2006). Despite widespread clinical use, performance status (PS) scoring systems are subjective, have poor inter-rate reliability, and are weak predictors of prognosis when PS is 'good' (i.e., KPS, ≥70%; ECOG, 0–1). Furthermore, these instruments do not adequately characterize functional capacity among lung cancer patients who present with a variety of comorbid conditions and other unique symptoms that influence QOL and prognosis. Thus, alternative methods that provide an objective assessment of physical functioning may allow for more accurate prognostication and personalized patient care (Jones et al. 2009b).

Over the past decade, VO_{2peak} as well as other measures of cardiorespiratory fitness (e.g., time to exercise exhaustion and 6-min walk distance [6MWD]) have become well established as strong, independent predictors of cardiovascular and all-cause mortality across a broad range of clinical populations (Myers et al. 2002; Prakash et al. 2001; Leeper et al. 2007; Gulati et al. 2003, 2005; Ghayoumi et al. 2002; Nishime et al. 2000; McAuley et al. 2007; Vanhees et al. 1994; Ekelund et al. 1988; Morise and Jalisi 2003; Sandvik et al. 1993). Moreover, VO_{2peak} has been shown to be the most important predictor of mortality even when controlling for the major cardiovascular disease risk factors (Myers et al. 2002; Gulati et al. 2005). Only two studies to date have evaluated the prognostic importance of cardiorespiratory fitness following a cancer diagnosis and both studies have been conducted in lung cancer. The first study, conducted by Kasymjanova et al. (2009), examined the prognostic value of the 6-min walk test (6MWT) in 45 patients diagnosed with inoperable non–small cell lung cancer. Median survival was 6.7 months (95% confidence interval 2.6–10.8) in patients walking <400 m compared with 13.9 months (95% confidence interval 10.0–17.8) in patients walking ≥400 m. A walk distance of ≥400 m was the only variable with a significant effect on survival in multivariate analyses.

In the second study, Jones et al. (Kohman et al. 2009) investigated the prognostic significance of preoperative cardiorespiratory fitness (VO_{2peak}) among operable candidates with non–small cell lung cancer. Using a prospective design, 398 patients with potentially resectable NSCLC enrolled in a Cancer and Leukemia Group B (CALGB) protocol; 9238 were recruited between 1993 and 1998. Participants performed a cardiopulmonary exercise test (CPET) to assess VO_{2peak} and were observed for death or until June 2008. Cox proportional models were used to estimate the risk of all-cause mortality according to cardiorespiratory fitness categories defined by VO_{2peak} tertiles (<0.96/0.96–1.29/>1.29 L/min) with adjustment for age, gender, and performance status. Median follow-up was 30.8 months; 294 deaths were reported during this period. Compared with patients achieving a VO_{2peak} <0.96 L/min, the adjusted hazard ratio (HR) for all-cause mortality was 0.64 (95% CI, 0.46–0.88) for a VO_{2peak} of 0.96–1.29 L/min and 0.56 (95% CI, 0.39–0.80) for a VO_{2peak} of >1.29 L/min ($p_{trend} = 0.0037$).

In totality, these data provide strong evidence that VO_{2peak} (cardiorespiratory fitness) is an attractive modifiable therapeutic target to improve surgical risk and/or recovery, symptom control, and possibly, cancer-specific outcomes following a lung cancer diagnosis. Chronic, repeated aerobic training (i.e., continuous activity involving large muscle groups) is widely established as the most effective method to improve VO_{2peak} in healthy humans. In the following sections, the available literature examining the role of exercise therapy in persons with a lung cancer diagnosis is reviewed. In this context, the role of exercise in three lung cancer settings will be reviewed: (1) operable disease – prior tosurgery, (2) operable disease – post surgery, and (3) inoperable disease. An overview of these studies is provided in Table 11.1.

11.4 Exercise Therapy Following a Cancer Diagnosis

As reviewed in other chapters, exercise therapy is becoming increasingly acknowledged as an integral component of survivorship across several different malignancies. Several excellent systematic reviews and one meta-analysis have summarized this literature (Jones and Demark-Wahnefried 2006; McNeely et al. 2006; Markes et al. 2006; Schmitz et al. 2005; Friendenreich and Courneya 1996; Stevinson et al. 2004) These reviews conclude that exercise therapy is associated with consistent and positive effects on measures of cardiorespiratory fitness, QOL, depression, anxiety, and fatigue (McNeely et al. 2006; Markes et al. 2006; Schmitz et al. 2005; Friendenreich and Courneya 1996; Stevinson et al. 2004), although all reviews state that the current putative literature provides promising preliminary evidence and additional large-scale, well-controlled intervention studies are required (McNeely et al. 2006; Schmitz et al. 2005).

11.5 Exercise Therapy Following a Lung Cancer Diagnosis

11.5.1 Exercise Therapy for Operable Lung Cancer – Prior to Surgical Resection

Surgery remains the best option for cure in operable lung cancer. Selection of patients for surgical resection must be weighed against the immediate risk of perioperative morbidity and long-term pulmonary disability and mortality (Beckles et al. 2003a, b). A wide number of general and pulmonary-specific evaluations are considered in determining the preoperative physiologic status of lung cancer patients. Among the wide range of preoperative physiologic evaluations, an incremental, symptom-limited cardiopulmonary exercise test (CPET) with gas exchange analysis to assess VO_{2peak} is a particularly useful assessment tool since it provides an objective measure of individual overall physical functioning (Jones et al. 2008a; Ross 2003). As discussed previously, VO_{2peak} has been shown to be the strongest independent predictor of surgical complication rate (Loewen et al. 2007; Benzo et al. 2007; Bobbio et al. 2008; Bolliger et al. 1994; Brutsche et al. 2000; Villani et al. 2003; Win et al. 2006). To this end, exercise training interventions that improve VO_{2peak} may, in turn, lower perioperative complications and improve postsurgical recovery in potentially resectable lung cancer patients.

Two small pilot studies have investigated the efficacy of presurgical exercise training on measures of cardiorespiratory fitness and other relevant endpoints in patients undergoing pulmonary resection for suspected lung cancer. The first study, conducted by Jones et al. (2007a), investigated the safety and feasibility of supervised aerobic training on VO_{2peak}, 6-min walk distance (6MWD), and QOL among 25 patients with suspected lung cancer scheduled for pulmonary resection. Aerobic training consisted of stationary cycling, five times a week at 60–100% of VO_{2peak} until surgical resection. Participants underwent CPET and 6-min walk test (6MWT) at baseline, immediately before and 30 days after surgical resection. Five patients were deemed ineligible prior to surgical resection and were removed from the analysis. Of the remaining 20 patients, follow-up assessments were obtained for 18 (90%) prior to resection and 13 (65%) patients post resection. Sixty-five percent were diagnosed with non–small cell lung cancer and 75% underwent a

Table 11.1 Exercise training studies following a lung cancer diagnosis in patients with operable and inoperable disease

Authors	Sample	Age	Design	Exercise intervention	Duration	Frequency/Intensity	Results
Operable-presurgery							
Jones et al.	25 patients with suspected operable lung cancer	65 ± 10 years	Single-group	Supervised, cycle ergometry	4–6 weeks	×5/week at 65–100% of baseline VO_{2peak} for 20–35 min/session	VO_{2peak} ↑ 2.4 mL kg min From baseline to presurgery. Presurgical VO_{2peak} decreased postsurgery, but not beyond baseline value
Bobbio et al.	12 patients with operable lung cancer	71 ± 4 years	Single-group	Combined aerobic, resistance, and flexibility program	4 weeks	×5/week for 90 min/session	VO_{2peak} ↑ 2.8 mL kg min From baseline to presurgery
Operable-postsurgery							
Spruit et al.	10 lung cancer patients with impaired pulmonary function	65 years	Single-group	Inpatient multi-component rehabilitation program after lung cancer therapy	8 weeks	×5/week at moderate intensity: Cycling: 20 min at 60% of baseline peak cycling load; Treadmill: 20 min 80% of baseline mean walking speed Resistance training: 3 × 15 reps at 60% of 1-repitetion maximum	↑ walk distance (145 m; 43.2% of baseline value) and peak exercise capacity (26 W; 34.4% of baseline value)

Cesario et al.	25 post-surgical lung cancer patients	–	Single-group	Inpatient multi-component pulmonary rehabilitation	3.7 weeks	Cycle ergometry at 70–80% of maximal work load; resistance training, and educational sessions	Functional parameters among treated patients improved as compared to control group from baseline to 1-month figures (6MWD 297.8 m versus 393.4 m; $p = <0.01$)
Jones et al.	20 patients with stage I–IIIB NSCLC after surgical intervention	62 ± 11 years	Single-group	Supervised, cycle ergometry	14 weeks	×3/week at 65–100% of baseline VO_{2peak} for 20–45 min/session	VO_{2peak} ↑ 1.1 mL kg min; peak workload ↑ 9 W; Quality of life ↑ 10 points and fatigue ↓ seven points
Inoperable							
Temel et al.	20 patients with newly diagnosed advanced NSCLC	–	Single-group	Physical therapist supervised aerobic and resistance training program	8 weeks	×2/week	44% Completed the study. Completers ↓ in lung cancer symptoms and maintenance of 6-min walk distance (6MWD)

11

lobectomy. At baseline, mean VO_{2peak} was 15.7 mL kg^{-1} min^{-1} (range: 9.4–23.1 mL kg^{-1} min^{-1}) equivalent to 70% of predicted for age and sex; mean 6MWD was 427 m (range: 220–606 m) equivalent to 68% predicted. Mean time from diagnosis to surgical resection was 67 ± 27 days and 51 ± 27 days from surgery to postsurgery follow-up. The overall adherence rate was 72% (range: 0–100%) with patients completing a mean of 30 ± 27 sessions (range: 0–75). Intention-to-treat analysis indicated that mean VO_{2peak} increased by 2.4 mL kg^{-1} min^{-1} ($p = 0.002$) and 6MWD increased 40 m ($p = 0.003$) from baseline to presurgery (see Fig. 11.2). Exploratory analyses indicated that presurgical VO_{2peak} decreased post surgery, but did not decrease beyond baseline values (Jones et al. 2007a).

As part of this study, Peddle et al. (2009) also examined the effect of exercise training on QOL, as measured by the Functional Assessment of Cancer Therapy – Lung scale. Paired analysis revealed that QOL did not change during the course of exercise training (i.e., baseline to presurgery), but there were significant and clinically meaningful declines from presurgery to postsurgery in several QOL sub domains. Finally, change in VO_{2peak} from presurgery to postsurgery was significantly associated with change in several QOL domains.

In the second study, Bobbio et al. (2008) investigated the impact of a short-term preoperative pulmonary rehabilitation program on VO_{2peak} in 12 patients with chronic obstructive pulmonary disease (COPD) undergoing lobectomy for non–small cell lung cancer. The pulmonary rehabilitation program consisted of physical therapy (breathing and coughing techniques) and a combined aerobic and resistance training program. Aerobic training was conducted at 50–80% of maximal work rate for 30 min, 5 days a week for 4 weeks. Resistance training included upper and trunk muscle exercises performed with free weights under the supervision of physical therapist. Results indicated a significant improvement in

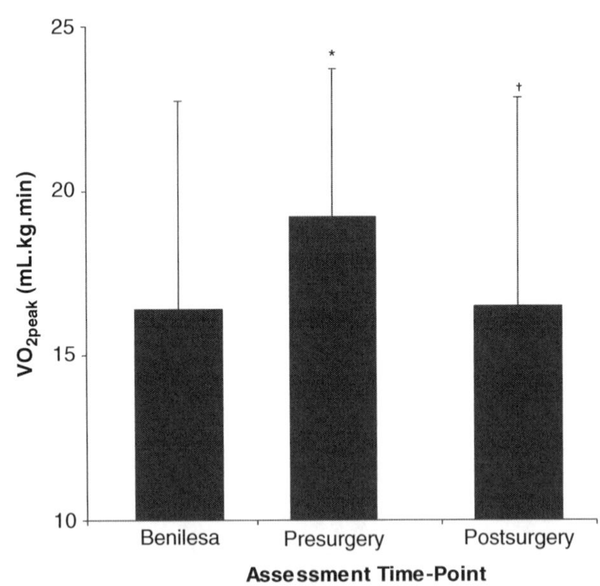

Fig. 11.2 Change in peak oxygen consumption (VO2peak) from baseline to presurgery to postsurgery among 20 patients with pulmonary malignancies (*p < 0.05 for baseline vs presurgery; *p < 0.05 for presurgery vs postsurgery)

VO_{2peak} of 2.8 mL kg^{-1} min^{-1} ($p < 0.001$). Significant improvements were also observed in several additional cardiopulmonary parameters including anaerobic threshold, peak workload capacity, and O_2 pulse (Bobbio et al. 2008).

The results of these studies provide 'proof of principle' that relatively short, high-intensity presurgical exercise training is associated with significant improvements in cardiorespiratory fitness among patients undergoing thoracic surgery for malignant lung lesions. These findings may have several implications for clinical practice. Most importantly, preoperative exercise training or rehabilitation could increase the numbers of candidates eligible for curative-intent pulmonary resection. Currently, pulmonary resection is standard care for patients diagnosed with operable lung cancer and other thoracic diseases but it is associated with significant complications (Beckles et al. 2003a; Semik et al. 2001). Patients with a VO_{2peak} ≤15 mL kg^{-1} min^{-1} or a 6MWD ≤250 m have a poor postoperative prognosis and are borderline surgical candidates (Win et al. 2006; Datta and Lahiri 2003). The results from the two published pilot studies (i.e., Jones et al. and Bobbio et al.) indicate that borderline surgical candidates can experience significant improvements in measures of cardiorespiratory fitness. Such improvements may in turn be associated with lower surgical complications and improved postoperative outcomes. Large, adequately powered trials are now required to formally address this question.

11.5.2 Exercise Therapy for Operable Lung Cancer – Postsurgical Resection

Surgery is the only curative-intent treatment for patients with localized lung cancer but postoperative morbidity is considerable, with an average reduction in VO_{2peak} being ~30% and 15–20% following pneumonectomy and lobectomy, respectively (Bolliger et al. 1996; Nagamatsu et al. 2007). Moreover, reductions in VO_{2peak} persist up to 3 years following resection remain significantly lower than preoperative values (Nagamatsu et al. 2007). The poor VO_{2peak} observed in postsurgical lung cancer may be caused by multiple mechanisms. Resection of the lung parenchyma reduces ventilatory capacity and reserve. In addition, lung cancer patients are typically older, are current or former smokers, deconditioned, and commonly present with other concomitant cardiovascular diseases. Also, up to 70% of lung cancer patients will receive either adjuvant locoregional and/or systemic therapy following resection (Jones et al. 2009a).

Physical inactivity is a strong determinant of cardiorespiratory fitness; inactivity due to pain, weakness, and locoregional and systemic therapy can exacerbate deconditioning throughout the entire cardiovascular system. To this end, Coups et al. (2009) examined changes in self-reported physical activity levels in 175 postsurgical lung cancer patients 1–6 years following initial diagnosis. Using a cross-sectional, retrospective design, participants were asked to report their physical activity levels at three different time periods: 6 months prior to diagnosis, 6 months following treatment, and at study recruitment. Results indicated that moderate and strenuous intensity exercise was lower during the post-treatment period compared with prior to diagnosis and at study entry. Approximately ~75% of participants were not meeting national physical activity recommendations at any of the three timepoints.

In light of the pathophysiologic mechanisms of poor VO_{2peak}, exercise training appears well placed to prevent and/or mitigate the observed poor VO_{2peak} in postsurgical lung cancer patients. To date, however, only three published studies have investigated the utility of exercise training in this setting.

Spruit et al. (2006) investigated the effects of an 8-week multidisciplinary inpatient

11

rehabilitation program among ten patients with severely impaired pulmonary function following treatment for operable lung cancer. Participants completed measures of cardiorespiratory fitness at baseline and the end of the intervention. The multidisciplinary rehabilitation program consisted of a multicomponent exercise training program including aerobic training (daily cycle ergometry, treadmill walking at 60% and 80% of baseline peak cycling load and baseline treadmill load, respectively), resistance training (upper and lower extremity exercises at 60% of one-repetition maximum), and general flexibility and mobilization exercises. At baseline, median 6MWD was 351 m, 64% of predicted while median peak cycling load was 82 W or 58% of predicted. Results indicated that the rehabilitation program was associated with significant improvements in measures of cardiorespiratory fitness (Spruit et al. 2006).

In the second study, Cesario et al. (2007) investigated the effects of a 28-day inpatient rehabilitation program among 25 patients following pulmonary resection. The rehabilitation program consisted of 5 weekly, 3-h sessions including incremental cycle ergometry (30 min/day at ~70% of maximal workload), resistance exercises and treadmill walking, and education. All patients underwent spriometry and 6MWT at baseline and post intervention. In comparison with patients who refused entry into the study ($n = 186$), inpatient rehabilitation was associated with significant improvements in 6 min walk distance with no changes in any pulmonary function outcomes (Cesario et al. 2007).

The final study, conducted by Jones et al. (2008b), examined the effects of supervised aerobic training on changes in VO_{2peak} and QOL among 20 newly diagnosed postsurgical non–small cell lung cancer patients (stage I–IIIB) 4–6 weeks post resection (Jones et al. in press). Aerobic training consisted of three endurance cycle ergometry sessions per week at 60–100% of baseline VO_{2peak} for 14 weeks. VO_{2peak} was assessed using a maximal CPET with expired gas analysis. Overall QOL and fatigue was assessed using the Functional Assessment of Cancer Therapy-Lung scale. Intention-to-treat analyses indicated that VO_{2peak} increased 1.1 mL kg^{-1} min^{-1} [95% CI, −0.3 to 2.5; $p = 0.109$] and peak workload increased 9 W [95% CI, 3–14; $p = 0.003$], whereas QOL increased 10 points [95% CI, −1 to 22; $p = 0.071$) and fatigue decreased 7 points [95% CI, −1 to −17; $p = 0.029$) from baseline to post intervention (Fig. 11.3). The investigators also conducted a per-protocol analysis that examined changes in study endpoints by treatment status (i.e., receiving chemotherapy vs no chemotherapy) (see Fig. 11.4). Exercise adherence was 93% and 72% for patients receiving and not receiving chemotherapy, respectively. For patients not receiving adjuvant chemotherapy ($n = 11$), VO_{2peak} increased 1.7 mL kg^{-1} min^{-1} whereas significant improvements were observed for the majority of QOL outcomes. Conversely, for patients receiving adjuvant chemotherapy ($n = 8$), there were no significant changes in any cardiopulmonary or QOL outcome.

Similar to the presurgical setting, results of these pilot studies provide 'proof of principle' that aerobic training is a safe and feasible intervention in lung cancer patients following pulmonary resection. Clearly, the research to date has a number of methodological limitations including single-sample designs, small sample sizes, and short-term follow-up. In addition, the improvements in measures of cardiorespiratory fitness were relatively modest (<10%), despite good exercise adherence rates (≥70% of planned sessions) when reported. Typical improvements in VO_{2peak} are ~15–20% following traditional aerobic training recommendations.

The reasons for the relatively modest improvements in cardiorespiratory fitness from exercise training in the postoperative setting are not known. An obvious potential explanation is a ventilatory limitation or inadequate gas exchange following removal of a substantial portion of lung parenchyma. However, several elegant studies have demonstrated that VO_{2peak} is not limited by

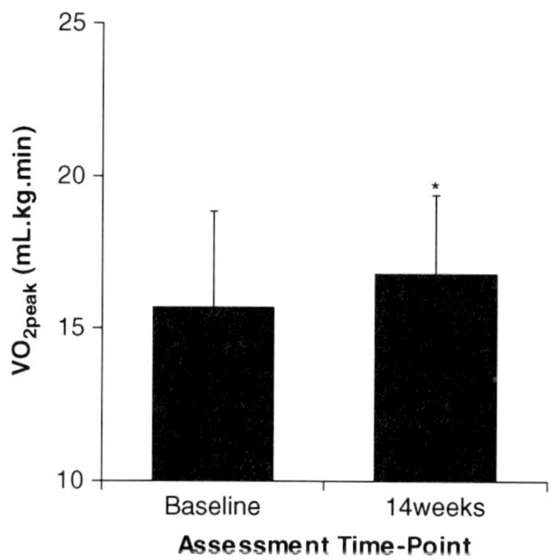

Fig. 11.3 Change in peak oxygen consumption (VO2peak) from baseline to post intervention (14 weeks) among 20 postsurgical non–small cell lung cancer patients (*p = 0.11)

ventilation or diffusion capacity (Degraff et al. 1965; Hsia et al. 1991, 1994, 2008) suggesting that exercise-induced adaptations (or lack thereof) in the other organ components that govern cardiorespiratory fitness (i.e., cardiac-vasculature–skeletal muscle axis) are responsible. In lung cancer patients, cardiorespiratory fitness is likely principally governed by poor cardiovascular O_2 delivery and oxidative capacity *as well as* unfavorable fiber type distribution and muscle atrophy/weakness similar to the limitations to exercise described in patients with chronic obstructive pulmonary disease (COPD). Major contributors to skeletal muscle dysfunction in postoperative lung cancer likely include direct skeletal myopathy (from the use of oral corticosteroids), deconditioning (from physical inactivity), and high levels of systemic inflammation (from underlying disease and therapy) (Wagner 2006).

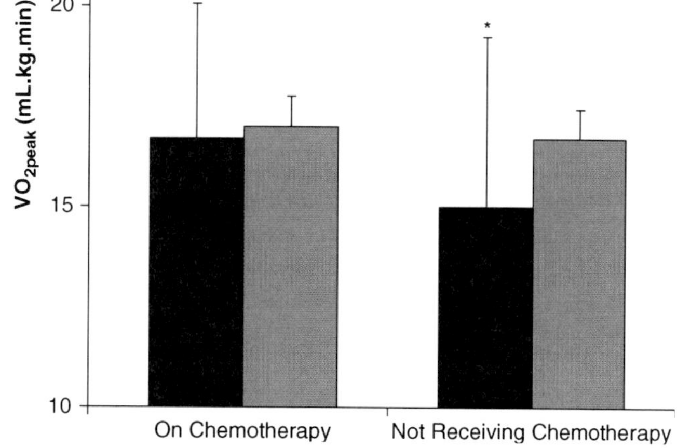

Fig. 11.4 Change in peak oxygen consumption (VO_{2peak}) by chemotherapy status (receiving chemotherapy, $n = 8$) versus no chemotherapy, $n = 11$) from baseline to postintervention (14 weeks) among 20 postsurgical non–small cell lung cancer patients (*$p < 0.05$)

11

The importance of central (e.g., cardiovascular O_2 delivery) and peripheral (e.g., skeletal muscle function) factors in determining cardiorespiratory fitness in postoperative lung cancer patients suggests that the combination of aerobic and resistance training may optimally augment changes in cardiorespiratory fitness in this setting more effectively than either exercise modality alone (see Fig. 11.5). An ongoing trial by Jones and colleagues will address this critical question. The Lung Cancer Exercise Training Study (LUNGEVITY) is a randomized trial designed to determine the efficacy of different types of exercise training on VO_{2peak} in 160 postoperative NSCLC patients. Eligible patients will be randomly assigned to one of four conditions: (1) aerobic training alone, (2) resistance training alone, (3) the combination of aerobic and resistance training, or (4) attention-control (progressive stretching) for 16 weeks. The primary study endpoint is VO_{2peak}. Secondary endpoints include: patient-reported outcomes (PROs) (e.g., quality of life, fatigue, depression, etc.) and organ components of the oxygen cascade (i.e., pulmonary function, cardiac function, skeletal muscle function). All endpoints will be assessed at baseline and post intervention (16 weeks).

This trial will address several key questions in this area of research including elucidation of the optimal type of exercise training as well as the physiological mechanisms underlying the effects of exercise on improvements in VO_{2peak}. In addition to translational research investigating the effect and underlying mechanisms of exercise on lung cancer biology and pathogenesis, such studies will provide the evidence base to design a mechanistically driven, adequately powered phase III trial investigating the effects of exercise on overall survival in postsurgical lung cancer patients.

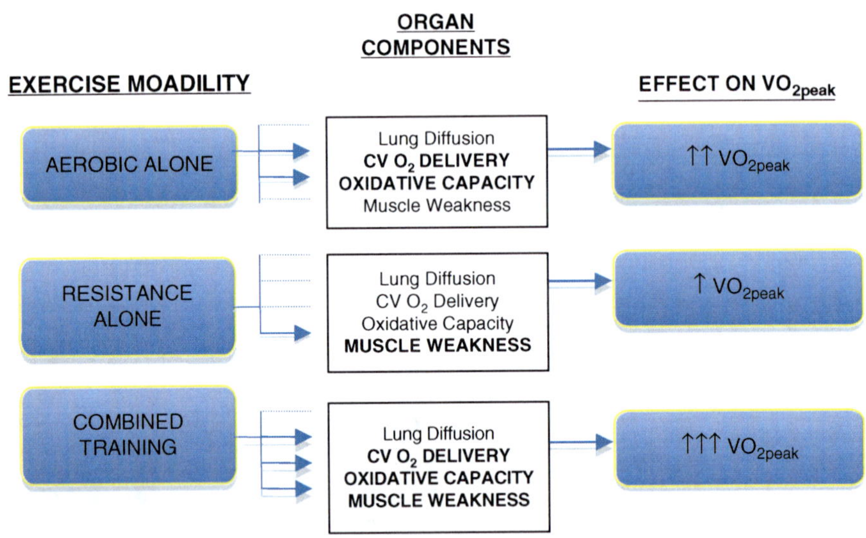

Fig. 11.5 Hypothesized effects of aerobic training alone, resistance training alone, and aerobic plus resistance training on the components of the oxygen cascade and resultant impact on peak oxygen consumption (VO2peak)

11.6 Exercise Therapy for Inoperable Lung Cancer

The majority of patients (~75%) diagnosed with lung cancer present with inoperable (advanced) disease. From an exercise therapy perspective, these patients present a unique challenge. Similar to the operable disease setting, patients with inoperable disease are often older and commonly present with a diverse range of cardiovascular and/or musculo-skeletal complications that may limit exercise tolerance. In addition, however, these patients present with diffuse tumor burden in the lungs as well as systemic metastatic disease commonly located in bone, kidney, liver, and brain. Furthermore, these patients receive aggressive therapy involving a combination of chemotherapy, radiotherapy, small molecule inhibitors, and supportive care therapies (e.g., decadron) that simultaneously adversely impact the ability to tolerate exercise and elevate the risk of an exercise-associated adverse event (Jones et al. 2007b).

In this context, symptom-limited, incremental exercise testing procedures will be critical to screen patients with exercise contraindications and to prescribe safe yet efficacious exercise prescriptions. As an initial step, Jones et al. evaluated the safety and feasibility of symptom-limited, incremental exercise testing in 46 patients with inoperable lung cancer (Jones et al. 2007b). Patients performed a CPET on a cycle ergometer with a 12-lead ECG. Only 105 of 470 (22%) screened patients were deemed to be 'physically able' to perform the CPET. Overall, there were two (4%) positive exercise tests and 11 (24%) indeterminate tests. One patient experienced an adverse event during exercise testing. Mean VO_{2peak} was 17.0 mL kg^{-1} min^{-1} which is 33% below age and sex-predicted. These preliminary findings indicate that a symptom-limited, individualized CPET is a relatively safe and feasible assessment tool to objectively evaluate physical functioning in *select* patients with inoperable NSCLC. Based on these results, particularly the low eligibility rate, exercise training interventions in this population will be challenging.

Not surprisingly, only one study to date has examined the role of exercise training in patients with inoperable lung cancer. Temel et al. (2009) examined the efficacy of an 8-week structured combined aerobic and resistance training hospital-based program among 20 patients with newly diagnosed inoperable lung cancer. Eleven patients (44%) completed the study. Significant reductions in lung cancer symptoms with maintenance of cardiorespiratory fitness, as measured by a 6-min walk test.

Clearly, the application of exercise interventions in patients with inoperable lung cancer will be limited to those with better performance status, less advanced disease, and less treatment-related complications. Nevertheless, given the significant number of individuals diagnosed with inoperable lung cancer annually, the relatively small proportion of patients who may be eligible for exercise interventions translates into a substantial number of individuals. In this context, future research is needed to examine the safety and efficacy of appropriate exercise interventions in *select* patients with inoperable disease.

11.7 Clinical Recommendations

The current literature base is insufficient to provide evidence-based, lung cancer-specific exercise prescription guidelines. Nevertheless, as reviewed in this chapter, emerging evidence corroborates work in other cancer populations that chronic (repeated) exercise therapy performed at least 3 days/week at a moderate intensity (e.g., 50–70% of heart rate reserve) is associated with improvements in cardiorespiratory fitness, QOL, and fatigue following a diagnosis of early-stage lung cancer. Exercise prescriptions guidelines are also informed by the results of recent landmark epidemiologic observational studies reporting that regular exercise (i.e., 3–5 days/week, ≥30 min/session, 50–70% of heart rate reserve) is associated with substantial reductions in cancer-specific mortality and all-cause mortality following a diagnosis of early-stage breast and colorectal cancer relative to those who were physically inactive (Meyerhardt et al. 2006, 2009; Holmes et al. 2005; Holick et al. 2008; Irwin et al. 2008; Haydon et al. 2006). Taken together, standard exercise prescription guidelines for healthy adults (i.e., 3–5 days/week, ≥30min/session, 50–70% of heart rate reserve) appear prudent for early-stage lung cancer patients both during and following adjuvant therapy until further evidence becomes available. As with any individual, when prescribing exercise it is important to consider several factors including exercise history, current exercise behavior, concomitant comorbid conditions, prior and current therapies, equipment/exercise availability, and exercise indication (e.g., strength, cardiorespiratory fitness, stress reduction). In most instances, exercise will need to be initiated at a lower level (i.e., 2 days/week, ≥10 min/session, 50–60% of heart rate reserve), particularly for sedentary individuals and those undergoing adjuvant therapies. This 'introductory' phase is important for individuals to become comfortable with the exercise prescription and incorporate exercise into their lives. After a period of 3–4 weeks in which the individual has experienced no exercise-related issues, the frequency, intensity, and duration of exercise can be gradually increased to workloads corresponding to the exercise prescription goal. The extent of progression will depend on the individual patient and will need to be modified based on response to therapy, medications, and other related factors. Exercise prescription guidelines are provided in Tables 11.2 and 11.3.

11.8 Future Directions

There are several recommendations for future investigation:

- Elucidation of the physiologic mechanisms underlying poor cardiorespiratory fitness in patients with early and advanced lung cancer is required. Current work indicates that lung cancer patients have markedly reduced cardiorespiratory fitness but the reason for this impairment is not known. Mechanistically driven studies are required to investigate which components of the cardiovascular system that govern cardiorespiratory fitness are primarily responsible for this impairment. Information gained from these studies will help refine exercise prescription guidelines for lung cancer patients.
- Investigation of the most appropriate exercise prescription for patients with early-stage lung cancer is warranted. Currently, the most appropriate and efficacious exercise prescription for cancer patients is not known. Adequately powered clinical trials are required to compare the effects of different exercise prescriptions on physiologic and psychosocial outcomes in patients with early-stage disease both during and following adjuvant therapy. For patients with inoperable disease, further research assessing the safety and feasibility of both cardiorespiratory testing and exercise therapy in this setting is warranted.
- Epidemiologic, observational studies examining the association between both self-reported and objective (e.g., VO_{2peak}, 6-min walk distance) measures of exercise capacity and cancer-specific mortality and all-cause mortality in patients with lung cancer is warranted. Such data will support the initiation of large-scale randomized trials investigating the effects of exercise therapy on disease

Table 11.2 Relative intensities for aerobic exercise prescription (for activities lasting up to 60 min) (Adapted from Warburton et al. 2006, Canada's Physical Activity Guide to Healthy Living (Canada Health 1998), ACSM's Guidelines for Exercise Testing and Prescription (Medicine ACoS 2000); and Howley 2001)

	Intensity	%HRR	$\%HR_{max}$	RPE	RPE	Breathing Rate	Body Temperature	Example Activity
	Very light effort	<20	<50	<10	<2	Normal	Normal	Dusting
Range Required for health	Light effort	20–39	50–63	10–11	2–3	Slight increase	Start to feel warm	Light gardening
	Moderate effort	40–59	64–76	12–13	4–6	Greater increase	Warmer	Brisk walking
	Vigorous effort	60–84	77–93	14–16	7–8	More out of breath	Quite Warm	Jogging
	Very hard effort	>84	>93	17–19	9	Greater increase	Hot	Running fast
	Maximal effort	100	100	20	10	Completely out of breath	Very hot/ Perspiring heavily	Sprinting All-out

Table 11.3 CSEP and health Canada's recommendations for aerobic physical activity (Health Canada and Canadian Society for Exercise Physiology 1998). Handbook for Canada's Physical Activity Guide to Healthy Active Living. Health Canada. Available: www.paguide.com)

Very Light Effort	Light Effort 60 min	Moderate Effort 30–60 min	Vigorous Effort 20–30 min	Maximum Effort 60 min
• Strolling • Dusting	• Light walking • Volleyball • Easy gardening • Stretching	• Brisk walking • Biking • Raking leaves • Swimming • Dancing • Water aerobics	• Aerobics • Jogging • Hockey • Basketball • Fast swimming • Fast dancing	• Sprinting • Racing
How does it feel? How warm am I? What is my breathing like?				
• No change from resting state	• Starting to feel warm	• Warmer	• Quite warm	• Very hot/perspiring heavily
• Normal breathing	• Slight increase in breathing rate	• Greater increase in breathing rate	• More out of breath	• Completely out of breath
Range needed to stay healthy				
Less than is required	Where you want to be			More than is required

outcomes in early-stage lung cancer. Of equal importance, parallel correlative science studies are required to elucidate the biologic mechanisms underlying the hypothesized beneficial effect of exercise therapy on recurrence and survival outcomes in cancer populations.

11.9 Summary

The pathophysiology of lung cancer together with conventional therapeutic management is associated with unique and varying degrees of adverse physiological impairments that dramatically reduce a patient's ability to tolerate exercise. Cardiorespiratory fitness is an attractive modifiable therapeutic target since it is a strong predictor of surgical risk and/or recovery, symptom control, and possibly, cancer-specific outcomes following a lung cancer diagnosis. On the basis of the literature reviewed in this chapter, research examining the role and efficacy of exercise in persons diagnosed with lung cancer is in its infancy relative to exercise research in the other major cancer diagnoses (i.e., breast, prostate, and colorectal cancer). Nevertheless, for patients with operable disease, both before and after pulmonary resection, the preliminary evidence suggests that supervised aerobic training is safe and feasible in these patients and potentially associated with improvements in several clinically relevant endpoints. Randomized trials are now required to address second generation questions in this setting, including elucidation of the optimal type and dose of exercise. Among patients with inoperable disease, further preliminary research assessing the safety and feasibility of exercise in this setting is warranted. Although much more work is required, exercise therapy may represent an important component of multidisciplinary management of patients diagnosed with lung cancer.

References

Arriagada R, Dunant A, Pignon JP et al (2009) Long-term results of the international adjuvant lung cancer trial evaluating adjuvant cisplatin-based chemotherapy in resected lung cancer. J Clin Oncol 28(1):35–42

Beckles MA, Spiro SG, Colice GL et al (2003a) The physiologic evaluation of patients with lung cancer being considered for resectional surgery. Chest 123(1 Suppl):105S–114S

Beckles MA, Spiro SG, Colice GL et al (2003b) Initial evaluation of the patient with lung cancer: symptoms, signs, laboratory tests, and paraneoplastic syndromes. Chest 123(1 Suppl): 97S–104S

Benzo R, Kelley GA, Recchi L et al (2007) Complications of lung resection and exercise capacity: a meta-analysis. Respir Med 101(8): 1790–1797

Blanchon F, Grivaux M, Asselain B et al (2006) 4-year mortality in patients with non-small-cell lung cancer: development and validation of a prognostic index. Lancet Oncol 7(10):829–836

Bobbio A, Chetta A, Carbognani P et al (2005) Changes in pulmonary function test and cardio-pulmonary exercise capacity in COPD patients after lobar pulmonary resection. Eur J Cardiothorac Surg 28(5): 754–758

Bobbio A, Chetta A, Ampollini L et al (2008) Preoperative pulmonary rehabilitation in patients undergoing lung resection for non-small cell lung cancer. Eur J Cardiothorac Surg 33(1): 95–98

Bolliger CT, Soler M, Stulz P et al (1994) Evaluation of high-risk lung resection candidates: pulmonary haemodynamics versus exercise testing. A series of five patients. Respiration 61(4): 181–186

Bolliger CT, Jordan P, Soler M et al (1996) Pulmonary function and exercise capacity after lung resection. Eur Respir J 9(3):415–421

Brundage MD, Davies D, Mackillop WJ (2002) Prognostic factors in non-small cell lung cancer: a decade of progress. Chest 122(3):1037–1057

Brutsche MH, Spiliopoulos A, Bolliger CT et al (2000) Exercise capacity and extent of resection as predictors of surgical risk in lung cancer. Eur Respir J 15(5):828–832

Butts CA, Ding K, Seymour L et al (2010) Randomized phase III trial of vinorelbine plus cisplatin compared with observation in completely resected stage IB and II non-small-cell

11

lung cancer: updated survival analysis of JBR-10. J Clin Oncol 28(1):29–34

Canada Health (1998) Canada's physical activity guide to healthy active living. Ottawa, 1998

Cesario A, Ferri L, Galetta D et al (2007) Pre-operative pulmonary rehabilitation and surgery for lung cancer. Lung Cancer 57(1):118–119

Clark MM, Novotny PJ, Patten CA et al (2008) Motivational readiness for physical activity and quality of life in long-term lung cancer survivors. Lung Cancer 61(1):117–22

Coups EJ, Park BJ, Feinstein MB et al (2009) Physical activity among lung cancer survivors: changes across the cancer trajectory and associations with quality of life. Cancer Epidemiol Biomarkers Prev 18(2):664–672

Datta D, Lahiri B (2003) Preoperative evaluation of patients undergoing lung resection surgery. Chest 123(6):2096–2103

Degraff AC Jr, Taylor HF, Ord JW et al (1965) Exercise limitation following extensive pulmonary resection. J Clin Invest 44:1514–1522

Douillard JY (2010) Adjuvant chemotherapy for non-small-cell lung cancer: it does not always fade with time. J Clin Oncol 28(1):3–5

Ekelund LG, Haskell WL, Johnson JL et al (1988) Physical fitness as a predictor of cardiovascular mortality in asymptomatic North American men. The lipid research clinics mortality follow-up study. N Engl J Med 319(21):1379–1384

Fan G, Filipczak L, Chow E (2007) Symptom clusters in cancer patients: a review of the literature. Curr Oncol 14(5):173–179

Friendenreich CM, Courneya KS (1996) Exercise as rehabilitation for cancer patients. Clin J Sport Med 6(4):237–244

Ghayoumi A, Raxwal V, Cho S et al (2002) Prognostic value of exercise tests in male veterans with chronic coronary artery disease. J Cardiopulm Rehabil Nov-Dec 22(6): 399–407

Gulati M, Pandey DK, Arnsdorf MF et al (2003) Exercise capacity and the risk of death in women: the St James Women Take Heart Project. Circulation 108(13):1554–1559

Gulati M, Black HR, Shaw LJ et al (2005) The prognostic value of a nomogram for exercise capacity in women. N Engl J Med 353(5): 468–475

Haydon AM, Macinnis RJ, English DR et al (2006) Effect of physical activity and body size on survival after diagnosis with colorectal cancer. Gut 55(1):62–67

Holick CN, Newcomb PA, Trentham-Dietz A et al (2008) Physical activity and survival after diagnosis of invasive breast cancer. Cancer Epidemiol Biomarkers Prev 17(2):379–386

Holmes MD, Chen WY, Feskanich D et al (2005) Physical activity and survival after breast cancer diagnosis. JAMA 293(20):2479–2486

Howley ET (2001) Type of activity: resistance, aerobic and leisure versus occupational physical activity. Med Sci Sports Exerc 33(6 Suppl): S364–369, discussion S419–S320

Hsia CC, Carlin JI, Ramanathan M et al (1991) Estimation of diffusion limitation after pneumonectomy from carbon monoxide diffusing capacity. Respir Physiol 83(1):11–21

Hsia CC, Herazo LF, Ramanathan M et al (1994) Cardiopulmonary adaptations to pneumonectomy in dogs IV. Membrane diffusing capacity and capillary blood volume. J Appl Physiol Aug 77(2):998–1005

Hsia CC, Dane DM, Estrera AS et al (2008) Shifting sources of functional limitation following extensive (70%) lung resection. J Appl Physiol 104(4): 1069–1079

Irwin ML, Smith AW, McTiernan A et al (2008) Influence of pre- and postdiagnosis physical activity on mortality in breast cancer survivors: the health, eating, activity, and lifestyle study. J Clin Oncol 26(24):3958–3964

Jemal A, Siegel R, Ward E et al (2009) Cancer statistics. CA Cancer J Clin 59(4):225–249

Jones LW, Demark-Wahnefried W (2006) Diet, exercise, and complementary therapies after primary treatment for cancer. Lancet Oncol 7(12): 1017–1026

Jones LW, Peddle CJ, Eves ND et al (2007a) Effects of presurgical exercise training on cardiorespiratory fitness among patients undergoing thoracic surgery for malignant lung lesions. Cancer 110(3):590–598

Jones LW, Eves ND, Mackey JR et al (2007b) Safety and feasibility of cardiopulmonary exercise testing in patients with advanced cancer. Lung Cancer 55(2):225–232

Jones LW, Eves ND, Haykowsky M et al (2008a) Cardiorespiratory exercise testing in clinical oncology research: systematic review and practice recommendations. Lancet Oncol 9(8): 757–765

Jones LW, Eves ND, Peterson BL et al (2008b) Safety and feasibility of aerobic training on cardiopulmonary function and quality of life in postsurgical nonsmall cell lung cancer patients: a pilot study. Cancer 113(12):3430–3439

Jones LW, Eves ND, Haykowsky M et al (2009a) Exercise intolerance in cancer and the role of exercise therapy to reverse dysfunction. Lancet Oncol 10(6):598–605

Jones LW, Cohen RR, Mabe SK et al (2009b) Assessment of physical functioning in recurrent glioma: preliminary comparison of performance status to functional capacity testing. J Neurooncol 94(1):79–85

Jones LW, Eves ND, Peterson BL et al. Safety and feasibility of aerobic training on cardiopulmonary function and quality of life in postsurgical non-small cell lung cancer patients: a pilot study. Cancer 2008; 113(11) 1410–9

Kasymjanova G, Correa JA, Kreisman H et al (2009) Prognostic value of the six-minute walk in advanced non-small cell lung cancer. J Thorac Oncol 4(5):602–607

Kavanagh T, Mertens DJ, Hamm LF et al (2002) Prediction of long-term prognosis in 12 169 men referred for cardiac rehabilitation. Circulation 106(6):666–671

Kenny PM, King MT, Viney RC et al (2008) Quality of life and survival in the 2 years after surgery for non small-cell lung cancer. J Clin Oncol 26(2):233–241

Kohman L, Watson D, Herndon JE et al (2009) CALGB 140803 – Association between cardiorespiratory fitness and overall survival in operable lung cancer patients: ancillary analysis of protocol 9238. J Clin Oncol 27(15s):(suppl; abstr 7518)

Leeper NJ, Dewey FE, Ashley EA et al (2007) Prognostic value of heart rate increase at onset of exercise testing. Circulation 115(4): 468–474

Li WW, Lee TW, Yim AP (2004) Quality of life after lung cancer resection. Thorac Surg Clin 14(3):353–365

Loewen GM, Watson D, Kohman L et al (2007) Preoperative exercise Vo2 measurement for lung resection candidates: results of Cancer and Leukemia Group B Protocol 9238. J Thorac Oncol 2(7):619–625

Markes M, Brockow T, Resch KL (2006) Exercise for women receiving adjuvant therapy for breast cancer. Cochrane Database Syst Rev (4): CD005001

McAuley PA, Myers JN, Abella JP et al (2007) Exercise capacity and body mass as predictors of mortality among male veterans with type 2 diabetes. Diab Care 30(6):1539–1543

McNeely ML, Campbell KL, Rowe BH et al (2006) Effects of exercise on breast cancer patients and survivors: a systematic review and meta-analysis. CMAJ 175(1):34–41

Medicine ACoS (2000) ACSM's guidelines for exercise testing and prescription. Lippincott, Williams & Wilkins, Philadelphia

Meyerhardt JA, Giovannucci EL, Holmes MD et al (2006) Physical activity and survival after colorectal cancer diagnosis. J Clin Oncol 24(22): 3527–3534

Meyerhardt JA, Giovannucci EL, Ogino S et al (2009) Physical activity and male colorectal cancer survival. Arch Intern Med 169(22): 2102–2108

Morise AP, Jalisi F (2003) Evaluation of pretest and exercise test scores to assess all-cause mortality in unselected patients presenting for exercise testing with symptoms of suspected coronary artery disease. J Am Coll Cardiol 42(5): 842–850

Myers J, Prakash M, Froelicher V et al (2002) Exercise capacity and mortality among men referred for exercise testing. N Engl J Med 346(11):793–801

Nagamatsu Y, Maeshiro K, Kimura NY et al (2007) Long-term recovery of exercise capacity and pulmonary function after lobectomy. J Thorac Cardiovasc Surg 134(5):1273–1278

Nishime EO, Cole CR, Blackstone EH et al (2000) Heart rate recovery and treadmill exercise score as predictors of mortality in patients referred for exercise ECG. JAMA 284(11):1392–1398

Paull DE, Thomas ML, Meade GE et al (2006) Determinants of quality of life in patients following pulmonary resection for lung cancer. Am J Surg 192(5):565–571

Peddle CJ, Jones LW, Eves ND et al (2009) Effects of presurgical exercise training on quality of life in patients undergoing lung resection for suspected malignancy: a pilot study. Cancer Nurs Mar-Apr 32(2):158–165

Prakash M, Myers J, Froelicher VF et al (2001) Clinical and exercise test predictors of all-cause mortality: results from > 6, 000 consecutive referred male patients. Chest 120(3): 1003–1013

Ross RM (2003) ATS/ACCP statement on cardiopulmonary exercise testing. Am J Respir Crit Care Med 167(2):211–277

11

Rumble ME, Keefe FJ, Edinger JD et al (2005) A pilot study investigating the utility of the cognitive-behavioral model of insomnia in early-stage lung cancer patients. J Pain Symptom Manage 30(2):160–169

Sandvik L, Erikssen J, Thaulow E et al (1993) Physical fitness as a predictor of mortality among healthy, middle-aged Norwegian men. N Engl J Med 328(8):533–537

Schmitz KH, Holtzman J, Courneya KS et al (2005) Controlled physical activity trials in cancer survivors: a systematic review and meta-analysis. Cancer Epidemiol Biomarkers Prev 14(7): 1588–1595

Semik M, Schmid C, Trosch F et al (2001) Lung cancer surgery–preoperative risk assessment and patient selection. Lung Cancer 33(Suppl 1): S9–15

Spruit MA, Janssen PP, Willemsen SC et al (2006) Exercise capacity before and after an 8-week multidisciplinary inpatient rehabilitation program in lung cancer patients: a pilot study. Lung Cancer 52(2):257–260

Stevinson C, Lawlor DA, Fox KR (2004) Exercise interventions for cancer patients: systematic review of controlled trials. Cancer Causes Control 15(10):1035–1056

Temel JS, Greer JA, Goldberg S et al (2009) A structured exercise program for patients with advanced non-small cell lung cancer. J Thorac Oncol 4(5):595–601

Vanhees L, Fagard R, Thijs L et al (1994) Prognostic significance of peak exercise capacity in patients with coronary artery disease. J Am Coll Cardiol 23(2):358–363

Villani F, De Maria P, Busia A (2003) Exercise testing as a predictor of surgical risk after pneumonectomy for bronchogenic carcinoma. Respir Med 97(12):1296–1298

Wagner PD (2006) Skeletal muscles in chronic obstructive pulmonary disease: deconditioning, or myopathy? Respirology 11(6):681–686

Wang JS, Abboud RT, Wang LM (2006) Effect of lung resection on exercise capacity and on carbon monoxide diffusing capacity during exercise. Chest 129(4):863–872

Warburton DE, Nicol CW, Bredin SS (2006) Prescribing exercise as preventive therapy. CMAJ 174(7):961–974

Win T, Jackson A, Groves AM et al (2006) Comparison of shuttle walk with measured peak oxygen consumption in patients with operable lung cancer. Thorax 61(1):57–60

Woodward RM, Brown ML, Stewart ST et al (2007) The value of medical interventions for lung cancer in the elderly: results from SEER-CMHSF. Cancer 110(11):2511–2518

Physical Activity and Hematological Cancer Survivorship

12

Claudio L. Battaglini

Abstract As previously presented in other chapters of this book, exercise has been shown through large scale studies to be associated with significant improvements in physical and psychological parameters in patients with one of several different tumor types (Galvao et al. 2010; Schwartz and Winters-Stone 2009; Galvao et al. 2009; Segal et al. 2009; Courneya et al. 2008a, b; Ligibel et al. 2008; Courneya et al. 2007; Schmitz et al. 2005a; Fairey et al. 2005). In addition, well conducted systematic reviews of the literature that have explored the effects of exercise before, during, or after anti-cancer therapy have consistently shown positive outcomes to patients treated for solid tumors. Consistent findings include an overall reduction in fatigue, depression, anxiety, and distress, paired with positive changes in fitness parameters such as aerobic capacity and overall muscle function (Speck et al. 2010; Jones et al. 2006; McNeely et al. 2006; Markes et al. 2006; Schmitz et al. 2005; Galvao and Newton 2005). However, a relative paucity of data exists in the area of exercise interventions for adult patients with hematological malignancies. This chapter reviews the current literature regarding the administration of exercise in adult patients diagnosed with hematological cancer. The few exercise intervention studies conducted in patients with hematological cancers suggest that it is feasible to administer exercise to most patients and that exercise should be considered as an intervention to alleviate treatment-related symptoms. Yet, efficacy along with the appropriate mode, intensity, and frequency of exercise training in different types of hematological cancers are yet to be established and require further research.

C.L. Battaglini
Department of Exercise and Sport Science and Lineberger Comprehensive Cancer Center, University of North Carolina at Chapel Hill, 25 C Fetzer Hall, Chapel Hill, North Carolina 27599-8700, USA
e-mail: claudio@email.unc.edu

12.1 Background and Significance of Hematological Cancers

Hematological cancers are types of cancer that develop in either the bone marrow or lymphatic tissues. Leukemia, myeloma, Hodgkin and non-Hodgkin lymphoma are the most common hematological cancers that interfere with the normal production of blood cells. They can lead to anemia, decreased immune response, and a predilection to bleeding.

K.S. Courneya and C.M. Friedenreich (eds.), *Physical Activity and Cancer*, Recent Results in Cancer Research 186, DOI: 10.1007/978-3-642-04231-7_12,

In the United States, it was estimated that in 2010, 137,260 men and women would be diagnosed with some form of hematological cancer and 53,240 men and women would die from them These hematological cancers account for approximately 9.0% of the total cancer deaths expected in 2009 (The Leukemia and Lymphoma Society 2010). The 5-year survival rate in adult patients diagnosed with hematological cancers varies from poor (acute leukemia patients) to modest-high (Hodgkin lymphoma) (The Leukemia and Lymphoma Society 2010), and any chance of survival hinges upon the ability to complete several courses of intensive treatment. While treatment protocols have increased survival rates (The Leukemia and Lymphoma Society 2010), these gains do not come without costs. A constellation of side effects resulting from intensive treatment compromises the patient's ability to live and function at precancer levels. In some cases, the side effects are severe enough to hinder administration of treatment, decreasing chances of survival.

12.2 Treatments for Hematological Cancers

Patients diagnosed with blood cancers, as patients diagnosed with any cancer, face difficult decisions about their treatment and care. From deciding where to which doctor to which type of treatment plan. and to type of treatment plan, patients face tremendous stress in addition to a very difficult diagnosis. Currently, treatment approaches for patients with blood cancers may include very high dose of chemotherapy, often combining different anticancer agents, radiation therapy, immunotherapy, and stem cell or marrow transplantation.

12.2.1 Chemotherapy

There are four types of chemotherapeutic drugs used for the treatment of different blood cancers; DNA-damaging agents, antimetabolites, antitumor antibiotics, and DNA-repair enzyme inhibitors. Common DNA-damaging agents, also known as alkylating agents, used to treat blood cancers include cyclophosphamide, chlorambucil, and melphalan; antimetabolites include methotrexate, fludarabine, and cytarabine; antitumor antibiotics include daunorubicin, doxorubicin, idarubicin, and mitoxantrone; and DNA-repair enzyme including etoposide or topotecan. For the treatment of lymphoma and lymphocytic leu-kemia, high doses of predisone and dexamethasone are also used (The Leukemia and Lymphoma Society 2010). Chemotherapy treatments are usually administered intravenously, orally, intramuscularly, or intrathecal. Due to the systemic nature of administration of chemotherapy treatment and the high dosages administered, a constellation of side effects impacting different physiological systems and tissues are very common. Pain and burning sensations in the mouth, nausea and vomiting, diarrhea, changes in cell count, fatigue, unfavorable body composition changes, and increased risk for infection are among the most common side effects. All of these reduce the ability of patients to function at a precancer level. The intensity of side effects can significantly impair physical and mental function and is dependant on the type and dosage of treatment and possibly the physical condition of the patient prior to treatment. Nevertheless, the majority of patients end up experiencing severe side effects and addressing these side effects may provide the opportunity to keep the patient on a planned course of treatment enhancing the chances for better overall treatment outcomes.

12.2.2 Radiation Therapy

Radiation therapy can be used alone or in combination with chemotherapy, depending on the type of disease and the reason for treatment. Cutaneous T-cell lymphoma, myeloma, acute lymphocytic leukemia, B-cell lymphoma, and

Hodgkin lymphoma are hematological diseases commonly treated with electron beam radiotherapy (The Leukemia and Lymphoma Society 2010). Radiation therapy is usually delivered in multiple bouts spread over weeks, averaging from 2 to 10 weeks of treatment. Even though the administration strategy of spreading the treatment over a period of a few weeks is done to minimize the development of side effects, common side effects including mucositis, loss of appetite, nausea, diarrhea, skin irritation, loss of hair on parts of the body exposed to the radiation, and fatigue occur in the majority of patients.

12.2.3 Immunotherapy

Immunotherapy is used for the treatment of leukemia, lymphoma, and myeloma cell residues that have remained after chemotherapy treatment. Immunotherapy can be used alone or in combination with other types of treatments. This type of treatment uses elements of the immune system (antibodies) that are directed to combat leukemia, lymphoma, and myeloma cells. Due to the targeted focus of this type of therapy, cancer cells and closely related cells are affected. However, differing from chemotherapy treatment, a wide variety of normal cells are not impacted by this treatment approach (The Leukemia and Lymphoma Society 2010).

12.2.4 Stem Cell and Marrow Transplantation

Autologous and allogenic are the two major types of stem cell transplantation. Autologous transplant uses the patient's own marrow while in allogenic transplants the marrow comes from a donor with the same type of tissue as the patient. The idea behind stem cell transplantation is that immune cells, as well as red and white cells, are produced from stem cells in the marrow, peripheral blood, and cord blood. With the transplant, there is hope that the marrow can restore the normal functioning that may have been compromised by marrow failure, destruction of marrow by disease, or exposure to intense chemicals and radiation. Prior to transplant, patients undergo high-dose chemotherapy and/or radiation therapy to ensure that no disease remains at the time of transplant. Patients with leukemia, lymphoma, myeloma, myelodysplastic syndrome or idiopathic myelofibrosis whose diseases do not respond well to standard chemotherapy, or patients who are at high risk for relapse or relapse after prior successful treatment are usually the candidates for stem cell or marrow transplantation.

Advancements in technology have improved the ability of physicians to treat hematological cancers. However, remission from the disease and perhaps survival comes with a debilitating treatment regiment. High doses of chemotherapy, in some cases administered in combination with radiation therapy, along with the in hospi tal treatment/recovery that can last numerous weeks are factors that contribute to physical and mental function decline, which can impact the ability of patients to complete the course of treatment as well as compromise tremendously the quality of life of these patients.

Nonpharmacological complementary therapies for the management of cancer treatment-related symptoms have gained and continue to gain traction within the medical community. As previously mentioned in this chapter, well established evidence and the continuous growth of scientific knowledge on the effects of exercise in certain cancer types continue to support the use of exercise as an effective complementary therapy in the management of cancer treatment-related symptoms (Galvão et al. 2010; Schwartz and Winters-Stone 2009; Galvão et al. 2009; Segal et al. 2009; Courneya et al. 2008b, 2008; Ligibel et al. 2008; Courneya et al. 2007; Schmitz et al. 2005a; Fairey et al. 2005). For some cancers, such as breast and colon, exercise has also been associated with decreased recurrence and mortality rates (Irwin et al. 2008; Meyerhardt et al. 2006; Demark-Wahnefried 2006). However, the examination of the potential benefits of exercise in hematological patients undergoing treatment or those in remission is scarce. Due to the nature of certain hematological cancers, treatment protocols, and some skepticism among hematology oncologists regarding the potential harm exercise can cause to their patients, opportunities to conduct research on the effects of exercise in this population can be challenging.

12.3 Exercise Intervention Studies on Adult Patients with Hematological Cancers

Most exercise intervention studies conducted in patients diagnosed with hematological cancers have focused on children. Currently there have been only 18 exercise intervention studies conducted in adult patients with hematological cancers (Cunningham et al. 1986; Decker et al. 1989; Dimeo et al. 1996; Dimeo et al. 2003; Mello et al. 2003; Oldervoll et al. 2003; Coleman et al. 2003; Hayes et al. 2004; Wilson et al. 2005; Carlson et al. 2006; Coleman et al. 2008; Chang et al. 2008; Battaglini et al. 2009; Elter et al. 2009; Shelton et al. 2009; Jarden et al. 2009; Courneya et al. 2009; Baumann et al. 2009). The first study using an exercise intervention program was conducted in 1986 by Cunningham and colleagues. Including the Cunningham et al. study, nine randomized controlled trials have been conducted to date (Cunningham et al. 1986; Mello et al. 2003; Coleman et al. 2003; Coleman et al. 2008; Chang et al. 2008; Shelton et al. 2009; Jarden et al. 2009; Courneya et al. 2009; Baumann et al. 2009), with only five having relatively large sample sizes (Coleman et al. 2008; Shelton et al. 2009; Jarden et al. 2009; Courneya et al. 2009; Baumann et al. 2009): one in patients diagnosed with multiple myeloma in 2008 (Coleman et al. 2008), three in patients diagnosed with different hematological malignancies (Shelton et al. 2009; Jarden et al. 2009; Baumann et al. 2009), and one involving patients diagnosed with lymphoma in 2009 (Courneya et al. 2009). To date, not one large randomized controlled clinical trial has examined the effect of exercise on a homogeneous sample of patients diagnosed with acute leukemia. Three studies identified in this review of literature, two of which were feasibility studies, specifically examined the effects of exercise on patients diagnosed with acute leukemia (Cunningham et al. 1986; Chang et al. 2008; Battaglini et al. 2009). As a point of clarification, this review includes only studies where the majority of the patients were adult patients diagnosed with hematological cancer.

The scientific exploration of the effects of exercise in patients with hematological malignancies started in the mid-1980s. Since then, most studies have used mixed hematological cancer populations in their study designs (Decker et al. 1989; Dimeo et al. 1996; Dimeo et al. 2003; Mello et al. 2003; Hayes et al. 2004; Wilson et al. 2005; Carlson et al. 2006; Elter et al. 2009; Shelton et al. 2009; Jarden et al. 2009; Baumann et al. 2009) and were conducted during or immediately following bone marrow transplantation. Less than half of the studies currently available in the literature have examined the effects of exercise while patients were undergoing treatment prior to qualifying for bone marrow transplantation. Among the different hematological cancer populations, cancer treatment protocols may present with many similarities. But, the timeline for administration of treatment, disease specific manifestations, differences in symptom development, the wide range of patient age, and the differences in treatment response hinder our ability to fully understand the true impact of exercise. Nevertheless, the aforementioned experiments provide valuable information necessary for subsequent research to be conducted in this area.

For organizational purposes, the following sections of this chapter are separated into studies conducted using mixed hematological patient populations followed by studies that use homogeneous sample of patients in their designs.

12.3.1 Studies Conducted with Mixed Patients with Different Hematological Cancer Diagnosis

Decker and colleagues conducted the first study examining the effects of exercise on a group of patients with different hematological cancers. This was a small trial with 12 patients. Five were able to complete the entire year of planned study protocol, which was administered after completion of bone marrow transplantation. In the brief report from Decker and colleagues, the authors reported that the 12 patients initially enrolled in the study were all able to tolerate a cardiopulmonary exercise test (CPET) without complications. Improvements in aerobic capacity were observed in each of the 5 patients who completed the 1 year trial, after participating in an unsupervised aerobic exercise training regiment on a cycle ergometer, 3 times per week for 30 min at an intensity of 85% of maximal heart rate. A small sample size, coupled with the brief nature of the published manuscript, leaves readers with unanswered questions regarding methodology. Therefore, not much can be concluded from this initial experiment, other than patients' tolerability to and absence of complications during the CPET tests.

In 1996, Dimeo and colleagues conducted a trial involving 20 patients with different hematological cancers. The report by Dimeo et al. presents a broader description of the study protocol. A detailed explanation of the aerobic training regiment used in the trial gives readers a better understanding not only of the exercise responses in this group of patients, but about patient tolerability of the intervention as well. Fourteen patients were able to complete the Dimeo et al. 6-week study protocol. The incidence of major complications in this group of patients appeared to be the same as that of similar patient populations undergoing otherwise typical care at the hospital where the study was conducted.

Another interesting point garnered from the Dimeo et al. study was that a treadmill was used instead of a cycle ergometer (used by Decker et al.). Dimeo and colleagues argued that the treadmill was more appropriate since it is adhered to a more natural form of exercise: walking. This suggestion can be debated, but knowing that patients were simply able to perform the exercise while on a treadmill gives future investigators additional options when selecting the most appropriate mode of exercise to be used.

Just as in the results presented by Decker et al. (1989), Dimeo et al. (1996) demonstrated significant improvements in patients' physical performance, specifically in training intensity, total walking distance per training session, and maximal performance (MET, Metabolic Equivalent) from baseline testing to the end of the exercise intervention. Although the small sample size and different hematological cancer diagnoses were major limitations in the Dimeo et al. study, the authors concluded that the results of the study were positive and that further investigation on the effects of aerobic exercise in patients with hematological cancer after bone marrow transplantation was warranted.

In 2003, Dimeo and colleagues conducted a significantly larger trial compared to their 1996 effort. Sixty-six patients with different hematological cancer diagnoses participated in a moderate-high intensity aerobic exercise training program for approximately 3 weeks (13 ± 9 days) while undergoing chemotherapy treatment. Patients underwent an aerobic protocol with interval training for 33 min on a treadmill, 3 times per week. The intensity during the interval training portion of the aerobic exercise session, which lasted 3 min per set, was performed with a speed corresponding to 70% of maximal heart rate. No significant improvement in walking speed at 80% of maximal heart rate or degree of perceived effort was observed from baseline to completion of the study protocol. One of the major contributions of this Dimeo et al. study was the fact that the study was conducted in patients undergoing treatment. However, regardless of the larger sample size and the fact that in-treatment patients exercised, the lack of a control group precludes the ability to interpret the efficacy of the aerobic exercise training program in the population studied. Also, the means of assessment for physical performance using a submaximal stress test to estimate maximal oxygen consumption based on the relationship between heart rate and workload was less than optimal and is another major limitation in the study. Dimeo et al. (2003) concluded that the high-intensity aerobic exercise training performed in combination with interval training reduced chemotherapy treatment-related decline in physical performance, which in this population is a tremendous accomplishment considering the harsh nature of the treatment protocol, and the difficulties associated with exercising during treatment, in-hospital.

In 2003, three other studies examined the effects of exercise training in patients diagnosed with hematological cancer (Mello et al. 2003; Oldervoll et al. 2003; Coleman et al. 2003). Attempting to address the methodological limitations from previous experiments, two of the studies conducted randomized trials including control groups in their design (treatment vs. control) (Mello et al. 2003; Coleman et al. 2003). The other single group study published in 2003 (Oldervoll et al. 2003), however, attempted to further scientific knowledge in the area by being the first one to examine a homogeneous sample which included only patients diagnosed with Hodgkin lymphoma. The 2003 studies that have examined specific groups of patients diagnosed with hematological cancer (Oldervoll et al. 2003; Coleman et al. 2003) are discussed later in this chapter.

In a randomized controlled clinical trial conducted by Mello et al. in 2003, 18 patients with different hematological diagnoses were assigned to either an exercise (n = 9) or control (n = 9) group after receiving bone marrow transplantation. The exercise group participated in an exercise program for 6 weeks, 3 times per week, which comprised a combination of a range of motion exercises, aerobic exercise training on a treadmill, and stretch exercises. The control group did not participate in any post transplant intervention. The aerobic program was similar to the previous protocol developed by Dimeo et al. (1996). This was the first study to measure muscular strength in patients with hematological cancers. The results of the Mello et al. (2003) study showed that an exercise regiment combining aerobic training, strength training, and stretching promoted improvements in muscular strength in patients with hematological malignancies after bone marrow transplantation. Regrettably, no exercise intensity or progression of training was presented for the resistance training portion of the exercise study protocol. The control group ended the study experiencing reduced muscular strength when compared to baseline values. Again, the authors reported that patients were able to tolerate the exercise intervention without adverse events due to exercise training.

Following the combined aerobic and strength exercise training approach and using a mixed hematological cancer population similar to the one used by Mello et al. (2003), Hayes et al. conducted a study in 2004 with a group of 12 patients. Patients were allocated to either a supervised exercise or control group in a non-randomized fashion. The exercise protocol in this study involved the participation in 12 weeks of moderate-high exercise intensity. The aerobic exercise portion of the protocol was administered 3 times per week with intensities increasing from 70% to 90% of maximal heart rate as the study progressed. The strength training portion of the exercise training protocol included 3–6 different strength exercises performed 2 times per week using weight training machines and free weights. All strength exercises were performed with weights set to induce fatigue between 8–20 repetitions. Using the gold standard measurement for the assessment of oxygen uptake (maximal oxygen consumption, CPET) and dynamometry for the assessment of muscular strength, Hayes et al. (2004) reported that hematological patients who undergo a combined aerobic and strength training program at moderate-high intensity following bone marrow transplantation can improve aerobic capacity and muscular strength, and that those changes could elicit values greater than prior to treatment.

The trend of studies using a mixed population of patients diagnosed with different types of hematological cancers after hematopoietic stem cell transplantation continued. Two small single arm studies, one in 2005 (Wilson et al. 2005) and another in 2006 (Carlson et al. 2006), were the only studies published during these years. These studies continued to examine the effects of aerobic exercise in patients with hematological cancer; however, the concept of using home-based exercise intervention in this population was introduced in a study conducted by Wilson and colleagues in 2005. In the Wilson et al. study (2005), 13 patients who had not received treatment for their disease for at least 6 months participated in a home-based aerobic exercise intervention for 12 weeks. The end points of the study included aerobic fitness, fatigue severity, and quality of life. This was the first study to examine the effects of exercise on psychological parameters in patients with hematological cancer. Patients were instructed to exercise 3 times per week at a target heart rate zone between 40–60% of heart rate reserve using their preferred mode of exercise (i.e. walking, cycling, swimming, and exercise tapes). Out of the 13 patients enrolled in the study, 9 returned their exercise logs for analyses of training, an 84% adherence rate. Improvements in aerobic fitness of 15%, reduction in fatigue symptom severity, and improvements in physical functioning and physical functioning subscale of the Medical Outcomes Study 36-Item Short Form (SF-36) were observed. Again, no adverse events were observed during the study. The authors concluded that this preliminary work supported the use of home-based aerobic training and that this type of training design can be utilized safely in this population of hematological cancer patients 6 months after transplantation. Again, the absence of a control group is a major limitation precluding an ability to confidently attribute the positive changes presented by Wilson and colleagues to the exercise protocol.

In the 2006 study of mixed population patients with hematological cancers, Carlson and colleagues also used aerobic exercise intervention with the goal of examining the effect of the exercise program on various psychological and physiological outcomes. The exercise intervention used a training methodology alternating days of light-moderate exercise sessions with high intensity workouts on the cycle ergometer 3 times per week for 12 weeks. Significant improvements in power output were observed along with significant reductions in fatigue at the end of the study as compared to baseline parameters. An adherence rate of approximately 90% was observed in this study. A follow up with patients who participated in the study at months 3, 6, 9, and 12 showed that a reduced level of fatigue was maintained during the year post exercise training. It is important to note that this study had many implications for future experiments. The well-controlled setting, where the study was associated with physiological markers of aerobic performance, allowed for a better understanding of the possible effects of exercise on aerobic capacity and, perhaps, on fatigue reduction. Again, no control group was available for comparison, which once again does not allow for definite conclusions to be made on the effect of the intervention, particularly on measures of psychological function. As mentioned by the authors, nevertheless, there is the need for larger randomized clinical trials to confirm or refute the findings of these initial studies.

The four most recent experiments examining the impact of exercise in groups of patients with mixed hematological cancers were conducted in 2009 (Elter et al. 2009; Shelton et al. 2009; Jarden et al. 2009; Baumann et al. 2009). The first one, a small trial including 12 patients with different hematological cancers while undergoing intense chemotherapy was conducted by Elter et al. (2009) Using a single arm design, this pilot study investigated the effects of a supervised aerobic training program administered on a cycle ergometer for 3 months, three times per week using submaximal exercise intensities. The uniqueness of this experiment lies in the attempt to examine the effects of exercise during treatment in patients with severe pancytopenia. Elter and colleagues' main goal was to examine the feasibility and safety of exercise for patients with pancytopenia during treatment as well as the effects of exercise on cardiovascular endurance and quality of life. The results once again demonstrated that most patients (8 out of 12) were able to complete the planned training protocol. For those who completed the training protocol, significant improvements in submaximal exercise capacity were attained. No changes in quality of life were observed at the end of the intervention. The Elter and colleagues study suggests that, even in patients with severe pancytopenia, exercise for patients with a thrombocyte count below 10,000 μL did not cause hemorrhage. The results are promising and have the potential to challenge current recommendations that patients with thrombocyte count below 20,000 should avoid exercise. Thus, future trials may consider maximizing patient participation in an exercise program by following the 10,000 μL thrombocytopenia count suggested by Elter and colleagues. Since this was a small trial, further studies are warranted to confirm or refute Elter and colleagues' preliminary results.

The last three studies conducted in 2009 (Shelton et al. 2009; Jarden et al. 2009; Baumann et al. 2009) were randomized controlled clinical trials with relatively larger sample sizes when compared to previous but similar trials. A study by Shelton and colleagues (2009) used a two-group design with a supervised vs. nonsupervised self-directed exercise intervention. Both groups participated in a 4-week exercise program composed of aerobic and resistance training designed by the research team. No significant differences between groups were observed for 6-min walking tests at the end of the study. For both groups, overall fatigue levels were initially similar to baseline, but decreased at the end of the study. The authors suggest that the homogeneity of the research sample, all patients having received allogenic stem cell transplant, was a strong point of the study indicating that the results could be generalized to this group of patients. The authors also concluded that an unsupervised self-directed exercise intervention may be as effective as a supervised training program in this population of post-transplant patients. This point is significant since it reflects a more practical approach to clinicians wanting to help their patients improve physical function during the recovery process after transplantation.

In a study by Jarden et al. (2009), a combination of aerobic and resistance exercises, relaxation techniques, and psychoeducation was administered to a treatment group in a randomized controlled clinical trial involving a group of patients with different hematological cancer diagnoses. The author's noble attempt to provide patients in the treatment group with a comprehensive intervention, aimed to cope with physical and psychological side effects of treatment, proved again that physical decline can be attenuated in patients undergoing treatment. Aside from the considerable treatment-related side effects observed in both groups during the course of the study, a slight, but nonsignificant improvement in fatigue and quality of life was observed in the treatment group upon completion. Just as in previous studies, the authors attributed the nonsignificant difference between groups to be due, in part, to the study's limitations in sample size. The authors concluded that it is feasible to combine both physical and psychological interventions during treatment and that multimodal intervention promotes the maintenance of aerobic fitness and muscle strength while minimizing loss of function performance. Furthermore, decreases in diarrhea were observed in the treatment group along with positive trends in improvements in quality of life, fatigue, and well being up to 6 months post transplantation.

The last study published to date using a design composed of a mixed group of patients diagnosed with different types of hematological cancers was conducted by Baumann and colleagues (2009). A randomized controlled clinical trial examined the effects of an aerobic exercise program conducted on a cycle ergometer combined with activities of daily living (walking and stepping activities) vs. a low-intensity hospital-based intervention composed of gymnastics, massage, and coordination training as part of the normal course of care given to bone marrow transplant recipients in the hospital where the study was conducted. Sixty-four patients undergoing stem cell transplantation were assessed for multiple physical and psychological parameters as well as for hematology prior to and after receiving a stem cell transplant. After the baseline assessment, patients participated in approximately three-and-a-half weeks of exercise training. The results of the study agree with previous research where exercise has shown to promote maintenance/improvement in aerobic capacity and strength in patients undergoing stem cell transplantation. The study also revealed that global quality of life and physical functioning, subdomains of the quality of life EORTC QLQ-C30 scale, were significantly different between the treatment and control groups, with the treatment group demonstrating a higher score at the end of the experiment. One of the major limitations of this study, however, was the fact that the treatment group received more training than the control group, which may help explain the difference in quality of life global and physical function domains. Because of this methodological limitation, conclusions regarding the true status of quality of life observed between intervention groups cannot be made. Nevertheless, this is yet another study where exercise has been demonstrated to be a suitable intervention for hematological patients undergoing bone marrow transplantation in order to prevent the adverse consequences of treatment, which result in poor physical and psychological functioning. Table 12.1 below presents, in chronological order from 1989 to date, the summary of exercise intervention studies conducted with mixed patients with different hematological cancer diagnosis.

The overall results of exercise intervention programs conducted in mixed patients with different hematological cancers revealed promising results. Those first experiments included in their designs exercise intensities for aerobic training varying from low intensity (40% of maximal heart rate) to high intensity (90% of Maximal Heart Rate). Aerobic exercise was performed continuously or through interval training. Exercise interventions varied from 3 to 16 weeks in duration. All had demonstrated the potential for positive changes in a variety of fitness and psychological measures. Positive changes in aerobic capacity, muscular strength, lean body mass, fatigue and quality of life was reported. Lastly, these studies demonstrated that it is not only feasible but also safe for patients with hematological cancer to exercise, with most trials reporting virtually no adverse effect due to exercise. It is important to note that only a few trials were conducted while patients were undergoing treatment and that many of the

Table 12.1 Exercise intervention studies conducted with mixed patients with different hematological cancer diagnosis

Authors	Sample	Age	Design	Exercise Intervention	Duration	Frequency/intensity	Results
Decker et al. (1989)	Five patients with hematological cancer (AML, CML, ALL) post-Treatment (post BMT)	43 (range 27–59) years	Single group	Unsupervised aerobic Ex training (Cycle ergometer)	12 weeks	30 min 3/week at 85% of HRmax (85% calculated from most recent aerobic test)	Patients were only able to perform aerobic test 4 months post BMT; however, all tolerated testing with no complications. Patients that did well 4 months post BMT ↑ VO2max
Dimeo et al. (1996)	14 patients with hematological cancer (ALL, AML, CML, HL, n-HL) Post-treatment and in clinical stable condition	36 ± 8 (range 22–55) years	Single Group	Supervised aerobic EX training + interval training (Treadmill walking)	6 weeks	30 min daily on weekdays. During week 1, 5 workloads (at 80% HR_{max}) of 3 min/day with 3 min walking half speed between workloads. Ex duration increased to 4 × 5 min on week 2, 3 × 8 min on week 3, 3 × 10 on week 4, and 2 × 15 on week 5. On week 6, patients trained continuously 30 min/day	↑ Physical performance (Training intensity improved (4.6 ± 1.1 km/h to 6 ± 0.6 km/h) from week 1 to week 6, Maximal performance improved from 4.7 ± 1.2 METs to 7.4 ± 2.5 METs) from baseline testing to the end of the training program. No major adverse events due to EX reported

Dimeo et al. (2003)	66 patients with hematological cancer (ALL, AML, CML, CLL, HL, n-HL, MM) in-treatment (HDC and ASCR)	48 ± 15 Years	Single group	Supervised aerobic EX training program with interval training (Treadmill walking)	~3 weeks (13 ± 9 days)	33 min daily (3 min warm-up, followed by 5 × 3 min at 70% HR_{max} by 3 min recovery period at half of the speed of the 3 min at 70% HR_{max})	No change in physical performance (mean walking speed at 80% of HR_{max}); No change in perceived exertion; ↓ hemoglobin concentration from baseline value. Two patients were not able to complete the study due to severe sepsis
Mello et al. (2003)	18 patients with (AML, CML, and n-HL) Post-treatment	Tx Group 27.9 (range18–39) years; C group 30.2 (range18–44) years	Two Groups RCT	Tx group: Supervised combined range of motion Ex, muscle stretching, and aerobic Ex training (walking on treadmill); C group: Usual care, no Ex	16 weeks study protocol (only 6 weeks of Ex training)	Tx group: 40 min total Ex daily on weekdays; First week aerobic training consisting of 5 sets of 3 min walking at a comfortable pace w/ 3 min rest between sets. Then progressed to 2 sets of 10 min walking at comfortable pace intercalated with 20 min walking at accelerated pace with HR no higher than 70% of HRR	Tx group ↑ in overall muscular strength; C group ↓ in overall muscular strength. No adverse events due to Ex reported

(continued)

Table 12.1 (continued)

Authors	Sample	Age	Design	Exercise Intervention	Duration	Frequency/intensity	Results
Hayes et al. (2004)	12 patients with hematological malignancies (AML, MM, n-HL, Lymphoblastic/ Lymphoma/ Leukemia, RHA), 4 solid; Post-treatment	Tx Group 54.5 (range 46–64) years; C group 39.5 (range16–64) years	Two Groups	Tx group: Supervised combined aerobic (treadmill walking and stationary cycle ergometer) and resistance Ex training (selectorized equipment and free weights); C group: Supervised stretching program	12 weeks	Tx group: 20–40min of aerobic Ex 3/week at 70–90% HR_{max}, 3–6 resistance exercises 2/ week with weights set to induce fatigue at 8–20 repetitions; C group: 20–30 different stretches Ex, 15–30 seconds 3/ week	Tx group: ↑ in VO_{2peak} of 9.17 mL.kg.min, and upper ↑ 0.29 kg/FFM (kg) and lower ↑ 0.71 kg/FFM (kg) body strength; C group: VO_{2peak} ↓ 1.4 mL.kg. min, upper body strength ↑ 0.02 kg/FFM (kg) and lower body strength and ↓ 0.71 kg/ FFM (kg). No adverse events due to Ex reported
Wilson et al. (2005)	13 patients (11 hematological (ALL, AML, n-HL), 6 solid; Post-treatment	48.9 (10.4) years	Single Group	Home-based aerobic Ex training (preferred mode of Ex, i.e: walking, cycling, swimming, exercise tapes)	12 weeks	20 min of continuous aerobic Ex at 40–60% of HRR al least 3/week	↑ MET (15%), ↓ fatigue symptom severity, QOL ↑ 4.5 points in the domain of physical functioning and↑ 4 points in role physical. No adverse events due to Ex reported

Carlson et al. (2006)	12 patients with hematological malignancies (CLL, CML, n-HL, AML, FL, MYE) Post-treatment	44.3 (8.7) years	Single Group	Supervised aerobic Ex training on stationary cycle ergometer	12 weeks	3/week; 1st workout 30 min at VT1 (RPE 2: light to moderate), 2nd workout 15 min at 20W above VT2 (RPE 6- hard to very hard), 3rd workout 20 min at V2 (RPE 4)	~ 90% Ex training compliance, ↑ VT2 power output 28% (26 W), ↑ 15% SV, ↓ RPE 1.5 points post intervention; ↓ fatigue (71.87%). No adverse events due to Ex reported
Elter et al. (2009)	12 patients with hematological malignancies (AML, ALL, n-HL) In-treatment	44.1 (14.0) Years	Single Group	Supervised aerobic Ex training on stationary cycle ergometer	12 weeks	3/week for 15 min at submaximal intensities WHO criteria THR of no more than 180 minus age	↑ in relative endurance capacity (W/BW), ↔ in QOL, 8 out 12 patients completed the protocol
Shelton et al. (2009)	61 patients with hematological malignancies (AML, ALL, CML, CLL, n-HL, HL) Post-treatment (Post-ASTC)	S Group; 43.6 (13.1) years; NS group; 48.9 (11.6) years	Two Groups (RCT)	S group: Supervised aerobic (upper and lower extremity cycle ergometer and treadmill) and resistance training weight machines) Ex training; NS group: Walking and resistance training with stretch bands with different resistance	4 weeks	S group: 3/week of aerobic Ex for 20–30 min at 60–75% of $HR_{max,}$ 7 different resistances EX, 1–3 sets of 10 repetitions to fatigue. NS group: 3/week of aerobic EX progressing to 30 min, 8 different EX 10–1–3 sets, 10–15 reps per Ex	S group ↑ 12% in the 6 min walking test, ↓ 21.2% in fatigue post-intervention; NS group: ↑ 9.8% in the 6 min walking test, ↓ 10.1in fatigue % post-intervention. No significant difference between groups for the 6 min walking test or fatigue. Fatigue was not significant different from baseline values

(continued)

Table 12.1 (continued)

Authors	Sample	Age	Design	Exercise Intervention	Duration	Frequency/intensity	Results
Jarden et al. (2009)	42 patiens with hematological malignancies (CML, AML, ALL, AA, MDS, WM, PNH, MF) In-treatment	Tx group: 40.9 (13.3) years C group: 37.4 (11.1) years	Two Groups (RCT)	Tx group: Aerobic EX on cycle ergometer, resistance training with dumbells + relaxation and psycho-education; C group: Usual care	4–6 weeks	Tx group: in-hospital, aerobic EX on cycle ergometer no higher than 75% HR_{max} (RPE between 10–13), 15–30 min daily. Resistance training 3/week, full body, 2 sets per EX, up to 12 reps max; C group: Standard Care (PT)	Significant ↑ in VO_{2max} and muscle strength favoring the Tx group at the end of study, No significant difference in QOL between groups at the end of study. Reduction in diarrhea was significant ↓ in TX group when compared to C
Baumman et al. (2009)	64 patients with hematological malignancies (AML, ALL, CML, MM, n-HL, MYE, MPS) In-treatment (prior to BMT)	Tx group: 44.9 (12.4) years C group: 44.1 (14.2) years	Two Groups (RCT)	Tx group: Aerobic EX on cycle ergometer plus ADL training. C group: Passive and active mobilization at low intensity	4 weeks	Tx group: 10–20 min of aerobic EX at 20% less W load than the results of the WHO-endurance test. 20 min per day of ADL including walking, stepping at RPE of strenuous level on Borg scale. C group: 10 min gymnastics, massages, and 5 min	Significant endurance performance difference between Tx and C groups was observed. ↔ in endurance performance in TX group (88.3 vs 86.5 W) and ↓ in C group (82.0 vs 60.0 W) from baseline to post-intervention. ↓ in muscular strength (10% Tx group vs 24% C group).

				coordination training at RPE below strenuous on Borg scale, 5 days a week starting 1 day post transplant	No significant difference in QOL between Tx and C; 15 patients deceased during study due to disease complications. All other patients completed study protocol

Ex Exercise, *BMT* Bone marrow transplant, *ASCT* Allogenic stem cell transplant, *ASCR* Allogenic stem cell rescue, *ALL* Acute lymphoblastic leukemia, *AML* Acute myelogenous leukemia, *CML* Chronic myelogenous leukemia, *HL* Hodgkin lymphoma, n-HL Non-hodgkin lymphoma, *MM* Multiple myeloma, RHA Rhabdomyosarcoma, *FL* Follicular lymphoma, *MYE* Myelodysplasia, *MPS* Myeloproliferative syndrome, *HDC* High-dose chemotherapy, HR_{max} Maximal heart rate, THR Target heart rate, *W* Watts, *BW* Body weight, *QOL* Quality of life, *Tx* Treatment, *C* Control, *S* Supervised, *NS* Non-supervised, *RCT* Randomized controlled clinical trial, VO_{2max} Maximal oxygen consumption, VO_{2peak} Maximal oxygen consumption patient attained during test, *MET* Metabolic equivalent, *RPE* Rate of perceived, HRR Heart rate reserve, *VT, FFM* Free fat mass, SV Stoke volume, *PT* Physical therapy, *ADL* Activities of daily living studies either used very small sample sizes or had no control group for comparison. Therefore, any interpretation from the above summary should be carefully made.

Supervised and home-based interventions including aerobic, strength, and stretching training protocols, along with some studies combining different modes of exercises with other forms of complementary therapies have been explored and open the doors for larger and better controlled trials necessary to elucidate the true effect of exercise on patients with different hematological diseases.

12.3.2 Studies Conducted in Patients with Multiple Myeloma

Two studies, both conducted by Coleman and colleagues (Coleman et al. 2003; Coleman et al. 2008) have examined the effects of an exercise intervention on patients with multiple myeloma. The first study, a feasibility study with 24 patients, was conducted in 2003. Coleman and colleagues randomized multiple myeloma patients undergoing treatment into a home-based aerobic, resistance training, and stretching exercise intervention, to be carried out 3 times per week versus a control group that received the usual care provided by their physicians. The aerobic intervention involved walking 18 min at a fast pace at a perceived exertion of 12–15 on the Borg Scale. After 24 weeks of the intervention, the group of patients assigned to the exercise intervention showed an average increase in lean body mass of 0.40 kg per month while the control group decreased approximately 0.44 kg per month. Changes in muscular strength were observed in both groups with significant increases observed in the exercise group (1 RM change from baseline of 2.4) while the control group experienced a decrease (1 RM change from baseline of 12.6). Decrease in total time on the treadmill test was observed in both groups; however, the control group had a more pronounced decline from baseline testing values. Mood was also examined in the Coleman et al. (2003) study with decreases observed in both groups throughout the study. Sleep patterns were also examined among this group of patients. At the end of the study, the exercise group showed a higher percentage of time asleep in bed at night when compared to the control group. Again, no adverse events due to exercise was reported.

Five years later, Coleman and colleagues (2008) conducted another trial in patients diagnosed with multiple myeloma. In one of the few larger randomized controlled clinical trials conducted, Coleman et al. examined the effect of a home-based exercise intervention similar to their study conducted in 2003. One-hundred-and-twenty patients participated in the trial, each receiving prophylactic EPO while undergoing high-dose chemotherapy and autologous peripheral-blood stem cell transplantation. The study end points included a physical performance measurement using the 6-min walk test and rate of perceived exercise (Borg Scale), red blood cell count, and the number of platelet transfusions. Once again, positive exercise responses were observed. As the treatment intensity increased, aerobic capacity decreased. However, the exercise group experienced significantly less of a decline when compared to the control group. No significant differences in red blood cell count was observed between groups; yet, it was suggested by the authors that the number of red blood cell and platelet transfusions were lower in the exercise group compared to the control group. Methodological issues, mainly surrounding the criteria for determining the number of red blood cell transfusions, preclude the ability to suggest the effects of exercise on this variable. However, in agreement with previous smaller studies, this first large randomized controlled trial confirms once again the feasibility and safety of using exercise in this population group. More studies must be conducted to verify the reproducibility of the results of this trial and to continue to explore different exercise intervention designs. Table 12.2 presents the summary of the exercise intervention studies conducted in patients with multiple myeloma.

12.3.3 Studies Conducted in Patients with Acute Leukemia

The standardized treatment protocol for patients diagnosed with acute leukemia is usually composed of high-dose chemotherapy (HDC) followed by bone marrow transplantation. During the first week of treatment, patients receive HDC daily. Next, patients remain in their hospital rooms and are advised to adhere to strict neutropenic procedures as an attempt to minimize the possibility of infection. The recovery period from the initial week of chemotherapy induction usually lasts from 3–5 weeks. After the initial hospital recovery phase, patients are discharged, and after two weeks of recovery at home, they return to the hospital for consolidated bouts of chemotherapy as an attempt to keep patients in remission until bone marrow transplant. Due to the nature of the treatment regiment, these patients are at increased susceptibility for severe treatment-associated complications. Reduced physical activity levels (bed rest), poor nutrition due to nausea, vomiting, diarrhea, and the effects of the high-dose chemotherapy are the perfect recipe for reduced physical functioning and perhaps poor treatment prognosis.

Exercise is an important intervention that has demonstrated in patients with solid tumors to assist in the management of treatment-related symptoms. As mentioned in this chapter, patients with hematological cancer, including those diagnosed with leukemia may also benefit from exercise. However, not until 2008 have studies tested this possibility in acute leukemia patients undergoing chemotherapy.

A major consideration when attempting to study the effects of exercise in acute leukemia patients during chemotherapy involves the logistics of the study design, since patients are usually admitted to the hospital to initiate treatment very quickly. Also, due to the nature of the disease and treatment, patients are confined to their hospital rooms and are advised to avoid contact with many people.

Three studies have examined the effects of exercise on acute leukemia patients undergoing treatment (Cunningham et al. 1986; Chang et al. 2008; Battaglini et al. 2009). Cunningham and colleagues (1986) conducted the first study examining the effects of a physical therapy program in patients undergoing bone marrow transplantation for acute leukemia. This small, randomized clinically controlled trial used three groups: a control group (no physical therapy), a physical therapy group twice a week (PT3), and a physical therapy group 5 times a week (PT5). Patients participated in the program for approximately 35 days. The physical therapy comprised resistive exercises. The main end point of the study was to examine the impact of resistive exercise on muscle protein status and turnover. The results showed that the exercise groups demonstrated a superior muscle protein status and turnover when compared to the control group. However, this pioneering study failed to demonstrate the real effect of the exercise intervention due to many limitations noted by the authors. Variability in the sample, improper nutritional support and control, a high patient dropout rate, and indirect measures of muscle protein were among the major study issues contributing to the difficulty in interpreting the results of the study.

The second exercise intervention study conducted in acute leukemia patients was a small randomized controlled clinical trial by Chang and colleagues (2008) who examined the effects of a walking protocol in a group of 22 patients diagnosed with and undergoing treatment for acute myelogenous leukemia (AML). Eleven

Table 12.2 Exercise intervention studies conducted in patients with multiple myeloma

Authors	Sample	Age	Design	Exercise Intervention	Duration	Frequency/intensity	Results
Coleman et al. (2003)	24 patients with MM in- treatment (HDC and PBST)	55 (range42–74) years	Two Groups RCT	Tx group: Home-based combined aerobic EX (walk, run, or cycling) and resistance Ex training (stretch bands with varying resistance); C group: Usual care	24 weeks	Tx group: 18 min of aerobic Ex (fast pace walk- primary Ex) at RPE between 12–15; resistance training at intensities based on different stretch bands with intensity adjusted based on patients' fatigue level; C group: walk 3/week for 20 min	Tx group improvement:↑ LBM (Average change) 0.1; ↑ 1RM (Average change) 2.4; ↓ total time on treadmill test (Average change) −0.6; and ↑ in sleep time. C group: ↓ LBM (Average change) −3.6; ↓ 1RM (Average change) −12.6; ↓ total time on treadmill test (Average change) −3.3. No adverse events due to Ex reported

Coleman et al. (2008)	120 patients with MM in-treatment (HDC and PBST). All patients received prophylactic EPO; In-treatment	55 (range32–74) years	Two Groups RCT	Tx group: Home-based combined stretching, aerobic, and resistance Ex training; UA group: Advised to walk 3/week	15 weeks	Tx group: Stretching (hamstring, shoulder, calves, hip flexors, and triceps), walking to tolerance, resistance training w/ stretch bands, and 1 chair exercise (chair stand) performed daily; UA group: walk 20 min/day	↓ in number of RBC transfusions and ↓ attempts at stem cell collection. Complications during the study reported but due to treatment and previous medical history and not directly associated with Ex

Ex Exercise, *MM* Multiple myeloma, *HDC* High-dose chemotherapy, *PBST* Peripheral blood stem cell transplantation ASCR, *Tx* treatment, *UC* Usual care, *RPE* Rate of perceived exertion, *LBM* Lean body mass, *EPO* Epoetin alfa, *RBC* Red blood cell, *RCT* Randomized controlled clinical trial patients were assigned to participate in a walking exercise program (treatment group) while the other 11 received usual care (the same amount of nurse visitations the walking group received but no intervention was administered). The walking program used as the intervention included 12 min of walking in the hospital hallway, 5 days per week for 3 weeks at an intensity of resting heart rate plus 30 beats per minute. Significant improvement in the distance walked during a 12-min walk test was observed for patients in the walking group while a decline was observed for the control group by the end of the study. A significant increase in fatigue level was observed in the control group throughout the study while no change was seen in the walking group. Also, symptom distress was significantly decreased in the walking group. Marginal differences in anxiety between groups were also observed with the walking group experiencing less than the control group. No difference in depressive status was observed between the groups. Chang and colleagues concluded that it was feasible to conduct a walking program in-hospital during the treatment of AML patients. The researches also suggested that a simple walking intervention may promote physical and psychological benefits and should be encouraged for AML patients undergoing treatment.

In the latest trial conducted in patients diagnosed with acute leukemia, Battaglini et al. (2009) examined the feasibility of administering a combined aerobic and resistance training exercise program in a group of 10 AML patients during the initial induction phase of treatment. The exercise program was administered 3–4 times per week with 36 hours of rest in between each training session for approximately 4 weeks in-hospital, and 3 times per week for 2 weeks at home. Each in-hospital exercise session was divided into 2 bouts. One bout was administered in the morning and the second late in the afternoon. A 30-min combination of aerobic exercise (performed on a recumbent cycle ergometer at low intensities varying from 40–50% of heart rate reserve) and resistance training using stretch bands, dumbbells, and free weights, with intensities monitored using the CR10 Borg modified perceived exertion scale never passing 5 (moderate), was used. Each patient's room was furnished with a recumbent cycle ergometer, treadmill, stretch bands, free weights, and a fitness ball. The equipment never left the room nor was it shared between patients. For the 2 week home-based intervention, patients were instructed to adhere to a walking protocol 3 times per week for a minimum of 10 and maximum of 30 min at a comfortable, moderate walking pace per exercise session. Not only did Battaglini et al. confirm the feasibility of AML patients exercising while receiving treatment as reported by Chang et al. (2008), but also reported significant improvement in total time on cycle ergometer, improvements in lower body muscular endurance, as well as reduction in fatigue and depression scores at the end of the study intervention. Contrary to Chang et al. (2008) a reduction in depression reported by Battaglini and colleagues may be explained by the more comprehensive, longer duration, and frequency of the exercise training protocol used in the study. In agreement with Chang's study, no major complications were observed during the exercise program. Table 12.3 presents the summary of the exercise intervention studies conducted in patients with acute leukemia.

The overall results presented by these three trials are promising and warrant further research. However, the need for more preliminary information regarding the effects of exercise in patients with other types of leukemia, for example, acute lymphoblastic leukemia (ALL), is needed. Now that the feasibility has been examined suggesting that acute leukemia patients can tolerate an exercise program and that they may even benefit from it, the exploration of direct measures of fitness performance such as maximal oxygen consumption tests, muscular strength tests, and precise evaluation of body

Table 12.3 Exercise intervention studies conducted in patients with acute leukemia

Authors	Sample	Age	Design	Exercise Intervention	Duration	Frequency/intensity	Results
Cunningham et al. (1986)	40 patients with AML and ALL During BMT	Tx groups: (PT3) 20.8 (Range14–33) Years (PT5) 26.0 (Range15–38) Years C group: 22.5 (Range15–41) Years	Three Groups RCT	Tx groups (PT3 and PT5): Physical therapy using resistive EX C group: UC, no Ex	4 weeks	Tx groups (Pt3 and PT5): Resistive exercise with 15 repetitions of 9 different exercises for approximately 30 min per Ex session	↓ in muscle protein in the control group. Protein-sparing effect observed in Tx groups; 10 patients at the end of the study were not able to be evaluated; 5 patients refused to continue on the study; 5 patients were not able to complete the study because of medical complications
Chang et al. (2008)	22 patients with AML; In-treatment	Tx group: 49.4 (15.3) years; C group: 53.3 (13.6) years	Two Groups RCT	Tx group: Walking Ex program; C group: UC, no Ex	3 weeks	Tx group: Walking Ex training program 5/ week at RHR + 30 BPM.	Tx group: ↑ in total distance walked, ↓ symptom distress ↔ of fatigue levels throughout study, C group: ↓ in total distance walked and ↑ in fatigue. Two patients dropped out from study because of disease complications. No adverse events due to Ex reported

(*continued*)

Table 12.3 (continued)

Authors	Sample	Age	Design	Exercise Intervention	Duration	Frequency/intensity	Results
Battaglini et al. (2009)	8 patients with AML; In-treatment	35.7 (8.9) years	Single Group	Supervised combined aerobic (cycle ergometer and/or treadmill) and resistance Ex training + home based aerobic exercise training (walking) during the last two weeks of study	6 weeks	Aerobic Ex training 4/ week 5–10 min in morning and 5–10 min in afternoon at 40–50% of HRR, resistance Ex training with dumbbells and resistance bands, exercise balls at RPE 5- moderate); home based walking Ex program for 2 weeks after hospital released (at conclu sion of first induction) for 10–30 min	↑ in total time of cycle ergometer, ↔ in overall muscular endurance, and ↓ fatigue and depression. Trend of ↓ in IL-6 and ↑ IL-10 with ↔ in IFN-γ. No adverse events due to Ex reported

Ex Exercise, *AML* Acute myelogenous leukemia, *Tx* treatment, *C* control, *PT3* Treatment group that received physical therapy 2/week, *PT5* Treatment group that received physical therapy 5/week, *UA* Usual activity, *UC* Usual care, *BMT* Bone marrow transplant, *HRR* Heart rate reserve, *RHR* Resting heart rate, *BPM* Beats per min, *RPE* Rate of perceived exertion; *RCT* Randomized controlled clinical trial; *IL-6* Interleukin 6, *IL-10* Interleukin 10 Interferon Gamma composition should be considered in the next generation of studies. The administration of different exercise modes and intensities would improve the current body of knowledge on the effects of exercise in acute leukemia patients undergoing treatment. Studies exploring different exercise protocols are needed before a large randomized controlled clinical trial can be conducted with the highest scientific rigor in this patient population.

12.3.4 Studies Conducted in Patients with Lymphoma

In 2003, Oldervoll and colleagues conducted the first trial examining the effects of an exercise program in patients with Hodgkin lymphoma. The purpose of this study was twofold: first, to compare the aerobic capacity between Hodgkin lymphoma patients with and without fatigue; second, to test the feasibility of administering a 20-week home-based aerobic exercise program at intensities between 65% and 80% of target heart rate. Patients could choose their exercise mode, which included brisk walking, jogging, bicycling, aerobics, cross-country skiing, or swimming. Even though the exercise intervention protocol in the study, as in any home-based protocol, may have lacked the rigorous control provided by a supervised intervention, significant improvements in aerobic capacity (VO_{2max}) and fatigue, approximately a 43% reduction, were observed post intervention. These results suggest that a home-based intervention may be a good venue for clinicians looking to improve aerobic fitness while reducing fatigue levels in patients. The small sample size, the unsupervised nature of the intervention, and the lack of a control group in the study design are all limitations that hinder the understanding of the effects of the exercise intervention on the endpoints of the study. Nevertheless, this study provided the initial information on the possible effects of a home-based exercise intervention in a group of patients with lymphoma.

In one of the most recent exercise studies involving patients with hematological cancer, Courneya et al. (2009) conducted the largest trial currently available in the literature; a randomized controlled clinical trial involving 122 patients diagnosed with Hodgkin and non-Hodgkin lymphoma. The patient-rated physical function was the primary endpoint of the study. Quality of life, fatigue, happiness, depression, anxiety, lymphoma symptoms, and general health were also analyzed. Fitness outcomes measured included maximal oxygen consumption (VO_{2peak}) and body composition. Patients were assigned to either a treatment group (aerobic exercise) or to a control group (no exercise above the baseline level). The aerobic exercise group performed on a recumbent cycle ergometer 3 times per week for 12 weeks. The exercise intensity progressed from 65% of peak power output, obtained from the VO_{2peak} test conducted at baseline, in increments of 5% weekly to 75% by week 4 of training. At the conclusion of aerobic training, a six-month-long follow-up was conducted. Superior improvements in VO_{2peak}, body composition (increase in lean body mass and reduction in fat mass) was observed in the exercise group when compared to the control group. The improvement in VO_{2peak} mediated changes in physical function measured by the TOI-An with borderline mediation on fatigue. No mediation of VO_{2peak} on happiness or depression was observed. The six-month follow up revealed that the effects of aerobic exercise appeared to favor the exercise group on patient-rated physical function when compared to the control group. However, no statistical significance was reached on changes in patient-rated physical function between groups. This is the largest trial conducted in patients with hematological cancer to date. The methodologically sound design and scientific rigor of this trial is a substantial step forward in the area of exercise and hematological cancers. Courneya and colleagues were able to demonstrate the positive impact of a supervised controlled aerobic exercise intervention on the alleviation of treatment-related side effects while improving overall physical function in lymphoma patients (those undergoing treatment and those who have completed treatment). The authors also suggested that the intervention used in the study did not interfere with medical treatment and should be considered as an intervention in lymphoma patients. Table 12.4 below presents the summary of the exercise intervention studies conducted in patients with lymphoma.

The results of these two trials presented above provide the evidence necessary for the development of future experiments examining the effects of exercise in lymphoma patients. Once again, more research is needed to continue exploring different exercise protocols. Perhaps the combination of aerobic exercise with resistance training, and exercise protocols designed with different intensities (mode, frequency, and duration) should be considered in future experiments involving lymphoma patients. Markers of inflammation associated with poor prognosis and the effects of exercise on immune function should also be considered.

12.4 Summary

Patients diagnosed with hematological cancers undergo heavy doses of chemotherapy, in some cases combined with radiation therapy, and ultimately bone marrow transplantation. The chance for relapse-free survival is dependant on the ability of the patients to tolerate treatment. Treatment is often associated with significant decline in physical and psychological function. This decline can greatly influence treatment prognosis and make it difficult for patients to resume physical and psychological activity after treatment completion. An attractive intervention that has proven to positively impact the physiology and psychology of cancer patients is exercise. However, the examination of its effects on patients with hematological cancers is in its infancy. Eighteen trials have been conducted to date examining the effects of exercise in such patients. Most studies, however, present methodological limitations including small sample sizes, indirect measures of physical fitness, and lack of true control groups for comparisons. Out of 18 studies, 11 have used a mixed population of patients with different hematological cancer, almost half of the studies have examined the effects of exercise post treatment, and only one has used a larger sample in a randomized controlled trial using objective/direct measures of physical and psychological function (Courneya et al. 2009). Nevertheless, the sparse literature currently available in the area of exercise and hematological cancer suggests that exercise can be safely administered and may positively impact aerobic condition, muscular fitness, body composition, fatigue, depression, and quality of life; all clinically relevant endpoints that may be associated with treatment tolerability and an increase in survival. Therefore, exercise training may prove in the future to be an important component in the overall care of patients diagnosed with hematological cancers. More research is needed to confirm or refute the results of these first 18 experiments.

12.5 Clinical Recommendations

As presented in this chapter, few studies have examined the effects of exercise in patients diagnosed with hematological cancers while undergoing treatment as well as those who have completed treatment and are in remission of

Table 12.4 Exercise intervention studies conducted in patients with lymphoma

Authors	Sample	Age	Design	Exercise intervention	Duration	Frequency/ intensity	Results
Oldervoll et al. (2003)	9 patients with HL; Post-treatment	41 ± 11.3 years	Single Group	Home-based aerobic Ex (brisk walk, jogging, cycling, or swimming)	20 weeks	40–60 min of continuous aerobic Ex at 65%–80% of TRH, 3/week	↓ in total fatigue (43% of baseline value); VO_{2max} ↑ 2.1 mL.kg.min and total time on treadmill ↑ 1min 50sec of baseline value. No adverse events due to Ex reported
Courneya et al. (2009)	122 patients with Lymphoma (n-RL and RL); Both, in and off-treatment	Tx Group 52.8 (Range 18–77) yearsUC group 53.5 (range18–80) years	Two Groups RCT	Tx group: Supervised aerobic Ex training on cycle ergometer; UC group: Usual care, no exercise beyond baseline	12 weeks	Tx group: Aerobic Ex training, 3/week initiated at 60% of VO_{2peak} and increased 5% each week to 75% by week 4. Duration of training started at 15–20 min	Superior improvement in physical function, LBM, fatigue, depression, happiness, overall QOL of Tx group over UC group. ↑ CF (VO_{2peak}) more than 20% observed in Tx

(continued)

Table 12.4 (continued)

Authors	Sample	Age	Design	Exercise intervention	Duration	Frequency/intensity	Results
						first 4 weeks and progressed 5 min per week to 40–45 min by week 9. Interval training above VT implemented on weeks 7 and 9.	group. No serious adverse events; however, 3 adverse events (orthopedic problems) were reported with one subject withdrawing from the study

Ex Exercise, *UC* Usual care, no Ex, *HL* Hodgkin lymphoma, *n-HL* Non-Hodgkin lymphoma, HR_{max} Maximal heart rate, *Tx* treatment, *UC* Usual care, VO_{2peak} Maximal oxygen consumption patient attained during test, *THR* Target heart rate, *VT* Ventilatory threshold, *RCT* Randomized controlled clinical trial, *CF* Cardiorespiratory fitness, *QOL* Quality of life, LBM Lean body mass their disease. Nevertheless, studies conducted to date are encouraging and present promising results regarding the possible benefits that exercise can provide to patients with hematological cancers. Below are recommendations for clinicians, health care providers, and exercise specialists on exercise specifics (mode, frequency, duration), and precautionary measures that should be taken into consideration when exercising patients with hematological cancers. The information below is based on current research findings and should be interpreted as preliminary recommendations only in an attempt for the administration of safe and effective exercise programs to patients with hematological cancers.

Most of the study findings have shown that administering exercise to patients with hematological cancers undergoing treatment or after treatment completion appears to be safe and that both physical and psychological benefits can be attained from a regular exercise training program. The frequencies of exercise training in the current literature vary from 2 to 5 days per week; however, the frequency should be adjusted based on the patient's health condition prior to each exercise training session. Exercise intensities should also be adjusted weekly or perhaps daily based on the physical health of the patient prior to each training session; since fatigue and physical complications commonly experienced by patients with hematological cancer is very likely to occur. Therefore, it is recommend that at the initiation of an exercise training program, health care providers should begin with 2 days per week, and as the patient improves physical fitness progress to more days of training per week. Even though a few trials have been conducted in an unsupervised setting (home-based interventions), for patients undergoing treatment (even for those treated as an outpatient) it is recommend that all exercise sessions should be supervised. Exercise intensities varying from 40–70% of maximum heart rate for cardiovascular workouts, and 7–10 different resistance exercises (targeting full body) with 2–3 repetitions between 8 and 12 (to fatigue) seems to elicit favorable outcomes. Based on empirical evidence, a combination of aerobic and resistance exercise should be considered helpful to mitigate the side effects of treatment. The mode of aerobic exercise can vary and should be considered based on the physical abilities and limitations of each patient. Treadmills, cycle ergometer, elliptical machines, and walking outdoors are great options for aerobic workouts. For patients' in-hospital/in-treatment, the use of resistance exercise should be used more often since resistance exercise in other clinical populations has been shown to minimize the loss of muscular mass and to maintain overall functionality – both conditions that commonly impact these patients during treatment. Since hematological cancer patients are confined to hospital rooms for weeks during specific phases of their treatment, resistance exercises could be performed in their own hospital rooms with dumbbells, resistance bands with different resistance, and through exercises using the patients' own body weight (Battaglini et al. 2009).

Although the recommendations above should give health care providers a starting point regarding the prescription of exercise for patients with hematological cancers, one needs to keep in mind that due to the nature of hematological cancers and harsh treatment protocols, these patients are at a very high risk for infection and other health complications. From a comprehensive screening process for participation in an exercise program (see Jones et al. 2008 for recommendations of health screening and fitness testing) to the administration of exercise prescription, strict neutropenic procedures, variation and adaptation of exercise prescription, and regular communication with the oncologist must be standard practice to ensure safety and hopefully a successful exercise program.

12

12.6 Future Research Directions

Large randomized controlled clinical trials are necessary to continue the exploration of the effects of exercise on patients with hematological malignancies. More specifically, studies designed to explore different modes, frequency, and intensity of exercise, using homogeneous samples of patients to allow for a better understanding of disease-specific responses to exercise, and objective and direct evaluation of physical parameters are needed. Investigations studying the effects of exercise on the duration of hospitalization, the number of blood transfusion and treatment complications, markers of inflammation associated with poor treatment outcomes, and the effects on immune function are also needed and should be considered in the next generation of studies. Furthermore, study protocols exploring the use of exercise in-hospital, while patients are undergoing treatment, in patients who have completed treatment and are waiting to receive bone marrow transplantation must be explored.

References

Galvão DA, Taaffe DR, Spry N et al (2010 Jan 10) Combined resistance and aerobic exercise program reverses muscle loss in men undergoing androgen suppression therapy for prostate cancer without bone metastases: a randomized controlled trial. J Clin Oncol 28(2):340–347

Schwartz AL, Winters-Stone K (2009 Oct) Effects of a 12-month randomized controlled trial of aerobic or resistance exercise during and following cancer treatment in women. Phys Sportsmed 37(3):62–67

Courneya KS, McKenzie DC, Mackey JR et al (2008a) Moderators of the effects of exercise training in breast cancer patients receiving chemotherapy: a randomized controlled trial. Cancer 112(8):1845–1853

Courneya KS, Segal RJ, Mackey JR et al (2007 Oct 1) Effects of aerobic and resistance exercise in breast cancer patients receiving adjuvant chemotherapy: A multicenter randomized controlled trial. J Clin Oncol 25(28):4396–4404

Galvão DA, Spry N, Taaffe DR et al (2009 Dec 2) A randomized controlled trial of an exercise intervention targeting cardiovascular and metabolic risk factors for prostate cancer patients from the RADAR trial. BMC Cancer 9:419

Segal RJ, Reid RD, Courneya KS et al (2009 Jan 20) Randomized controlled trial of resistance or aerobic exercise in men receiving radiation therapy for prostate cancer. J Clin Oncol 27(3): 344–351

Courneya KS, Jones LW, Peddle CJ et al (2008b) Effects of aerobic exercise training in anemic cancer patients receiving darbepoetin alfa: a randomized controlled trial. Oncologist 13(9): 1012–1020

Ligibel JA, Campbell N, Partridge A et al (2008 Feb 20) Impact of a mixed strength and endurance exercise intervention on insulin levels in breast cancer survivors. J Clin Oncol 26(6):907–912

Schmitz KH, Ahmed RL, Hannan PJ et al (2005a) Safety and efficacy of weight training in recent breast cancer survivors to alter body composition, insulin, and insulin-like growth factor axis proteins. Cancer Epidemiol Biomark Prev 14(7): 1672–80

Fairey AS, Courneya KS, Field CJ et al (2005 Apr) Randomized controlled trial of exercise and blood immune function in postmenopausal breast cancer survivors. J Appl Physiol 98(4): 1534–1540

Speck RM, Courneya KS, Mâsse LC, et al. (2010) An update of controlled physical activity trials in cancer survivors: a systematic review and meta-analysis. *J Cancer Surviv*. Jan 6 [Epub ahead of print]

Jones LW, Demark-Wahnefried W (Dec 2006) Diet, exercise, and complementary therapies after primary treatment for cancer. Lancet Oncol 7(12): 1017–1026

McNeely ML, Campbell KL, Rowe BH et al (Jul 4 2006) Effects of exercise on breast cancer patients and survivors: a systematic review and meta-analysis. CMAJ 175(1):34–41

Markes M, Brockow T, Resch KL. Exercise for women receiving adjuvant therapy for breast cancer. Cochrane Database Syst Rev 2006(4): CD005001

Schmitz KH, Holtzman J, Courneya KS et al (Jul 2005b) Controlled physical activity trials in cancer survivors: A systematic review and meta-analysis. Cancer Epidemiol Biomark Prev 14(7): 1588–1595

Galvão DA, Newton RU (2005 Feb 1) Review of exercise intervention studies in cancer patients. J Clin Oncol 23(4):899–909

The Leukemia and Lymphoma Society Website [Internet]. White Plains, NY: The Leukemia & Lymphoma Society, Accessed on 01/09/2010

Irwin ML, Smith AW, McTiernan A et al (2008 Aug 20) Influence of pre- and postdiagnosis physical activity on mortality in breast cancer survivors: the health, eating, activity, and lifestyle study. J Clin Oncol 26(24):3958–3964

Meyerhardt JA, Heseltine D, Niedzwiecki D et al (2006 Aug 1) Impact of physical activity on cancer recurrence and survival in patients with stage III colon cancer: Findings from CALGB 89803. J Clin Oncol 24(22):3535–3541

Demark-Wahnefried W (2006 Aug 1) Cancer survival: Time to get moving? Data accumulate suggesting a link between physical activity and cancer survival. J Clin Oncol 24(22):3517–3518

Cunningham BA, Morris G, Cheney CL et al (1986 Nov–Dec) Effects of resistive exercise on skeletal muscle in marrow transplant recipients receiving total parenteral nutrition. J Parenter Enteral Nutr 10(6):558–563

Decker WA, Turner-McGlade J, Fehir KM (1989) Psychosocial aspects and the physiological effects of a cardiopulmonary exercise program in patients undergoing bone marrow transplantation (BMT) for acute leukemia (AL). Transplant Proc 21(1 Pt 3):3068–3069

Dimeo F, Bertz H, Finke J et al (1996) An aerobic exercise program for patients with hematological malignancies after bone marrow transplantation. Bone Marrow Transplant 18(6): 1157–60

Dimeo F, Schwartz S, Fietz T et al (2003 Oct) Effects of endurance training on the physical performance of patients with hematological malignancies during chemotherapy. Support Care Cancer 11(10):623–628

Mello M, Tanaka C, Dulley FL (2003 Oct) Effects of an exercise program on muscle performance in patients undergoing allogeneic bone marrow transplantation. Bone Marrow Transplant 32(7): 723–728

Oldervoll LM, Kaasa S, Knobel H et al (2003 Jan) Exercise reduces fatigue in chronic fatigued Hodgkins disease survivors–results from a pilot study. Eur J Cancer 39(1):57–63

Coleman EA, Coon S, Hall-Barrow J et al (2003 Oct) Feasibility of exercise during treatment for multiple myeloma. Cancer Nurs 26(5): 410–419

Hayes SC, Davies PS, Parker TW et al (2004 Jun) Role of a mixed type, moderate intensity exercise programme after peripheral blood stem cell transplantation. Br J Sports Med 38(3):304–309, discussion 309

Wilson RW, Jacobsen PB, Fields KK (2005 Apr) Pilot study of a home-based aerobic exercise program for sedentary cancer survivors treated with hematopoietic stem cell transplantation. Bone Marrow Transplant 35(7):721–727

Carlson LE, Smith D, Russell J et al (2006 May) Individualized exercise program for the treatment of severe fatigue in patients after allogeneic hematopoietic stem-cell transplant: A pilot study. Bone Marrow Transplant 37(10): 945–954

Coleman EA, Coon SK, Kennedy RL et al (2008 May) Effects of exercise in combination with epoetin alfa during high-dose chemotherapy and autologous peripheral blood stem cell transplantation for multiple myeloma. Oncol Nurs Forum 35(3):E53–E61

Chang PH, Lai YH, Shun SC et al (2008 May) Effects of a walking intervention on fatigue related experiences of hospitalized acute myelogenous leukemia patients undergoing chemotherapy: A randomized controlled trial. J Pain Symptom Manage 35(5):524–534

Battaglini CL, Hackney AC, Garcia R et al (2009 Jun) The effects of an exercise program in leukemia patients. Integr Cancer Ther 8(2):130–138

Elter T, Stipanov M, Heuser E et al (2009) Is Physical exercise possible in patients with critical cytopenia undergoing intensive chemotherapy for acute leukaemia or aggressive lymphoma? Int J Hematol 90:199–204

Shelton ML, Lee JQ, Morris GS et al (2009 Apr) A randomized control trial of a supervised versus a self-directed exercise program for allogeneic stem cell transplant patients. Psychooncology 18(4):353–359

Jarden M, Baadsgaard MT, Hovgaard DJ et al (2009 May) A randomized trial on the effect of

12

a multimodal intervention on physical capacity, functional performance and quality of life in adult patients undergoing allogenic SCT. Bone Marrow Transplant 43(9):725–737

Courneya KS, Sellar CM, Stevinson C et al (2009 Sep 20) Randomized controlled trial of the effects of aerobic exercise on physical functioning and quality of life in lymphoma patients. J Clin Oncol 27(27):4605–4612

Baumann FT, Kraut L, Schüle K, et al. A controlled randomized study examining the effects of exercise therapy on patients undergoing haematopoietic stem cell transplantation. *Bone Marrow Transplant*. 2009 Jul 13 [Epub ahead of print]

Jones LW, Eves ND, Haykowsky M, Joy AA, Douglas PS (2008 Aug) Cardiorespiratory exercise testing in clinical oncology research: systematic review and practice recommendations. Lancet Oncology 9(8): 757–65

Physical Activity and Gynecologic Cancer Survivorship

13

Karen M. Gil and Vivian E. von Gruenigen

Abstract Gynecologic oncology involves the study of preinvasive disease and cancers of the vulva, vagina, cervix, uterus, ovaries, and gestational trophoblastic disease. Endometrial cancer is the most common of the pelvic malignancies however, ovarian cancer is the most lethal. The other gynecologic cancers have not been studied in relation to physical activity (PA) and prognosis, and therefore are not included. Research addressing the relationship between PA and ovarian and endometrial cancer is sparse nevertheless, there are some emerging concepts. Studies suggest that overweight/obesity is associated with reduced survival from ovarian cancer, but the role that PA plays in these results, and whether survival can be altered by changes in body weight and/or PA following diagnosis is unknown. Limited research reveals that increased PA in older ovarian cancer patients is feasible and safe. The majority of endometrial cancer patients are overweight or obese. Obesity is associated with higher mortality, probably from cardiovascular disease and not cancer. Research reveals that increasing PA in overweight/obese endometrial cancers is feasible and successful. The effects of increased PA on recurrence or survival in gynecological cancers are not yet established, and randomized controlled trials are needed for definitive data.

K.M. Gil
Akron General Medical Center, Akron, OH, USA and Northeastern Ohio Universities College of Medicine and Pharmacy, Rootstown, OH, USA

V.E. von Gruenigen (✉)
Northeastern Ohio Universities College of Medicine and Pharmacy, Rootstown, OH, USA and
Chair, Obstetrics and Gynecology,
Akron City and St. Thomas Hospitals, System Medical Director for Women's Health, Summa Health System Akron , OH, USA
e-mail: vongruev@summahealth.org

13.1 Introduction

Gynecologic oncology involves the study of preinvasive disease and cancers of the vulva, vagina, cervix, uterus, ovaries, and gestational trophoblastic disease. Endometrial cancer is the most common of the pelvic malignancies, however, ovarian cancer is the most lethal. Research addressing the relationship between physical activity (PA) and ovarian and endometrial cancer is sparse, nevertheless, there are some emerging concepts.

K.S. Courneya and C.M. Friedenreich (eds.), *Physical Activity and Cancer*, Recent Results in Cancer Research 186, DOI: 10.1007/978-3-642-04231-7_13,

13.2 Ovarian Cancer

In 2008, an estimated 21,650 new cases of ovarian cancer were diagnosed in the USA (www.cancer.org, accessed January 12, 2010). Ovarian cancer is primarily a disease of postmenopausal women and has an age-related increase in incidence; the median age of a patient with ovarian cancer is about 63 years (www.cancer.org, accessed January 12, 2010). Epithelial ovarian cancer is rarely diagnosed at an early stage because the disease causes few specific symptoms, particularly when it is localized to the ovary. Unlike breast and cervical cancers, there is no currently accepted screening tool to detect ovarian cancer at an early stage. The majority of patients present with a pelvic mass and undergo surgery. Surgery includes a total abdominal hysterectomy, bilateral salpin-go-oophorectomy, omentectomy, retroperitoneal lymph node sampling, inspection under the diaphragms, random biopsies, and peritoneal cavity washes. Premenopausal women, therefore, undergo surgical menopause.

Prognosis. Two conditions that affect prognosis are stage of disease and success in removing visible tumor (cytoreduction). The 5-year survival rates for women with Stages I, II, III and IV disease are 89%, 66%, 34% and 18%, and the majority are diagnosed with advanced stage disease (www.cancer.org, accessed January 12, 2010; Pomel et al. 2007). Survival is also greatly increased if only very small (less than 1 cm) amounts of tumor remain following surgery (Pomel et al. 2007; Winter et al. 2007). Thus, only 34% of women with Stage III disease will live for longer than 5 years, but prognosis is improved in those with success in removing visible tumor is removed successfully. These distinctions are important in discussing the potential effects of PA on survival as behavioral changes may be more likely to exert an effect in the setting of a more favorable prognosis.

First-Line Chemotherapy. Ovarian cancer is one of the most chemotherapy-sensitive malignancies, and adjuvant treatment has a strong impact on survival. Two adjuvant chemotherapy options include intravenous (IV) and intraperitoneal (IP) chemotherapy. A standard-dose regimen includes six cycles of outpatient IV chemotherapy with carboplatin and paclitaxel, every 21 days (Ozols 2006). Cisplatin-based IP chemotherapy has a demonstrated survival benefit in optimally cytoreduced patients with advanced ovarian cancer and is gradually becoming a standard of care (Armstrong et al. 2006). Median survival time for women treated with IV chemotherapy is approximately 40 months; for women receiving IP chemotherapy, it is around 66 months. Approximately 60–80% of women will respond to chemotherapy and experience a remission of disease (Markman 2008).

13.2.1 Recurrence and Survival

Unfortunately, the majority of patients will face a recurrence of disease (Markman 2008). Management may include surgery but typically involves several chemotherapy options. Although stage, histological type and degree of cytoreduction affect outcome (Pomel et al. 2007; Winter et al. 2007), these variables do not completely account for the differences in recurrence and ultimate survival, suggesting other variables are involved. A major research focus is to identify interactions between different types of tumors and chemotherapeutic agents in order to determine which agents are more likely to be effective for individual patients; however, another potentially important contributor to variability in time to recurrence is lifestyle factors (Bandera et al. 2009).

Obesity. The effects of obesity, level of PA, and exercise on survival are beginning to be explored, with much of the research conducted in breast cancer survivors (Irwin and Mayne

2008 ; Speed-Andrews and Courneya 2009; Speck et al. 2010). Physical activity and being overweight/obese are linked and often difficult to separate (Colditz and Coakley 1997). In a prospective study of women free from cancer at enrollment, the relative risk of death from ovarian cancer was increased in women who were overweight or obese (Calle et al. 2003; Rodriguez et al. 2002, Table 13.1). Obesity was found to be independently associated with reduced time to recurrence and shorter overall survival in women diagnosed with ovarian cancer in the USA (Pavelka et al. 2006). A prospective study of women with ovarian cancer conducted in Sweden found that women who had remained obese throughout life had a 68% increased risk of death (Yang et al. 2008 Table 13.1). A study of Danish women diagnosed with ovarian cancer found that women who had been overweight during the previous 5 years had an increased risk of death compa-red with normal weight women (Kjaerbye–Thaygesen et al. 2006, Table 13.1). A prospective study in China of women diagnosed with ovarian cancer also found that increased body mass index (BMI) 5 years prior to diagnosis was associated with reduced survival (Zhang et al. 2005, Table 13.1). These studies suggest that overweight/obesity is associated with reduced survival from ovarian cancer, but the role that PA plays in these results, and whether survival can be altered by changes in body weight and/or PA following diagnosis is unknown.

Health and Prognosis. Two additional areas related to PA that may affect survival are health related quality of life (QOL) and morbidity during treatment. A study examining ovarian cancer survivors found that those meeting public health guidelines for PA had lower self reported levels of fatigue, and better scores for peripheral neuropathy, depression, anxiety, and sleep quality than women not meeting guidelines (Stevinson et al. 2009). This study suggests that PA improves QOL, but this improved QOL may have greater consequences. QOL measured during treatment has been found to be a prognostic indicator for overall survival in women receiving chemotherapy for ovarian cancer (Wenzel et al. 2005). Women whose QOL scores were in the lowest quartile had reduced overall survival compared to women in the higher three quartiles (Wenzel et al. 2005). It is unknown if response to chemotherapy toxicity or continued underlying disease was responsible for this effect; however, a study of women undergoing gynecologic surgery found that baseline characteristics such physical and mental health, age, and body weight affect QOL scores (Gil et al. 2007). Thus, improved QOL, which is affected by overall health, may signal an increased ability to tolerate or respond to chemotherapy. To the extent that regular PA increases QOL and ability to tolerate surgery and chemotherapy, then enhanced PA may affect survival.

von Gruenigen presented results regarding newly diagnosed ovarian or peritoneal cancer patients receiving adjuvant IP or IV chemotherapy on a QOL lifestyle intervention trial (von Gruenigen et al. 2010). A registered dietitian met individually with patients at every chemotherapy visit for six cycles. They were counseled in PA and nutrition quality. Patients were given pedometers and instructed to walk and increase their PA every day. Assessments were obtained at entry to the study (postoperative visit), during chemotherapy (cycle 3), and after chemotherapy. QOL was measured with the Functional Assessment of Cancer Therapy-Ovarian (FACT-O), PA with the Leisure Score Index (LSI), symptom severity/distress by the Memorial symptom assessment scale (MSAS) and diet quality by 3-day food records. The mean age of the patients was 60 (SD = 9.2, range 45–76). The median number of minutes/week spent in PA was 150 min during chemotherapy (range: 45–350 min/week). Following chemotherapy, patients reported a median of 130 min of PA/week. Median LSI score was 6 at baseline and increased to 12 during chemotherapy and 18 following

13

Table 13.1 Effect of BMI on mortality from ovarian cancer

Authors (reference)	Sample	Design	Results
Calle et al. (2003); Rodriguez et al. (2002) (Data from Rodriguez et al. 2002)	300,537 US women who were free of cancer at enrollment in 1982; followed for 16 years. There were 1,511 deaths from ovarian cancer	Prospective study	Ovarian cancer mortality rates were higher among overweight (BMI ≥ 25: RR, 1.16, 95% CI, 1.04–1.30) and obese women (BMI ≥ 30: RR, 1.26, 95% CI, 1.07–1.48) compared with women with BMI < 25, p for trend = 0.001
Pavelka et al. (2006)	216 women undergoing primary cytoreductive surgery for EOC in Los Angeles, CA between 1996 and 2003	Retrospective review	In a subcohort of 146 patients with Stage III or IV disease, a significant trend was identified, favoring increased BMI as an independent negative factor for disease free (p = 0.02) and overall (p = 0.02) survival
Yang et al. (2008)	635 women with a new histologically confirmed diagnosis of EOC in Sweden between 1993 and 1995; followed for 7–9 years	Prospective follow-up of women indentified in a national wide, population-based case-control study	Women who remained obese throughout life had a 68% increased risk of death (HR, 1.7, 95% CI, 1.1–2.6) relative to women who remained normal weight throughout life
Kjaerbye-Thygesen et al. (2006)	295 Danish women with stage III EOC diagnosed between 1994 and 1999; followed for a median of 7.3 years	Prospective follow-up of women identified in a population-based case-control study	Women who were overweight (BMI ≥ 25) over the 5 years prior to diagnosis had an increased risk of ovarian cancer death (HR, 1.83, 95% CI, 1.38–2.42) compared with normal weight women (BMI 18.5–24.9)
Zhang et al. (2005)	207 women from Hangzhou, China diagnosed with EOC after surgery in 1999–2000; followed for 3–4 years	Prospective follow-up of women identified in a population-based case-control study	Reduced survival was observed among patients with BMI ≥ 25 versus <25 at 5 years before diagnosis (p = 0.001)

EOC Epithelial ovarian cancer, *RR* Relative risk, *CI* Confidence interval, *HR* Hazard ratios

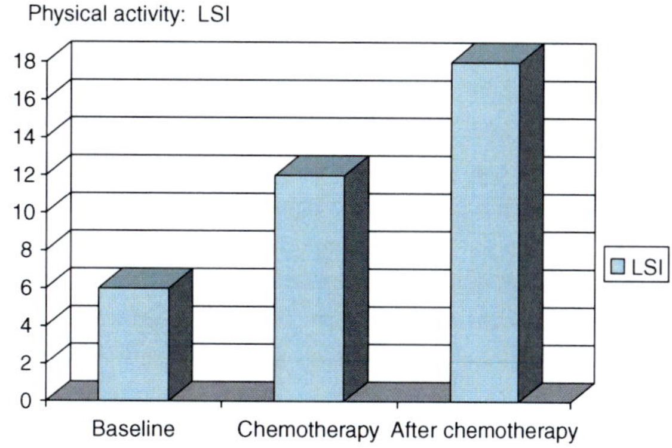

Fig. 13.1 Physical activity as measured by the Leisure Score Index (LSI)

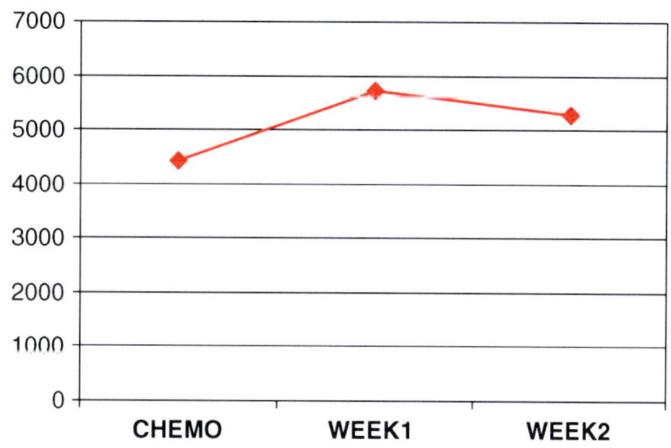

Fig. 13.2 Pedometer steps during chemotherapy cycled every 21 days

chemotherapy (Fig. 13.1). Median number of steps during the chemotherapy administration week was 4,433, week 1 following chemotherapy was 5,738, and 2 weeks following chemotherapy 5,287 ($p = 0.05$ for change from week 1–3) (Fig. 13.2). Median number of steps during cycles 1–5 was 4,235, 5,161, 6,123, 5,611 and 5,256. Emotional and functional well-being scores increased linearly during chemotherapy and following chemotherapy compared to baseline ($p = .021$). Total FACT-G increased in a similar fashion ($p = .05$).

13.2.2 Clinical Recommendations

While PA and cancer outcomes are more prominent in other primary cancers, it could be inferred that ovarian cancer patients may derive the same benefits. Certainly, the above study supports the feasibility of exercise during adjuvant chemotherapy in an elderly population. In addition, since QOL is a predictor for survival and PA has the potential to increase QOL, the question remains as to whether increased PA could improve overall survival (Wenzel et al. 2005). Therefore, ovarian cancer patients should follow the American Cancer Society's guidelines to accumulate at least 150 min of moderate-to-strenuous, or 60 min of strenuous, PA per week (Doyle et al. 2006) .

13.2.3 Future Research Directions

While ovarian cancer is very responsive to chemotherapeutic agents, an important component of survival is recurrence. Development of biologic targeted treatment modalities to prevent recurrence is a key line of research; however, modifications in lifestyle that could affect recurrence are also being investigated, especially as the time in remission increases due to effective first-line treatments. Understanding that all women are not equally able to tolerate treatment and providing support during what is often very rigorous treatment may increase treatment effectiveness. A promising line of research is the identification of QOL items that may signal reduced ability to optimally undergo treatment (Gil et al. 2007; von Gruenigen et al. 2009).

13.3 Endometrial Cancer

Endometrial carcinoma is the most common gynecologic malignancy in the USA with 40,100 woman diagnosed and 7,470 dying of this disease in 2008 (www.cancer.org, accessed January 12, 2010). Half of all cases are diagnosed in women aged 50–69 (www.cancer.org, accessed January 12, 2010).

Risk Factor. The main risk factor is obesity; about half of all cases in postmenopausal women are attributable to being overweight or obese (Reeves et al. 2007). In a study of 1.2 million women enrolled in the Million Women Study in the UK, the relative risk of developing endometrial cancer was 2.73 (95% CI, 2.55–2.92) in women with a BMI ≥ 30 relative to women of normal weight (BMI between 22.5 and 24.9) (Reeves et al. 2007). Data from over 32,000 women ≥45 years old participating in the Women's Health Study confirmed the relationship between BMI and risk of endometrial cancer (Conroy et al. 2009). The authors of this study also found that leisure time PA and walking were unrelated to risk, although women reporting any vigorous activity had lower risk than those reporting none. A large, prospective cohort study of over 250,000 women 35–70 years old at enrollment from nine European countries found little association between PA and endometrial cancer risk, although a potential risk reduction in premenopausal women was identified (Friedenreich et al. 2007). Data from the NIH-AARP Diet and Health Study of over 100,000 women 50–71 years old were analyzed to examine the relationship between PA and risk for endometrial cancer (Gierach et al. 2009). The authors found a dose-response relationship between vigorous activity and endometrial cancer risk but no association with light/moderate, daily routine, or occupational physical activities. The association between vigorous PA and endometrial cancer risk was more pronounced among women who were overweight or obese (RR, 0.61, 95% CI: 0.47–0.79 for women with BMI ≥ 25 who exercised vigorously five or more times/week versus never or rarely). The relationship between PA and endometrial cancer risk was also examined in the American Cancer Society Cancer Prevention Study II Nutrition Cohort of over 40,000 postmenopausal women (Patel et al. 2008). They found that light and moderate Physical activities (PA) were associated with lower endometrial cancer risk, although BMI attenuated the association. Physical activity was strongly associated with reduced risk in overweight and obese women in this study (RR, 0.59, 95% CI 0.42 – 0.83 for > 17.5 MET-h/week versus < 7 MET-h/week).

The extent to which differences in level of PA contribute to endometrial cancer risk are not clear, nor is the relationship between PA, BMI and risk of endometrial cancer. In contrast, the relationship with BMI is clear. Regardless of the direct effect of PA on endometrial cancer risk, women should be encouraged to maintain appropriate levels of PA to help maintain body weight (Conroy et al. 2009).

Prognosis. In contrast to ovarian cancer, endometrial cancer is typically found at early stages due to early onset of symptoms, notably postmenopausal bleeding, and the 5-year survival rate for women diagnosed at this early stage is over 95% (www.cancer.org, accessed January 12 2010). Treatment is primarily surgical (hysterectomy, bilateral salpingo-oophorectomy, washing, and lymph node sampling) followed in some cases with adjuvant radiotherapy and/or chemotherapy. As the majority of cases are diagnosed in the early stage, surgical treatment is generally curative and recurrence is rare. However, obesity is still associated with reduced survival (Table 13.2). The highest relative risk of death identified in women was from endometrial cancer for women with a BMI greater than 40 relative to normal weight women in a prospective study of women who were free of cancer at enrollment (Calle et al. 2003, Table 13.2). Data from the Million Women Study supported this relationship (Reeves et al. 2007, Table 13.2).

A recent Gynecologic Oncology Group study examined this relationship in women with early-stage endometrial cancer and found obesity was associated with higher mortality (Table 13.2); however, it appeared to be due to causes other than endometrial cancer and not disease recurrence (von Gruenigen et al. 2006). A review of five Gynecologic Oncology Group trials in women with advanced or recurrent endometrial cancer found increasing BMI was associated with increased risk of death in women with Stage III/IV disease (Table 13.2), but not in women with recurrent disease (Modesitt et al. 2007). Many endometrial patients suffer from obesity related comorbidities such as diabetes, hypertension, heart disease, and pulmonary disease, which may lead to increased mortality following surgical treatment (Fader et al. 2009).

13.3.1 Quality of Life

Quality of life is compromised in endometrial cancer survivors, but not for the same reasons as ovarian cancer patients. A recent ancillary analysis of two prospective endometrial cancer QOL trials revealed scores were similar to normative data in age-matched women without cancer (Fader et al. 2008). When considering increasing BMI, analysis revealed a significant decrease in the physical component and the functional domains based on increasing weight. BMI was inversely correlated with functional, physical, and social well-being and with several decreases in line items within the functional domain, including ability at work and being content. BMI also had an inverse relationship with the "lack of energy" item in the physical domain. Fatigue was present in nearly 30% of survivors and increased as weight increased.

Lack of exercise and obesity are associated with lower QOL in endometrial cancer survivors. A survey of 386 Canadian endometrial cancer survivors found lack of exercise and excess body weight exacerbated treatment-related declines in QOL (Courneya et al. 2005). Roughly 70% of the women surveyed were obese and were not meeting public health exercise guidelines. Multiple linear regression analysis demonstrated that both exercise ($p < 0.001$) and BMI ($p < 0.001$) were independently associated with QOL. A survey of 120 endometrial cancer survivors diagnosed within 5 years in the USA demonstrated that reports of pain and fatigue decreased linearly, while physical functioning increased linearly, with level of PA (Basen-Engquist et al. 2009).

von Gruenigen and colleagues conducted a prospective observational trial in 43 newly diagnosed endometrial patients, 86% of whom were obese, which assessed diet, exercise, and complementary medicine use preoperatively and 6 months postoperatively (von Gruenigen et al. 2005). No study interventions were performed to modify behaviors. Weight, exercise, and fruit and vegetable intake did not change over time; however, complementary/alternative medicine use increased significantly at 6 months ($P = 0.008$). Although small, this study highlighted an important observation that may apply

13

Table 13.2 Effect of BMI on mortality from endometrial cancer

Authors (Ref)	Sample	Design	Results
Calle et al. (2003)	495,477 women US women who were free of cancer at enrollment in 1982 and were followed for 16 years. There were 704 deaths from endometrial cancer	Prospective study	Endometrial cancer mortality rates were higher among overweight and obese women relative to normal weight women: (BMI 25.0–29.9, RR 1.50, 95% CI 1.26–1.78; BMI 30.0–34.9, RR 2.53, 95% CI 2.02–3.18; BMI 35.0–39.9, RR 2.77, 95% CI 1.83–4.18; BMI ≥ 40.0, RR 6.25, 95% CI 3.75–10.42), p for trend < 0.001
Reeves et al. (2007)	1, 222, 630 UK women aged 50–64 during 1996–2001, and followed up, on average, for 7.0 years for cancer mortality. There were 236 deaths from endometrial cancer	Prospective study	Endometrial cancer mortality rates were higher among overweight and obese women relative to normal weight women: (BMI 25–27.4, FAR 1.09, 95% FCI 0.82–1.45; BMI 27.5–29.5, FAR 1.21, 95% FCI 0.85–1.71; BMI ≥ 30, FAR 2.28, 95% FCI 1.81–2.87), $p < 0.001$
von Gruenigen et al. (2006)	380 women with early-stage endometrial cancer in a randomized trial of surgery with or without adjuvant radiation therapy between 1987–1995	Retrospective review	Compared with patients with BMI <30, survival time was shorter in morbidly obese (BMI ≥ 40) patients (HR 2.77, 95% CI, 1.21–6.36, $p = 0.016$)
Modesitt et al. (2007)	949 women who participated in one of five prospective, randomized Phase III treatment trials for advanced stage or recurrent endometrial cancer	Retrospective review	After adjusting for age, pretreatment performance status, disease stage, histological type, tumor grade, and protocol, BMI was associated with survival (BMI 25.0–29.9, HR = 0.96, 95% CI, 0.69–1.33; BMI 30.0–39.9, HR = 1.33, 95% CI, 0.96–1.84; BMI ≥40.0, HR = 1.86, 95% CI, 1.16–2.99), $p = 0.02$ for global variable test

RR Relative risk, *CI* Confidence interval, *FAR* Floating absolute risk, *FCI* Floated confidence interval, *HR* Hazard ratios to endometrial cancer patients – without intervention, survivors of endometrial cancer who are sedentary and/or obese are unlikely to spontaneously modify their exercise and nutrition behaviors after diagnosis and treatment.

It is important to implement lifestyle interventions to improve survivorship of endometrial cancer patients who are at an increased risk for poor QOL and premature death. A recent randomized controlled study of an interventional lifestyle program in 45 endometrial cancer survivors demonstrated that patients can lose weight, and improve their exercise for 6 months following the intervention (von Gruenigen et al. 2008). At 12 months, the intervention group lost 3.5 kg compared to 1.4-kg gain in the control group and had increased LSI score of 16.4 versus 1.3 in the control group from baseline. A lifestyle intervention program in obese endometrial cancer patients is feasible and can result in sustained behavior change and weight loss over a 1-year period. This same research group is presently enrolling 110 endometrial cancer survivors to a lifestyle intervention trial that includes not only aerobic exercise but has added a strength training component.

13.3.2 Clinical Recommendations

This population is quite different from ovarian cancer patients with regard to patient characteristics and outcomes. The majority of these patients present with early-stage disease and should survive. However, a significant number of patients have premature death secondary to their obesity comorbidities.

13.3.3 Future Research Directions

Behavioral models have been developed and used to enhance the ability to make changes in lifestyle that will have long-term effects on health. Survivors of endometrial cancer who are overweight or obese need to make changes in diet and level of PA to increase their QOL and decrease the likelihood of significant morbidity and mortality. Development and implementation of effective modifications will be increasingly needed as the incidence of this obesity-related disease increases (Mokdad et al. 2003).

13.4 Summary: Lifestyle and Ovarian and Endometrial Cancer

In summary, obesity is a risk factor for endometrial cancer and is a risk factor for poor outcome for both cancers. The increase in prevalence in obesity in the USA (Mokdad et al. 2003) suggests that incidence of endometrial cancer and outcomes for both these diseases may worsen. The extent to which PA independently affects outcome of these diseases is unknown. Prospective trials to explore factors that influence recurrence of ovarian cancer should include lifestyle. Identification of successful interventions to decrease obesity and increase levels of PA to prevent the occurrence of endometrial cancer is needed. Finally, interventions to help women who are diagnosed with this obesity-related disease to alter their lifestyle will affect not only QOL but survival.

References

American Cancer Society, www.cancer.org, accessed January 12, 2010

Pomel C, Jeyarajah A, Oram D, Shepherd J, Milliken D, Dauplat J, Reynolds K (2007) Cytoreductive surgery in ovarian cancer. Cancer Imaging 7: 210–215

Winter WE, Maxwell GL, Tian C, Carlson JW, Ozols RF, Rose PG, Markman M, Armstrong DK, Muggia F, McGuire WP (2007) Gynecologic

Oncology Group Study. Prognostic factors for stage III epithelial ovarian cancer: a Gynecologic Oncology Group Study. J Clin Oncol 25(24): 3621–3627

Ozols RF (2006) Challenges for chemotherapy in ovarian cancer. Ann Oncol 17(Suppl 5): v181–v187

Armstrong DK, Bundy B, Wenzel L, Huang HQ, Baergen R, Lele S, Copeland LJ, Walker JL, Burger RA (2006) Gynecologic Oncology Group. Intraperitoneal cisplatin and paclitaxel in ovarian cancer. N Engl J Med 354(1):34–43

Markman M (2008) Pharmaceutical management of ovarian cancer: current status. Drugs 68(6): 771–789

Bandera EV, Kushi LH, Rodriguez-Rodriguez L (2009) Nutritional factors in ovarian cancer survival. Nutr Cancer 61(5):580–586

Irwin ML, Mayne ST (2008) Impact of nutrition and exercise on cancer survival. Cancer J 14(6): 435–441

Speed-Andrews AE, Courneya KS (2009) Effects of exercise on quality of life and prognosis in cancer survivors. Curr Sports Med Rep 8(4):176–181

Speck RM, Courneya KS, Mâsse LC, Duval S, Schmitz KH (2010). An update of controlled physical activity trials in cancer survivors: a systematic review and meta-analysis. J Cancer Surviv 4(2):87–100

Colditz GA, Coakley E (1997) Weight, weight gain, activity, and major illnesses: the Nurses' Health Study. Int J Sports Med 18(Suppl 3): S162–170

Calle EE, Rodriguez C, Walker-Thurmond K, Thun MJ (2003) Overweight, obesity, and mortality from cancer in a prospectively studied cohort of U.S. adults. N Engl J Med 348(17): 1625–1638

Rodriguez C, Calle EE, Fakhrabadi-Shokoohi D, Jacobs EJ, Thun MJ (2002) Body mass index, height, and the risk of ovarian cancer mortality in a prospective cohort of postmenopausal women. Cancer Epidemiol Biomarkers Prev 11(9): 822–828

Pavelka JC, Brown RS, Karlan BY, Cass I, Leuchter RS, Lagasse LD, Li AJ (2006) Effect of obesity on survival in epithelial ovarian cancer. Cancer 107(7):1520–1524

Yang L, Klint A, Lambe M, Bellocco R, Riman T, Bergfeldt K, Persson I, Weiderpass E (2008) Predictors of ovarian cancer survival: A population-based prospective study in Sweden. Int J Cancer 123:672–679

Kjaerbye-Thygesen A, Frederiksen K, Høgdall EV, Glud E, Christensen L, Høgdall CK, Blaakaer J, Kjaer SK (2006) Smoking and overweight: negative prognostic factors in stage III epithelial ovarian cancer. Cancer Epidemiol Biomarkers Prev 15(4):798–803

Zhang M, Xie X, Lee AH, Binns CW, Holman CD (2005) Body mass index in relation to ovarian cancer survival. Cancer Epidemiol Biomarkers Prev 14(5):1307–1310

Stevinson C, Steed H, Faught W, Tonkin K, Vallance JK, Ladha AB, Schepansky A, Capstick V, Courneya KS (2009) Physical activity in ovarian cancer survivors: associations with fatigue, sleep, and psychosocial functioning. Int J Gynecol Cancer 19(1):73–8

Wenzel L, Huang HQ, Monk BJ, Rose PG, Cella D (2005) Quality-of-life comparisons in a randomized trial of interval secondary cytoreduction in advanced ovarian carcinoma: A Gynecologic Oncology Group study. J Clin Oncol 23(24): 5605–5612

Gil KM, Gibbons HE, Jenison EL, Hopkins MP, von Gruenigen VE (2007) Baseline characteristics influencing quality of life in women undergoing gynecologic oncology surgery. Health Qual Life Outcomes 5:25

von Gruenigen V, Frasure H, Kavanagh M, Nieves-Arriba L, Lerner E, Waggoner S, Courneya K (2010) Physical activity may improve quality of life in women with ovarian cancer on adjuvant chemotherapy. Gynecol Oncol 116(3):S140

Doyle C, Kushi L, Byers T et al (2006) Nutrition and physical activity during and after cancer treatment: An American Cancer Society guide to informed choices. CA Cancer J Clin 56: 323–353

von Gruenigen VE, Huang HQ, Gil KM, Gibbons HE, Monk BJ, Rose PG, Armstrong DK,Cella D, Wenzel L (2009). Assessment of factors that contribute to decreased quality of life in Gynecologic Oncology Group ovarian cancer trials. Cancer 15;115(20):4857–4864

Reeves GK, Pirie K, Beral V, Green J, Spencer E, Bull D (2007) Million Women Study Collaboration. Cancer incidence and mortality in relation to body mass index in the Million Women Study: cohort study. BMJ 335(7630): 1134

Conroy MB, Sattelmair JR, Cook NR, Manson JE, Buring JE, Lee IM (2009) Physical activity, adiposity, and risk of endometrial cancer. Cancer Causes Control 20(7):1107–1115

Friedenreich C, Cust A, Lahmann PH et al (2007) Physical activity and risk of endometrial cancer: the European prospective investigation into cancer and nutrition. Int J Cancer 121(2):347–355

Gierach GL, Chang SC, Brinton LA, Lacey JV Jr, Hollenbeck AR, Schatzkin A, Leitzmann MF (2009) Physical activity, sedentary behavior, and endometrial cancer risk in the NIH-AARP Diet and Health Study. Int J Cancer 124(9): 2139–2147

Patel AV, Feigelson HS, Talbot JT, McCullough ML, Rodriguez C, Patel RC, Thun MJ, Calle EE (2008) The role of body weight in the relationship between physical activity and endometrial cancer: results from a large cohort of US women. Int J Cancer 123(8):1877–1882

von Gruenigen VE, Tian C, Frasure H, Waggoner S, Keys H, Barakat RR (2006) Treatment effects, disease recurrence, and survival in obese women with early endometrial carcinoma: A Gynecologic Oncology Group study. Cancer 107(12): 2786–2791

Modesitt SC, Tian C, Kryscio R, Thigpen JT, Randall ME, Gallion HH, Fleming GF (2007) Gynecologic Oncology Group. Impact of body mass index on treatment outcomes in endometrial cancer patients receiving doxorubicin and cisplatin: A Gynecologic Oncology Group study. Gynecol Oncol 105(1):59–65

Fader AN, Arriba LN, Frasure HE, von Gruenigen VE (2009) Endometrial cancer and obesity: epidemiology, biomarkers, prevention and survivorship. Gynecol Oncol 114(1)):121–127

Fader AN, Gibbons H, Gil K (2008) von Gruenigen. The impact of obesity on health-related quality of life in endometrial cancer survivors. Gynecol Oncol 108(3):S7–S8

Courneya KS, Karvinen KH, Campbell KL, Pearcey RG, Dundas G, Capstick V, Tonkin KS (2005) Associations among exercise, body weight, and quality of life in a population-based sample of endometrial cancer survivors. Gynecol Oncol 97(2):422–430

Basen-Engquist K, Scruggs S, Jhingran A, Bodurka DC, Lu K, Ramondetta L, Hughes D, Taylor CC (2009). Physical activity and obesity in endometrial cancer survivors: Associations with pain, fatigue, and physical functioning. Am J Obstet Gynecol 200(3):288.e1–8

von Gruenigen VE, Gil KM, Frasure HE, Jenison EL, Hopkins MP (2005) The impact of obesity and age on quality of life in gynecologic surgery. Am J Obstet Gynecol 193(4):1369–1375

von Gruenigen VE, Courneya KS, Gibbons HE, Kavanagh MB, Waggoner SE, Lerner E (2008) Feasibility and effectiveness of a lifestyle intervention program in obese endometrial cancer patients: A randomized trial. Gynecol Oncol 109(1):19–26

Mokdad AH, Ford ES, Bowman BA, Dietz WH, Vinicor F, Bales VS, Marks JS (2003) Prevalence of obesity, diabetes, and obesity-related health risk factors, 2001. JAMA 289(1): 76–79

Part III

Physical Activity and Cancer Special Topics

Physical Activity and Pediatric Cancer Survivorship 14

Alejandro F. San Juan, Kathleen Wolin, and Alejandro Lucía

Abstract Owing to improved treatment protocols in the last 25 years there have been dramatic improvements in the 5-year relative survival rate of the most prevalent childhood cancers. For instance, the 5-year relative survival rate among children for all cancer sites combined, improved from 58% to 80% in patients diagnosed in 1975–1977 and in 1996–2004 respectively. However, as survival rates have improved, there has been an increasing recognition of adverse short and longer term effects associated with treatment and cancer itself, which we describe in detail in this chapter. There is growing interest in those interventions that can counteract the adverse effects of treatment and cancer. Because such adverse effects are further aggravated by physical inactivity, a special emphasis is being placed on physical activity (PA) interventions. Results are promising: there is increasing evidence that regular PA can improve the overall health status, functional capacity, and quality of life (QOL) of children with cancer as well as of older survivors of childhood cancer.

A.F. San Juan (✉)
Department of Education, International University of Rioja, Avenida de la Gran Vía Rey Juan Carlos I, 41, 26002 Logroño' Spain
e-mail: alejandro.ferrer@unir.net

K. Wolin
Department of Surgery, Washington University School of Medicine, 660 South Euclid Avenue, Box 8100, St. Louis, MO 63110, USA
e-mail: wolink@wustl.edu

A. Lucía
Departamento de Biomedicina (Polideportivo, Laboratorio P-102), Universidad Europea de Madrid, c/Tajo S/N, 28670 Villaviciosa de Odón, Madrid, Spain
e-mail: alejandro.lucia@uem.es

14.1 Medical Overview of Pediatric Cancer

Cancer is a major public health concern worldwide. The recent Cancer Statistics report by the American Cancer Society has indentified cancer as the second leading cause of death (~12% of total) among children aged 1–14 years, surpassed only by accidents (unintentional injuries) (~36%) (Jemal et al. 2009). Leukemia (particularly acute lymphocytic leukemia, ALL) is the most common type of cancer in children aged 0–14 years, followed by cancers of the nervous system, soft tissue sarcomas, renal (Wilms) tumors, and non-Hodgkin lymphoma (Ries et al. 2008).

In this chapter we will put a special emphasis in ALL given its prevalence and the fact that it

K.S. Courneya and C.M. Friedenreich (eds.), *Physical Activity and Cancer*, Recent Results in Cancer Research 186, DOI: 10.1007/978-3-642-04231-7_14,

is the most commonly studied pediatric cancer in terms of exercise research. We will also describe in detail the different phases of ALL treatment because the standard multiagent chemotherapy treatment for other hematologic malignancies is often similar, e.g. the so-called 'induction' phase (see below).

14.1.1 B Cell Acute Lymphoblastic Leukemia (ALL)

This is the most common type of cancer in childhood, representing 23% of all cancers among children of less than 15 years of age (National Cancer Institute 2010). Patients usually present with signs of bone marrow failure, e.g. bleeding, infection, and abnormal blood counts. As for treatment, contemporary multiagent chemotherapy regimen is composed of four phases: (i) *induction*, (ii) *central nervous system (CNS)-directed treatment and consolidation*, (iii) *reinduction*, and (iv) *maintenance* (Pieters and Carroll 2008).

The goal of the induction phase is to induce morphological remission and to restore normal hematopoiesis (Fauci et al. 2008). Three drugs are commonly used: vincristine, prednisone/dexamethasone and L-asparaginase, in conjunction with intrathecal therapy (IT, including methotrexate, cytarabine, and hydrocortisone) (Pui and Evans 2006). More drugs [anthracyclines (daunomycin), vincristine, prednisone/dexamethasone, L-asparaginase] are used in patients at high risk for treatment failure (LeClerc et al. 2002). This induction phase aims to induce complete remission in 4–6 weeks (Pieters and Carroll 2008).

The second phase, CNS-directed therapy, aims to prevent CNS relapses and to reduce the systemic minimal residual leukemia burden (Fauci et al. 2008). It consists of weekly or biweekly IT therapy alone (Pieters and Carroll 2008). The consolidation phase includes administration of high-dose systemic therapy, including intermediate- or high-dose methotrexate (Mahoney et al. 2000; Schrappe et al. 2000), drugs similar to those used to achieve remission (Schrappe et al. 2000), the combination of different drugs with little-known cross-resistance to the drug combination applied in the induction phase (Richards et al. 1998; Schrappe et al. 2000), the extended use of high-dose L-asparaginase (Silverman et al. 2001), or combinations of the above (Richards et al. 1998; Rizzari et al. 2001).

The third phase of treatment (reinduction, also termed delayed (re)intensification), which commonly uses drugs similar to those applied during the previous induction and consolidation phases, has clearly shown its efficacy to reduce the risk of relapse (Pieters and Carroll 2008). Finally, the last phase of treatment, the maintenance phase, is prolonged, lasting 2–3 years. It consists of daily oral 6-Mercaptopurine and weekly oral methotrexate. In some protocols, pulsed applications of glucocorticoids, vincristine, and IT chemotherapy are also administered (Pieters and Carroll 2008).

14.1.2 Other Types of Hematological Malignancies in Children

These include B-cell chronic lymphoid leukemia / small lymphocytic lymphoma, which is the most common type of lymphoid leukemia, with a clinical presentation as either leukemia or lymphoma (Fauci et al. 2008); B-cell prolymphocytic leukemia, with usually poor chances of complete remission response to therapy; precursor T cell ALL, of which the majority of patients ≤10 years can be cured with very intensive induction and consolidation regimens; precursor T-cell lymphoblastic lymphoma, which is often treated with 'leukemia-like' regimens (Fauci et al. 2008); acute myeloid leukemia, (AML), for which up to 65% of pediatric patients experience long-term survival (Kaspers and Creutzig 2005); acute promyelocytic leukemia, which is frequently characterized by a severe coagulopathy at the time of diagnosis (Tallman et al. 1993) and a worse prognosis than ALL or AML owing to potential bleeding complications; and chronic myeloid leukemia, [which is usually associated with the so-called Philadelphia chromosome, and for which allogeneic hematopoietic cell transplant is the treatment of choice when feasible and the only curative therapy (Fauci et al. 2008).

14.1.3 Other Types of Pediatric Cancer

14.1.3.1 Tumors of the Central Nervous System (CNS)

Cancer of the CNS is the second most common cancer primary site (~21%) in children aged 0–14 years (National Cancer Institute 2010). Taken as a group, CNS tumors represent the most common solid tumor in childhood. Though they have a 5-year relative survival rate of 74% (Jemal et al. 2009), they also have the highest mortality (~30%) of all cancer primary sites (National Cancer Institute 2010). The therapy options include surgery alone, surgery plus local radiotherapy, radiotherapy alone, and adjuvant chemotherapy (vincristine, carboplatin) (National Cancer Institute 2010). Recurrence may occur many years after initial treatment in low grade and malignant childhood CNS tumors (Matsutani et al. 1997).

14.1.3.2 Soft Tissue Sarcomas

Soft tissue sarcomas account for ~7% of the primary cancer sites in children (aged 0–14 years) (National Cancer Institute 2010), and they account for ~4% of the mortality of all cancer primary sites (National Cancer Institute 2010). Soft tissue sarcomas have now a 5-year relative survival rate of 74% (Jemal et al. 2009). More than 50% of soft tissue sarcomas in children are rhabdomyosarcomas, tumors of striated muscle, and undifferentiated sarcomas. The remaining are nonrhabdomyosarcomatous soft tissue sarcomas, i.e., tumors of adipose and fibrous tissue and of blood and lymph vessels (Ferrari et al. 2006).

The therapy options are similar in children and adults, yet the morbidity with radiation therapy is much greater in infants and young children than in adults (Suit and Spiro 1995). Moreover, in pediatric soft tissue sarcomas the efficacy of adjuvant chemotherapy (vincristine, dactinomycin, cyclophosphamide, and doxorubicin) is lower than in adults (Pratt et al. 1999). Surgery alone can cure a significant number of nonmetastatic tumors, particularly fibrosarcoma (Neville et al. 2003).

14.1.3.3 Renal (Wilms) Tumors

This type of cancer accounts for ~6% of the primary cancer sites in children (aged 0–14 years) (National Cancer Institute 2010). Wilms tumors have now a 5-year relative survival rate of 92% (Jemal et al. 2009), and they account for ~4% of mortality of all cancer primary sites (National Cancer Institute 2010). Approximately 10% of patients have histopathological characteristics associated with a poorer prognosis, i.e., higher incidence of relapse and death. The standard treatment for Wilms tumor in the USA includes surgery followed by chemotherapy (e.g. vincristine, dactinomycin, doxorubicin, cyclophosphamide) and radiation therapy in some cases (Green 2004).

14.1.3.4 Non-Hodgkin Lymphoma (NHL)

This tumor accounts for ~6% of the primary cancer sites in children aged 0–14 years (National Cancer Institute 2010) and has a 5-year relative survival rate of 86% (Jemal et al.

2009). Pediatric NHL has a different form (i.e., high grade) compared with common lymphomas in adults (i.e., low or intermediate grade) (Sandlund et al. 1996). NHL is more prevalent in males and in the second decade of life (especially in children aged 15–19 years). Patients with CNS involvement have the worst outcome, i.e., event-free survival at 6 years of 64%, vs. 86% in CNS-negative patients (Cairo et al. 2007; Salzburg et al. 2007).

Combination chemotherapy (e.g. vincristine, doxorubicin, cyclophosphamide, prednisone, mercaptopurine, and methotrexate) (Link et al. 1997) is recommended for most pediatric patients with NHL (Patte et al. 2007).

14.2 Side Effects of Treatment

14.2.1 Early Side Effects

Cancer treatment, i.e., surgery, radiotherapy, and chemotherapy, may affect numerous body tissues and functions. Early side effects in pediatric malignancies are experienced during or shortly after treatment and include increased risk of infections, hemorrhagic and thromboembolic complications, nausea and vomiting, loss of appetite, allergic reactions, skin changes, fatigue, pain, or temporary hair loss (Lucia et al. 2003; Pieters and Carroll 2008).

14.2.2 Late Side Effects: Opposite Effects of Cancer/Treatment and Regular PA

Late side effects occur after months or years, though they can also be permanent, and affect most body systems (Table 14.1) (American Academy of Pediatrics 2009; Lucia et al. 2003; Pieters and Carroll 2008). Besides impairing patients' health-related QOL, late adverse effects of treatment may also exacerbate the risk for secondary malignancies (American Academy of Pediatrics 2009).

Interest in PA interventions (Section 14.3) for survivors of childhood cancer has largely focused on its potential to ameliorate the side effects of treatment. Regular PA (i.e. in children, moderate-intense exercise such as 'active playing', swimming, ball games, physical education classes or brisk walking for a total of at least 60 min on most days of the week) has a beneficial effect on the chain of interactive events between the CNS and the contraction of the skeletal muscle that are involved in most types of PA. These events include blood oxygenation (which depends on pulmonary function), blood oxygen-carrying capacity, supply of oxygenated blood to the working muscles (which depends on cardiac output), and muscles' ability to consume oxygen and to produce force while contracting. Thus, regular PA increases the ability to cope with activities of daily living, as well as the peak cardiorespiratory capacity (commonly expressed as peak oxygen uptake, VO_{2peak}), of virtually all population groups (Lucia et al. 2003).

Anticancer treatment has however the opposite effect. Radiotherapy, cyclophosphamide or lung infections during or subsequent to treatment (e.g. bacterial, or due to respiratory syncytial virus, candida, pneumocystis or cytomegalovirus) can impair lung function (Jenney et al. 1995). For instance, pulmonary function impairment is reflected in ALL survivors by the occurrence of arterial desaturation (oxygen saturation values <90%) during exercise (Matthys et al. 1993). Besides causing anemia, which decreases blood oxygen transport capacity, chemotherapy (particularly anthracyclines) may affect cardiac output, and thus blood supply to body tissues, particularly exercising muscles (Edwards et al. 2000). Higher chemotherapy doses are associated with lower cardiac function (Turner-Gomes et al. 1996). Boys and

Table 14.1 Potential late effects of selected therapeutic interventions for childhood cancer

Organ/system	Therapeutic exposures			Potential late effect
	Chemotherapy	Radiation therapy	Surgery	
Cardio-vascular	Anthracycline agents (e.g. doxorrubicin, daunorubicin)	Chest (e.g. Mantle, mediastinal); upper abdominal	–	Cardiomyopathy, congestive heart failure, arrhythmia, subclinical left ventricular dys-function. XRT only: valvular disease, atherosclerotic heart disease, myocardial infarction, pericarditis, pericardial fibrosis
Pulmonary	Bleomycin, busulfan, carmustine, lomustine	Chest (e.g. Mantle, mediastinal, whole lung), TBI	Pulmonary resection, lobectomy	Pulmonary fibrosis, interstitial pneumonitis, restrictive/obstructive lung disease, pulmonary dysfunction
Liver	Antimetabolites (mercaptopurine, thioguanine, methotrexate)	Abdominal (doses ≥ 30 Gy)	–	Hepatic dysfunction, veno-occlusive disease, hepatic fibrosis, cirrhosis, cholelithiasis
Renal	Cisplatin, carboplatin, isofosfamide, methotrexate,	Abdominal (including kidney)	Nephrectomy	Glomerular toxicity, tubular dysfunction, renal insufficiency, hypertension
Bladder	Cyclophosphamide, isofosfamide	Pelvic (including bladder), lumbar-sacral spine	Spinal surgery, cystectomy	Hemorrhagic cystitis, bladder fibrosis, dysfunctional voiding, neurogenic bladder, bladder malignancy (cyclophosphamide, XRT)
Endocrine/ metabolic	–	Hypothalamic-pituitary, neck (thyroid)	Thyroidec tomy	Growth hormone deficiency, precocious puberty, hypothyroidism, thyroid nodules/cancer, XRT doses ≥ 40 Gy: hyperprolactinemia, central adrenal insufficiency, gonadotropin deficiency, hyperthyroidism

(*continued*)

14

Table 14.1 (continued)

Organ/system	Therapeutic exposures			Potential late effect
	Chemotherapy	Radiation therapy	Surgery	
Musculoskeletal	Corticosteroids, methotrexate	–	–	Osteopenia/osteoporosis, osteonecrosis
	–	All fields	–	Reduced/uneven growth, reduced function/mobility, hypoplasia, fibrosis, radiation-induced fracture (doses ≥ 40 Gy), scoliosis/kyphosis (trunk fields only), secondary benign or malignant neoplasm
	–	–	Amputation, limb sparing	Reduced/uneven growth, reduced function/mobility
Neurocognitive	Methotrexate (intrathecal administration or IV doses ≥ 1,000 mg/m^2), cytarabine (IV doses ≥ 1,000 mg/m^2)	Craneal, ear/infratemporal, total body irradiation	Neurosurgery	Neurocognitive deficits (executive function, attention, memory processing speed, visual motor integration), learning deficits, diminished intellectual quotient
Central nervous system	Methotrexate, cytarabine (IV doses ≥ 1,000 mg/m^2)	Doses ≥ 18 Gy to: cranial, orbital/eye, ear/infratemporal, nasopharyngeal	Neurosurgery	Leukoencephalopathy (spasticity, ataxia, dysarthria, dysphagia, hemiparesis, seizures (chemotherapy and XRT), motor and sensory deficits, cerebrovascular complications (stroke, Moya moya disease, occlusive cerebral, vasculopathy (XRT and surgery)), brain tumor (any XRT dose)
Peripheral nervous system	Plant alkaloids (vincristine, vinblastine), cis platin, carboplatin	–	Spinal surgery	Peripheral sensory or motor neuropathy

Table 14.1 (continued)

Organ/system	Therapeutic exposures			Potential late effect
	Chemotherapy	Radiation therapy	Surgery	
Psychosocial	Any	Any	Any	Social withdrawal, educational problems, depression, anxiety, post-traumatic stress.

Adapted from American Academy of Pediatrics, Children's Oncology Group. Long-term follow-up care for pediatric cancer survivors. Pediatrics 2009; 123:906–915

girls (7–19 years) who are long-term ALL survivors (>1.5 years post-treatment) have significantly reduced cardiorespiratory fitness and this reduction is correlated with cumulative chemotherapy dose (Warner et al. 1997). In fact, the impairment in the cardiorespiratory fitness of ALL survivors already starts in the early phases of life – 3–7 years of age; these are the years during which treatment protocols are usually applied (a total of ~30 months of therapy) (Oeffinger et al. 2001).

In addition to having low levels of cardiorespiratory fitness (Warner et al. 1997), children undergoing cancer treatment can experience fatigue even during normal activities of daily living (Felder-Puig et al. 2006). Chemotherapy induces gastrointestinal toxicities which can interfere with nutrition and thus with energetic supply to muscles (Duggan et al. 2003; White et al. 2005). Glucocorticoid therapy can decrease muscle mass while increasing adiposity and total body mass in children receiving treatment for ALL (Oeffinger et al. 2001).

Other late side effects of treatment that can further deteriorate the physical function of survivors of childhood cancer include, among others, diminished neurological function, growth problems, altered endocrine function, and physical inactivity (which in turn is associated with increased risk for numerous chronic diseases) (Tillmann et al. 2002). Cranial radiotherapy, which was used in the last two decades for high-risk ALL (typically at 18 Gy dose) is strongly associated with physical inactivity during adulthood (Florin et al. 2007). Long-term survivors of ALL are more likely to be obese than the general population, which is itself a risk factor for adverse postdisease outcomes (Florin et al. 2007). Finally, long-term ALL survivors are at increased risk of having other physical inactivity-related diseases such as cardiovascular disease or osteoporosis (Davies 1993; Nysom et al. 1998; Reinders-Messelink et al. 1999).

14.2.3 HSCT Further Impairs Children's Physical Function

Hematopoietic stem cell transplantation (HSCT) includes both bone marrow (BMT) and peripheral blood stem cell transplantation and typically occurs following radiation or chemotherapy in the more severe hematologic malignancies, as well as in the treatment of refractory solid tumors. This therapy further impairs children's physical functioning owing to a loss of muscle mass/strength (Felder-Puig et al. 2006). Muscle atrophy is indeed associated with several transplant-related problems, including immunosuppressive therapy, bed rest, and drug toxicities (e.g. oral intestinal mucositis and diarrhea) (Duggan et al. 2003; White et al. 2005).

14

14.2.4 Cancer Fatigue

Adult patients report fatigue as a loss of physical function during daily tasks: walking a short distance, climbing a few stairs, or completing household tasks (Lucia et al. 2003). Such severe activity-limiting fatigue is caused by extreme muscular deconditioning related to both the disease and its treatment but also to the sedentary habits commonly adopted by patients and survivors (Lucia et al. 2003). Compared with adults, less data are available on cancer-related fatigue in the pediatric literature. It is nevertheless known that fatigue can have a negative impact on the QOL of young cancer survivors, particularly with regard to physical, sentimental, and emotional domains (Hockenberry-Eaton et al. 1998; Meeske et al. 2005). Children often complain of early fatigue during games and outdoor activities common to their age, which makes them feel frustrated and unhealthy (San Juan et al. 2007a, b). This feeling of frustration may detract them from achieving high enough levels of PA, further aggravating their physical status. Preliminary recent data (Keats and Culos-Read 2008) shows that PA has a moderate to strong correlation with fatigue, and may be used as a modifiable tool (i.e. by improving the lifestyle behavior) to help young cancer patients and survivors cope with cancer-related fatigue.

14.3 Physical Activity and Fitness Levels in Children with Cancer and in Survivors of Childhood Cancer

[Note: As for the potential distinction between a cancer patient and a cancer survivor, for simplicity purposes in Sections 14.3 and 14.4, we applied the North American definition of survivor, which includes individuals from the time of diagnosis onward (http://www.canceradvocacy.org)].

The harmful effects of treatment that we described above (Section 14.2) are further aggravated by the typically low PA levels of childhood cancer survivors, as shown by extensive observational research (Table 14.2). The cumulative effects of the disease and the treatment, together with the poor PA habits of survivors of childhood cancer negatively affects their musculoskeletal and cardiorespiratory systems; this further reduces their functional capacity and physical fitness in comparison with their healthy peers and/or pretreatment conditions (Table 14.3).

Most published data are in ALL survivors. This is due (i) to the fact that it is the most common type of pediatric cancer, and (ii) its high survival rate, i.e. more than 70% of children with standard risk disease can now expect to be cured. This type of cancer thus represents an excellent model to recognise the adverse late effects associated with treatment and cancer itself and how these adverse effects could be further aggravated by physical inactivity. In ALL survivors, low PA levels begin during the first two decades of life. Child survivors of ALL have lower PA levels than their healthy referents (Mayer et al. 2000; Reilly et al. 1998; Tillmann et al. 2002; Warner et al. 1998), leading to worse cardiorespiratory fitness (Bell et al. 2006; Jenney et al. 1995; Ness et al. 2007; San Juan et al. 2008a; b; van Brussel et al. 2006; Warner et al. 1997), physical function (Ness et al. 2007), balance, and coordination (Wright et al. 1998). Children with nonhematologic cancer (i.e. CNS tumors) are also less active than their healthy referents (Harz et al. 2003). Though Finnegan et al. (2007) recently showed that the majority of survivors of childhood cancer (hematologic and non-hematologic) reported that they met PA recommendations, studies using objective methods for PA quantification (particularly, accelerometry) have largely demonstrated that survivors of childhood cancer rarely meet PA recommendations and are less active than their healthy

Table 14.2 Observational studies reporting physical activity levels (PA) or related variables in children with cancer and in survivors of childhood cancer

Citation	Demographics	Type of cancer	Setting	Results
Reilly et al. (1998)	n = 40, 45% male; mean age 11	ALL		Observed that energy expended on PA was significantly higher in healthy controls than in ALL survivors largely due to lower PA among survivors
Warner et al. (1998)	n = 56 cancer survivors (45% male) and n = 32 sibling controls (56% male); age 7–18	Mixed (62% hematologic cancers)		Total EE significantly lower in ALL than participants without cancer. No differences observed for other malignancies; PAL significant lower in survivors with ALL than survivors with other cancers and controls.
Mayer et al. (2000)	n = 39; mean age 10.7–20.5	ALL	Outpatient	Lower self-reported PA self and RMR significantly lower in survivors irradiated compared to nonirradiated (chemotherapy alone). Higher prevalence of obesity in survivors after treatment than before treatment.
Oeffinger et al. (2001)	n = 26; age 18–32 42% male	ALL	Post treatment	PA was not associated with treatment-related cardiovascular risk factors (obesity, dyslipidemia, blood pressure, insulin resistance).
Tillmann et al. (2002)	n = 28 survivors 61% male n = 28 age/sex matched controls, 61% male; age 5–15	ALL	Post treatment	No difference found between ALL and controls for bone mineral content, bone area, area BMD, and percent fat mass. Significantly lower lumbar BMD volume and weekly PA score in ALL vs control. In ALL, PA correlated with total BMD, lumbar BMD, and percent FM
Harz et al. (2003)	n = 45; 7–16 years; 49% male	CNS tumors	Inpatient and outpatient	Significantly lower PA levels in patients than in controls, especially during leisure time. The daily energy intake was not higher in patients.

(*continued*)

14

Table 14.2 (continued)

Citation	Demographics	Type of cancer	Setting	Results
Demark-Wahnefried et al. (2005)	N = 389; age 11–33	ALL, lymphoma, CNS tumors	Post treatment	59% ALL Survivors, 40% CNS-Tumor Survivors, and recommendations. 45% Lymphoma Survivors met PA recommendations. No difference between cancer groups.
Aznar et al. (2006)	n = 14; 57% male; mean age 5.6	ALL	Outpatient	Survivors with ALL had significantly similar levels of total PA, though lower levels of moderate/vigorous PA, than controls. No significant difference observed in the percentage of time spent in sedentary behavior between ALL survivors and controls.
Keats et al. (2006)	n = 97; mean age 17.3 years	Mixed	Post treatment	In a self-reported questionnaire, patients did not achieve prediagnosis levels after treatment.
Tercyak et al. (2006)	n = 75, mean age 14.2 (range 11–21)	Mixed	Post treatment	20% of cancer survivors reported to be insufficiently active.
Finnegan et al. (2007)	N = 47, mean age 24	ALL, lymphoma, CNS and bone tumours	Post treatment	According to a self-report, web-based survey, >87% ALL survivors, >91% CNS-tumor survivors, >70% lymphoma survivors, and >61% bone tumor survivors met PA recommendations.
Florin et al. (2007)	n = 2658; mean age 28.7; 50.4% female	ALL	Outpatient	Greater proportion of survivors did not meet CDC recommendations and a greater number of survivors were inactive when compared to the general population.
Jacob et al. (2007)	n = 49; mean age 12,5 %male?	Mixed	Inpatient	25% Patients reported low activity levels. No correlation between PA and pain.
Reeves et al. (2007)	N = 28; mean age 21 52% male	ALL, lymphoma, CNS tumours	Post treatment	33% of ALL survivors, 8% of CNS-tumor survivors, and 86% of lymphoma survivors respectively, reported they met PA recommendations.

Table 14.2 (continued)

Citation	Demographics	Type of cancer	Setting	Results
Arroyave et al. (2008)	n = 118, 45% male; age 13–35	ALL, lymphoma, CNS tumors	Outpatient	Barriers to exercise include being too tired or busy, not belonging to a gym, or preferring to do other activities. Barriers did not greatly differ among cancer types; younger cancer survivors reported more barriers.
Sanford et al. (2008)	N = 88 (61% male)	ALL (maintenance treatment)	Outpatient	Though girls with ALL napped more and had less fragmented night sleep than boys with ALL, no gender differences were observed for subjective fatigue or daytime activity in the total sample.
Winter et al. (2009)	80 patients (59 %male) and 45 age and gender-matched controls; age 5–18	ALL (induction-consolidation) and bone tumors (during treatment	Inpatient/ Outpatient	Lower levels of total PA and moderate/vigorous PA in ALL and bone tumor patients than in controls. Lower PA levels in ALL and bone tumor patients during inpatient than during outpatient (home) stays
Heath et al. (2010)	19 children (53%male) age 6–15	ALL (6 months–5 years after treatment)	Outpatient	Survivors of ALL spent an average of 141 ± 74 min/day engaged in moderate to vigorous physical activity (MVPA), an amount similar to that previously documented in healthy children [only three of the 19 subjects averaged less MVPA than the recommended amount (at least 60 min/day)].
				Overall, boys engaged in significantly more MVPA than girls (P = 0.029).

(*continued*)

14

Table 14.2 (continued)

Citation	Demographics	Type of cancer	Setting	Results
Norris et al. (2010)	19 families with 17 survivors (47% male) age 10–17	Mixed including ALL, CNS, lymphoma; 11–127 months since diagnosis	Outpatient	Survivors reported an average of 59+/– 55 MET hours/week of PA. Survivor PA was significantly correlated with maternal PA ($r = 0.52$), but not sibling's or father's PA. PA was not correlated with survivor self reported QOL, but was correlated with maternally ($r = 0.48$) and paternally ($r = 0.55$) rated total QOL.

ALL, acute lymphoblastic leukemia; AML, acute myelogenous leukemia; BMD, bone mineral density; CNS, central nervous system; EE, energy expenditure; MVPA, moderate to vigorous physical activity; PA, physical activity; RMR, resting metabolic rate
Note: only published studies (excluding meeting abstracts) were included

Table 14.3 Observational studies reporting functional capacity variables and fitness levels in children with cancer and survivors of childhood cancer

Citation	Demographics	Type of cancer	Setting	Results
Jenney et al. (1995)	n = 70 survivors (60%) male, n = 146 controls (58% male) mean age 5.8	ALL, AML	Post treatment	There were significant reductions in lung function in survivors who had been treated for leukemia compared to controls.
Warner et al. (1997)	n = 56 cancer survivors (45% male) and n = 32 sibling controls, (56% male); age 7–19	Mixed (63% hematologic cancers)	Post treatment	Observed a reduced VO_2 peak in male and female survivors of ALL compared to controls. This reduction was associated with chemo therapy cumulative dose and inversely associated with fat free mass.
Wright et al. (1998)	n = 36, 69% male; age 5–14	ALL	Post treatment	ALL survivors had high gross motor function scores but these were significantly lower than those for the general population. Balance and coordination were found to be significantly lower in ALL.

Table 14.3 (continued)

Citation	Demographics	Type of cancer	Setting	Results
Hogarty et al. (2000)	n = 33, 39% female; age 7–34	Tumors requiring BMT (52% hematologic cancer)	Outpatient	VO_2 max increased, on average, with time since BMT
White et al. (2005)	n = 99 cancer survivors (56% male, mean age 12) and n = 89 matched controls (51% male, mean age 12)	ALL	Post treatment	ALL survivors had poorer balance, lower self-perceptions of adequacy and predilection for PA, and lower health-related QOL than healthy controls.
Bell et al. (2006)	n = 67 (35 ALL survivors, 32 controls); 48% male; age 11–12	ALL	Outpatient	VO_2 peak was smaller in survivors than in controls. No significant interaction for any variables in males when evaluating interactions (Intensity x group). However VO_2 peak was significant in females. Main effect for intensity was significant in all variables for boys and girls. There was a small nonsignificant correlation observed between length of time off treatment and relative VO_2 peak and relative HR values for males but these were not significant for females. Length of time off treatment and perceived effort had no significant correlation in either gender group.
DeCaro et al. (2006)	N = 163 (84 survivors, 79 control); 68% male, age 7–21	Mixed (76% hematologic cancer)	Outpatient	Survivors treated with anthracyclines did not differ from controls in response to exercise testing
van Brussel et al. (2006)	n = 13; 46% male; age 8–24	ALL plus one Non-Hodgkin Lymphoma	Post treatment	Anaerobic indicators and knee extensor were found to be significantly lower in ALL than in healthy controls. No significant differences observed between the two groups for strength for any of the five muscle groups: handgrip, shoulder, foot, wrist, and hip.

(*continued*)

14

Table 14.3 (continued)

Citation	Demographics	Type of cancer	Setting	Results
Ness et al. (2007)	n = 75; 41.3% male. Mean age 30.2	ALL	Post treatment	BMI and bone mineral count did not differ between study participants and the expected values for the normal population. Percent fat mass was higher in the study population. Fitness levels were significantly lower for the study population than those expected for the normative population. Study group took significantly longer to complete the TUG and walked a significantly shorter distance than expected for the normal population. TUG completion time had a significant positive correlation with BMI.
San Juan et al. (2008a)	n = 15, 60% male, mean age 7 Matched healthy controls (60% male, mean age 7)	ALL		Significantly lower levels of VO_2 peak, active ankle dorsiflexion range of motion, and also significantly lower values of QOL items (self-report of satisfaction, comfort, and resilience) in patients compared with controls

ALL, acute lymphoblastic leukemia; BMI, body mass index; BMT, bone marrow transplant; HR, heart rate; QOL, quality of life; TUG, time up and go; QOL, quality of life; VO_2 max, maximal oxygen consumption (i.e., an indicator of maximal cardiorespiratory fitness); VO_2 peak, peak oxygen consumption (this term is more commonly applied in patients whereas VO_{2max} is more commonly applied in athletes or healthy young people)

Note: only published studies (excluding meeting abstracts) were included

referents (Harz et al. 2003; Aznar et al. 2006; Winter et al. 2009). However, a recent study using accelerometers found activity levels in ALL survivors similar to healthy peers and most (84%) recorded at least 60 min/day of moderate or vigorous PA (Heath et al. 2010). It seems that among children with cancer, the lowest PA levels are found in those with bone tumors (Finnegan et al. 2007; Winter et al. 2009). Future interventions aiming at increasing PA and fitness levels in pediatric cancer patients should thus focus in this special type of malignancy, which limits yet does not preclude, exercise participation. For instance, one of our patients was missing the lower part of a leg due to surgical removal; this condition did not preclude her from performing upper-body exercises (weightlifting) and aerobic activities (one-leg stationary cycling) during inpatient stay for HSCT (Chamorro-Vina et al. 2010).

Though pediatric leukemia and lymphoma survivors might perceive barriers to be physically active, e.g. being tired and busy, difficult access to facilities (Arroyave et al. 2008), their usually low PA levels largely reflect an overprotective attitude of parents and educators (Aznar et al. 2006). On the other hand, the low levels of PA observed in pediatric cancer survivors may highlight a particular need. Most pediatric cancers tend to peak in incidence between age 2 and 5 years and involve an average of 2.5 years of therapy (Oeffinger et al. 2001). This is the time when many children are introduced to leisure time PA. Thus, their disease may preclude them from establishing interest in playing with their peers. The PA habits established during this early phase of life 'track into adulthood'; as such, this may represent an important window of opportunity to prevent the occurrence of physical inactivity-related diseases (notably, obesity) in later phases of life.

14.4 Exercise Interventions in Children with Cancer

Intervention studies are summarized in Table 14.4.

14.4.1 Children not Receiving HSCT

Evaluating the effects of exercise interventions in pediatric populations poses numerous challenges compared with research on adult patients. The fact that pediatric tumors are relatively rare and involve debilitating treatment results in recruitment challenges. Fourteen published studies (Hartman et al. 2009; Keats and Culos-Reed 2008; Ladha et al. 2006; Marchese et al. 2004; Moyer-Mileur et al. 2009; Oldervoll et al. 2003; Ruiz et al. 2010; San Juan et al. 2007a; b; Sharkey et al. 1993; Shore and Shepard 1999; Takken et al. 2009) including three randomized controlled trials (RCT) (Hartman et al. 2009; Moyer-Mileur et al. 2009) have evaluated the effects of PA interventions on diverse physical fitness and health-related outcomes in children with pediatric cancer who did not undergo HSCT. Except in the study by Sharkey et al. (1993), most (when not all) patients recruited for these studies had hematologic cancer, particularly ALL. One study evaluated the effects of a single (30 min) exercise bout (Ladha et al. 2006).

14.4.1.1 Home-based, Physical-therapy Derived Interventions

Several of the programs reported in the literature derive from physical therapy programs that are standard care in many non-US countries, especially for children with ALL. These programs typically involve limited doses of supervised outpatient PA (generally very light resistance training) supplemented with home-based activities (usually aerobic activity). These interventions have typically not demonstrated significant benefit in children surviving ALL, especially those that are home-based.

A small, pioneering intervention study that included supervised and home-based exercise increased PA levels, but had no effect on body fat, lung function, muscle strength or flexibility (Sharkey et al. 1993). A more recent 20-week aerobic intervention of thrice weekly activity for 30–40 min following treatment improved fitness and reduced fatigue, but had no effect on body mass index in Hodgkin lymphoma survivors (Oldervoll et al. 2003). In a 12-week intervention in the physical therapy setting following treatment, Marchese et al. (2004) reported that supervised resistance training with home-based aerobic activity resulted in improved ankle dorsiflexion range of motion, yet induced no change in hemoglobin, ankle strength, physical function, endurance or QOL in ALL survivors (4–15 years). In a similar intervention lasting 12 weeks and involving 45 min of supervised resistance training twice a week followed by twice weekly home-based aerobic activity, others (Takken et al. 2009) found no effect on strength, functional mobility, or fatigue in ALL survivors (6–14 years). A physical therapy-based RCT that called for sessions of resistance and aerobic

Table 14.4 Intervention studies of exercise in children with cancer

Citation	Design	Demographics	Type of cancer	Setting	Aerobic or resistance	Intervention length	Results
Sharkey et al. (1993)	UCT	N = 12;50% female; mean age 19	Mixed (50% hematologic cancers, Ewing's and Wilms tumor, neuroblastoma, rhabdomyosarcoma)	Outpatient and home-based	Aerobic	12 week	No significant change in body fat, spirometry, heart rate, peak cardiac index, peak stroke volume index, or vascular resistance. Exercise time significantly increased from pretest to posttest.
Shore and* Shephard (1999)	CC/ CCT/ UCT	n = 6 survivors; age 13–14	Mostly ALL	Inpatient and outpatient	Aerobic	12 week	Significant pre- and post difference in fitness, fat and anxiety in the intervention group. Exercise impaired immune function.
Oldervoll et al. (2003)	UCT	n = 27 59% male	Hodgkin Lymphoma	Home	Aerobic	20 week	Observed no significant difference between nonfatigued and fatigued survivors in max and resting HR, fitness, BMI, and resting blood pressure. Total fatigue score was found to be. significantly reduced in the intervention group. The intervention group significantly increased fitness and time to exhaustion on treadmill but had no significant changes in BMI, resting or target HR

Marchese et al. (2004)	CCT	n = 28; 71% male; age 8.3–7.5	ALL	Home-based and outpatient	Aerobic and resistance	12 week	Hemoglobin did not change significantly in either group. A significant increase was observed in ankle dorsiflexion active range of motion in the intervention group. No significant between-groups difference was observed in: ankle dorsiflexion strength, physical function, 9-min run-walk, QOL from pretest to post-test.
Ladha et al. (2006)	UCT	n = 10; all male; age 7–18	ALL	Inpatient	Aerobic	30 min	Observed no acute effect on white blood cells, absolute lymphocyte count, monocyte, eosinophil or basophil count
Hinds et al. (2007)	RCT	n = 29; mean age 12.5 %male	Mixed (86% solid tumors, test AML)	Inpatient	Aerobic	Two 30-min sessions	Improved sleep efficiency with enhanced PA
San Juan et al. (2007b)	UCT	n = 7; 57% male; age 4–7	ALL	Intrahospital	Aerobic and resistance	16 week plus 20 week detraining	Significant improvement in fitness, functional mobility and strength endurance from pretraining to post-training. Only the increased strength endurance remained significant after detraining. No significant effect on range of motion, mean fitness, and QOL.
San Juan et al. (2007b)	UCT	n = 7; 57% male; age 4–7	ALL	Intrahospital	Aerobic and resistance	8 week	Significant improvements in strength and physical function.

(*continued*)

Table 14.4 (continued)

Citation	Design	Demographics	Type of cancer	Setting	Aerobic or resistance	Intervention length	Results
Keats et al. 2008	POC/UCT	n = 10, 20% male; age14–18	Mixed (80% hematologic cancers)	Outpatient	Aerobic, resistance, and flexibility	16 week	Although improvements in total PA, physical fitness, and QOL were noted across the intervention, the follow-up data revealed that participants failed to maintain their postintervention PA levels at both the 3- and 12-month follow-up assessments
San Juan et al. 2008a	CCT	N = 8; 50% female; age 8–16	ALL and AML	Outpatient	Aerobic and resistance	8 week	Significant effect on functional mobility and VO_2 peak. Observed no significant change in range of motion, VT, or HR max.
Chamorro-Vina et al. (2010)	CCT	N = 20 (7 survivor, 13 control), 70% male, mean age 8	Mixed (90% hematologic cancer)	Inpatient	Aerobic and resistance	13 days	Significant increase in fitness. Significant intervention effect on body composition (i.e., increased body mass). No significant effect (after multivariable adjustment) on immune cell recovery.
Hartman et al. (2009)	RCT	n = 51, mean age 5.4 59% male	ALL	Inpatient and home-based	Aerobic and resistance	2 years	BMI significantly increased but there were no significant changes in body fat in either group during treatment. 1 year after finishing treatment body fat significantly decreased in both groups but was more prominent and significant in the intervention group. No

							significant differences found in LBM between both groups. BMD decreased significantly in both groups between the start and end of treatment. No significant difference found in changes in motor performance, which increased and passive ankle dorsiflexion which significantly decreased in both groups
Moyer-Mileur et al. (2009)	RCT	N = 1; 53% male; age 4–10	ALL	Home	Aerobic and resistance	12 months	No significant differences in food intake, height, weight, BMI between groups. At 12 months a significant increase was observed in self-reported PA but not in pedometer recorded steps. Significant increase was also observed in fitness at 12 months. From 6 months to 12 months and from 0 to 12 months found a significant difference in percent change in steps but not in self-reported PA or fitness. Observed no intervention effect on strength or flexibility.
Takken et al. (2009)	UCT	n = 9, 33% male; age: 6–14	ALL	Home-based and outpatient	Aerobic and resistance	12 week	Majority of trainers were satisfied with the program. There were no significant findings observed in muscle strength, exercise

(*continued*)

Table 14.4 (continued)

Citation	Design	Demographics	Type of cancer	Setting	Aerobic or resistance	Intervention length	Results
							capability, functional mobility, and fatigue between the evaluations conducted before and after the training.
Ruiz et al. (2010)	UCT	n = 7; 57% male; age 4–7	ALL	Intrahospital	Aerobic and resistance	16 week plus 20 week detraining	No significant changes observed over the study period in GH, IGFs, and IGPBP.
Children							

ALL, acute lymphoblastic leukemia; AML, acute myelogenous leukemia; BMD, bone mineral density; BMI, body mass index; CCT, Controlled clinical trial; CML, chronic myelogenous leukemia; GH, growth hormone; IGF; insulin growth factor, IGFBPs, insulin growth factor binding protein; PA, physical activity; RCT: Randomized controlled trial; UCT, Uncontrolled trial (pre–post); ROC, retrospective observational cohort; HR, heart rate; QOL, quality of life; UCT, Uncontrolled trial (pre–post); VT, ventilatory threshold; VO_2 max, maximal oxygen consumption; VO_2 peak, peak oxygen consumption

*Study stated to participant diagnosis was "predominantly lymphoblastic leukemia"

Note: only published studies (excluding meeting abstracts) were included training every 6 weeks with home-based exercises for 2 years found no effect on body composition (Hartman et al. 2008). Finally, in another recent RCT (12-month home-based aerobic and resistance training intervention), (Moyer-Mileur et al. 2009) found a significant increase in self-reported PA and fitness, yet no increase in objectively measured PA levels (pedometer measured steps).

Individual supervision of exercise sessions in children seems necessary for maximizing fitness improvements. In a pilot study, Shore et al. reported that a 12-week aerobic intervention of 30 min of aerobic exercise that was partially supervised (i.e. by a fitness professional once per week and by parents twice per week) significantly improved fitness and anxiety (pre–post comparison) in three pediatric ALL survivors (13–14 years) within 4 weeks of the conclusion of induction therapy. Though this intervention tended to decrease CD3, CD4, and CD8 cell counts, the change was not clinically significant.

14.4.1.2 Community-based Interventions

Scarce data are available with regards to outpatient, group-based exercise interventions for children and adolescent survivors of cancer. This is a potential area of interest; as the number of pediatric survivors continues to grow strong emphasis should be placed on all possible types of fitness and health-promoting behavioral interventions. For instance, it could be useful to encourage childhood cancer survivors to engage in group activities after their physical fitness levels have returned to predisease levels with a short-term (e.g. few months), more specific (i.e. individually supervised) intra-hospital program as those described in the next section (Section 14.4.1.3). A recent community-based intervention showed improvements in PA levels, physical fitness, and QOL in adolescent survivors, though they returned to low PA levels shortly after they finished the program (Keats and Culos-Reed 2008).

14.4.1.3 Intra-hospital, Individually Supervised interventions with a Strong Emphasis on Resistance (Weight Lifting) Training

Intra-hospital, individually supervised training programs appear beneficial for young ALL survivors. [See next session (Section 14.4.2) for supervised, intra-hospital interventions in children undergoing HSCT]. Especially beneficial are resistance (weight lifting) training interventions. Despite earlier concerns regarding the safety and efficacy of youth strength training, current public health objectives now aim to increase the number of boys and girls (age 6 and older) who regularly participate in PA that enhances and maintains muscular fitness (Faigenbaum et al. 2009). If appropriate training guidelines are followed (i.e. qualified instruction, competent supervision, and appropriate progression of the volume and intensity of training), regular participation in a strength-training program has the potential to increase bone mineral density, improve motor performance skills, enhance children's physical capacity, and overall health and fitness status (Faigenbaum et al. 2009). Children and adolescents cannot only learn advanced strength training exercises but can feel good about their performances, and have fun. San Juan et al. (2007b) reported that a 16-week combined aerobic and medium-intensity resistance training intervention of thrice weekly activity for 90–120 min significantly improved aerobic fitness, muscle strength, and functional mobility in very young (4–7 years) pediatric ALL survivors in the maintenance treatment phase. Improvements in muscle strength were already evident after the first 8 weeks of training (San Juan et al. 2007a).

14.4.2 Children Undergoing HSCT

As mentioned above (Section 14.2), HSCT further aggravates the decline in patients' physical functioning owing to a further loss of muscle mass/strength (Felder-Puig et al. 2006); this poses an additional challenge for patient recruitment and exercise designs. Only two intervention studies are available in pediatric HSCT patients (Chamorro-Vina et al. 2010; San Juan et al. 2008b) (Table 14.4). Though more research is needed, the existing preliminary data are promising. In ALL and acute myeloid leukemia survivors in the outpatient setting (8–16 years) who received HSCT within the previous year, an 8-week aerobic and resistance exercise intervention resulted in a significant improvement in muscle strength, functional mobility, aerobic fitness, and QOL (San Juan et al. 2008b). A recent brief aerobic and resistance training intervention during inpatient hospitalization for HSCT resulted in significantly increased fitness and body mass with no deleterious effect on immune cell recovery (Chamorro-Vina et al. 2010).

14.4.3 Follow-Up Assessment

Some studies performed a follow-up assessment of exercise outcomes after the intervention had been completed (Blaauwbroek et al. 2009; Keats and Culos-Reed. 2008; San Juan et al. 2007b); the results supported the notion that exercise-induced gains are maintained, at least partly, over time (months) and over a wide age span of childhood cancer survivors. Keats and Culos-Reed (2008) observed that pediatric cancer survivors (age 14–18 years) maintained improvements in cardiorespiratory endurance, strength, flexibility, QOL, and fatigue at 3 and 12 months post intervention. Similar findings for muscle strength were obtained by San Juan et al. (2007b) in very young ALL survivors after 20 weeks (age: 4–7 years). In adult survivors of pediatric cancer, training-induced gains in PA levels persist 26 weeks after the intervention (Blaauwbroek et al. 2009).

14.4.4 Safety and Side Effects

More research is needed to establish the minimum platelet count and hemoglobin levels needed to ensure safety of training interventions, especially in inpatients. Preliminary data by Chamorro-Vina et al. (2010) in seven exercised inpatients (compared with 13 matched controls) of very young age (mean 8 years) suggest that training during the neutropenic phase following HSCT (neutrophil count $< 0.5*10^9 \cdot L^{-1}$) does not increase risk of adverse events. In a sample of older (7–18 years) ALL survivors, Ladha et al. (2006) reported no effect of a single acute exercise bout on white blood cells, monocytes or eosinophils, indicating no adverse immune response. Large studies are however necessary with immunocompromised patients to establish the safety of exercise with regard to infection risk. Though larger trials are needed, resistance exercise, even at relatively high loads (i.e. with weight training machines, and well above the loads used in physical therapy, home-based programs) appears safe even in the youngest patients. Ruiz et al. (in press) recently found no changes in growth hormone, insulin-like growth factor (IGF)-1, and IGF binding proteins in a combined (aerobic and resistance) training program in very young (4–7 years) ALL survivors during maintenance treatment. Elevated levels of IGF-1 have been previously linked with increased cancer risk (Chan et al. 1998; Hankinson et al. 1998) including leukemia (Tower and Spector 2007).

14.5 Practical Clinical Recommendations

Exercise interventions are safe in this pediatric population and there is strong evidence for a benefit on cardiorespiratory fitness and, especially, muscle strength (Wolin et al. 2010). That said, individually supervised interventions have shown a greater benefit than home-based programs. Particularly, the physical therapy programs bridging the inpatient and outpatient settings, that are the standard of care in many settings, appear to have less benefit than the supervised programs that have been applied in relatively recent studies. Based on the available research data (which are still small compared with published data on adulthood cancer), we conclude than supervised exercise interventions should be ideally performed inside the treating hospital, in part to overcome the safety concerns expressed by some parents. Programs can start not only during the maintenance phase, but also earlier in the treatment protocol (with more gradual habituation to exercise in the more debilitated children). Each session should be closely supervised by instructors (at least one instructor for every two children). We recommend that instructors are qualified professionals who can be classified as 'fitness specialists', i.e., professionals involved in prescription of PA for preventive and rehabilitative purposes (see for example www.acsm.org). Given the emphasis that should be put on strength exercises, hospitals should ideally be equipped with a gymnasium specially built for children (see Fig. 14.1 for an example).

Once children have reached normal (or close to normal levels) of muscle strength for their age (which can be reasonably achieved within 2–3 months of inpatient training), children should be encouraged to follow an active lifestyle on their own in the transition from the inpatient to the outpatient condition. We believe

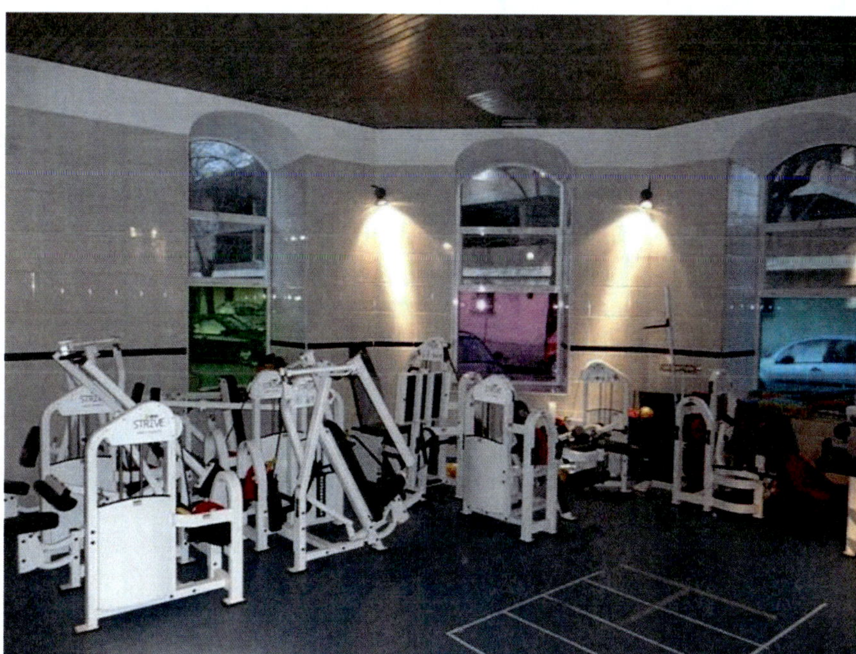

Fig. 14.1 Example of intrahospital gymnasium in the Children's Hospital Niño Jesús (Madrid, Spain). The weight training machines are specially built for children and were donated by Strive Inc (Canonsburg, PA, USA)

14

that an overprotective attitude of parents/guardians and teachers (especially in Physical Education classes) is detrimental for children who are in the last phases of treatment or have completed the treatment.

Finally, clinicians should emphasize the role that families can play in promoting PA for the pediatric cancer survivor. A recent study (Norris et al. 2010) reported a significant correlation between the PA levels of parents and those of child survivors.

14.6 Research Gaps and Future Research Directions

Several specific limitations in the available literature should be noted to improve the quality and level of evidence of future research. In general this is a quasi-experimental field due to a lack of control groups, incomplete randomization, or failure to conduct intent-to-treat analyses following participant drop out. This may explain the lack of statistically significant findings in the outcome variables assessed in several reports. Study populations are often small and mix populations both on diagnosis and treatment. Further, some studies recruited based on treatment modality (e.g. HSCT or not) while others based on primary tumor. Though both treatment modality and diagnosis likely influence children's initial physical condition and may also modify intervention effectiveness, no studies have been large enough to evaluate the interaction. Given the difficulty of gathering large population samples (as opposed to adult cancer), multicenter studies should be performed. We also propose that future RCTs reach at least four of the following criteria to ensure high quality (Schmitz et al. 2005): randomization, appropriate statistical testing (i.e. intent-to-treat analysis, statistical significance reported), concurrent comparison group, at least 70% adherence to the intervention prescription, less than 20% of participants lost to follow up, documented reliability/validity of the exposure assessment, documented reliability/validity of the outcome, and blinded measurement.

Finally, the molecular mechanisms by which exercise training exerts its beneficial effects in the pediatric cancer population remain to be clearly elucidated. For instance, whether the beneficial effects of regular physical exercise in cancer patients/survivors are associated with decreased production of pro-inflammatory cytokines remains to be determined. This is a question of medical relevance given the relationship between circulating cytokines and cancer symptoms and outcome (Seruga et al. 2008).

References

American Academy of Pediatrics (2009) Long-term follow-up care for pediatric cancer survivors. Pediatrics 123:906–915

Arroyave WD, Clipp EC, Miller PE, Jones LW, Ward DS, Bonner MJ, et al. (2008) Childhood cancer survivors' perceived barriers to improving exercise and dietary behaviors. Oncol Nurs Forum 35:121–130.

Aznar S, Webster AL, San Juan AF, Chamorro-Vina C, Mate-Munoz JL, Moral S, Perez M, Garcia-Castro J, Ramirez M, Madero L, Lucia A (2006) Physical activity during treatment in children with leukemia: a pilot study. Appl Physiol Nutr Metab 31:407–413

Bell W, Warner JT, Evans WD, Webb DK, Mullen RH, Gregory JW (2006) Perception of effort at low and moderate intensity exercise in survivors of childhood acute lymphoblastic leukaemia. Ann Hum Biol 33:357–371

Blaauwbroek R, Bouma MJ, Tuinier W, Groenier KH, de Greef MH, Meyboom-de Jong B, Kamps WA, Postma A (2009) The effect of exercise counselling with feedback from a pedometer on fatigue in adult survivors of childhood cancer: a pilot study. Support Care Cancer 17: 1041–1048

Bluhm EC, Ronckers C, Hayashi RJ, Neglia JP, Mertens AC, Stovall M, Meadows AT, Mitby PA, Whitton JA, Hammond S, Barker JD,

Donaldson SS, Robison LL, Inskip PD (2008) Cause-specific mortality and second cancer incidence after non-Hodgkin lymphoma: a report from the Childhood Cancer Survivor Study. Blood 111:4014–4021

Burkhardt B, Woessmann W, Zimmermann M, Kontny U, Vormoor J, Doerffel W, Mann G, Henze G, Niggli F, Ludwig WD, Janssen D, Riehm H, Schrappe M, Reiter A (2006) Impact of cranial radiotherapy on central nervous system prophylaxis in children and adolescents with central nervous system-negative stage III or IV lymphoblastic lymphoma. J Clin Oncol 24: 491–499

Cairo MS, Gerrard M, Sposto R, Auperin A, Pinkerton CR, Michon J, Weston C, Perkins SL, Raphael M, McCarthy K, Patte C (2007) Results of a randomized international study of high-risk central nervous system B non-Hodgkin lymphoma and B acute lymphoblastic leukemia in children and adolescents. Blood 109:2736–2743

Chamorro-Vina C, Ruiz JR, Santana-Sosa E, Gonzalez Vicent M, Madero L, Perez M, Fleck SJ, Perez A, Ramirez M, Lucia A (2010) Exercise during Hematopoietic Stem Cell Transplant Hospitalization in Children. Med Sci Sports Exerc 42(6):1045–1053

Chan JM, Stampfer MJ, Giovannucci E, Gann PH, Ma J, Wilkinson P, Hennekens CH, Pollak M (1998) Plasma insulin-like growth factor-I and prostate cancer risk: a prospective study. Science 279:563–566

Coppes MJ, Arnold M, Beckwith JB, Ritchey ML, D'Angio GJ, Green DM, Breslow NE (1999) Factors affecting the risk of contralateral Wilms tumor development: a report from the National Wilms Tumor Study Group. Cancer 85:1616–1625

Davies HA (1993) Late problems faced by childhood cancer survivors. Br J Hosp Med 50: 137–140

De Caro E, Fioredda F, Calevo MG, Smeraldi A, Saitta M, Hanau G, et al (2006). Exercise capacity in apparently healthy survivors of cancer. Arch Dis Child 91: 47–51

Demark-Wahnefried W, Werner C, Clipp EC, Guill AB, Bonner M, Jones LW, Rosoff PM (2005). Survivors of childhood cancer and their guardians. Cancer. 103:2171–2180

Duggan C, Bechard L, Donovan K, Vangel M, O'Leary A, Holmes C, Lehmann L, Guinan E (2003) Changes in resting energy expenditure among children undergoing allogeneic stem cell transplantation. Am J Clin Nutr 78:104–109

Edwards MR, Hunte GS, Belzberg AS, Sheel AW, Worsley DF, McKenzie DC (2000) Alveolar epithelial integrity in athletes with exercise-induced hypoxemia. J Appl Physiol 89: 1537–1542

Faigenbaum AD, Kraemer WJ, Blimkie CJ, Jeffreys I, Micheli LJ, Nitka M, Rowland TW (2009) Youth resistance training: updated position statement paper from the national strength and conditioning association. J Strength Cond Res 23: S60–79

Fauci A, Kasper D, Braunwald E, Hauser S, Longo D, Jameson J (2008) Harrison's principles of internal medicine, 17 edn. McGraw-Hill Medical Publishing Division, New York

Felder-Puig R, di Gallo A, Waldenmair M, Norden P, Winter A, Gadner H, Topf R (2006) Health-related quality of life of pediatric patients receiving allogeneic stem cell or bone marrow transplantation: results of a longitudinal, multi-center study. Bone Marrow Transplant 38: 119–126

Ferrari S, Briccoli A, Mercuri M, Bertoni F, Cesari M, Longhi A, Bacci G (2006) Late relapse in osteosarcoma. J Pediatr Hematol Oncol 28: 418–422

Finnegan L, Wilkie DJ, Wilbur J, Campbell RT, Zong S, Katula S (2007) Correlates of physical activity in young adult survivors of childhood cancers. Oncol Nurs Forum 34:E60–69

Florin TA, Fryer GE, Miyoshi T, Weitzman M, Mertens AC, Hudson MM, Sklar CA, Emmons K, Hinkle A, Whitton J, Stovall M, Robison LL, Oeffinger KC (2007) Physical inactivity in adult survivors of childhood acute lymphoblastic leukemia: a report from the childhood cancer survivor study. Cancer Epidemiol Biomarkers Prev 16:1356–1363

Green DM (2004) The treatment of stages I–IV favorable histology Wilms' tumor. J Clin Oncol 22:1366–1372

Hankinson SE, Willett WC, Colditz GA, Hunter DJ, Michaud DS, Deroo B, Rosner B, Speizer FE, Pollak M (1998) Circulating concentrations of insulin-like growth factor-I and risk of breast cancer. Lancet 351:1393–1396

Hartman A, van den Bos C, Stijnen T, Pieters R (2008) Decrease in peripheral muscle strength and ankle dorsiflexion as long-term side effects of treatment for childhood cancer. Pediatr Blood Cancer 50:833–837

Hartman A, te Winkel ML, Van Beek RD, de Muinck Keizer-Schrama SM, Kemper HC, Hop WC, Van den Heuvel-Eibrink MM, Pieters R (2009) A randomized trial investigating an exercise program to prevent reduction of bone mineral density and impairment of motor performance during treatment for childhood acute lymphoblastic leukemia. Pediatr Blood Cancer 53: 64–71

Harz KJ, Muller HL, Waldeck E, Pudel V, Roth C (2003) Obesity in patients with craniopharyngioma: assessment of food intake and movement counts indicating physical activity. J Clin Endocrinol Metab 88:5227–5231

Heath JA, Ramzy JM, Donath SM (2010) Physical activity in survivors of childhood acute lymphoblastic leukaemia. J Paediatr Child Health 46: 149–153

Hinds PS, Hockenberry M, Rai SN, Zhang L, Razzouk BI, Cremer L, McCarthy K, Rodriguez-Galindo C (2007) Clinical field testing of an enhanced-activity intervention in hospitalized children with cancer. J Pain Symptom Manage 33:686–697.

Hockenberry-Eaton M, Hinds PS, Alcoser P, O'Neill JB, Euell K, Howard V, Gattuso J, Taylor J (1998) Fatigue in children and adolescents with cancer. J Pediatr Oncol Nurs 15:172–182

Hogarty AN, Leahey A, Zhao H, Hogarty MD, Bunin N, Cnaan A, et al (2000). Longitudinal evaluation of cardiopulmonary performance during exercise after bone marrow transplantation in children. J Pediatr 136: 311–317.

Jacob E, Hesselgrave J, Sambuco G, Hockenberry M (2007). Variations in pain, sleep, and activity during hospitalization in children with cancer. J Pediatr Oncol Nurs 24:208–219.

Jemal A, Siegel R, Ward E, Hao Y, Xu J, Thun MJ (2009) Cancer statistics, 2009. CA Cancer J Clin 59:225–249

Jenney ME, Faragher EB, Jones PH, Woodcock A (1995) Lung function and exercise capacity in survivors of childhood leukaemia. Med Pediatr Oncol 24:222–230

Kaspers GJ, Creutzig U (2005) Pediatric acute myeloid leukemia: international progress and future directions. Leukemia 19:2025–2029

Keats MR, Culos-Reed SN (2008) A community-based physical activity program for adolescents with cancer (project TREK): program feasibility and preliminary findings. J Pediatr Hematol Oncol 30:272–280

Keats MR, Culos-Reed SN, Courneya KS, McBride M (2006). An examination of physical activity behaviors in a sample of adolescent cancer survivors. J Pediatr Oncol Nurs. 23: 135–142.

Ladha AB, Courneya KS, Bell GJ, Field CJ, Grundy P (2006) Effects of acute exercise on neutrophils in pediatric acute lymphoblastic leukemia survivors: a pilot study. J Pediatr Hematol Oncol 28:671–677

LeClerc JM, Billett AL, Gelber RD, Dalton V, Tarbell N, Lipton JM, Barr R, Clavell LA, Asselin B, Hurwitz C, Schorin M, Lipshultz SE, Declerck L, Silverman LB, Cohen HJ, Sallan SE (2002) Treatment of childhood acute lymphoblastic leukemia: results of Dana-Farber ALL Consortium Protocol 87-01. J Clin Oncol 20: 237–246

Link MP, Shuster JJ, Donaldson SS, Berard CW, Murphy SB (1997) Treatment of children and young adults with early-stage non-Hodgkin's lymphoma. N Engl J Med 337: 1259–1266

Lucia A, Earnest C, Perez M (2003) Cancer-related fatigue: can exercise physiology assist oncologists? Lancet Oncol 4:616–625

Mahoney DH Jr, Shuster JJ, Nitschke R, Lauer S, Steuber CP, Camitta B (2000) Intensification with intermediate-dose intravenous methotrexate is effective therapy for children with lower-risk B-precursor acute lymphoblastic leukemia: A Pediatric Oncology Group study. J Clin Oncol 18:1285–1294

Marchese VG, Chiarello LA, Lange BJ (2004) Effects of physical therapy intervention for children with acute lymphoblastic leukemia. Pediatr Blood Cancer 42:127–133

Matsutani M, Sano K, Takakura K, Fujimaki T, Nakamura O, Funata N, Seto T (1997) Primary intracranial germ cell tumors: a clinical analysis of 153 histologically verified cases. J Neurosurg 86:446–455

Matthys D, Verhaaren H, Benoit Y, Laureys G, De Naeyer A, Craen M (1993) Gender difference in aerobic capacity in adolescents after cure from malignant disease in childhood. Acta Paediatr 82:459–462

Mayer EI, Reuter M, Dopfer RE, Ranke MB (2000) Energy expenditure, energy intake and prevalence of obesity after therapy for acute lymphoblastic leukemia during childhood. Horm Res 53:193–199

Meeske KA, Siegel SE, Globe DR, Mack WJ, Bernstein L (2005) Prevalence and correlates of fatigue in long-term survivors of childhood leukemia. J Clin Oncol 23:5501–5510

Moyer-Mileur LJ, Ransdell L, Bruggers CS (2009) Fitness of children with standard-risk acute lymphoblastic leukemia during maintenance therapy: response to a home-based exercise and nutrition program. J Pediatr Hematol Oncol 31: 259–266

National Cancer Institute (2010) United States of America. Last access Feb 2010. http://www.cancer.gov/ Statistical data obtained from: http://www.seer.cancer.gov/ and www.seer.gov/csr/1975-2006/results_merged/sect_28childhood_cancer.pdf.

Ness KK, Baker KS, Dengel DR, Youngren N, Sibley S, Mertens AC, Gurney JG (2007) Body composition, muscle strength deficits and mobility limitations in adult survivors of childhood acute lymphoblastic leukemia. Pediatr Blood Cancer 49:975–981

Neville H, Corpron C, Blakely ML, Andrassy R (2003) Pediatric neurofibrosarcoma. J Pediatr Surg 38:343–346, discussion 343–346

Norris JM, Moules N, Pelletier G, Culos-Reed SN (2010) Families of young pediatric cancer survivors: A cross-sectional survey examining physical activity behavior and health-related quality of life. J Pediatr Oncol Nurs 27(4): 196–208

Nysom K, Molgaard C, Holm K, Hertz H, Michaelsen KF (1998) Bone mass and body composition after cessation of therapy for childhood cancer. Int J Cancer Suppl 11:40–43

Oeffinger KC, Buchanan GR, Eshelman DA, Denke MA, Andrews TC, Germak JA, Tomlinson GE, Snell LE, Foster BM (2001) Cardiovascular risk factors in young adult survivors of childhood acute lymphoblastic leukemia. J Pediatr Hematol Oncol 23:424–430

Oldervoll LM, Kaasa S, Knobel H, Loge JH (2003) Exercise reduces fatigue in chronic fatigued Hodgkins disease survivors–results from a pilot study. Eur J Cancer 39:57–63

Patte C, Auperin A, Gerrard M, Michon J, Pinkerton R, Sposto R, Weston C, Raphael M, Perkins SL, McCarthy K, Cairo MS (2007) Results of the randomized international FAB/LMB96 trial for intermediate risk B-cell non-Hodgkin lymphoma in children and adolescents: it is possible to reduce treatment for the early responding patients. Blood 109: 2773–2780

Pieters R, Carroll WL (2008) Biology and treatment of acute lymphoblastic leukemia. Pediatr Clin North Am 55:1–20, ix

Pratt CB, Pappo AS, Gieser P, Jenkins JJ, Salzbergdagger A, Neff J, Rao B, Green D, Thomas P, Marcus R, Parham D, Maurer H (1999) Role of adjuvant chemotherapy in the treatment of surgically resected pediatric nonrhabdomyosarcomatous soft tissue sarcomas: A Pediatric Oncology Group Study. J Clin Oncol 17:1219

Pui CH, Evans WE (2006) Treatment of acute lymphoblastic leukemia. N Engl J Med 354: 166–178

Reilly JJ, Ventham JC, Ralston JM, Donaldson M, Gibson B (1998) Reduced energy expenditure in preobese children treated for acute lymphoblastic leukemia. Pediatr Res 44:557–562

Reinders-Messelink H, Schoemaker M, Snijders T, Goeken L, van Den Briel M, Bokkerink J, Kamps W (1999) Motor performance of children during treatment for acute lymphoblastic leukemia. Med Pediatr Oncol 33:545–550

Reeves M, Eakin E, Lawler S, Demark-Wahnefried W (2007). Health behaviours in survivors of childhood cancer. Aust Fam Physician 36:95–96.

Richards S, Burrett J, Hann I, Chessells J, Hill F, Bailey C (1998) Improved survival with early intensification: combined results from the Medical Research Council childhood ALL randomised trials UKALL X and UKALL XI. Medical Research Council Working Party on Childhood Leukaemia. Leukemia 12: 1031–1036

Ries LAG, Melbert D, Krapcho M (2008) SEER Cancer Statistics Review, 1975–2005. Bethesda, MD: National Cancer Institute; Available at: http://seer.cancer.gov/ csr/1975_2005/. .

Rizzari C, Valsecchi MG, Arico M, Conter V, Testi A, Barisone E, Casale F, Lo Nigro L, Rondelli R, Basso G, Santoro N, Masera G (2001) Effect of protracted high-dose L-asparaginase given as a second exposure in a Berlin-Frankfurt-Munster-based treatment: results of the randomized 9102 intermediate-risk childhood acute lymphoblastic leukemia study – a report from the Associazione

Italiana Ematologia Oncologia Pediatric. J Clin Oncol 19:1297–1303

Ruiz JR, Fleck SJ, Vingren JL, Ramirez M, Madero L, Fragala MS, Kraemer WJ, Lucia A (2010) Preliminary findings of a 4-month intrahospital exercise training intervention on IGFs and IGFBPs in children with leukemia. J Strength Condition Res 24:1292–1297

Salzburg J, Burkhardt B, Zimmermann M, Wachowski O, Woessmann W, Oschlies I, Klapper W, Wacker HH, Ludwig WD, Niggli F, Mann G, Gadner H, Riehm H, Schrappe M, Reiter A (2007) Prevalence, clinical pattern, and outcome of CNS involvement in childhood and adolescent non-Hodgkin's lymphoma differ by non-Hodgkin's lymphoma subtype: a Berlin-Frankfurt-Munster Group Report. J Clin Oncol 25:3915–3922

Sanford SD, Okuma JO, Pan J, Srivastava DK, West N, Farr L, Hinds PS (2008). Gender differences in sleep, fatigue, and daytime activity in a pediatric oncology sample receiving dexamethasone. J Pediatr Psychol 33:298–306.

San Juan AF, Fruleck SJ, Chamorro-Vina C, Mate-Munoz JL, Moral S, Garcia-Castro J, Ramirez M, Madero L, Lucia A (2007b) Early-phase adaptations to intrahospital training in strength and functional mobility of children with leukemia. J Strength Cond Res 21:173–177

San Juan AF, Fleck SJ, Chamorro-Vina C, Mate-Munoz JL, Moral S, Perez M, Cardona C, Del Valle MF, Hernandez M, Ramirez M, Madero L, Lucia A (2007b) Effects of an intrahospital exercise program intervention for children with leukemia. Med Sci Sports Exercise 39: 13–21

San Juan AF, Chamorro-Vina C, Mate-Munoz JL, Fernandez del Valle M, Cardona C, Hernandez M, Madero L, Perez M, Ramirez M, Lucia A (2008a) Functional capacity of children with leukemia. Int J Sports Med 29:163–167

San Juan AF, Chamorro-Vina C, Moral S, Fernandez del Valle M, Madero L, Ramirez M, Perez M, Lucia A (2008b) Benefits of intrahospital exercise training after pediatric bone marrow transplantation. Int J Sports Med 29: 439–446

Sandlund JT, Downing JR, Crist WM (1996) Non-Hodgkin's lymphoma in childhood. N Engl J Med 334:1238–1248

Schmitz KH, Holtzman J, Courneya KS, Masse LC, Duval S, Kane R (2005) Controlled physical activity trials in cancer survivors: a systematic review and meta-analysis. Cancer Epidemiol Biomarkers Prev 14:1588–1595

Schrappe M, Reiter A, Ludwig WD, Harbott J, Zimmermann M, Hiddemann W, Niemeyer C, Henze G, Feldges A, Zintl F, Kornhuber B, Ritter J, Welte K, Gadner H, Riehm H (2000) Improved outcome in childhood acute lymphoblastic leukemia despite reduced use of anthracyclines and cranial radiotherapy: results of trial ALL-BFM 90 German-Austrian-Swiss ALL-BFM Study Group. Blood 95:3310–3322

Seruga B, Zhang H, Bernstein LJ, Tannock IF (2008) Cytokines and their relationship to the symptoms and outcome of cancer. Nat Rev Cancer 8:887–899

Sharkey AM, Carey AB, Heise CT, Barber G (1993) Cardiac rehabilitation after cancer therapy in children and young adults. Am J Cardiol 71: 1488–1490

Shore S, Shepard RJ (1999) Immune responses to exercise in children treated for cancer. J Sports Med Phys Fitness 39:240–243

Silverman LB, Gelber RD, Dalton VK, Asselin BL, Barr RD, Clavell LA, Hurwitz CA, Moghrabi A, Samson Y, Schorin MA, Arkin S, Declerck L, Cohen HJ, Sallan SE (2001) Improved outcome for children with acute lymphoblastic leukemia: results of Dana-Farber Consortium Protocol 91-01. Blood 97:1211–1218

Suit H, Spiro I (1995) Radiation as a therapeutic modality in sarcomas of the soft tissue. Hematol Oncol Clin North Am 9:733–746

Takken T, van der Torre P, Zwerink M, Hulzebos EH, Bierings M, Helders PJ, van der Net J (2009) Development, feasibility and efficacy of a community-based exercise training program in pediatric cancer survivors. Psychooncology 18: 440–448

Tallman MS, Hakimian D, Kwaan HC, Rickles FR (1993) New insights into the pathogenesis of coagulation dysfunction in acute promyelocytic leukemia. Leuk Lymphoma 11:27–36

Tercyak KP, Donze JR, Prahlad S, Mosher RB, Shad AT (2006). Multiple behavioral risk factors among adolescent survivors of childhood cancer in the Survivor Health and Resilience Education

(SHARE) program. Pediatr Blood Cancer. 47:825–830.

Tillmann V, Darlington AS, Eiser C, Bishop NJ, Davies HA (2002) Male sex and low physical activity are associated with reduced spine bone mineral density in survivors of childhood acute lymphoblastic leukemia. J Bone Miner Res 17: 1073–1080

Tower RL, Spector LG (2007) The epidemiology of childhood leukemia with a focus on birth weight and diet. Crit Rev Clin Lab Sci 44:203–242

Turner-Gomes SO, Lands LC, Halton J, Hanning RM, Heigenhauser GJ, Pai M, Barr R (1996) Cardiorespiratory status after treatment for acute lymphoblastic leukemia. Med Pediatr Oncol 26: 160–165

van Brussel M, Takken T, van der Net J, Engelbert RH, Bierings M, Schoenmakers MA, Helders PJ (2006) Physical function and fitness in long-term survivors of childhood leukaemia. Pediatr Rehabil 9:267–274

Warner JT, Bell W, Webb DK, Gregory JW (1997) Relationship between cardiopulmonary response to exercise and adiposity in survivors of childhood malignancy. Arch Dis Child 76:298–303

Warner JT, Bell W, Webb DK, Gregory JW (1998) Daily energy expenditure and physical activity in survivors of childhood malignancy. Pediatr Res 43:607–613

White AC, Terrin N, Miller KB, Ryan HF (2005) Impaired respiratory and skeletal muscle strength in patients prior to hematopoietic stem-cell transplantation. Chest 128:145–152

Winter C, Muller C, Brandes M, Brinkmann A, Hoffmann C, Hardes J, Gosheger G, Boos J, Rosenbaum D (2009) Level of activity in children undergoing cancer treatment. Pediatr Blood Cancer 53:438–443

Wolin KY, Ruiz JR, Tuchman H, Lucia A (2010) Exercise in adult and pediatric hematological cancer survivors: an intervention review. Leukemia 24:1113–1120

Wright MJ, Halton JM, Martin RF, Barr RD (1998) Long-term gross motor performance following treatment for acute lymphoblastic leukemia. Med Pediatr Oncol 31:86–90

Wright MJ, Galea V, Barr RD (2005). Proficiency of balance in children and youth who have had acute lymphoblastic leukemia. Phys Ther. 85:782–890.

Physical Activity and Palliative Cancer Care

15

Sonya S. Lowe

Abstract Palliative care is an interdisciplinary and holistic approach aimed at alleviating suffering from physical, psychosocial, and spiritual issues in progressive, advanced disease. Progressive fatigue and anorexia–cachexia syndrome can contribute to loss of physical function in the palliative cancer patient, to the detriment of overall quality of life. Physical activity is one potential intervention, which may address these needs in the palliative cancer patient. There is preliminary evidence that at least some palliative cancer patients are willing and able to tolerate physical activity interventions, with some patients demonstrating improvement in select supportive care outcomes postintervention. Methodologically rigorous studies and consensus on common definitions are required to advance this area of research.

S.S. Lowe (✉)
Department of Symptom Control and Palliative Care, Cross Cancer Institute, 11560 University Drive NW, Edmonton T6G 1Z2, Alberta
e-mail: Sonya.Lowe@albertahealthservices.ca

15.1 Introduction

The World Health Organization defines palliative care as "an approach which improves the quality of life of patients and their families facing life-threatening illness, through the prevention and relief of suffering by means of early identification and impeccable assessment and treatment of pain and other problems, physical, psychological, and spiritual" (Sepulveda et al. 2002). In its broadest sense, this definition is applicable throughout the disease trajectory as part of comprehensive and integrated medical care. The primary goal of palliative care is to maximize overall quality of life for patients and their families (Borgsteede et al. 2006).

According to the Canadian Hospice Palliative Care Association, it is estimated that more than 65% of all deaths annually in Canada require access to hospice palliative care services (CHPCA 2007). When applying this principle to the cancer population, of the approximately 75,300 deaths from cancer that occurred in Canada in 2009, one can postulate that more than 49,000 cancer-related deaths would have required access to hospice palliative care services (Canadian Cancer Society 2009). In conjunction with an aging population, and the

K.S. Courneya and C.M. Friedenreich (eds.), *Physical Activity and Cancer*,
Recent Results in Cancer Research 186, DOI: 10.1007/978-3-642-04231-7_15,

15

projected increase in rate of deaths in Canada by 33% by the year 2020, the demand for hospice palliative care will inevitably increase. The need for hospice palliative care services applies across all cancer diagnoses at any point during the disease trajectory.

As methods of cancer detection and treatment improve, survival is prolonged and lifetime burden of distressing physical and psychosocial symptoms increases. Palliative care increasingly encompasses a wide chronological range within the spectrum of cancer control, from those who are newly diagnosed with life-threatening disease (i.e., Stage IV lung cancer), to those who are undergoing chemotherapy and radiotherapy for symptom management (i.e., breast cancer with bone metastases), and those who are eligible for hospice care or who are actively dying. Although the mandate of palliative care can apply throughout the cancer trajectory, its greatest impact is associated with the end stages of life (Bakitas et al. 2006).

Given these broadly inclusive aims, the lack of uniform criteria for defining palliative care populations is a well-recognized limitation in oncological research (Borgsteede et al. 2006); there is no consensus as to what time point in life expectancy the cancer patient can be considered "palliative" or "terminal" (Stone and Lund 2007). The U.S. National Cancer Institute defines advanced cancer as "cancer that has spread to other places in the body and usually cannot be cured or controlled with treatment" (National Cancer Institute: Dictionary of Cancer Terms 2007). Despite these challenges, it is recognized that the closer the patient is toward death, the greater the disease and symptom burden becomes, thus making palliation the sole focus of care (Cohen and Leis 2002). For the purposes of this review, the palliative cancer patient will be defined as a patient who has progressive, incurable, and locally recurrent or metastatic cancer, with a clinician-estimated survival of less than 12 months.

15.2 Fatigue in the Palliative Cancer Patient

The most common symptom reported by palliative cancer patients is cancer-related fatigue (CRF) (Del Fabbro et al. 2006). Fatigue is defined as a subjective sensation of tiredness, weakness, or lack of energy (Radbruch et al. 2008). Fatigue (69%), weakness (66%), and lack of energy (61%) were among the five most prevalent symptoms in a retrospective study of 1,000 patients in an American palliative medicine program (Walsh et al. 2000). Between 60 and 90% of advanced cancer patients report experiencing CRF, and rate CRF as the symptom with the most negative impact on overall quality of life (Munch et al. 2006).

Pathophysiologically, primary fatigue is postulated to be related to the tumor itself, either peripherally through energy depletion or centrally through the hypothalamic–pituitary–adrenal axis or serotonin dysfunction (Barnes and Bruera 2002). Tumor load and subsequent proinflammatory cytokine production, including interleukin-1, interleukin-6, and tumor necrosis factor-α, interact to contribute to CRF in the end stages of cancer. In combination with progressive metabolic abnormalities and autonomic failure, these cytokines are key mediators of anemia, anorexia–cachexia, and fever, all of which contribute to CRF. Psychologically, the high prevalence of depression and anxiety in palliative cancer patients may compound the cognitive and affective difficulties as a result of CRF. The increasing use of medications, such as opioid analgesics and anxiolytics, to palliate these individual symptoms may likewise worsen CRF.

One of the devastating repercussions of CRF is loss of physical function, which has been reported by palliative cancer patients as one of their primary concerns at the end of life (Axelsson and Sjoden 1998). Neurohormonal

Table 15.1 Characteristics of studies examining physical activity in palliative cancer patients

Study	Features	Participants	Diagnoses	Intervention	Outcomes	Comments
Porock et al. (2000) (Australia)	Unsupervised home-based physical activity program in home hospice care patients	9 patients 3 male, 6 female Mean age 59.87 years (SD 9.77)	Bowel (n = 4) Pancreas (n = 2) Melanoma (n = 1) Breast (n = 1) Oral (n = 1) Metastases (n = 7) Active RT (n = 1) Active chemo (n = 2)	Individualized "Duke Energizing Exercise Plan" with a range of physical activities throughout the day, frequency and duration set according to Winningham's half rule of thumb for 28 days.	(1) Fatigue via MFI (2) Anxiety and Depression via HADS (3) Symptom Distress via McCorkle and Young's SDS (4) QOL via Graham and Longman's QOL scale	Single group pre–post intervention study. No staging information available. Incomplete data for HADS, adherence and withdrawals.
Crevenna (2003a) (*Wien Med Wschr*) (Austria)	Supervised aerobic exercise program during palliative thalidomide therapy	1 man, age 55 years old	Advanced hepatocellular cancer with lung and brain metastases	(1) Bicycle ergometer cycling with workload systematic increase to maintain training HR at 60% of maximum workload of first symptom-limited exercise test. 60 min per session, 2 sessions per week for 6 weeks.	(1) Symptom-limited ergometric bicycle exercise test: peak work capacity, endurance capacity and HR (2) 6-min walk (3) Grimsby's self-reported physical performance questionnaire (4) QOL via SF-36	Case report. Partially reported baseline performance status. No adverse events reported. 100% compliance with training sessions. Participant commented on "being persistently and positively motivated by the physicians".

(*continued*)

Table 15.1 continued

Study	Features	Participants	Diagnoses	Intervention	Outcomes	Comments
					(5) Self-reported benefit in physical performance, mental state, satisfaction and QOL	
Crevenna (2003b) (*Support Care Cancer*) (Austria)	Supervised aerobic exercise program during palliative chemotherapy (gemcitabine, epirubicin, paclitaxel) and palliative radiotherapy	1 female, age 48 years old	Advanced breast cancer with lung, liver and bone metastases	(1) Bicycle ergometer cycling with workload increased to maintain training HR at 60% of maximum workload of first symptom-limited exercise test. 60 min per session, 3 sessions per week for 52 weeks.	(1) Symptom-limited ergometric bicycle exercise test: VO_2max, peak work capacity, and HR (2) Lung function via respiratory quotient (3) QOL via SF-36 (4) Self-reported benefit in physical performance, mental state, fatigue, sleep, satisfaction and QOL	Case report. Baseline performance status not reported. No adverse events reported. Participant attributed benefit to persistent and positive motivation by the physicians.
Kelm et al. (2003) (Germany)	Supervised whole body strength and endurance training during postoperative intrahepatic chemotherapy	1 man, age 58 years old	Rectal adenocarcinoma (pT3N0M1) with liver metastases	(1) Strength training machines at 40–60% of 1-repetition maximum up to 5 series of 20 repetitions.	(1) Upper extremity and Lower extremity strength: 1RM	Case report. Unknown baseline performance status.

				(2) Treadmill/ bicycle/ upper body ergometer 10 min each with resistance and speed controlled to HR between 130–150bpm. 6-weeks postop and every 2 weeks between chemotherapy cycles for total of 13 weeks	(2) Endurance by reduction in HR and lactate concentration (3) Lung function by FEV_1, FVC and VC (4) QOL by GIQLI score (5) Immune function by NK cell count	Unable to determine whether functional gains secondary to post-operative recovery or intervention.
Headley et al. (2004) (USA)	Unsupervised home-based seated exercise program in stage IV breast cancer patients receiving chemotherapy	38 women Mean age 51 years (SD 9.43)	Stage IV breast cancer (n = 38)	Seated exercise program using Armchair Fitness: Gentle Exercise video, 30 min per session, 3 sessions per week for 12 weeks	(1) Fatigue and QOL via the FACIT-F (2) Perceived intensity via the Borg Rating of Perceived Exertion scale	Randomized controlled longitudinal trial. Incomplete data for adherence, intensity and frequency of activity.
Oldervoll et al. (2005) (2006) (Norway)	Supervised group exercise program in palliative patients from outpatient clinic and hospice	34 patients 15 males, 19 females Mean age 55 years (SD 11.5) Mean KPS 83 (SD 13.2)	Gastrointestinal (n = 16) Breast (n = 5) Genitourinary (n = 5) Lung (n = 1) Miscellaneous (n = 7) Metastases (n = 27) Active chemo (n = 9) Active hormone therapy (n = 3)	Group exercise program (3–8 patients per group) with personalized circuit training stations focused on UE/LE muscle strength, standing balance and aerobic endurance with 50 min per session, 2 sessions per week for 6 weeks.	(1) Physical performance via 6-min walk, timed sit-to-stand, functional reach (2) Fatigue via FQ (3) QOL via EORTC QLQ-C30	Single group pre–post intervention study. No progression of workload reported. Adherence rate to exercise sessions 10.6/12. 46% attrition rate.

(*continued*)

Table 15.1 continued

Study	Features	Participants	Diagnoses	Intervention	Outcomes	Comments
Dahele et al. (2007) (United Kingdom)	Pilot accelerometry study of ambulatory outpatients with GI cancer versus age-matched healthy controls	20 patients (18 male, 2 female; mean age 62) and 13 age-matched controls (9 male, 4 female; mean age 59)	Esophagus (n = 8) Gastric (n = 6) Esophagogastric junction (n = 2) Pancreatic (n = 2) Other (n = 2)	No physical activity intervention. Free-living physical activity was measured for 1 week using the activPAL™ meter	(1) Anorexia/cachexia via FAACT (2) Fatigue via FACIT-F (3) QOL via EORTC QLQ-C30	No physical activity intervention. Query precision of standardized MET values in capturing actual energy expended. Query clinically significant magnitude of change in physical activity.
Clark et al. (2007) (USA)	Pilot survey of convenience sample of advanced cancer patients receiving outpatient chemotherapy	128 patients (42 male, 58 female; mean age 59.8 (SD 13.4))	Breast (n = 21) Digestive (n = 17) Lung (n = 13) Gynecological (n = 12) Genitourinary (n = 9) Neurological (n = 5) Head and neck (n = 4) Other (n = 21)	No physical activity intervention. Cross-sectional survey assessing physical activity levels, mood and quality of life variables.	(1) Self-efficacy for PA via Likert scale (2) Outcome expectations, perceived barriers and benefits. interest in and plans for PA via closed and open-ended items (3) PA via GLTEQ (4) Mood via PA-NAS (5) QOL via FACT-G	No physical activity intervention. Estimated life expectancy of less than 5 years and greater than 6 months. Lack of objective measurement of activity level in patients.

Lowe (2009b) (Canada)	Pilot survey of palliative cancer patients from palliative home care and outpatient clinics	50 patients (20 male, 30 female; mean age 61.5 (SD 13.1)) Median survival from time of survey to time of death was 104 days.	Lung (n = 15) Genitourinary (n = 11) Breast (n = 8) Gastrointestinal (n = 8) Hematological (n = 4) Head and neck (n = 2) Other (n = 2)	No physical activity intervention. Cross-sectional survey assessing self-reported QOL, physical function, symptoms and physical activity behavior.	(1) QOL via MQOL (2) Symptoms via ESAS (3) PA via modified items from PASE (4) Abbreviated version of the Late-Life Function and Disability Instrument (LLFDI)	No physical activity intervention. Lack of objective measurement of activity level in patients.
Kasymjanova et al. (2009) (Canada)	6MW in advanced NSCLC patients before and after two cycles of chemotherapy	45 completer patients (25 male, 20 female; mean age 62.8 (SD 10.6)) 19 dropout patients (4 male, 15 female; mean age 60.2 (SD 10.9))	Lung (n = 64)	6 MW once on initial assessment, once prechemotherapy and once after two cycles of chemotherapy.	(1) Survival (2) Change in 6MW	No physical activity intervention.

SD, standard deviation; *RT*, radiotherapy; *MFI*, multidimensional fatigue inventory; *HADS*, hospital anxiety and depression scale; *SDS*, symptom distress scale; *QOL*, quality of life; *HR*, heart rate; *SF-36*, short form 36 survey; VO_2max, peak oxygen uptake; *GIQLI*, gastrointestinal quality of life index; *1-RM* = 1-repetition maximum; FEV_1, forced expiratory volume in 1 s; *FVC*, forced vital capacity; *VC*, vital capacity; *NK*, natural killer cell; *FACIT-F*, functional assessment of chronic illness therapy – fatigue version IV; *KPS*, Karnofsky performance score; *UE/LE*, upper extremity/lower extremity; *FQ*, fatigue questionnaire; *EORTC QLQ-C30* = European organization for research and treatment of cancer core quality of life questionnaire; *GI* , gastrointestinal; *FAACT*, functional assessment of anorexia and cachexia therapy; *MET*, metabolic equivalents; *PA*, physical activity level; *GLTEQ*, Godin Leisure-time exercise questionnaire; *PA-NAS*, positive affect negative affect scales; *FACT-G*, functional assessment of cancer therapy-general; *MQOL*, McGill quality of life questionnaire; *ESAS*, Edmonton symptom assessment system; *PASE*, physical activity scale for the elderly; *LLFDI*, late-life function and disability instrument; *6MW*, 6-min walk test; *NSCLC*, nonsmall cell lung cancer

15

Table 15.2 Patient-reported outcomes of studies examining physical activity in palliative cancer patients

Study	Quality of life (tool/score)	Physical function (tool/score)	Fatigue (tool/score)	Symptoms (tool/score)
Porock et al. (2000) (Australia)	Graham & Longman's Scale Mean QOL rating: 5.3 (Day 0) 6.1 (Day 7) 6.6 (Day 14)	None reported	Incomplete data for all time points	Incomplete data
Crevenna (2003a) (*Wien Med Wschr*) (Austria)	SF-36 General health perception subscale: Pre: 65, Post: 62	SF-36 Physical functioning subscale: Pre:65, Post:85	SF-36 Vitality/fatigue subscale: Pre:25, Post:50	SF-36 Pain subscale: Pre: 22, Post: 41
Crevenna (2003b) (*Support Care Cancer*) (Austria)	None reported	None reported	None reported	SF-36 Incomplete data
Kelm et al. (2003) (Germany)	GIQLI Pre:106, Post:129 +21.6% difference	None reported	None reported	None reported
Headley et al. (2004) (USA)	FACIT-F Total scores: t[49] = 2.31; p = 0.0254 Experimental group decline in total-wellbeing, slower rate than in control group	FACIT-F Functional well-being subscale: no significant difference between groups at any time point	FACIT-F Fatigue subscale: t[49] = 2.78; p = 0.0078 Experimental group decline in fatigue slower rate than in control group	None reported
Oldervoll et al. (2006) (Norway)	EORTC QLQ-C30 Global QOL subscale: Pre:61(21), Post:64(20) p = 0.26	EORTC QLQ-C30 Physical functioning subscale: Pre:65(20), Post:67(22) p = 0.62	Fatigue Questionnaire Total fatigue subscale: Pre:17.5(4.7), Post:15.5(5.8) p = 0.06 Mental fatigue subscale: Pre:5.3(1.7), Post:5.1(2.0) p = 0.42 Physical fatigue subscale: Pre:12.2(3.6), Post:10.4(4.1) p = 0.04	EORTC QLQ-C30 Nausea/vomiting: Pre:18(25), Post:14(19) p = 0.26 Pain: Pre:41(35), Post:37(34) p = 0.36 Dyspnea: Pre: 42(33), Post:30(31) p = 0.006 Appetite loss: Pre:37(38), Post:28(35) p = 0.07

Study	Quality of life (tool/score)	Physical function (tool/score)	Fatigue (tool/ score)	Symptoms (tool/score)
Dahele et al. (2007) (United Kingdom)	EORTC QLQ-C30 Global health/ QOoL subscale Correlation between estimated total energy expenditure (r = −0.029, P = 0.905) or average steps per day (r = 0.047, P = 0.848)	EORTC QLQ-C30 Physical functioning subscale Correlation between estimated total energy expenditure (r = 0.352, P = 0.139) or average steps per day (r = 0.370, P = 0.113)	FACIT-F Trial outcome index Correlation between estimated total energy expenditure (r = 0.59, P = 0.009) or average steps per day (r = 0.59, P = 0.008) EORTC QLQ-C30 Fatigue subscale Correlation between estimated total energy expenditure (r = −0.281, P = 0.244) or average steps per day (r = −0.398, P = 0.091)	FAACT (anorexia/ cachexia) Trial outcome index Correlation between estimated total energy expenditure (r = 0.40, P = 0.089) or average steps per day (r = 0.41, P = 0.080)
Clark et al. (2007) (USA)	FACT-G Physical well-being subscale (t = 0.63, p = 0.53) Overall QOL Rating Mean 7.1 (1.9)	None reported	None reported	PA-NAS Positive affect (t = 2.18, p <0.05) Negative affect (t = 0.59, p = 0.58)
Lowe (2009b) (Canada)	MQOL Total score Walking ≥ 30 min per day (d = 0.59, P = 0.046) PA ≥ 60 min per day (d = 0.16, P = 0.543)	LLFDI Total function score Walking ≥ 30 min per day (d = −0.32, P = 0.261) PA ≥ 60 min per day (d = −0.18, P = 0.530)	ESAS Fatigue subscale Walking ≥ 30 min per day (d = −0.31, P = 0.273) PA ≥ 60 min per day (d = 0.04, P = 0.895)	ESAS Pain subscale Walking ≥ 30 min per day (d = 0.15, P = 0.590) PA ≥ 60 min per day (d = −0.22, P = 0.443)
Kasymjanova et al. (2009) (Canada)	None reported	None reported	None reported	None reported

QOL, quality of life; *SF-36*, short form 36 survey; *GIQLI*, gastrointestinal quality of life index; *FACIT-F*, functional assessment of chronic illness therapy – fatigue version IV; *EORTC QLQ-C30*, European Organization for Research and Treatment of Cancer Core Quality of Life Questionnaire; *PA*, physical activity; *FAACT*, functional assessment of anorexia and cachexia therapy; *FACT-G*, functional assessment of cancer therapy – general; *PA-NAS*, positive affect negative affect scales; *MQOL*, McGill quality of life questionnaire; *LLFDI*, late life function and disability instrument; *ESAS*, Edmonton symptom assessment system

Table 15.3 Objective outcomes of studies examining physical activity in palliative cancer patients

Study	Physical function (tool/score)	Physical fitness (tool/score)
Dahele et al. (2007) (United Kingdom)	Cancer patients undergoing palliative chemotherapy spent more time lying/sitting ($p = 0.0005$) and less time in stepping ($p = 0.003$) than controls. Median number of total steps taken during week by cancer patients approximately 43% fewer than healthy controls ($p = 0.002$).	None reported
Dahele et al. (2007) (USA)	None reported	None reported
Lowe (2009b) (Canada)	None reported	None reported
Kasymjanova et al. (2009) (Canada)	Patients with initial 6MW 400m ≤ had significantly greater survival time than those with initial 6MW < 400m (hazard ratio 0.44; 95% CI; 0.23–0.83 ($p = 0.001$)	None reported

(6MW = 6-min walk test)

abnormalities and anorexia–cachexia result in extensive loss of skeletal muscle mass in the advanced cancer patient. Progressive deconditioning and impaired mobility lead to a loss of independence in activities of daily living; this decline in physical function thus compounds the fear of becoming a burden to others, which can trigger severe emotional distress in the advanced cancer patient (Cheville 2001). Optimizing physical function with the aim of maintaining autonomy is therefore critical in maximizing overall quality of life in palliative cancer patients. Not only does loss of physical functioning impede the patient's ability to perform activities of daily living, but increasing physical dependence on caregivers and loved ones for support causes an additional emotional and psychological burden on the patient as well (Chochinov et al. 2007). The desire of advanced cancer patients to keep mobile is fundamentally linked to the desire to remain as independent as possible. Participation in daily activities was identified as a significant factor in patients living with terminal illness (Carter et al. 2004). Functional disability can result in devastating impact on the advanced cancer patient's quality of life (Dahlin and Heiwe 2009).

Physical activity is one potential intervention that can address this need in palliative cancer patients. Physical activity is defined as any bodily movement produced by the skeletal muscles which results in a substantial increase in energy expenditure over resting levels (Bouchard and Shephard 1994). Currently, there are no physical activity recommendations specific for palliative cancer patients. For individuals with low functional status in general, Drouin et al. proposed a model of exercise prescription such that patients who are bedbound or experience fatigue on mild exertion may benefit from short sessions of low-intensity activity several times per week, in order to maintain physical functioning and prevent deconditioning (Drouin and Lucinda 2006).

In our recent systematic review, few studies had examined physical activity in palliative cancer patients, and the current evidence is limited largely to case reports and uncontrolled trials (Lowe et al. 2009a). These preliminary studies did provide some evidence that at least some palliative cancer patients are willing and able to tolerate physical activity interventions, with some patients demonstrating improvement in some supportive care outcomes post intervention.

The purpose of this review is to summarize the major evidence, to date, of physical activity in palliative cancer patients, in order to evaluate future direction of research in this area. We have excluded studies that involved a mixed population of different stages of disease, including palliative cancer patients, if they did not report data or analyze data separately for advanced stage.

15.3 State of the Evidence

Porock et al. conducted a pilot study of nine home care hospice cancer patients in Australia who were administered an unsupervised home-based physical activity program based on the Duke Energizing Exercise Plan, with a range of different physical activities prescribed according to the patient's individual condition and tolerability. Forty-six percent (11/24) of the patients approached agreed to participate. Their study sample was composed of six females and three males, with a mean age of 60 ± 10 years. The most common cancer diagnosis was bowel cancer, with seven participants having metastases. Two participants reported undergoing concurrent chemotherapy, whereas one participant reported undergoing concurrent radiotherapy. Despite the trend toward increased quality of life scores, it was unclear if the program took the participant's exercise preferences or interests into account, and the authors concluded that the optimal type of physical activity program for this population is still unknown (Porock et al. 2000).

Crevenna et al. examined supervised ergometer bicycling interventions in two case reports: the first was a 55-year-old male with hepatocellular carcinoma metastasized to lung and brain (Crevenna et al. 2003a), and the second was a 48-year-old female with breast cancer metastasized to liver, lung, and bone (Crevenna et al. 2003b). The former participant was undergoing concurrent thalidomide treatment, and participated in twice weekly sessions for a total of 6 weeks, with increasing workload to maintain heart rate at 60% of maximum workload for 60-min sessions. Hundred percent adherence was reported from this single participant. The latter participant was undergoing concurrent palliative chemotherapy and radiotherapy, and participated in 60-min sessions three times per week for a 52-week program while systematically increasing workload according to the same criteria.

Kelm et al. examined a 13-week whole body strength and endurance training program in a 58-year-old male with rectal adenocarcinoma metastatic to the liver undergoing concurrent intrathecal chemotherapy (Kelm et al. 2003). The participant completed biweekly sessions involving both strength training machines at 40–60% of 1-repetition maximum, and treadmill walking or ergometer cycling with resistance and speed controlled to maintain a heart rate of between 130 and 150 beats per minute.

Headley et al. conducted a randomized controlled trial of an unsupervised, home-based seated exercise program in Stage IV breast cancer patients receiving chemotherapy (Headley et al. 2004). The control group had more participants with higher baseline physical activity levels, which were not adjusted for in their analysis. Their study sample was composed of 38 females, with a mean age of 51 ± 9 years. The participants performed a 30-min seated exercise program using the Armchair Fitness: Gentle Exercise video in their own homes three times per week for a total of 12 weeks. Self-reported intensity was assessed using Borg Ratings of Perceived Exertion; however, no method of progression of intervention workload was reported. The experimental group had a statistically significant slower decline in total well-being scores than the control group ($p = 0.03$). In addition, the experimental group showed a statistically significant slower rate of increase in fatigue ($p = 0.01$) compared to the control group. There was no significant difference in patient-reported physical functioning scores between groups at any time point.

Oldervoll et al. conducted a prospective phase II pilot study to examine the effects of a structured physical activity program on 34 advanced cancer patients with clinician-estimated survival between 3 and 12 months (Oldervoll et al. 2005). The authors reported a 62% (63/101) recruitment rate. Participants were recruited from both outpatient clinic and hospice sites, with hospice participants having a statistically significant lower baseline Karnofsky Performance Scores than outpatient participants ($p = 0.003$), which was not accounted for in subsequent data analysis. The mean age of their study sample was 65 ± 12 years, and the mean baseline Karnofsky Performance Score was 83 ± 13. The most common diagnosis was gastrointestinal cancer ($n = 16$), with 79% of participants reporting metastases. Twenty-six percent of participants were undergoing concurrent chemotherapy, and 9% of participants were undergoing concurrent hormone therapy during the intervention period. Sixty-three percent of the incurable cancer patients invited to the study were willing to participate in a physical activity intervention, and 54% of those who agreed to participate actually completed the intervention. Patients who did not want to participate, however, identified limitations of fatigue, lack of mobility, and the burden of physically getting to the hospital gym where the group exercise intervention took place. The authors concluded that these limitations "might indicate a need for specially tailored interventions…in the form of home-based exercises adjusted to for the individual patient" (Oldervoll et al. 2005).

In their subsequent pilot intervention, groups of between three to eight participants performed a series of personalized circuit training stations focused on whole body muscle strength, standing balance, and aerobic endurance for 50-min sessions twice per week. The authors reported that an average of 10.6 out of 12 (88%) prescribed sessions were completed. In all, 34/47 (72%) of participants completed the exercise intervention with all 34 (100%) participants completing follow-up assessments. Oldervoll et al. reported a significant improvement in both the emotional and social functioning subscores ($p < 0.01$) of the EORTQ QLQ-C30. They found a statistically significant improvement in the 6-min walk ($p = 0.007$) and timed sit-to-stand ($p = 0.001$) pre- to postintervention, although the global QOL and physical functioning scores remained unchanged. There was a statistically significant improvement pre- to postintervention in the dyspnea subscore ($p = 0.006$). There was a borderline significant decrease in total fatigue subscale scores ($p = 0.06$) (Oldervoll et al. 2006).

Clark et al. conducted a cross-sectional survey on 128 patients with advanced-stage cancer receiving chemotherapy (Clark et al. 2007). Eligibility criteria included an estimated life expectancy of less than 5 years but greater than 6 months. Breast cancer was the most common diagnosis among the study participants, although no information was given regarding presence or location of metastatic disease, and actual survival of participants was not measured. Positive outcome expectations for physical activity, positive mood, and higher current exercise level were related to self-efficacy. Fatigue or low energy was identified as the most significant barrier to physical activity. Altogether, 89% of participants intended to either increase or maintain their physical activity level, and 47% of participants were probably or definitely interested in receiving professional support for physical activity.

Given the limited functional data linking advanced cancer to physical activity, Dahele et al. conducted a pilot accelerometry study of 20 patients with upper gastrointestinal cancer receiving palliative chemotherapy, compared to 13 age-matched healthy controls (Dahele et al. 2007). No information was provided about whether the patients had metastatic disease, and actual survival of participants was not reported. Patients receiving palliative chemotherapy were less active than healthy controls; however, there was no correlation between average number of steps taken per day and global QOL scores of the EORTC QLQ-C30 in advanced gastrointestinal cancer patients undergoing chemotherapy (Dahele et al. 2007).

Most recently, we conducted a cross-sectional pilot survey of fifty advanced cancer patients aged 18 years or older with clinician-estimated life expectancy of between 3 and 12 months and palliative performance status scale scores of greater than 30% (Lowe et al. 2009b). The median survival of participants was 104 days from time of survey to time of death. Walking was the most common reported physical activity. Our sample demonstrated a significant positive association between physical activity and quality of life scores as measured by the McGill Quality of Life Questionnaire (MQOL). In particular, participants who reported walking more than 30 min per day reported higher existential subscores, support subscores, and total scores on the MQOL. Overall, there appeared to be an advantage in quality of life for those palliative cancer patients who reported greater levels of walking and total physical activity over the past week.

In our pilot study, a majority of palliative cancer patients in this sample were interested in and felt able to participate in a physical activity program, with the majority of participants indicating a preference to perform physical activity alone and in their own homes (Lowe et al. 2009c). Walking was identified as the preferred modality of physical activity by the majority of our sample (Table 15.4). Examining these unique physical activity interests and preferences may aid in the development of an appropriate physical activity program for palliative cancer patients that could be tested in future research.

Kasymjanova et al. conducted a study examining the 6-min walk test as a prognostic tool in of forty-five advanced nonsmall cell lung cancer patients both before and after two cycles of chemotherapy (Kasymjanova et al.

Table 15.4 Descriptive statistics for physical activity preferences of palliative cancer patients

Preference variable	N (%)
Is being physically active important to you now?	
Yes	47 (94%)
No	3 (6%)
Are you interested in a physical activity program now?	
Yes	39 (78%)
No	4 (8%)
Maybe	7 (14%)
Do you think you would be able to participate in a physical activity program now?	
Yes	29 (58%)
No	4 (8%)
Maybe	17 (34%)
If you were to begin a physical activity program, who would you like to participate with?	
Alone	27 (54%)
With caregiver/spouse	5 (10%)
With family/friends	3 (6%)
With other cancer patients	0
No preference	15 (30%)
If you were to begin a physical activity program, where would you like to participate?	
At home	42 (84%)
At a hospital-based center	0
At a cancer center	0
At a local fitness center	0
No preference	8 (16%)

(n = 50) (Lowe 2009)

15

2009). All participants had Stage IIIA or higher nonsmall cell lung cancer, and overall median survival of all participants was 11.1 months. The authors reported a statistically significant decline in distance on 6-min walk after two cycles of chemotherapy, with a distance of greater than or equal to 400 m on initial 6-min walk being the only variable with significant effect on survival after adjusting for covariates.

15.4 Summary and Future Perspectives

Future research is required to establish a standardized definition of palliative patients in oncology. Defining a "palliative" population has been identified as one of the top methodological challenges of conducting palliative care research; with respect to cancer, there is no standardized definition of a palliative patient, and multiple terms such as "advanced cancer", "end stage cancer", and "terminal cancer" have been used without uniform consensus as to the description of the eligible populations (Addington-Hall 2002). In their survey study of Dutch general practitioners, Borgsteede et al. demonstrated significant differences in the elicited patient populations based on the different inclusive criteria of "non-curative treatment", "palliative care", and "death was expected"; the authors recommended that future research should include a combination of different criteria, including the intent of the palliative care provided as well as an assessment of the participant's life expectancy as an indicator of their chronological status along the cancer trajectory (Borgsteede et al. 2006). Consensus on the description of palliative research populations is crucial in order to facilitate interstudy comparison and quantitative analysis. In lieu of clinician estimates, use of a validated prognostic tool may aid in defining the patient population more precisely.

Other than defining the participant inclusion criteria by life expectancy, it may be worthwhile to categorize participants by palliative performance status level. The palliative performance status (PPS) scale has been widely used and validated in palliative care and has been shown to be predictive of prognosis in palliative cancer populations (Lau et al. 2007). Hence, targeting cancer patients with a specific PPS level, irrespective of cancer diagnosis or estimated life expectancy, may facilitate recruitment and add a unique dimension to physical activity intervention research in cancer.

The physical ability to participate in a physical activity program may decline rapidly in patients with short-life expectancy, and symptom burden and physical well-being of end stage cancer patients can fluctuate on a daily basis, such that both adherence and retention to a physical activity program can be affected. In a multicenter randomized, controlled trial comparing the effects of cannabinoids on appetite and quality of life in 164 advanced cancer patients, Strasser et al. reported a 33% dropout rate over the course of their 6-week intervention; the most common reason for dropout was withdrawn consent, which the authors partially attributed to "the clinical reality of interfering symptoms and complications" in this patient population (Strasser et al. 2006). Given the challenges of patient attrition within this population, future physical activity intervention trials may benefit from a multicenter approach in order to be adequately powered to determine efficacy for the outcomes of interest.

In a recent systematic review, Jordhoy et al. showed that physical functioning is a neglected dimension in palliative care quality of life measures, and that there is little consensus as to how physical functioning should be assessed or what components of physical functioning should be elicited in palliative cancer patients (Jordhoy et al. 2007). Consensus is also required on standardized physical function assessment tools for the palliative cancer population. In a recent evaluation study of the development of an international self-report instrument for physical functioning in palliative cancer care, mobility and self-care subdimensions were identified as being particularly relevant for this population (Helbostad et al. 2009). Correlation with objective tests of physical functioning would also minimize the potential for error and bias in outcome measurement.

Key future research directions for the palliative cancer population would include more thorough characterization of the functional trajectory of disease, as well as increasing focus on what interventions could be performed in patients who have extremely limited mobility or are bedbound. Determining the optimal type of physical activity interventions at each level of palliative performance status would be a priority so as to include as many patients of varying functional abilities for as long as possible during their disease course. Rather than targeting a small subset of palliative cancer patients, future research should aim toward encouraging mobility in as many palliative cancer patients as possible, in view of decreasing symptom burden and maintaining overall quality of life.

In summary, the potential role for physical activity as a supportive care intervention is promising; however, further feasibility studies are needed to substantiate preliminary findings and further advance this emerging area of research. Consensus is required to develop common definitions for palliative cancer populations, interventions, and outcomes to validate findings, justify interpretations, and make meaningful recommendations to patients and their families.

15.5 Clinical Recommendations

Based on the current evidence, palliative cancer patients are encouraged to consider physical activity as a supportive care intervention under the specific direction and guidance of their attending medical team. As described in Lowe et al.'s study, walking is reported to be among the most preferred activities by this cancer population (Lowe et al. 2009c) and can be performed to tolerance in most individuals. Repetition of specific physical function tasks may be more beneficial in light of preserving basic activities of daily living and independence for the palliative cancer patient. Rather than improving fitness, the overall goal of physical activity would be to maintain or even slow the decline in physical functioning for as long as possible.

Although the optimal types of physical activity interventions for this population are yet to be determined, intervention goals may be shifted from energy expenditure to that of energy conservation. The loss of lean body mass tissues at the end stages of cancer may be accelerated by progressive anorexia–cachexia syndrome, and gentler forms of physical activity interventions, such as tai chi or qi gong, may be preferable. Even in patients with poor palliative performance status, active and assisted range of motion exercises should be encouraged to minimize muscle contractures and to slow muscle deconditioning. Given the heterogeneity of this cancer population in terms of cancer diagnoses, disease, and medical variables, physical activity interventions should be individually prescribed and regularly monitored by the patient's attending medical team.

References

Addington-Hall J (2002) Research sensitivities to palliative care patients. Eur J Cancer Care 11: 200–224

Axelsson B, Sjoden PO (1998) Quality of life of cancer patients and their spouses in palliative home care. Palliat Med 12:29–39

Bakitas MA, Lyons KD, Dixon J et al (2006) Palliative care program effectiveness research:

15

developing rigor in sampling design, conduct, and reporting. J Pain Symptom Manage 31(3): 270–284

Barnes EA, Bruera E (2002) Fatigue in patients with advanced cancer: a review. Int J Gynecol Cancer 12(5):424–428

Borgsteede SD, Deliens L, Francke AL et al (2006) Defining the patient population: one of the problems for palliative care research. Palliat Med 20:63–68

Bouchard C, Shephard RJ (1994) Physical activity, fitness and health: the model and key concepts. In: Bouchard C, Shephard RJ, Stephens T (eds) Physical activity, fitness, and health. international proceedings and consensus statement. Human Kinetics Publishers, Champaign, IL, pp 77–88

Canadian Cancer Society's Steering Committee: Canadian Cancer Statistics (2009); Toronto: Canadian Cancer Society, 2009

Canadian Hospice Palliative Care Association (2007) Hospice palliative care in Canada: a brief to the special senate committee on aging [cited April 29, 2010]; Available from: http://www.chpca.net/public_policy_advocacy/special_committee_on_aging/Brief_to_Spec_Sen_Comm_on_Aging-HPC_in_Canada.pdf

Carter H, MacLeod R, Brander P et al (2004) Living with a terminal illness: patient's priorities. J Adv Nurs 45(6):611–620

Cheville A (2001) Rehabilitation of patients with advanced cancer. Cancer 92:1039–1048

Chochinov HM, Kristjanson LJ, Hack TF et al (2007) Burden to others and the terminally ill. J Pain Symptom Manage 34(5):463–471

Clark MM, Vickers KS, Hathaway JC et al (2007) Physical activity in advanced-stage cancer actively receiving chemotherapy. J Support Oncol 5(10):487–493

Cohen SR, Leis A (2002) What determines quality of life of terminally ill cancer patients from their own perspective? J Palliat Care 18(1):48–58

Crevenna R, Schmidinger M, Keilani M et al (2003a) Aerobic exercise as additive palliative treatment for a patient with advanced hepatocellular cancer. Wien Med Wochenschr 115(19–20): 710–714

Crevenna R, Schmidinger M, Keilani M et al (2003b) Aerobic exercise for a patient suffering from metastatic bone disease. Support Care Cancer 11:120–122

Dahele M, Skipworth RJE, Wall L et al (2007) Objective physical activity and self-reported quality of life in patients receiving palliative chemotherapy. J Pain Symptom Manage 33(6): 676–685

Dahlin Y, Heiwe S (2009) Patient's experiences of physical therapy within palliative cancer care. J Pall Care 25(1):12–20

Del Fabbro E, Dalal S, Bruera E (2006) Symptom control in palliative care – part II: cachexia/anorexia and fatigue. J Palliat Med 9(2): 409–421

Drouin J, Lucinda P (2006) Physical activity and disability. National Center on Physical Activity and Disability [cited August 21, 2006]; Available from:http://www.ncpad.org/disability/fact_sheet.php?sheet=195&section=1463.

Headley JA, Ownby KK, John LD (2004) The effect of seated exercise on fatigue and quality of life in women with advanced breast cancer. Oncol Nurs Forum 31(5):977–983

Helbostad JL, Holen JC, Jordhoy MS et al (2009) A first step in the development of an international self-report instrument for physical functioning in palliative cancer care: a systematic literature review and an expert opinion evaluation study. J Pain Symptom Manage 37(2): 196–205

Jordhoy MS, Inger Ringdal G, Helbostad JL et al (2007) Assessing physical functioning: a systematic review of quality of life measures developed for use in palliative care. Palliat Med 21(8):673–682

Kasymjanova G, Correa JA, Kreisman H et al (2009) Prognostic value of the six-minute walk in advanced non-small cell lung cancer. J Thorac Oncol 4(5):602–607

Kelm J, Ahlhelm F, Weibenbach P et al (2003) Physical training during intrahepatic chemotherapy. Arch Phys Med Rehabil 84(5): 687–690

Lau F, Cloutier-Fisher D, Kuziemsky C et al (2007) A systematic review of prognostic tools for estimating survival time in palliative care. J Palliat Care 23(3):93–112

Lowe SS, Watanabe SM, Courneya KS (2009a) Physical activity as a supportive care intervention in palliative cancer patients: a systematic review. J Support Oncol 7(1):27–34

Lowe SS, Watanabe SM, Baracos VE et al (2009b) Associations between physical activity and quality of life in cancer patients receiving palliative care: a pilot survey. J Pain Symptom Manage 38(5):785–796

Lowe SS, Watanabe SM, Baracos VE et al (2009c) Physical activity interests and preferences in palliative cancer patients. Support Care Cancer 2009 Nov 10 [Epub ahead of print]

Munch TN, Stromgren AS, Pedersen L et al (2006) Multidimensional measurement of fatigue in advanced cancer patients in palliative care: an application of the multidimensional fatigue inventory. J Pain Symptom Manage 31(6): 533–541

National Cancer Institute: Dictionary of cancer terms (2007) [cited January 5, 2008]; Available from: http://www.cancer.gov/dictionary/

Oldervoll LM, Loge JH, Paltiel H et al (2005) Are palliative cancer patients willing and able to participate in a physical exercise program? Palliat Support Care 3:281–287

Oldervoll LM, Loge JH, Paltiel H et al (2006) The effect of a physical exercise program in palliative care: a phase II study. J Pain Symptom Manage 31:421–430

Porock D, Kristjanson LJ, Tinnelly K et al (2000) An exercise intervention for advanced cancer patients experiencing fatigue: a pilot study. J Palliat Care 16(3):30–36

Radbruch L, Strasser F, Elsner F et al (2008) Fatigue in palliative care patients – an EAPC approach. Palliat Med 22:13–32

Sepulveda C, Marlin A, Yoshida T et al (2002) Palliative care: the World Health Organization's global perspective. J Pain Symptom Manage 24(2):91–96

Stone PC, Lund S (2007) Predicting prognosis in patients with advanced cancer. Ann Oncol 18(6):971–976

Strasser F, Luftner D, Possinger K et al (2006) Comparison of orally administered cannabis extract and delta-9-tetrahydrocannabinol in treating patients with cancer-related anorexia-cachexia syndrome: a multicenter, phase III, randomized, double-blind, placebo-controlled clinical trial from cannabis-in-cachexia study-group. J Clin Oncol 24(21):3394–3400

Walsh D, Donnelly S, Rybicki L (2000) The symptoms of advanced cancer: relationship to age, gender, and performance status in 1, 000 patients. Support Care Cancer 8(3): 175–179()

Physical Activity Motivation and Cancer Survivorship 16

Bernardine M. Pinto and Joseph T. Ciccolo

Abstract Physical activity (PA) participation has been shown to be helpful in improving physical and mental well-being among cancer survivors. The purpose of this chapter is to review the literature on the determinants of physical activity motivation and behavior among cancer survivors. Using theories of behavior change, researchers have sought to identify the correlates of motivation that predict the participation in regular physical activity in observational studies, while intervention studies have focused on manipulating those factors to support the initiation of physical activity. The majority of this work has been conducted with breast cancer survivors, and there is an interest in expanding this work to survivors of others cancers (e.g., prostate, lung, and colorectal cancer). Results suggest that constructs from the Theory of Planned Behavior (TPB), Transtheoretical Model (TTM), and Social Cognitive Theory (SCT) are associated with greater motivation for physical activity, and some of these constructs have been used in interventions to promote physical activity adoption. There is scope for understanding the determinants of physical activity adoption in various cancer survivor populations. Much more needs to done to identify the determinants of maintenance of physical activity.

B.M. Pinto (✉)
Centers for Behavioral and Preventive Medicine, Coro Bldg, Suite 500, One Hoppin Street, Providence, RI 02903
e-mail: Bpinto@lifespan.org

J.T. Ciccolo
Miriam Hospital and W. Alpert Medical School of Brown University, Providence, RI, USA
e-mail: jciccolo@lifespan.org

16.1 Introduction

Over the past decade, there has been a burgeoning interest in examining lifestyle behaviors among those diagnosed with cancer (Pinto et al. 2000). Examining the prevalence of health risk behaviors such as smoking, sedentary behavior, unhealthy food intake, alcohol use and associated factors have led to efforts to modify these behaviors among these individuals. It is estimated that there are over 12 million cancer survivors (survivorship is defined from the time of diagnosis through the balance of life, National

Dr. Pinto is supported by grants from the National Cancer Institute (CA 132854, CA 101770). Dr. Ciccolo is supported by a grant from the National Cancer Institute (CA 132475).

K.S. Courneya and C.M. Friedenreich (eds.), *Physical Activity and Cancer*,
Recent Results in Cancer Research 186, DOI: 10.1007/978-3-642-04231-7_16,

Cancer Institute Office of Cancer Survivorship, and the National Coalition for Cancer Survivorship), and this population is expected to increase steadily (Smith et al. 2009). With the increased number of survivors, there is a growing understanding of their risks for chronic diseases such as cardiovascular disease, diabetes, and the like, and the relevance of modifying unhealthy behaviors in this population.

Examining the prevalence of healthy behaviors such as regular physical activity (PA) among US cancer survivors has revealed that approximately 30% of cancer survivors met PA guidelines (Bellizi et al. 2005; Blanchard et al. 2008). Using National Health Interview Survey 2000 data, prevalence of regular physical activity was found to vary by age from 20.6% among older adult survivors (aged 65 years and over) to 40.7% among 18–39 year olds (Coups and Ostroff 2005). However, the prevalence levels did not differ from noncancer controls. Among the 40–64 year olds, there was a lower prevalence among cancer survivors (25.2%) versus noncancer controls (30.8%).

Beginning a PA program can be a significant challenge for anyone, and it can be even more difficult for those dealing with the lingering effects of a chronic illness such as cancer. The motivation to be physically active can be described as a process in which internal and external factors direct and energize the thoughts, feelings, and actions around PA (Lewthwaite 1990). Although only in its infancy, research with cancer survivors has now shown motivation to be a strong predictor of PA participation. In this chapter, we provide an overview of the research focused on the determinants of PA motivation and behavior among cancer survivors. The literature on the determinants is largely theory based. Hence, we first review the theories used to assess motivation, we then provide a summary of the observational and intervention studies conducted to date (also see Tables 16.1 and 16.2), and we end with the clinical implications of this work.

Searches of electronic databases (PubMed, PsychInfo, Web of Science) for papers published through January 2010 were used as the sources for this chapter. Only studies specifically focusing on the determinants of PA motivation and behavior were used. These included primarily adults of either sex, diagnosed with any type or stage of cancer, in current treatment or in posttreatment. Studies of relaxation exercises such as yoga or tai chi, physical therapy, or rehabilitation were excluded if they did not include a PA component. It should be noted that, although there have been over 77 PA intervention trials (Speck et al. 2010) for cancer survivors, only a subgroup of these interventions have been based on theories of motivation for behavior change and it is these studies that were reviewed for this chapter.

16.2 Cognitive Behavioral Theory

Cognitive Behavior Theory (CBT) is widely accepted as an effective evidence-based psychotherapy for numerous psychological disorders. The theory asserts that thoughts, feelings, and behaviors are all interconnected and mutually influence one another (Beck 1993). The goal of therapy is to modify cognitions, assumptions, and beliefs to ameliorate disturbed emotions or problematic behaviors. CBT emphasizes a collaborative relationship between the patient and practitioner and requires the patient to practice learned techniques outside of treatment. Techniques often include goal setting, self-monitoring, analyzing behavioral antecedents, building coping skills, and social skills training.

A number of intervention studies have used CBT or its techniques as a method to improve quality of life, physical functioning and increase PA participation in cancer survivors (Culos-Reed et al. 2009; Daley et al. 2007b; Duijts et al.

2009; May et al. 2008, 2009; Korstjens et al. 2008). For example, CBT education was provided as part of an intervention that included 4–6-weeks on-site structured exercise and progressive relaxation to 42 patients who were undergoing myeloablative allogeneic hematopoietic stem cell transplantation (Jarden et al. 2009). In another randomized controlled trial (RCT) among patients with various cancer diagnosis, 12-week programs of group exercise training

Table 16.1 Motivational theories of behavior change and observational studies among cancer survivors

Theory	Observational Studies (Type of Cancer; Treatment/ Survivorship Phase)
Social Cognitive Theory (SCT)	Rogers et al. 2004 (BCa; mixed: receiving treatment, >12 months posttreatment)
	Rogers et al. 2005 (BCa; receiving treatment)
	Rogers et al. 2007 (BCa; Stages I–III)
	Rogers et al. 2008 (BCa; Stages I–IV)
	Karvinen et al. 2006 (endometrial; long-term survivors > 4 years post-diagnosis)
Theory of Planned Behavior (TPB)	Hunt-Shanks et al. 2006 (BCa and prostate; receiving treatment)
	Karvinen et al. 2009 (bladder; long-term survivors >5 years post-diagnosis)
	Courneya et al. 2005b (non-Hodgkin's lymphoma; long-term survivors >5 years post-diagnosis)
	Jones et al. 2006 (multiple myeloma; long-term survivors >5 years post-diagnosis)
	Stevinson et al. 2009 (ovarian; long-term survivors >6 years post-diagnosis)
	Jones et al. 2007 (brain; currently receiving or posttreatment)
	Keats et al. 2007 (mixed, adolescents; >24 months post-diagnosis)
	Courneya et al. 2000 (mixed; receiving treatment)
Transtheoretical Model (TTM)	Clark et al. 2008 (lung; long-term survivors ≥5 years post-diagnosis)
Self-determination Theory (SDT)	Milne et al. 2008a (BCa; 24 months post-diagnosis)
	Peddle et al. 2009 (lung; awaiting surgery)
	Lauver et al. 2007 (mixed, female only; ≥1 month posttreatment)
	Wilson et al. 2006 (mixed; unreported)
Interaction Model of Client Health Behavior (IMCHB)	Cox et al. 2009 (childhood cancer; long-term survivors ≥5 years post-diagnosis)
	Finnegan et al. 2007 (childhood cancer; ≥24 months posttreatment)
Five Factor Model (FFM) of Personality	Rhodes et al. 2001 (BCa; 20 months post-diagnosis)
	Rhodes and Courneya 2003 (mixed; postsurgery and adjuvant therapy)

Note: *BCa* Breast cancer

16

Table 16.2 Motivational theories and intervention studies during and after cancer treatment

Theory	Study	Type of Cancer, Treatment/Survivorship Phase
Cognitive Behavior Therapy (CBT)	Culos-Reed et al. 2009	Prostate cancer, receiving androgen deprivation therapy
	Daley et al. 2007b	BCa, posttreatment (12–36 months)
	Duijts et al. 2009	BCa, posttreatment (4 months–5 years)
	May et al. 2008	Mixed cancers, posttreatment (≥3 months)
	Korstjens et al. 2008	Mixed cancers, posttreatment (≥3 months)
	Jarden et al. 2009	Mixed cancers, before myeloblative allogeneic hematopoietic stem cell transplantation
Social Cognitive Theory (SCT)	Basen-Engquist et al. 2006 with TTM	BCa, posttreatment (<7 years post-diagnosis)
	Campbell et al. 2009	Colorectal cancer, posttreatment (2.5 years post-diagnosis)
	Demark-Wahnefried et al. 2003 with TTM	BCa, Prostate cancer diagnosed in previous 9 months
	Matthews et al. 2007	Bca, posttreatment (<12 months)
	Morey et al. 2009 with TTM	BCa, prostate and colorectal cancer, long-term survivors (≥5 years post-diagnosis)
	Pinto et al. 2005 with TTM	BCa, posttreatment (<5 years post-diagnosis)
	Pinto et al. 2009a with TTM and MI	BCa, posttreatment (<5 years post-diagnosis)
	Rogers et al. 2009a	BCa, posttreatment
	Taylor et al. 2006 with TTM	Prostate cancer, receiving androgen ablation treatment
Theory of Planned Behavior (TPB)	Cadmus et al. 2009 with TTM, IMPACT study	BCa, recently diagnosed, not yet begun or recently begun adjuvant treatment
	Jones et al. 2004	BCa, recently diagnosed
	Vallance et al. 2007	BCa, posttreatment
Transtheoretical Model (TTM)	Mutrie et al. 2007	BCa, during adjuvant treatment (radiation or chemotherapy)

Table 16.2 (continued)

Theory	Study	Type of Cancer, Treatment/Survivorship Phase
Self-Determination Theory (SDT)	Milne et al. 2008b	Bca, posttreatment (≥1 month)
Motivational Interviewing (MI)	Bennett et al. 2007	Mixed cancers, posttreatment (≥6 months after treatment)
Roy Adaptation Model	Mock et al. 1994	BCa, receiving chemotherapy
	Mock et al. 1997	BCa, prior to starting radiation treatment
Levine Conservation Model	Mock et al. 2005	BCa, prior to starting radiation or chemotherapy

Note: *BCa* Breast cancer

plus CBT were compared to group exercise training (group format) and to no intervention (Korstjens et al. 2008; May et al. 2008; 2009). The CBT program focused on problem solving and structured self-management skills training. Despite high program attendance rates (>80%), there was no additional benefit of adding CBT toward outcomes of fitness and PA activity at post-intervention and at follow-ups (May et al. 2008, 2009). In another RCT (Daley et al. 2007b) women treated for breast cancer were randomly assigned to a supervised aerobic exercise, exercise-placebo (body conditioning), or usual care over 8 weeks. CBT techniques were used to promote exercise during the exercise group sessions. Seventy-seven percent of the aerobic exercise group and 89% of the exercise-placebo group attended at least 70% of the scheduled sessions. This group of researchers conducted analyses on the determinants of session adherence (e.g., recruitment method, socioeconomic characteristics). However, they were not able to identify any factors but acknowledged that other psycho-cognitive factors may have played a contributing role (Daley et al. 2007a).

CBT techniques (goal setting, monitoring behavior, overcoming barriers, role of a positive attitude and social support, and relapse prevention) were also used in a 16-week RCT among 100 prostate cancer patients receiving androgen deprivation therapy (Culos-Reed et al. 2009). The men were randomly assigned to an individually tailored home-based aerobic and light resistance training program and weekly group sessions versus wait-list control. Although there were significant increases in PA in the exercise group and adherence rates were 78%; overall attrition was 34%.

Findings suggest that this may be a viable guiding theory to support PA adoption among cancer survivors and CBT techniques have been applied among patients with various cancer diagnoses. However, in the one study that compared the additional benefits of CBT to an exercise program did not find that it led to superior outcomes (May et al. 2008, 2009).

16.3 Social Cognitive Theory

Social Cognitive Theory (SCT) (Bandura 1986) is based upon the principle of triadic reciprocal causation, which states that behavior, environmental factors, and personal factors of the individual, such as cognitions, emotions, and physical characteristics are mutually influential.

This theory has provided a useful framework for understanding PA behavior in cancer survivors, as previous research has shown multiple SCT-based cross-sectional studies and interventions to explain and promote PA participation. Self-efficacy, a central concept within SCT, is consistently identified as a psychosocial determinant of adherence to PA among cancer survivors (e.g., Pinto et al. 2009b; Rogers et al. 2004). Outcome expectations, another major component of SCT, can also alter PA participation. The expectations may be oriented toward positive or negative self-evaluations (e.g., an emotional response), physical outcomes (e.g., pain or pleasure), or social outcomes (e.g., dis/approval by peers).

In observational studies, the specific relationship each of the SCT constructs has with motivation for cancer survivors, however, is not entirely clear. The motivation to engage in a behavior such as PA has been shown to be related to self-efficacy, as those with higher self-efficacy (i.e., confidence that a behavior can be completed successfully) are more likely to be motivated to complete that behavior, as has been found among breast cancer survivors (e.g., Rabin et al. 2006; Rogers et al. 2004, 2005, 2008). The motivation to participate in PA has also been closely linked to outcome expectations, specifically in cancer survivors who perceive more positive outcomes with PA (Rogers et al. 2007). Non-Hodgkin's lymphoma and endometrial cancer survivors have reported that they expected PA to provide them with improved mental attitude, physical function, increased energy, and reduced stress (Courneya et al. 2005b; Karvinen et al. 2006). Examining the role of these constructs in PA motivation among patients treated for other cancers (e.g., lung, prostate, or colorectal) is needed. It is also worthwhile to examine the dynamic relationship between motivation and other chief constructs of SCT (e.g., the environment) (Rogers et al. 2009b).

Several interventions used SCT to guide their interventions targeting sedentary behavior (Matthews et al. 2007; Pinto et al. 2005) and unhealthy diet and sedentary behavior (Demark-Wahnefried et al. 2003; Morey et al. 2009). Patients treated for breast (Demark-Wahnefried et al. 2003; Matthews et al. 2007; Morey et al. 2009; Pinto et al. 2005), prostate (Morey et al. 2009; Taylor et al 2006) and colorectal cancer (Morey et al. 2009) have participated in these trials. As with observational studies, SCT-based interventions often focus on the construct of "self-efficacy." Self-efficacy can be enhanced by encouraging participants to set realistic, easily attainable goals, particularly at the outset of the intervention (Pinto et al. 2005), choosing specific physical activities as opposed to prescribed exercise or dietary regimens (Basen-Engquist et al. 2006) , focusing on participants' progress, and reinforcing successes (Demark-Wahnefried et al. 2003). Efforts are also made to strengthen outcome expectations. SCT techniques used in these studies included the use of decisional balance (explained later in this chapter), social modeling, self-regulation strategies, and building social support for PA (Matthews et al. 2007; Taylor et al. 2006).

Interventions based on SCT constructs and techniques have been effective. For example, significant increases have been reported in exercise activities such as walking (Matthews et al. 2007; Pinto et al. 2005). However, there has not been an extensive examination of whether these interventions had an effect on underlying SCT constructs. In one of the trials that did so, Taylor and colleagues (2006) did not find changes in social support at 6 or 12 months. Consistent with the literature on behavior change in noncancer populations that has shown self-efficacy to be a strong predictor of behavior change, Demark-Wahnefried and colleagues (2006) found significant increases in self-efficacy for exercise adoption at 6 months following an intervention that targeted both exercise and diet. Mediator analyses of SCT constructs in intervention trials among cancer patients have not been conducted.

Using baseline data from an RCT for prostate cancer survivors wherein a lifestyle PA program was compared to that of an education support program and a standard care condition, education, vitality, and bodily pain were associated with self-efficacy for PA (Perkins et al. 2009) (note that this intervention did not produce significant improvements in PA).

In another study, Rogers and colleagues (2009a) assigned 41 breast cancer patients on hormone therapy to a 12-week multidisciplinary PA behavior change intervention or usual care. The specific SCT constructs addressed in six discussion group sessions included self-efficacy, emotional coping, reciprocal determinism, perceived barriers, outcome expectations, behavioral capability, goal setting, environment, observational learning, and self-control. Many of these constructs were also addressed in individual sessions (three in-person sessions with an exercise specialist). The intervention was effective in increasing accelerometer counts, aerobic fitness, and similar outcomes but intervention effects on the underlying determinants of PA were not reported.

In sum, there is some support for SCT constructs for PA both in observational and intervention studies. The interventions based on these motivational variables have generally been effective in increasing PA but the effects of the intervention on the determinants of PA require further examination.

16.4 Theory of Planned Behavior

The Theory of Planned Behavior (TPB) (Ajzen and Madden 1986) is the most widely used theory within the area of PA motivation for cancer survivors. The theory posits that behavior is directly predicted by intention, which in turn, is directly predicted by attitude, subjective norm, and perceived control. Perceived control is the belief that a behavior can be performed with ease or difficulty and it may directly predict the behavior; attitude is the personal evaluation of performing the behavior; and subjective norm is the perceived normative beliefs of relevant others regarding the behavior. Thus, according to the theory, an individual will intend, and be motivated to, perform a behavior when they view it favorably, believe that important others think they should perform it, and believe that the behavior is under their control and can be carried out (see Fig. 16.1).

The vast majority of studies assessing the motivation to be physically active and the determinants of being physically active have used the TPB, either alone or in conjunction with another theory. Many of these studies have been cross-sectional and most have focused on breast cancer survivors (c.f., Vallance et al. 2008; Courneya et al. 2001), with at least one or more studies

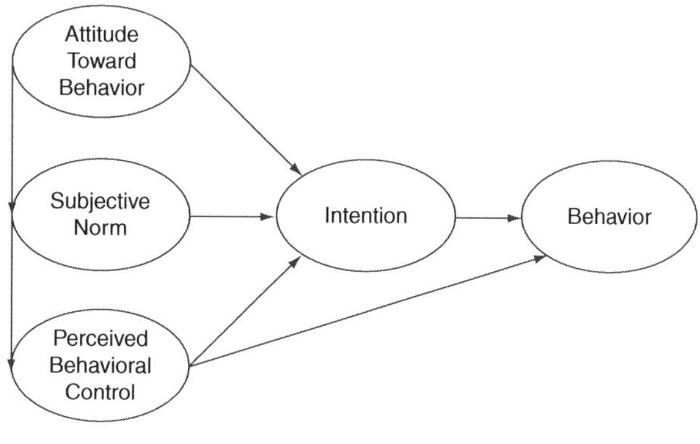

Fig. 16.1 Theory of Planned Behavior (TPB)

conducted among colorectal (Courneya et al. 2004b), prostate (Hunt-Shanks et al. 2006), bladder (Karvinen et al. 2009), non-Hodgkins lymphoma (Courneya et al. 2005b), multiple myeloma (Jones et al. 2006), endometrial (Karvinen et al. 2006), ovarian (Stevinson et al. 2009), brain (Jones et al. 2007), or child/adolescent cancer survivors (Keats et al. 2007). Of note, as described by the TPB, the intention to perform a behavior is considered a proxy for the motivation to perform that behavior, and the measurement of each is one and the same. Overall, there appears to be great utility in using the TPB to understand PA motivation for any group of cancer survivors, as studies have reported capturing 32–68% of the variance in intention to be active (Jones et al. 2007; Courneya et al. 2000). Although the strength of the relationship between intention and each specific antecedent (i.e., attitude, social norm, perceived control) has varied among studies, and among different cancer groups, all antecedents have been shown to significantly contribute (e.g., Karvinen et al. 2009; Jones et al. 2007). It should be noted that some cross-sectional studies have focused on intention rather than the behavior as the primary outcome (e.g., Jones et al. 2007; Hunt-Shanks et al. 2006), but it is important to establish the link to the behavioral outcome.

In a small sample of 24 breast cancer survivors who attended a twice weekly 12-week training program to prepare for a dragon boat race (single group, pre-post design), the predictors of adherence and intention were examined (Courneya et al. 2001). Analyses showed intention to exercise to be the sole determinant of program attendance (attendance was at 66%, intention accounted for 35% of the variance). TPB constructs explained almost half the variance in intention with subjective norm as the strongest determinant. The researchers identified other key beliefs such as support from important others and confidence in being able to attend the training despite barriers as correlates of program attendance.

In another study among 52 breast cancer patients, the 24 patients randomized to the exercise intervention (15 weeks, on-site supervised exercise) completed measures based on the TPB (Courneya et al. 2006). At post-intervention, attitudes and perceptions of control were higher in the exercise group compared to pre-intervention (the wait list control group did not complete the measures at post-intervention). Specifically, among the perceived benefits of the exercise program, the participants reported that exercise helped them maintain a normal lifestyle more than they had anticipated at pre-randomization. Among beliefs focused on the extent to which certain barriers would interfere with attendance at the program (i.e., control beliefs), they reported less interference from other medical problems, pain, and family responsibility. Both instrumental attitudes and affective attitudes improved from pre-randomization to post-intervention. Significant improvements in perceptions of perceived control were also noted. However, no changes were reported for self-efficacy, and scores on injunctive (belief that important others would approve of their participation in the program) and descriptive norms (belief that important others also exercised) for exercise decreased compared to pre-randomization scores.

TPB constructs have also been assessed in intervention studies among patients with other types of cancer. For example, in a pilot single group study, 19 patients awaiting surgical resection of suspected malignant lung lesions were offered an onsite supervised exercise training program (Peddle et al. 2009). Although the intervention components were not based on TPB, perceived behavioral control and subjective norm were significantly correlated with exercise adherence (73% mean adherence).

The application of the TPB in an intervention, in contrast to observational studies, has been limited. Jones and colleagues (2004) conducted an RCT developed within the tenets of the TPB. Recently diagnosed breast cancer survivors ($N = 450$) were randomly assigned to receive an oncologist exercise recommendation only, an oncologist recommendation plus referral to an exercise specialist or to usual care at their first adjuvant treatment consultation. In support of the TPB, results demonstrated that perceived behavioral control had a direct effect on exercise and it mediated the effect of the recommendation-only intervention on exercise (Jones et al. 2005). Also in support of the TPB, the direct effects of attitude, subjective norm, and perceived behavioral control on intention were upheld. However, in contrast with the theory's prediction, no direct effects of intention on exercise were found.

In another RCT among breast cancer survivors, interventions based on the TPB were found to increase PA significantly at 12 weeks (approximately 40–60 min/week) (Vallance et al. 2007). There were small increases in specific TPB constructs (instrumental attitude, intention, and planning) in the intervention groups versus the comparison group. It is noteworthy that mediator analyses were conducted which showed that both planning and intention partially mediated the effects of the intervention on PA (Vallance et al. 2008).

A few studies have combined variables from the Transtheoretical Model (TTM) (see below) with TPB to promote self-efficacy for PA and overcome barriers to exercise (Cadmus et al. 2009) but the effects of these variables have generally not been examined. An exception can be found in an exercise trial offered to 82 prostate cancer patients receiving androgen deprivation therapy, wherein Courneya and colleagues (2004c) examined predictors of adherence to supervised resistance exercise training. They found that exercise stage of change at baseline was the strongest predictor of exercise adherence; while higher age predicted lower adherence. Intention was also an independent predictor of adherence.

Overall, there has been support for TPB variables as related to motivation for PA among various cancer populations. However, less is known about how to develop interventions based on these variables and to test their meditational role in changing sedentary behavior. Another challenge lies in continuing to test the TPB in conjunction with or against other pertinent theories. This will likely provide unique contributions and clarity into understanding the motivational determinants of PA.

16.5 Transtheoretical Model

The TTM of health behavior change (Prochaska and DiClemente 1983) postulates that individuals move through a series of six stages of motivational readiness while making a behavior change (i.e., precontemplation, contemplation, preparation, action, maintenance, and termination) and this approach has been applied to PA (Marcus and Simkin 1993) (see Fig. 16.2). While progressing through these stages, the individual engages in ten different cognitive and behavioral processes of change (e.g., self-reevaluation, contingency management) that are important in the adoption and maintenance of a new behavior. For example, research on exercise adoption suggests that cognitive processes of change (e.g., setting realistic goals)

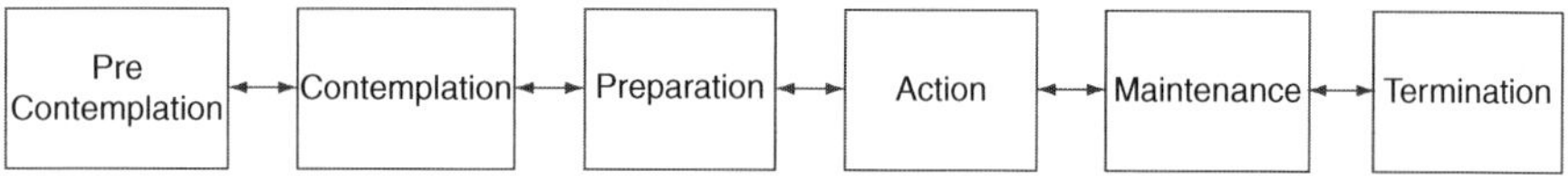

Fig. 16.2 Transtheoretical Model (TTM)

should be encouraged among those in precontemplation and contemplation, while behavioral processes (e.g., placing reminders to exercise at work or home) should be promoted among those in the more advanced stages of motivational readiness (Marcus et al. 1992b). The concepts of decisional balance (e.g., pros and cons of initiating the behavior) and self-efficacy are also used in conjunction with the stages of change in terms of both intervention content and outcomes.

Although the model has received a considerable amount of criticism (e.g., Bridle et al. 2005), PA research among breast, prostate, and lung cancer survivors using the TTM or a mixed model of TTM and SCT (e.g., Clark et al. 2008; Basen-Engquist et al. 2006; Morey et al. 2009; Pinto et al. 2005, 2009a) have revealed some key findings. In cross-sectional analyses, significant correlations were found between stage of readiness for PA, quality of life, and symptom management (Clark et al. 2008).

TTM-based interventions attempt to tailor the recommendations to a participant's motivational readiness to change. Hence, in interventions for exercise adoption, participants who are ready to start exercising (e.g., those in contemplation or preparation) receive appropriate guidance on setting exercise goals (e.g., choosing specific types of exercise, deciding where to exercise, setting up reminders to exercise and the like). Conversely, the TTM would suggest that such action-oriented recommendations would be ineffective for those who have no intention to adopt exercise (e.g., those in precontemplation).

Another construct that is used with the TTM, is that of decisional balance (taken from decision theory; Janis and Mann 1977). This construct refers to the balance between the advantages or "pros" of the behavior change compared to the disadvantages or "cons" of behavior change. In general, the balance tends to favor the "pros" among those in action and maintenance, while the "cons" dominate among those in earlier stages of motivational readiness (Bock et al. 2001; Marcus et al. 1992a, b). When applied in interventions, efforts are made to help the patient to identify the advantages and drawbacks for behavior change. Assistance is provided to overcome the drawbacks and when appropriate, information is provided on potential advantages so as to strengthen motivation to change.

Constructs from the TTM (Prochaska and DiClemente 1983; Prochaska et al. 1992) were used in several trials targeting a single behavior such as sedentary behavior alone (Basen-Engquist et al. 2006; Mutrie et al. 2007; Pinto et al. 2005; Taylor et al. 2006) or multiple behaviors such as diet and sedentary behavior (Demark-Wahnefried et al. 2003, 2004; Morey et al. 2009). The patient groups in these trials included those treated for breast cancer (Basen-Engquist et al. 2006; Demark-Wahnefried et al. 2003; Mutrie et al. 2007; Pinto et al. 2005), prostate cancer (Demark-Wahnefried et al. 2003; Taylor et al. 2006), and various cancers (Morey et al. 2009). Several of these trials were effective in increasing PA in the intervention group (e.g., Pinto et al. 2005; Mutrie et al. 2007; Morey et al. 2009).

Apart from assessing outcomes, a few studies examined the effects of the intervention on the underlying determinants of behavior change. Taylor and fellow researchers (2006) found a significantly greater use of cognitive and behavioral processes in the TTM-intervention group at 6 and 12 months and decisional balance components at 6 months (pros of exercise significantly increased in the TTM-intervention arm). In post hoc analyses of the effects of a 12-week home-based PA intervention based on the TTM (Pinto et al 2005), behavioral processes were found to increase significantly at post-intervention. However, TTM constructs were not found to be mediators of the intervention effects on PA (Rabin et al. 2006).

It should be noted that in some of these RCTs, constructs from TTM have been used along with SCT (e.g., Basen-Engquist et al. 2006; Demark-Wahnefried et al. 2003; Morey et al. 2009; Pinto et al. 2005; 2009a). For example, in a study promoting both dietary change and PA to improve physical functioning among breast, prostate, and colorectal cancer survivors (Snyder et al. 2009), SCT was used to overcome barriers, achieve incremental behavioral goals, monitor progress, provide reinforcement for goal achievement and TTM was used for tailored progress reports that were provided every 12 weeks to participants in the intervention arm. Interestingly in an earlier study, the same group of researchers offered a 10-month program of tailored mailed print materials that aimed at improving dietary intake and exercise (based on TTM and SCT), and found that the intervention was found not to significantly affect self-efficacy for exercise, but there was a significant positive relationship between self-efficacy and exercise duration at 12 months (Mosher et al. 2008).

Thus, whether used alone or in conjunction with another theory, the TTM can provide important information on PA motivation and appears to be useful for cancer survivorship research. More research with other subgroups of cancer survivors is needed as well as an examination of the determinants of exercise.

16.6 Self-determination Theory

The Self-determination Theory (SDT) posits that behaviors are regulated by motives that range on a continuum from highly controlled (extrinsically motivated) to fully autonomous (intrinsically motivated) (see Fig. 16.3). Extrinsically motivated behaviors are performed in response to the avoidance of something negative such as emotions, a threat, or a demand. Intrinsically motivated behaviors are typically those behaviors that are done to provide the individual inherent enjoyment, satisfaction, or pleasure. A state of amotivation also exists, whereby the individual has no motivation to engage in a specific behavior. It is thought that intrinsic motivation leads to greater interest, more confidence and longer persistence of a behavior (Deci and Ryan 1985).

With just a handful of studies conducted thus far (Milne et al. 2008a, b; Peddle et al. 2008; Lauver et al. 2007; Wilson et al. 2006), SDT has recently been used as a new guiding theory for research with cancer survivors. The evidence collected to date suggests that it can be just as useful as other theories in explaining the motivation to engage in PA. For example, a recent set of cross-sectional studies (Milne et al. 2008a;

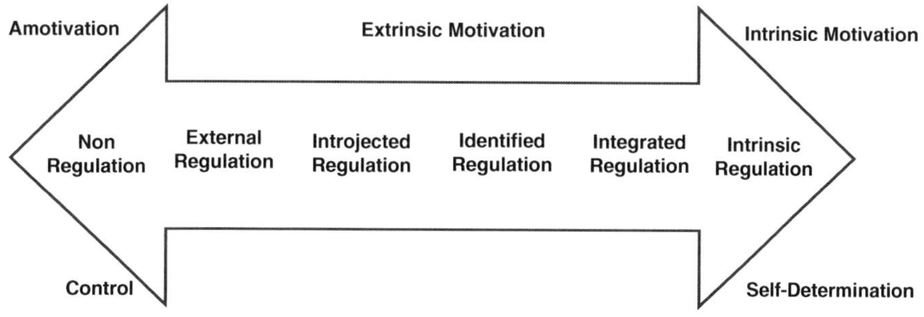

Fig. 16.3 Self-Determination Theory (SDT)

16

Wilson et al. 2006) has shown that SDT may capture variance unexplained by the TPB. Specifically, the TPB uses subjective norm (a variable that measures the perceived pressure from relevant others to perform a behavior), but this factor has been shown to impede motivation (Milne et al 2008a). In comparison, SDT uses an autonomously supported social influence construct, and it has been reported to enhance motivation (Wilson et al. 2006; Milne et al. 2008a). Other factors unique to using SDT include the measurement of autonomous (or intrinsic) motivation, as was reported by Wilson and colleagues (2006) who found autonomous motivation to predict the number of minutes engaged in moderate-to-vigorous (MVPA) intensity PA in a sample of 220 cancer survivors and a similar size noncancer cohort (it should be noted that cancer status did not moderate the motivation–PA relationship). This is similar to another study that found the constructs of SDT to be independently associated with PA participation in a sample of 414 colorectal cancer survivors (Peddle et al. 2008). Most recently, however, SDT constructs were able to explain 20.2% of the variance in PA in a sample of 558 breast cancer survivors (Milne et al. 2008a).

There has been recent interest in using this theory to inform interventions. Milne and colleagues (2008b) randomized 60 breast cancer survivors to an immediate or delayed 12-week aerobic and resistance training program and found significant group by time interactions for almost all psychological needs and motivations that favored the exercise intervention (Milne et al. 2008b). In this RCT, the investigators reported 61% adherence, and less than 5% attrition. The researchers found an increase in self-determined regulations for exercise (identified regulation and intrinsic motivation, and in perceived autonomy, competence, and relatedness). They found positive associations between psychological needs (autonomy, competence, and relatedness) and autonomous regulations. These results suggest that participants were no longer exercising simply for extrinsic reasons but developed an interest in exercise. This type of motivated state may be achieved by offering interventions designed to support autonomy (e.g., providing a noncontrolling environment to exercise, allowing participants flexibility in choosing activities, attendance time, and length of stay), develop perceived competence (e.g., by teaching correct techniques), and enhance relatedness (e.g., by offering group classes).

In sum, there is much scope to use SDT constructs in predicting PA both in observational and intervention studies. In addition, the implementation of these constructs to enhance motivation for PA in interventions for cancer survivors can be a promising avenue to advance the field (Milne et al. 2008b).

16.7 Other Theories and Approaches

16.7.1 Attribution Theory

Attribution Theory (AT) (Weiner 1985) posits that the attributions individuals make to explain outcomes (e.g., achievement) will influence future behavior. Specifically, it is hypothesized that individuals process attributions using varying dimensions of locus (internal/external), stability (stable/unstable), and control (controllable/uncontrollable). Although not widely used, Courneya and associates (2004a) have suggested that AT may be useful for understanding PA motivation and adherence in cancer survivors.

Constructs based on this approach were used to examine predictors of exercise at posttreatment and at a 5-week follow-up of cancer survivors who participated in group psychotherapy and home-based physical exercise (Courneya et al. 2004a). Although the intervention was not based on AT, adherence during the intervention phase and perceived success were the strongest predictors of exercise at post-intervention. Additionally, perceived success (vs objective success) interacted with personal control to influence expected success and negative affect. These results suggest that high perceptions of success attributed to personal control may foster expected success and positive affective reactions to an exercise program. Many more studies will be needed to confirm these hypotheses; however, as there has yet to be an RCT testing this specific theory.

16.7.2 Motivational Interviewing

Motivational interviewing (MI) (Miller and Rollnick 2002) is an individually administered, client-centered approach to bring about behavior change. MI seeks to reduce resistance to change by developing a discrepancy between an individual's current behavior and his or her values and goals. There are four general principles that underlie this approach: (1) express empathy, (2) develop discrepancy, (3) roll with resistance, and (4) support self-efficacy.

To date, just a few studies (Bennett et al. 2007; Pinto et al. 2009a) have used MI with TTM and SCT to increase PA effectively among cancer survivors. It appears that MI is most successful when key psychosocial determinants of change (i.e., self-efficacy) are affected (e.g., Bennett et al 2007). However, another study using MI along with TTM and SCT among colorectal cancer survivors and adults without a cancer history did not show intervention effects on PA (Campbell et al. 2009). However, given the small number of studies using this approach, it is unclear what specific mediators and moderators could be responsible for a change in motivation. Future studies are therefore needed to fully examine the utility of the MI approach.

16.7.3 Roy Adaptation Model and the Levine Conservation Model

Mock and her colleagues (1994, 1997) used the Roy Adaptation model (Roy and Andrews 1991) and the Levine Conservation Model of adaptation (Levine 1973, 1989) to guide their exercise interventions for women treated for breast cancer. These rehabilitation models focused on physiological and psychosocial interventions to promote positive, adaptive responses to a cancer diagnosis and treatment.

In the Roy model, adaptation is viewed as an active process initiated by the individual of adjusting to environmental changes through physiological or psychological modes and in turn, affecting the environment. The walking intervention that was offered to breast cancer patients was conceptualized as a physiological intervention with psychosocial effects that had the potential to promote adaptive responses among women undergoing chemotherapy (Mock et al. 1994) or radiation treatment for breast cancer (Mock et al. 1997). The physiological mode was assessed via tests of physical functioning and symptom assessments and the psychosocial modes were assessed via measures of self concept, body image, and adjustment.

The Levine Conservation Model is based on conserving individual integrity for the maintenance of life. According to the theory, the goal of the individual is to conserve or preserve an integrated and balanced whole (Levine 1973). There are four principles that underlie the model: conservation of energy, structural integrity, personal integrity and social integrity (Levine 1989). Mock and associates have proposed that this is a useful framework for guiding a PA intervention for fatigue and physical function in cancer survivors (Mock et al 2007, 2005). Specifically, constructing an intervention that balances energy resources with energy expenditure, promotes the benefits of using PA to reduce fatigue, uses personalized feedback

16

and motivation, and focuses on the importance of a supportive environment; each principle of the model is utilized. Although initial results have been promising (Mock et al. 2007), there is a lack of research using this model and more studies will be needed.

16.7.4 Interaction Model of Client Health Behavior

The Interaction Model of Client Health Behavior (IMCHB) proposed by Cox (2003) is a nursing-based model that has been proposed as a heuristic for studies of childhood cancer survivors. It has three major elements that mutually influence one another during a client–provider interaction: intrapersonal characteristics, patient and health-care provider interaction, and behavior-related health outcome. Overall, the IMCHB identifies background, cognitive, affective, motivational, and contextual variables that explain health-related behaviors. The model defines the interactive and collective contributions of a survivor, family, and provider to adherence to protocols, reduction of risk behavior, and promotion of health-protective behavior. The model can identify new determinants of health-related behavior that can be targeted by specific inter- or intrapersonal interventions to protect the health of childhood cancer survivors (Cox 2003). Thus far, cross-sectional studies using this model have shown motivation, in addition to numerous other factors (e.g., gender, physician advice), to be an important predictor of PA participation in childhood cancer survivors (Cox et al. 2009; Finnegan et al. 2007). Given that only two cross-sectional studies have used this model, and all data are self-reported, there are limitations regarding the findings. Nonetheless, it is likely that interventions considering multiple factors (i.e., those identified by this model) and the interaction among those factors will have the greatest potential to influence motivation for, and participation in, PA for this population.

16.7.5 Five Factor Model of Personality

The Five Factor Model (FFM) is a leading framework for studying personality (Digman 1990; McCrae and John 1992). The FFM is a broad-level categorization of personality traits, which are neuroticism, extraversion, openness, conscientiousness, and agreeableness. A relationship between personality and PA has long been known, and a 2006 meta-analysis identified extraversion, neuroticism and conscientiousness as key correlates to PA participation (Rhodes and Smith 2006). Personality and PA has been studied among breast cancer survivors (Rhodes et al. 2001; Courneya et al. 2002; Rhodes and Courneya 2003), and it has been hypothesized that individuals of a particular personality structure may be more inherently motivated to participate in PA or to continue to participate in PA once started (Rhodes and Courneya 2003; Courneya et al. 1999). For example, even after controlling for the constructs of the TPB, extraversion has been shown to predict PA participation (Courneya et al. 1999). Thus, future research would benefit from including an assessment of personality attributes, as it carries the potential to capture an aspect of motivation that may not be measured with other approaches. The FFM has not yet been used in intervention development (e.g., tailoring the intervention to the personality type).

16.8 Other Determinants

The work reviewed in this chapter exemplifies the growing interest in understanding PA behavior among cancer survivors, the constructs that predict PA and how these variables can be manipulated in interventions to promote PA. It would be important, however, to attend to any cancer-specific variables that may affect PA motivation and behavior. Some of these variables related to treatment, time since diagnosis and the like, are reviewed below.

In a small sample of breast cancer patients assessed at 3-month intervals for a year following treatment, younger age, longer time since diagnosis, being partnered, having greater social support and higher depression at baseline predicted participation in vigorous-intensity PA (Pinto et al. 2002). In a longitudinal study of 287 breast cancer patients assessed at 6, 12, and 18 months post-diagnosis, only two factors showed statistically significant relationships to change in PA from 6 to 18 months: baseline PA was a negative predictor (those with higher values declined or regressed to the mean) and treatment-related complications: those who experienced one or more complication showed a modest decline in total PA (Harrison et al. 2009). Cross-sectional studies have revealed that preoperative pulmonary function and number of surgical complications have inverse relationships with PA among lung cancer survivors (e.g., Coups et al. 2009). In a population-based cohort of colorectal cancer survivors, having a stoma, having adjuvant therapy, and experiencing fatigue negatively affected PA (e.g., Lynch et al. 2007). Among several motivational and informational variables examined in a cross-sectional study among Danish cancer patients undergoing chemotherapy, Midtgaard and colleagues (2009) noted that those who stated that they had been informed about exercise were more likely to exercise. These data suggest the important role that healthcare providers may play in promoting PA among those diagnosed with cancer. Finally, in one of the only observational studies to track survivors over 5 years, Emery and his team (2009) found a curvilinear pattern in PA over time. The researchers found that poor physical health, depressive symptoms and lower emotional well-being were associated with less PA. However, higher family support was associated with a slower decline in PA over time.

In secondary analyses of an intervention study of a 16-week home-based exercise trial for colorectal cancer patients, the reasons for not meeting the minimum exercise goals were obtained on a weekly basis from the 69 patients assigned to the exercise arm (Courneya et al. 2005a). Participants reported 37 different exercise barriers: the three most common were lack of time/too busy, treatment side-effects, and fatigue. The top seven barriers (included surgical complications, work responsibilities, progressing toward the exercise prescription, and getting enough activity elsewhere) accounted for 70–80% of weeks in which exercise goals were not met. Medical, demographic, and past exercise variables were not consistently related to the number and frequency of exercise barriers with the exception of treatment protocol. Patients who received adjuvant therapy (chemotherapy, radiation) were more likely to report treatment side effects, diarrhea, and nausea as barriers to exercise compared to those who received surgery alone.

PA interventions have been offered to individuals undergoing treatment, those in the post-treatment phase and those who are long-term survivors (see Table 16.2). To date, there has not been an examination of intervention efficacy for patients at various points in the cancer diagnosis and treatment trajectories. It is likely that patients receiving adjuvant treatments may experience more immediate treatment side-effects (e.g., nausea, fatigue) that can interfere in becoming physically active compared to patients who have completed such treatments. In sum, apart from the theory-based constructs that related to PA motivation and behavior, cancer-specific factors (e.g., treatment regimen and toxicities), demographics (e.g., older age), and medical history (e.g., co-morbid illnesses) may also influence PA adoption and should be considered when promoting PA among cancer survivors.

16.9 Clinical Implications

Clinicians and practitioners working with cancer survivors can draw on the theories of behavior change reviewed in this chapter. Key constructs that have been used in several interventions include social-cognitive techniques for self-management, strengthening self-efficacy (or behavioral control) for becoming physically active, developing realistic expectations for outcomes, strengthening the intention to exercise, and developing plans that are appropriate to an individual's readiness to become active. Promising approaches such as MI techniques and helping sedentary individuals develop intrinsic motivation to become active are also worthy of consideration. In the absence of studies that compare PA adoption among cancer survivors versus patients with other chronic disease such as cardiovascular disease, diabetes and the like versus the general population (two exceptions are the study by Wilson et al. 2006 that compared cancer and noncancer cohorts in applying the SDT; and the PA and dietary intervention among colorectal cancer survivors and adults without cancer, Campbell et al. 2009), it is premature to make conclusions about whether these factors are unique to cancer survivors or apply in unique ways. We have provided descriptions of how these variables were implemented in interventions to enable practitioners to use these techniques. However, it should be reiterated that although some of the interventions were effective in promoting PA and/or in improving health outcomes, the number of theory-based interventions are limited, and fewer still have examined the contributions of these variables or techniques on outcomes. On similar lines, there has not yet been a comparison of interventions based on different theories to promote exercise among cancer survivors to answer questions such as which theory or combinations of theories are the most effective in promoting behavior change (i.e., adoption of regular exercise) and in affecting other outcomes such as physical functioning, quality of life, and the like.

Clinicians should recognize that much of the work promoting PA has focused on individual-level variables. In the past several years, there is growing recognition of the role of "macro" variables in promoting PA among the general populations such as social support in the family and/or the community, the built environment, perceived access to exercise facilities, and neighborhoods and areas that facilitate PA. Finally, the focus of PA interventions among cancer survivors thus far has been to promote the *adoption* of PA and less attention has been paid to the challenges of *maintaining* such activity.

16.10 Conclusions

Understanding the motivation for PA adoption among cancer survivors has revealed many similarities between these populations and noncancer populations. Much work has been done among survivors (primarily those diagnosed with early-stage breast cancer) during treatment and in the posttreatment phase. Examining the motivations for PA among people diagnosed with other types of cancer or at other points in the cancer continuum (post-diagnosis, long-term survivorship, palliative and end of life) remains to be examined. It should be noted that there is much scope in intervention studies for manipulating the variables that have already been identified as PA correlates from observational studies. Practitioners should be aware that there has been little examination of PA interventions on the corresponding constructs and the mediational role of these variables on changing sedentary lifestyles. These types of analyses will be important in developing effective interventions that are cost-effective and can contribute to improved health and well-being of the burgeoning population of cancer survivors in the twenty-first century.

References

Ajzen I, Madden TJ (1986) Prediction of goal-directed behavior: attitudes, intentions, and perceived behavioral control. J Exp Soc Psychol 22: 453–474

Beck A (1993) Cognitive therapy and the emotional disorders. Penguin, New York, NY

Bandura A (1986) Social foundations of thought and action: a social cognitive theory. Prentice-Hall, Englewood Cliffs, NJ

Basen-Engquist K, Taylor CL, Rosenblum C et al (2006) Randomized pilot test of a lifestyle physical activity intervention for breast cancer survivors. Patient Educ Couns 64(1–3):225–34

Bellizi KM, Rowland JH, Jeffrey DD, McNeel T (2005) Health behaviors of cancer survivors: examining opportunities for cancer control intervention. J Clin Oncol 23(34):8884–93

Bennett JA, Lyons KS, Winters-Stone K et al (2007) Motivational interviewing to increase physical activity in long-term cancer survivors: a randomized controlled trial. Nurs Res 56:18–27

Blanchard CM, Courneya KS, Stein K (2008) Cancer survivors' adherence to lifestyle behavior recommendations and associations with health-related quality of life: results from the American Cancer Society's SCS-II. J Clin Oncol 26(13):2198–204

Bock BC, Marcus BH, Pinto BM et al (2001) Maintenance of physical activity following an individualized motivationally tailored intervention. Ann Behav Med 23(2):79–87

Bridle C, Riemsma RP, Pattenden J et al (2005) Systematic review of the effectiveness of health behavior interventions based on the transtheoretical model. Psychol Health 20:283–301

Cadmus LA, Salovey P, Yu H et al (2009) Exercise and quality of life during and after treatment for breast cancer: results of two randomized controlled trials. Psychooncology 18:343–352

Campbell MK, Carr C, DeVellis B, Switzer B, Biddle A, Amamoo A et al (2009) A randomized trial of tailoring and motivational interviewing to promote fruit and vegetable consumption for cancer prevention and control. Ann Behav Med 38: 71–85

Clark MM, Novotny PJ, Patten CA et al (2008) Motivational readiness for physical activity and quality of life in long-term lung cancer survivors. Lung Cancer 61:117–122

Coups EJ, Ostroff JS (2005) A population-based estimate of the prevalence of behavioral risk factors among adult cancer survivors and noncancer controls. Prev Med 40(6):702–711

Coups EJ, Park BJ, Feinstein MB et al (2009) Correlates of physical activity among lung cancer survivors. Psychooncology 18:396–404

Courneya KS, Blanchard CM, Laing DM (2001) Exercise adherence in breast cancer survivors training for a dragon boat race competition: a preliminary investigation. Psychooncology 10: 444–452

Courneya KS, Bobick TM, Schinke RJ (1999) Does the theory of planned behavior mediate the relationship between personality and exercise behavior. Basic Appl Soc Psychol 21:317–324

Courneya KS, Friedenreich CM, Sela RA et al (2002) Correlates of adherence and contamination in a randomized controlled trial of exercise in cancer survivors: an application of the theory of planned behavior and the five factor model of personality. Ann Behav Med 24:257–268

Courneya KS, Friedenreich CM, Sela RA et al (2004a) Exercise motivation and adherence in cancer survivors after participation in a randomized controlled trial: an attribution theory perspective. Int J Behav Med 11:8–17

Courneya KS, Friedenreich CM, Quinney HA et al (2004b) Predictors of adherence and contamination in a randomized trial of exercise in colorectal cancer survivors. Psychooncology 13: 857–866

Courneya KS, Friedenreich CM, Quinney HA et al (2005a) A longitudinal study of exercise barriers in colorectal cancer survivors participating in a randomized controlled trial. Ann Behav Med 29: 147–153

Courneya KS, Jones LW, Mackey JR et al (2006) Exercise beliefs of breast cancer survivors before and after participation in a randomized controlled trial. Int J Behav Med 13:259–264

16

Courneya KS, Keats MR, Turner AR (2000) Physical exercise and quality of life in cancer patients following high dose chemotherapy and autologous bone marrow transplantation. Psychooncology 9:127–136

Courneya KS, Segal RJ, Reid RD et al (2004c) Three independent factors predicted adherence in a randomized controlled trial of resistance exercise training among prostate cancer survivors. J Clin Epidemiol 57:571–579

Courneya KS, Vallance JK, Jones LW et al (2005b) Correlates of exercise intentions in non-Hodgkin's lymphoma survivors: An application of the theory of planned behavior. J Sport Exerc Psychol 27:335–349

Cox CL (2003) Online exclusive: a model of health behavior to guide studies of childhood cancer survivors. Oncol Nurs Forum 30:92–99

Cox CL, Montgomery M, Oeffinger KC et al (2009) Promoting physical activity in childhood cancer survivors: results from the Childhood Cancer Survivor Study. Cancer 115:642–654

Culos-Reed N, Robinson JW, Lau H et al (2009) Physical activity for men receiving androgen deprivation therapy for prostate cancer: benefits from a 16-week intervention. Support Care Cancer. doi:10.1007/s00520-009-0694-3

Daley AJ, Crank H, Mutrie N et al (2007a) Determinants of adherence to exercise in women treated for breast cancer. Eur J Oncol Nurs 11: 392–399

Daley AJ, Crank H, Saxton JM et al (2007b) Randomized trial of exercise therapy in women treated for breast cancer. J Clin Oncol 25: 1713–1721

Deci EL, Ryan RM (1985) Intrinsic motivation and self-determination in human behavior. Plenum Publishing Co., New York

Demark-Wahnefried W, Clipp EC, Morey MC et al (2006) Lifestyle intervention development study to improve physical function in older adults with cancer: outcomes from Project LEAD. J Clin Oncol 24(21):3465–73

Demark-Wahnefried W, Morey MC, Clipp EC et al (2003) Leading the way in exercise and diet (Project LEAD): intervening to improve function among older breast and prostate cancer survivors. Control Clin Trials 24(2):206–23

Digman JM (1990) Personality structure: emergence of the five-factor model. Annu Rev Psychol 41:417–440

Duijts SF, Oldenburg HS, van Beurden M et al (2009) Cognitive behavioral therapy and physical exercise for climacteric symptoms in breast cancer patients experiencing treatment-induced menopause: design of a multi-center trial. BMC Womens' Health 6:9–15

Emery FF, Yang HC, Frierson GM et al (2009) Determinants of physical activity among women treated for breast caner in a 5-year longitudinal follow-up investigation. Psychooncology 18: 377–386

Finnegan L, Wilkie DJ, Wilbur J et al (2007) Correlates of physical activity in young adult survivors of childhood cancers. Oncol Nurs Forum 34:60–69

Harrison S, Hayes SC, Newman B (2009) Level of physical activity and characteristics associated with change following breast cancer diagnosis and treatment. Psychooncology 18: 387–394

Hunt-Shanks TT, Blanchard CM, Baker F et al (2006) Exercise use as complementary therapy among breast and prostate cancer survivors receiving active treatment: examination of exercise intention. Integ Cancer Ther 5:109–116

Janis I, Mann L (1977) Decision making: a psychological analysis of conflict, choice and commitment. Collier Macmillan, New York

Jarden M, Nelausen K, Hovgaard D et al (2009) The effect of a multimodal intervention on treatment-related symptoms in patients undergoing hematopoietic stem call transplantation: a randomized controlled trial. J Pain Symptom Manage 38:174–190

Jones LW, Courneya KS, Fairey AS et al (2004) Effects of an oncologist's recommendation to exercise on self-reported exercise behavior in newly diagnosed breast cancer survivors: a single-blind, randomized controlled trial. Ann Behav Med 28(2):105–13

Jones LW, Courneya KS, Fairey AS et al (2005) Does the theory of planned behavior mediate the effects of an oncologist's recommendation to exercise in newly diagnosed breast cancer survivors? Results from a randomized controlled trial. Health Psychol 24(2):189–97

Jones LW, Courneya KS, Vallance JK et al (2006) Understanding the determinants of exercise intentions in multiple myeloma cancer survivors: an application of the theory of planned behavior. Cancer Nurs 29:167–175

Jones LW, Guill B, Keir ST et al (2007) Using the theory of planned behavior to understand the determinants of exercise intention in patients diagnosed with primary brain cancer. Psychooncology 16:232–240

Karvinen KH, Courneya KS, Campbell KL et al (2006) Exercise preferences of endometrial cancer survivors: a population-based study. Cancer Nurs 29:259–265

Karvinen KH, Courneya KS, Plotnikoff RC et al (2009) A prospective study of the determinants of exercise in bladder cancer survivors using the theory of planned behavior. Support Care Cancer 17:171–179

Keats MR, Culos-Reed SN, Courneya KS et al (2007) Understanding physical activity in adolescent cancer survivors: an application of the theory of planned behavior. Psychooncology 16:448–457

Korstjens I, May AM, van Weert E et al (2008) Quality of life after self-management cancer rehabilitation: a randomized controlled trial comparing physical and cognitive-behavioral training versus physical training. Psychosom Med 70:422–429

Lauver DR, Connolly-Nelson K, Vang P (2007) Stressors and coping strategies among female cancer survivors after treatments. Cancer Nurs 30:101–111

Lewthwaite R (1990) Motivational considerations in physical activity involvement. Phys Ther 70: 808–819

Levine M (1989) The conservation principles of nursing: twenty years later. In: Riehl-Sisca H (ed) Conceptual models for nursing practice. Appleton-Lange, Norwalk, CT

Levine ME (1973) Introduction to clinical nursing, 2nd edn. FA Davis, Philadelphia, PA

Lynch BM, Cerin E, Newman B et al (2007) Physical activity, activity change and their correlates in a population-based sample of colorectal cancer survivors. Ann Behav Med 34:135–143

May AM, Korstjens I, van Weert E et al (2009) Long-term effects on cancer survivors' quality of life of physical training versus physical training combined with cognitive-behavioral therapy: results from a randomized trial. Support Care Cancer 17:653–663

May AM, Van Weert E, Korstjens I et al (2008) Improved physical fitness of cancer survivors: a randomised controlled trial comparing physical training with physical and cognitive-behavioural training. Acta Oncol 47:825–834

Matthews CE, Wilcox S, Hanby CL et al (2007) Evaluation of a 12-week home-based walking intervention for breast cancer survivors. Support Care Cancer 15(2):203–11

Marcus BH, Simkin LR (1993) The stages of exercise behavior. J Sports Med Phys Fitness 33(1): 83–88

Marcus BH, Rakowski W, Rossi JS (1992a) Assessing motivational readiness and decision making for exercise. Health Psychol 11(4): 257–61

Marcus BH, Rossi JS, Selby VC et al (1992b) The stages and processes of exercise adoption and maintenance in a worksite sample. Health Psychol 11(6):386–395

McCrae RR, John OP (1992) An introduction to the five-factor model and its applications. J Pers 60:175–215

Miller WR, Rollnick S (2002) Motivational interviewing: preparing people for change. Guilford Press, New York

Milne HM, Wallman KE, Guilfoyle A et al (2008a) Self-determination theory and physical activity among breast cancer survivors. J Sport Exerc Psychol 30:23–38

Milne HM, Wallman KE, Gordon S et al (2008b) Impact of a combined resistance and aerobic exercise program on motivational variables in breast cancer survivors: a randomized controlled trial. Ann Behav Med 36:158–166

Midtgaard J, Baadsgaard MT, Moller TM et al (2009) Self-reported physical activity behavior; exercise motivation and information among Danish adult caner patients undergoing chemotherapy. Eur J Oncol Nurs 13:116–121

Mock V, Burke MB, Sheehan P et al (1994) A nursing rehabilitation program for women with breast cancer receiving adjuvant chemotherapy. Oncol Nurs Forum 21(5):899–907

Mock V, Dow KH, Meares CJ et al (1997) Effects of exercise on fatigue, physical functioning, and emotional distress during radiation therapy for breast cancer. Oncol Nurs Forum 24(6): 991–1000

Mock V, Frangakis C, Davidson NE et al (2005) Exercise manages fatigue during breast cancer treatment: a randomized controlled trial. Psychooncol ogy 14:464–477

Mock V, St Ours C, Hall S et al (2007) Using a conceptual model in nursing research-mitigating fatigue in cancer patients. J Adv Nurs 58: 503–512

Morey MC, Snyder DC, Sloane R et al (2009) Effects of home-based diet and exercise on functional outcomes among older, overweight long-term cancer survivors: RENEW: a randomized controlled trial. J Am Med Assoc 301(18): 1883–91

Mosher CE, Fuemmeler BF, Sloane R et al (2008) Changes in self-efficacy partially mediates the effects of the FRESH START intervention on cancer survivors' dietary outcomes. Psycho oncology 17:1014–1023

Mutrie N, Campbell AM, Whyte F et al (2007) Benefits of supervised group exercise programme for women being treated for early stage breast cancer: pragmatic randomized controlled trial. British Medical J, 334 (doi:10.1136/bmj.39094.648553.AE)

Perkins HY, Baum GP, Taylor DL et al (2009) Effects of treatment-related factors, comorbidities and health-related quality of life on self-efficacy for physical activity in cancer survivors. Psychooncology 18:405–411

Peddle CJ, Au HJ, Courneya KS et al. (2008) Associations between exercise, quality of life, and fatigue in colorectal cancer survivors. Dis Colon Rectum 51(8):1242–8

Peddle CJ, Jones LW, Eves ND et al (2009) Correlates of adherence to supervised exercise in patients awaiting surgical removal of malignant lung lesions: results of a pilot study. Oncol Nurs Forum 36:287–295

Pinto BM, Eakin E, Maruyama NC (2000) Health behavior changes after a cancer diagnosis: what do we know and where do we go from here? Ann Behav Med 22:38–52

Pinto BM, Frierson GM, Rabin C et al (2005) Home-based physical activity intervention for breast cancer patients. J Clin Oncol 23: 3577–3587

Pinto BM, Goldstein MG, Papandonatos GD (2009a) Promoting physical activity in follow-up care for breast cancer patients. Ann Behav Med 37:S233

Pinto BM, Rabin C, Dunsiger S (2009b) Home-based exercise among cancer survivors: adherence and its predictors. Psychooncology 18 :369–376

Pinto BM, Trunzo JJ, Reiss P et al (2002) Exercise participation after diagnosis of breast cancer: trends and effects on mood and quality of life. Psychooncology 11:389–400

Prochaska JO, DiClemente CC (1983) Stages and processes of self-change of smoking: toward an integrative model of change. J Consult Clin Psychol 51:390–395

Prochaska JO, DiClemente CC, Norcross JC (1992) In search of how people change. Applications to addictive behaviors. Am Psychol 47(9): 1102–14

Rabin C, Pinto B, Frierson G (2006) Mediators of a randomized controlled physical activity intervention of breast cancer survivors. J Sport Exerc Psychol 28:269–284

Rhodes RE, Courneya KS (2003) Relationships between personality, an extended theory of planned behaviour model and exercise behaviour. Br J Health Psychol 8:19–36

Rhodes RE, Courneya KS, Bobick TM (2001) Personality and exercise participation across the breast cancer experience. Psychooncology 10: 380–388

Rhodes RE, Smith NE (2006) Personality correlates of physical activity: a review and meta-analysis. Br J Sports Med 40:958–965

Rogers LQ, Courneya KS, Shah P et al (2007) Exercise stage of change, barriers, expectations, values and preferences among breast cancer patients during treatment: a pilot study. Eur J Cancer Care 16:55–66

Rogers LQ, Hopkins-Price VS et al (2009a) A randomized trial to increase physical activity in breast cancer survivors. Med Sci Sports Exerc 41:935–946

Rogers LQ, McAuley E, Courneya KS et al (2008) Correlates of physical activity self-efficacy among breast cancer survivors. Am J Health Behav 32:594–603

Rogers LQ, Markwell SJ, Courneya KS et al (2009b) Exercise preference patterns, resources, and environment among rural breast cancer survivors. J Rural Health 25:388–391

Rogers LQ, Matevey C, Hopkins-Price P et al (2004) Exploring social cognitive theory constructs for promoting exercise among breast cancer patients. Cancer Nurs 27:462–473

Rogers LQ, Shah P, Dunnington G et al (2005) Social cognitive theory and physical activity during breast cancer treatment. Oncol Nurs Forum 32:807–815

Roy C, Andrews HA (1991) The Roy adaptation model. The definitive statement. Appleton & Lange, Norwald, CT

Smith BD, Smith GL, Huria A et al (2009) Future of cancer incidence in the United States: burdens upon an aging changing nation. J Clin Oncol 27:2758–2765

Speck RM, Courneya KS, Mâsse LC et al (2010) An update of controlled physical activity trials in cancer survivors: a systematic review and meta-analysis. J Cancer Surviv 4(2):87–100

Stevinson C, Tonkin K, Capstick V et al (2009) A population-based study of the determinants of physical activity in ovarian cancer survivors. J Phys Act Health 6:339–346

Snyder DC, Morey MC, Sloane R et al (2009) Reach out to ENhancE Wellness in older cancer survivors (RENEW): design, methods and recruitment challenges of a home-based exercise and diet intervention to improve physical function among long-term survivors of breast, prostate and colorectal cancer. Psychooncology 18: 429–439

Taylor CL, Demoor C, Smith MA et al (2006) Active for life after cancer: a randomized trial examining a lifestyle physical activity program for prostate cancer patients. Psychooncology 15(10):847–62

Vallance JK, Courneya KS, Plotnikoff RC et al (2007) Randomized controlled trial of the effects of print materials and step pedometers on physical activity and quality of life in breast caner survivors. J Clin Oncol 17:2352–2359

Vallance JK, Courneya KS, Plotnikoff RC et al (2008) Analyzing theoretical mechanisms of physical activity behavior change in breast cancer survivors: results from the activity promotion (ACTION) trial. Ann Behav Med 35: 150–158

Weiner B (1985) An attributional theory of achievement motivation and emotion. Psychol Rev 92:548–573

Wilson PM, Blanchard CM, Nehl E et al (2006) Predicting physical activity and outcome expectations in cancer survivors: an application of self-determination theory. Psychooncology 15: 567–578